D., J.D.

CHALLENGING CASES IN ENDOCRINOLOGY

CONTEMPORARY ENDOCRINOLOGY

P. Michael Conn, SERIES EDITOR

CHALLENGING CASES IN ENDOCRINOLOGY

Edited by

MARK E. MOLITCH, MD

Center for Endocrinology, Metabolism, and Molecular Medicine, Northwestern University Medical School, Chicago, IL

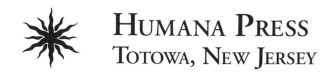

HUMANA PRESS
TOTOWA, NEW JERSEY

© 2002 Humana Press Inc.
999 Riverview Drive, Suite 208
Totowa, New Jersey 07512
humanapress.com

For additional copies, pricing for bulk purchases, and/or information about other Humana titles,
contact Humana at the above address or at any of the following numbers: Tel: 973-256-1699;
Fax: 973-256-8341; E-mail: humana@humanapr.com; Website: http://humanapress.com

Cover Illustration: Left: Cohesive groups of benign follicular cells. (*See* Fig. 1, p. 69.) Center: Coronal section
through the pituitary from a T1-weighted MRI image. (*See* Fig. 1, p. 39.) Right: CT scan of a 7.2. cm adrenal
mass. (*See* Fig. 1, p. 157.)

Cover design by Patricia F. Cleary.

Production Editor: Mark J. Breaugh.

All articles, comments, opinions, conclusions, or recommendations are those of the author(s), and do not necessarily reflect
the views of the publisher.

This publication is printed on acid-free paper. ∞
ANSI Z39.48-1984 (American National Standards Institute)
Permanence of Paper for Printed Library Materials.

Printed in the United States of America. 10 9 8 7 6 5 4 3 2 1

Library of Congress Cataloging-in-Publication Data
Challenging cases in endocrinology/edited by Mark E. Molitch.
     p. cm. — (Contemporary endocrinology)
   Includes bibliographical references and index.
   ISBN 0-89603-914-5 (alk. paper)
   1. Endocrinology--Case studies. I. Molitch, Mark E. II. Contemporary endocrinology
(Totowa, NJ)
   [DNLM: 1. Endocrine Diseases--diagnosis. 2. Endocrine Diseases--therapy. WK 140
D569 2002]
   RC649.5 .D544 2002
   616.4--dc21

PREFACE

I enjoy seeing patients, as I think most endocrinologists do. One of the things I believe we enjoy most is seeing patients who provide challenges to us, so that we have to think a little harder to find the diagnosis and to be creative in our disease management. Going to the literature and textbooks—often via the computer—to look up the latest information, discussing cases with colleagues, reaching for help by way of telephone or email from more distant colleagues with greater expertise, are part of what we do on an everyday basis to provide the best care for our patients and also to provide intellectual stimulation for ourselves. This continued desire on our part to meet such challenging cases head-on and to stimulate ourselves intellectually are the reasons I am confident readers will like *Challenging Cases in Endocrinology*.

I have asked experts in their fields to provide for us accounts of those difficult cases that have required of them extra effort and creative thinking in diagnosis and management. You will be able to follow with them how they did what they did, and why. They have also provided detailed, up-to-date, referenced discussions to put their cases into context. In this way, you will be able to bring much of this information into daily use in your own practices, and the references we have provided will allow you to look up additional material as needed. As editor, I have read all of these cases and have personally picked up information and a number of tips that I have already put to use in my own practice.

This, therefore, is a book for the *practicing endocrinologist*, whether a fellow still in training, a full-time clinician out in practice for 25 years, or a clinician/academic who only sees patients one-half day per week. You can take it on the airplane with you or read a case at a time when you can fit it in. Very few of the cases are straightforward and many provide twists or turns—almost as if you were reading a novel.

I wish to thank the authors of these chapters for taking the time out of their busy schedules to write up their cases and for sharing their clinical expertise with us. I also wish to thank Ms. Joella Ackerman for helping me keep things organized and helping with the editing. Mr. Paul Dolgert and the editorial and production staff at Humana Press have been very supportive. Finally, I would like to thank my family—Susan, Tamara, Ethan, and Michael—who are used to seeing me at home working at the computer in the evenings and on weekends, for supporting me in this endeavor.

Mark E. Molitch, MD

CONTENTS

* Deceased

CONTRIBUTORS

LOUIS AFONSO, MD, *Division of Cardiology, Veterans Administration Medical Center, Wayne State University, Detroit, MI*

ERIK K. ALEXANDER, MD, *Division of Endocrine–Hypertension, Harvard Medical School, Brigham and Women's Hospital, Boston, MA*

HISHAM ALREFAI, MD, *Division of Endocrinology, Wayne State University, Detroit, MI*

BAHA M. ARAFAH, MD, *Division of Clinical and Molecular Endocrinology, Case Western Reserve University; University Hospitals of Cleveland, Cleveland, OH*

ELENA I. BARENGOLTS, MD, *University of Illinois Medical School, Medical Service, VA Chicago Health Care System–West Side Division, Chicago, IL*

SHALENDER BHASIN, MD, *Division of Endocrinology, Metabolism and Molecular Medicine, Charles R. Drew University of Medicine and Science, Los Angeles, CA*

PHILLIP BUKBERG, MD, *St. Vincent's Hospital, New York, NY*

ROBERT CHRISTIANSEN, MD, *Department of Pediatrics, Charles R. Drew University of Medicine and Science, Los Angeles, CA*

NEELIMA V. CHU, MD, *Division of Endocrinology and Metabolism, University of California–San Diego Medical School, La Jolla, CA*

BART L. CLARKE, MD, *Mayo Medical School, Mayo Clinic and Foundation, Rochester, MN*

DAVID S. COOPER, MD, *Division of Endocrinology, Sinai Hospital of Baltimore; The Johns Hopkins Hospital; Johns Hopkins Medical School, Baltimore, MD*

ROBERT DLUHY, MD, *Division of Endocrine–Hypertension, Brigham and Women's Hospital, Harvard Medical School, Boston, MA*

DOUGLAS B. EVANS, MD, *Department of Surgical Oncology, The University of Texas M.D. Anderson Cancer Center, Houston, TX*

JAMES W. FINDLING, MD, *Medical College of Wisconsin, Endocrine Diabetes Center, St. Luke's Medical Center, Milwaukee, WI*

ROBERT F. GAGEL, MD, *Section of Endocrine Neoplasia and Hormonal Disorders, Division of Internal Medicine, The University of Texas M.D. Anderson Cancer Center, Houston, TX*

MARY P. GILLAM, MD, *Center for Endocrinology, Metabolism and Molecular Medicine, Northwestern University Medical School, Chicago, IL*

HELMUTH GOEPFERT, MD, *Department of Head and Neck Surgery, The University of Texas M.D. Anderson Cancer Center, Houston, TX*

IRA J. GOLDBERG, MD, *Division of Preventive Medicine and Nutrition, Columbia University College of Physicians and Surgeons, New York, NY*

ROBERT R. HENRY, MD, *Division and Endocrinology and Metabolism, University of California–San Diego Medical School, Section of Diabetes, Endocrinology & Metabolism, Veterans Administration San Diego Healthcare System, La Jolla, CA*

MICHAEL M. KAPLAN, MD, *Associated Endocrinologists, West Bloomfield, MI; Departments of Nuclear Medicine and Internal Medicine, William Beaumont Hospital, Royal Oak, MI*

SUNDEEP KHOSLA, MD, *Mayo Medical School, Mayo Clinic and Foundation, Rochester, MN*

MICHAEL KLEEREKOPER, MD, *Division of Endocrinology, Wayne State University, Detroit, MI*

RICHARD T. KLOOS, MD, *Divisions of Endocrinology, Diabetes, and Metabolism & Nuclear Medicine, Departments of Internal Medicine and Radiology, Arthur G. James Cancer Hospital and Richard J. Solove Research Institute, Ohio State University School of Medicine, Columbus, OH*

SUBHASH C. KUKREJA, MD, *University of Illinois Medical School, Medical Service, VA Chicago Health Care System–West Side Division, Chicago, IL*

LEWIS LANDSBERG, MD, *Northwestern University Medical School, Chicago, IL*

JEFFREY E. LEE, MD, *Department of Surgical Oncology, The University of Texas M.D. Anderson Cancer Center, Houston, TX*

ERNEST L. MAZZAFERRI, MD, *Department of Internal Medicine, Ohio State University School of Medicine, Columbus, OH*

DONALD A. MEIER, MD, *Associated Endocrinologists, West Bloomfield, MI; Departments of Nuclear Medicine, William Beaumont Hospital, Royal Oak, MI*

MOISES MERCADO, MD, *Endocrinology Section, Hospital de Especialidades, Centro Medico Nacional, México City, México*

BOYD E. METZGER, MD, *Center for Endocrinology, Metabolism and Molecular Medicine, Northwestern University Medical School, Chicago, IL*

MARK E. MOLITCH, MD, *Center for Endocrinology, Metabolism and Molecular Medicine, Northwestern University Medical School, Chicago, IL*

MONA P. NASRALLAH, MD, *Division of Clinical and Molecular Endocrinology, Case Western Reserve University; University Hospitals of Cleveland, Cleveland, OH*

NEENA NATT, MD, *Division of Endocrinology, Diabetes and Metabolism, Mayo Medical School, Mayo Clinic and Foundation, Rochester, MN*

LISA P. PURDY, MD, CM, *Center for Endocrinology, Metabolism, Molecular Medicine, Northwestern University Medical School, Chicago, IL*

BHARAT RAMAN, MD, *Department of Medicine, University of North Dakota, Grand Forks, ND*

ROBERT REBAR, MD, *American Society for Reproductive Medicine, Birmingham, AL*

ERICK J. RICHMOND, MD, *Division of Pediatric Endocrinology, University of Virginia School of Medicine, Charlottesville, VA*

JARED C. ROBINS, MD, *Department of Obstetrics and Gynecology, University of Cincinnati Medical School, Cincinnati, OH*

ALAN D. ROGOL, MD, PhD, *Insmed Incorporated, Glen Allen, VA; Medical College of Virginia, Virginia Commonwealth University, Richmond, VA; Division of Pediatric Endocrinology, University of Virginia School of Medicine, Charlottesville, VA*

F. JOHN SERVICE, MD, PhD, *Mayo Medical School, Division of Endocrinology, Diabetes and Metabolism, Mayo Clinic and Mayo Foundation, Rochester, MN*

ATAM B. SINGH, MD, *Division of Endocrinology, Metabolism and Molecular Medicine, Charles R. Drew University of Medicine and Science, Los Angeles, CA*

J. WOODY SISTRUNK, MD, *Mississippi Baptist Medical Center, Jackson, MS*

DENNIS M. STYNE, MD, *Section of Pediatric Endocrinology, University of California–Davis Medical School, Davis, CA*

JOSEPH G. VERBALIS, MD, *Division of Endocrinology, Georgetown University Medical Center, Washington, DC*

KELLY L. WIRFEL, MD, *Department of Endocrinology, The University of Texas Medical School, Houston, TX*

LISA L. WONG, MD, *Division of Endocrinology, Georgetown University Medical Center, Washington, DC*

BRUCE ZIMMERMAN, MD, *Deceased, formerly of Division and Endocrinology and Metabolism, Mayo Medical School, Mayo Clinic and Foundation, Rochester, MN*

1

Pituitary Tumors

Moises Mercado, MD and Mark E. Molitch, MD

CONTENTS

CASE #1: ADOLESCENT WITH A PROLACTINOMA

Case Description

A 27-yr-old woman initially presented to the emergency room in 1988 at age 16 with increasing headaches and decreased visual acuity and was found to have a visual field defect. She also had primary amenorrhea. A computed tomography (CT) scan showed a 2 × 3-cm suprasellar mass and she was admitted to the neurosurgery service. She was operated on for what was thought then to be a craniopharyngioma. Her examination at that time showed a modestly obese young girl of normal height with Tanner Stage IV breast and pubic hair development. Preoperative laboratory results that were not available at the time of the surgery showed a serum PRL of 1270 ng/mL, a cortisol of 6.6 μg/dL, a T4 of 4.8 μg/dL, a growth hormone (GH) of 1.4 ng/mL, a luteinizing hormone (LH) of 3.8 mIU/mL, and a follicle-stimulating hormone (FSH) of 17.4 mIU/mL. Postoperatively, her PRL was 415 ng/mL and she was referred to the endocrine service where testing showed panhypopituitarism. A postoperative MRI showed little change in the tumor size. She was begun on l-thyroxine, prednisone, and bromocriptine.

Over the course of the next 2 yr, despite many attempts, the bromocriptine dose could not be increased sufficiently to normalize PRL levels without causing severe nausea. The highest dose she was able to tolerate was 10 mg/d with a resultant PRL of 95 ng/mL, but because of nausea she rarely stayed on this dose. She tried intravaginal bromocriptine but refused to take it regularly via this route and her PRL levels increased to over 600 ng/dL.

From: *Contemporary Endocrinology: Challenging Cases in Endocrinology*
Edited by: M. E. Molitch © Humana Press Inc., Totowa, NJ

Table 1
Stepwise Decrease in Prolactin Levels
with Stepwise Increase in Cabergoline Dose/Wk in Case 1

Date	11/13/96	5/5/97	8/4/97	12/15/97	3/30/98	7/20/98	10/7/98	11/16/98	4/12/99	7/9/99
PRL (ng/dL)	655	288	329	311	172	127	109	96	65	38
Dose (mg/wk)	0	0.5	0.5	1.0	2.0	3.0	4.0	6.0	8.0	8.0

Because of her psychological refusal to accept her illness and need for medication, as well as the nausea that occurred on taking bromocriptine, she stopped all her medication frequently for months at a time with failure to return for follow-up visits. She was also tried on pergolide in doses up to 0.25 mg/d but her PRL remained over 100 ng/mL and attempts to increase the dose resulted in nausea and stopping medication. Off medication, her PRL would rise to levels in the 1600 ng/mL range. Her parents divorced shortly after her surgery and were unable to provide adequate emotional support and direction. She was advised to seek psychiatric counseling many times, but did not do so.

Despite the poor medication compliance, with intermittently quite high PRL levels, periodic magnetic resonance imaging (MRI) scans showed no change in tumor size. However, in 1995, after not being seen for 8 mo and off dopamine agonists during all that time, her PRL was 7101 ng/mL and an MRI showed a considerable enlargement of the residual tumor with suprasellar extension bowing the optic chiasm and she had a right visual field defect. She underwent transsphenoidal surgery with improvement in her visual fields and her postoperative PRL level was 1123 ng/mL. Postoperatively, she was again noncompliant with bromocriptine and her other medications with a rise in PRL to 1838 ng/mL. In March 1997, she was started on cabergoline and experienced a stepwise reduction in PRL levels with each stepwise increase in her cabergoline dose (see Table 1). Finally, on a dose of 8 mg/wk, her PRL levels reached 38 ng/mL and an MRI showed a marked decrease in the size of her residual tumor. However, despite near normalization of her PRL levels, she remained amenorrheic and a dual X-ray absorptiometry study showed that her bone mineral density at the lumbar spine was 74% of normal young women. In July 1999, she was started for the first time on oral contraceptives for estrogen replacement along with her 8 mg/wk of cabergoline. As of November 1999, she has missed two return visits.

Discussion

This case illustrates a number of important features of the management of a patient with a prolactinoma. First, is her initial presentation at age 16 with amenorrhea and a large macroadenoma. Children and adolescents may present with growth arrest, pubertal delay, or primary amenorrhea in addition to the more standard presentations of galactorrhea and/or oligo/amenorrhea (1–4). In contrast to the tumor size distribution of patients in adults, almost two-thirds of children with prolactinomas have large macroadenomas in reported series, even allowing for possible selection bias because of reporting from neurosurgical units. Furthermore, the percentage of patients resistant to dopamine agonists may be higher than in adults, with Colao et al. (4) reporting that PRL levels were normalized in only 10/26 children and adolescents taking bromocriptine, 5/15 taking quinagolide, and 15/20 taking cabergoline. The reasons for the high percentage of large macroadenomas and the relative resistance to dopamine agonists are not known, but it is tempting to speculate that the tumor growth may be linked to resistance to endogenous dopamine.

Her initial referral to neurosurgery was unusual and was caused, in part, by her being admitted to the neurosurgery service from the emergency room and then not waiting for the results of hormone testing before going to surgery. Generally, most patients with prolactinomas now do not have surgery; rather, they are treated with dopamine agonists, especially those with large tumors. In a compilation of data from 34 published series, it was shown that 973/1321 (73.7%) microadenomas and 415/1279 (32.4%) macroadenomas were reported as being curatively resected, i.e., having PRL levels normalized by 1–12 wk following surgery (5). From these series, recurrence rates for microadenomas (114/544 = 21.0%) and macroadenomas (50/253 = 19.8%) are similar (5). Thus, the long-term surgical cure rate for microadenomas is 58%, and that for macroadenomas is 26%, understanding that these numbers are derived from patients in whom the neurosurgeon thought there was a possibility of cure. For patients with giant prolactinomas and those with considerable cavernous sinus invasion, the chance for surgical cure is essentially zero.

Complications from transsphenoidal surgery for microadenomas are quite infrequent, the mortality rate being 0.5–0.9%, and the major morbidity rate being about 1.5–6% (6,7). Transient diabetes insipidus (DI) is quite common with transsphenoidal surgery for both micro- and macroadenomas, but permanent DI occurs in only about 1% of surgeries on macroadenomas (6,7). Hypopituitarism is common in patients with macroadenomas prior to surgery as a result of mass effects, occurring in more than 50% of patients (6,7). With surgery, both further worsening or improvement may occur (6,7). Surgery involving craniotomy is much more hazardous. It is clear that the less experienced the surgeon, the greater the rate of complications (7).

In contrast, bromocriptine generally restores normal PRL levels in about 80–85% of patients with prolactinomas of all sizes, usually with a reduction in tumor size. In a compilation of several series with a total of 302 patients with macroadenomas, 76.8% had some tumor size decrease in response to bromocriptine with periods of observation ranging from 6 wk to more than 10 yr (5). Ten series quantitated their tumor size reductions in a total of 112 patients; 45 (40.2%) had a >50% reduction in tumor size, 32 (28.6%) had a 25–50% reduction in tumor size, 14 (12.5%) had a <25% reduction, and 21 (18.7%) had no evidence of any reduction in tumor size (5).

Thus, it would have been expected that she would not be cured by surgery, and she was not. Furthermore, it was expected that bromocriptine would cause her PRL levels to return to normal with tumor shrinkage, but this also did not happen. Because of her resistance to bromocriptine, she required high doses, which she could not tolerate and she became noncompliant with therapy. One of the problems with intermittent therapy is that the patient may restart again at the dose at which they stopped, probably a relatively high dose, and get side effects immediately, whereas if they restarted at a low dose they might tolerate the drug better. As aforementioned, tumors in the pediatric population tend to be more resistant to dopamine agonists.

She was also tried on intravaginal bromocriptine but was even more noncompliant with this route of administration. Several years ago, Vermesh et al. (8) reported that similar reductions in PRL levels are achieved with oral and intravaginal administration of oral bromocriptine tablets. However, the drug effect lasts for up to 24 h with a single dose administered intravaginally and gastrointestinal side effects are much less with the intravaginal route (8). Women intolerant of oral bromocriptine with macroadenomas may respond well with tumor shrinkage to intravaginal bromocriptine *(9)*. However, not all are willing to try this route, and some who do, develop local vaginal irritation. She was also tried on pergolide with results similar to those for bromocriptine, as could be predicted from earlier studies *(10)*.

She finally responded to cabergoline, which is different from other dopamine agonists in that it has a very long half-life and can be given orally once or twice weekly. The long duration of action stems from its slow elimination from pituitary tissue *(11)*, its high affinity binding to pituitary dopamine receptors *(12)*, and extensive enterohepatic recycling *(13)*. A number of studies have now shown that cabergoline is at least as effective as, and perhaps more effective, than bromocriptine in lowering PRL levels but with substantially fewer side effects *(14–20)*. Rare patients experience limiting nausea and vomiting with cabergoline, and they may be treated with intravaginal cabergoline as well *(15)*.

Several studies have assessed the effect of cabergoline on macroadenoma size *(14–20)*. A total of 130 patients in these series had their tumor size assessed in a semiquantitative way in studies ranging from 3 to 24 mo duration of treatment with 25% experiencing a >50% tumor size reduction, 47% experiencing a 25–50% reduction, 7% having a < 25% reduction, and 21% having no change in tumor size. In a recent series of 27 patients who had all been previously shown to be resistant to bromocriptine or quinagolide (CV205-502), Colao et al. *(20)* showed that cabergoline was able to normalize PRL levels in 15 of 19 patients with macroadenomas and all 8 patients with microadenomas; tumor shrinkage was documented in 9 of the 19 macroadenomas and 4 of the 8 microadenomas *(20)*.

Thus, our patient was finally able to tolerate cabergoline in a dose sufficient to normalize PRL levels. Most patients have a rapid fall in PRL with just modest doses of dopamine agonist. However, a small percentage, perhaps <5%, experience small stepwise reductions in PRL in response to stepwise increases in medication dose, as in our patient. Although 3 mg/wk is the maximum dose recommended in the package insert, it should be remembered that patients with Parkinson's disease often take doses as high as 5–6 mg *daily (21)* and, as long as the patient is not having adverse effects, I have no qualms in increasing the dose as long as the PRL continues to come down.

Because of her loss of thyroid-stimulating hormone (TSH) and adrenocorticotropic hormone (ACTH) functions, it was expected that she would not have return of function of her gonadotropins even after the PRL was normalized. However, because of her resistance to the dopamine agonists and the known effects of estrogen in decreasing dopamine inhibition of lactotrophs *(22)*, including the known effects of pregnancy in inducing tumor-size increase *(23)*, estrogens were withheld until it was felt that her tumor had been brought under control with cabergoline. It should be mentioned, however, that in patients with microadenomas and those with small macroadenomas, the administration of estrogens has not generally been reported to cause an increase in tumor size *(24,25)*. However, because of the previously demonstrated propensity of this young woman's tumor to grow, we were hesitant to start her on estrogen replacement until we felt her tumor size had finally come under control with cabergoline.

REFERENCES

1. Partington MD, Davis DH, Laws ER Jr, Scheithauer BW. Pituitary adenomas in childhood and adolescence. Results of transsphenoidal surgery. J Neurosurg 1994;80:209–216.
2. Mindermann T, Wilson CB. Pediatric pituitary adenomas. Neurosurgery 1995;36:259–269.
3. Artese R, D'Osvaldo DH, Molocznik I, et al. Pituitary tumors in adolescent patients. Neurol Res 1998; 20:415–417.

4. Colao AM, Loche S, Cappa M, et al. Prolactinomas in children and adolescents. Clinical presentation and long-term follow-up. J Clin Endocrinol Metab 1998;83:2777–2780.
5. Molitch ME. Prolactinoma. In: Melmed S, ed. The Pituitary. 2nd ed. Blackwell Scientific, Boston, MA, in press.
6. Laws ER Jr, Thapar K. Pituitary surgery. Endocrinol Metab Clin North Am 1999;28:119–131.
7. Ciric I, Ragin A, Baumgartner C, Pierce D. Complications of transsphenoidal surgery: results of a national survey, review of the literature, and personal experience. Neurosurgery 1997;40:225–236.
8. Vermesh M, Fossum GT, Kletzky OA. Vaginal bromocriptine: pharmacology and effect on serum prolactin in normal women. Obstet Gynecol 1988;72:693–698.
9. Katz E, Schran HF, Adashi EY. Successful treatment of a prolactin-producing pituitary macroadenoma with intravaginal bromocriptine mesylate: a novel approach to intolerance of oral therapy. Obstet Gynecol 1989;73:517–520.
10. Freda PU, Andreadis CI, Khandji G, et al. Long-term treatment of prolactin-secreting macroadenomas with pergolide. J Clin Endocrinol Metab 2000;85:8–13.
11. DiSalle E, Ornati G, Giudici D. A comparison of the *in vivo* and *in vitro* duration of prolactin lowering effect in rats of FCE 21336, pergolide and bromocriptine. J Endocrinol Invest 1984;7(Suppl1):32.
12. Strolin BM, Doster P, Barone D, Efthymiopoulos C, Peretti G, Roncucci R. *In vivo* interaction of CAB with rat brain dopamine receptors labelled with 3H-N-n-propylinorapomorphine. Eur J Pharmacol 1990;187:399–408.
13. Andreotti AC, Pianezzola E, Persiani S, et al. Pharmacokinetics, pharmacodynamics, and tolerability of cabergoline, a prolactin-lowering drug after administration of increasing oral doses (0.5, 1.0, and 1.5 milligrams) in healthy male volunteers. J Clin Endocrinol Metab 1995;80:841.
14. Webster J, Piscitelli G, Polli A, Ferrari CI, Ismail I, Scanlon MF for the Cabergoline Comparative Study Group. N Engl J Med 1994;331:904–909.
15. Motta T, Colombo N, de Vincentiis S, D'Alberton A, Marchini M. Vaginal cabergoline in the treatment of hyperprolactinemic patients intolerant to oral dopaminergics. Fertil Steril 1996;65:440–442.
16. Biller BMK, Molitch ME, Vance ML, Cannistraro KB, Davis KR, Simons JA, Schoefelder JR, Klibanski A. Treatment of prolactin-secreting macroadenomas with the once-weekly dopamine agonist cabergoline. J Clin Endocrinol Metab 1996;81:2338–2343.
17. Delgrange E, Maiter D, Donckier J. Effects of the dopamine agonist cabergoline in patients with prolactinoma intolerant or resistant to bromocriptine. Eur J Endocrinol 1996;134:454–456.
18. Colao A, DeSarno A, Landi ML, et al. Long-term and low-dose treatment with cabergoline induces macroprolactinoma shrinkage. J Clin Endocrinol Metab 1997;82:3574–3579.
19. Ferrari CI, Abs R, Bevan JS, et al. Treatment of macroprolactinoma with cabergoline: a study of 85 patients. Clin Endocrinol 1997;46:409–413.
20. Colao A, DiSarno A, Sarnacchiaro S, Ferone D, DiRenzo G, Annunziato L, Merola B, Lombardi G. Prolactinomas resistant to standard dopamine-agonists respond to chronic cabergoline treatment. J Clin Endocrinol Metab 1997;82:876–883.
21. Inzelberg R, Nisipeanu P, Rabey JM, et al. Double-blind comparison of cabergoline and bromocriptine in Parkinson's disease patients with motor fluctuations. Neurology 1996;47:785–788.
22. Shull JD, Gorski J. Regulation of prolactin gene transcription in vivo: Interactions between estrogen, pimozide, and ergocryptine. Molec Pharmacol 1989;37:215–221.
23. Molitch ME. Management of prolactinomas during pregnancy. J Reprod Med 1999;44(Suppl):1121–1126.
24. Corenblum B, Donovan L. The safety of physiological estrogen plus progestin replacement therapy and with oral contraceptive therapy in women with pathological hyperprolactinemia. Fertil Steril 1993;59:671–673.
25. Testa G, Vegetti W, Motta T, et al. Two-year treatment with oral contraceptives in hyperprolactinemic patients. Contraception 1998;58:69–73.

CASE #2: ACROMEGALY
WITH MINIMAL GROWTH HORMONE ELEVATION

Case Description

A 46-yr-old female sought medical attention because of generalized athralgias, headaches and excessive sweating of 2 yr duration. She also stated that for the past 7 yr she

Table 2
GH Levels During an Oral Glucose
Tolerance Test and IGF-1 Levels in Case 2

| | December 1999 | | January 2000 | |
	GH (ng/mL)	Glucose (mg/dL)	GH (ng/dL)	Glucose (mg/dL)
0 min	1.9	126	3.5	117
30 min	1.9	183	2	151
60 min	1.7	233	1.4	224
90 min	1.3	235	1.2	205
120 min	1.3	192	1	218
IGF-1 (ng/mL)	444*		306*	

*Age and sex adjusted normal 100–300 ng/mL.

had been noticing a progressive increase in shoe size, as well as "swelling" of her hands and coarsening of her facial features. One year before, she had been diagnosed with high blood pressure and glucose intolerance, but did not follow any specific treatment for these conditions. She had a positive family history of type 2 diabetes. She also complained of occasional hot flushes but her menses were regular. She has had four uneventful term pregnancies (the last one 15 yr ago), and none of her children had been macrosomic.

On physical examination, her blood pressure was 130/90 without postural changes, pulse 85 and regular, temperature 36°C, weight 80 Kg, and height 1.60 m. She appeared older than her stated age. Her head examination was remarkable for prognathism and macroglossia, as well as striking dental separation. A normal-sized nodular thyroid gland was palpated. No adenopathy was found. More than 30 skin tags were counted over the anterior neck and chest, and there was acanthosis nigricans in both axillae and posterior neck. The cardiopulmonary examination was normal. The abdomen was obese but no visceromegaly was encountered. Both hands and feet were bulky and large, but no signs of synovitis were found. The CNS exam was nonfocal, including visual fields.

Laboratory evaluation showed normal BUN, creatinine, electrolytes, calcium, and phosphorus with a fasting plasma glucose of 128 mg/dL. Colonoscopy revealed diverticular disease but no polyps or bleeding lesions. Her electrocardiogram was remarkable for evidence of left ventricular hypertrophy.

Hormonal work-up showed a PRL of 60 ng/mL, LH < 3 mIU/mL, FSH 10 mIU/mL, cortisol 13 µg/dL, estradiol 7 pg/mL, TSH 1.8 mU/mL, free T4 0.4 ng/dL, T4 5.5 µg/dL, and T3 70 ng/dL. Evaluation of the somatotropic axis was performed twice 1 mo apart and showed GH suppression by a 100-g glucose load, but elevated insulin-like growth factor 1 (IGF-1) measurements (see Table 2).

A pituitary MRI showed gland asymmetry with displacement of the pituitary stalk to the right (see Fig. 1). A computerized visual field examination was normal. She was started on 0.05 mg daily of levothyroxine. Because of the equivocal biochemical and imaging data, the case was brought to the neuroendocrine tumor board. Upon reviewing the MRI, it was felt that the pituitary gland asymmetry was a result of the presence of a 6–8-mm microadenoma that displaced the stalk to the right. It was decided to proceed

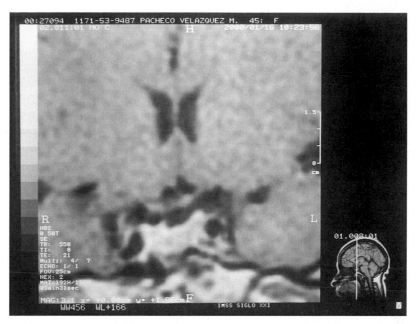

Fig. 1. MRI scan in Case 2. The stalk appears to be deviated to the right. No clear adenoma is seen.

with a transsphenoidal exploration. A distinct microadenoma was found that immuno-stained for PRL and GH.

Discussion

Acromegaly is a rare disease, with an estimated annual incidence of 2–3 per million, that in more than 95% of the cases results from a GH-secreting pituitary adenoma *(1,2)*. Most endocrinologists are familiar with the clinical manifestations of the disease and with the rather peculiar physical appearance of these patients *(2,3)*. The diagnosis is usually confirmed by the demonstration of an elevated GH level that is not suppressed by glucose loading and by the finding of an increased serum concentration of IGF-1 *(2,4)*. Almost all of these patients have an easily demonstrable pituitary adenoma, which in 60–70% of the cases is larger than 1 cm *(1,2)*.

What should be done when the clinical suspicion is not clearly confirmed by biochemical and imaging studies? Good medicine calls for a reconsideration of the clinical diagnosis. Severe hypothyroidism can cause coarsening of facial features because of edema, macroglossia, and diastolic hypertension *(5)*. Although this patient had evidence of mild central hypothyroidism, her skin was moist, she had acanthosis nigricans and definite acral enlargement not resulting from myxedema. Also, her glucose intolerance cannot be explained by hypothyroidism, which in its severe form is accompanied by a tendency to hypoglycemia *(6)*. The absence of a clear-cut pituitary adenoma on the MRI in a patient with the clinical features of acromegaly should raise the suspicion of ectopic GH-releasing hormone (GHRH) secretion. Ectopic GHRH secretion is extremely rare and is usually caused by carcinoid tumors and other neuroendocrine tumors of the pancreas and the pituitary pathology is almost always hyperplasia rather than true adenoma *(7)*. Recently, a well-documented case of acromegaly caused by the ectopic secretion of GH by a lymphoma has been reported *(8)*. However, in ectopic GHRH secretion producing acromegaly, there is always biochemical evidence of GH excess *(7,8)*.

The only other entity in which acral enlargement coexists with glucose intolerance and hypertension with normal GH and IGF-1 levels is acromegaloidism or pseudoacromegaly. Pseudoacromegaly can be considered a state of extreme but selective postreceptor insulin resistance *(9)*. In this condition, insulin-mediated glucose uptake is impaired but the mitogenic and growth-promoting activities of this hormone are retained *(9)*. Patients with pseudoacromegaly are usually young, tall females with large hands and feet, acanthosis nigricans, polycystic ovaries, and varying degrees of hyperandrogenism *(9)*. Molecular studies have shown that the insulin receptor *(10)* and *GLUT*-4 genes *(11)* are normal. More recent studies have found an impaired activation of the IRS-I-associated phosphoinositide 3-kinase in cultured fibroblasts from these patients *(12)*.

Ten yr ago, the degree of GH suppression by glucose found in our patient would have been considered "normal" *(4)*. The latter, along with an almost normal IGF-1 value and a borderline MRI with respect to the presence of an adenoma, would have raised a serious suspicion of pseudoacromegaly. The patient had a normal fasting insulin value (data not shown in the summary), which, in essence, rules out this condition. The development of ultrasensitive GH assays has changed the way we look at GH secretory dynamics, particularly the degree of suppression that should be achieved with a glucose load. With a glucose load, normal individuals should suppress their GH levels to about 0.25 ng/mL in females and 0.075 ng/mL in males *(13)*. Therefore, a GH suppression by glucose to just 1 ng/mL should be considered abnormal. Indeed, a recent abstract by Dimaraki et al coined the term "micromegaly" to describe five patients with active acromegaly and GH suppression to less than 2 ng/mL, but with elevated age- and sex-adjusted IGF-1 levels *(14)*. IGF-1 was determined twice in our patient, the first time the result was clearly, though not strikingly, above the normal range for age- and sex-matched controls; in the second measurement, IGF-1 was at the upper limit of normal. Why there is such variation in the ratio of GH to IGF-1 levels between individuals is not clear and aspects of GH binding to its receptor and signal transduction have not been investigated in such patients. Finally, the MRI was considered abnormal enough to merit transsphenoidal exploration. The patient did have a GH-producing microadenoma, that cosynthesized PRL as well (a mammosomatotropic tumor). One month postoperatively, she has noticed a significant reduction in the size of her hands and feet, a normalization of her blood pressure without antihypertensive medications, and a normalization of her fasting blood glucose. She will undergo full biochemical assessment of her somatotropic axis next month.

REFERENCES

1. Melmed S, Ho K, Klibanski A, et al. Recent advances in pathogenesis, diagnosis and management of acromegaly. J Clin Endocrinol Metab 1995;80:3395–3402.
2. Ezzat S, Forster MJ, Berchtold P, et al. Acromegaly: clinical and biochemical features in 500 patients. Medicine 1994;73:233–240.
3. Molitch ME. Clinical manifestations of acromegaly. Endocrinol Metab Clin North Am 1992;21:597–614.
4. Chang-DeMoranville BM, Jackson IMD. Diagnosis and endocrine testing in acromegaly. Endocrinol Metab Clin North Am 1992;21:649–668.
5. Klein I, Levey GS. Unusual manifestations of hypothyroidism. Arch Intern Med 1984;144:123–128.
6. Samaan NA. Hypoglycemia secondary to endocrine deficiencies. Endocrinol Metab Clin North Am 1989;18:145–154.
7. Faglia G, Arosio M, Bazzoni M. Ectopic acromegaly. Endocrinol Metab Clin North Am 1992;21:575–596.

8. Beuschlein F, Strasburger CJ, Siegerstetter V, et al. Acromegaly caused by secretion of growth hormone by a non-Hodgkin's lymphoma. N Engl J Med 2000;342:1871–1876.

9. Flier JS, Moller DE, Moses AC, et al. Insulin-mediated pseudoacromegaly: clinical and biochemical characterization of a syndrome of selective insulin resistance. J Clin Endocrinol Metab 1993;76:1533–1541.

10. Krook AS, Kumar I, Laing AJM, et al. Molecular scanning of the insulin receptor gene in syndromes of insulin resistance. Diabetes 1994;43:357–368.

11. Kumar S, Durrington PM, O'Rahilly S, et al. Severe insulin resistance, diabetes mellitus, hypertriglyceridemia and pseudoacromegaly. J Clin Endocrinol Metab 1996;81:3465–3468.

12. Dib K, Whitehead JP, Humphreys PJ, et al. Impaired activation of phosphoinositide 3-kinase by insulin in fibroblasts from patients with severe insulin resistance and pseudoacromegaly. A disorder characterized by selective postreceptor insulin resistance. J Clin Invest 1998;101:1111–1120.

13. Chapman IM, Hartman ML, Straume M, et al. Enhanced sensitivity growth hormone (GH) chemiluminescence assay reveals lower post-glucose nadir GH concentrations in men than women. J Clin Endocrinol Metab 1994;78:1312–1319.

14. Dimaraki EV, Jaffe CA, DeMott-Frieberg R, et al. Micromegaly: Active acromegaly with normal GH levels. Implications for diagnostic and follow-up criteria. Abstract P3-658, 81st Ann Meet Endocrine Soc, San Diego, CA, 1999.

CASE #3: 31-YR-OLD MAN WITH HYPERTHYROIDISM AND HYPOKALEMIC PERIODIC PARALYSIS AS A RESULT OF THYROTROPINOMA

Case Description

A 31-yr-old male was admitted to the hospital because of recurrent episodes of profound lower limb weakness over the previous month. These episodes developed acutely, without any apparent triggering event, and had made him fall on several occasions. On a previous admission to the emergency room he had been given the diagnosis of hypokalemic periodic paralysis and he improved with intravenous KCl administration. Upon direct questioning, he reported a 5-mo history of weight loss (10 Kg), palpitations, diaphoresis, diarrhea, and increasing anxiety. On physical examination, his blood pressure was 110/70, pulse 120 and regular, and temperature 37.5°C. He appeared anxious with a stare and his skin was moist and warm. There was lid-lag bilaterally but no proptosis was found and extraocular muscles were normal. His neck examination showed a small diffuse goiter with no bruits and no adenopathy. Deep tendon reflexes were brisk and he had a fine distal tremor.

Initial laboratory evaluation was remarkable only for a serum potassium level of 2.7 mEq/L. Thyroid function tests (TFT) revealed a T3 of 534 ng/dL (normal 90–190), T4 24 µg/dL (normal 5–12), free T4 7.7 ng/dL (normal 0.7–2) and TSH 5.4 mU/L (normal 0.3–5). A radioiodine scan showed a diffusely enlarged thyroid gland with a homogeneous uptake of 40%. GH, PRL, LH, FSH, morning cortisol, and total testosterone levels were all within normal limits.

Repeated testing showed apparently normal TSH levels in the presence of high circulating T3 and T4 levels. The patient was treated with methimazole and propranolol and his symptoms of hyperthyroidism improved; however, the TSH rose to 7.5 mU/L and his free T4 remained elevated. Methimazole was discontinued and 3 wk later, dynamic tests were performed. TSH levels did not change upon stimulation with 500 µg of TRH, nor could they be suppressed with the administration of increasing doses of T3 (50 µg for 3 d, 100 µg for 3 d, 200 µg for 3 d). Chromatography of the patient's serum revealed that approximately 75% of the TSH immunoreactivity eluted in the fraction that corresponds to the

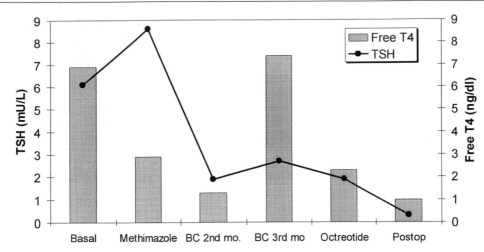

Fig. 2. TSH response to treatment in Case 3. Free T4 levels are shown by the bars and TSH levels by the line. Treatments are shown on the abscissa. BC-Bromocriptine treatment.

alpha subunit. Pituitary MRI revealed a right 4-mm hypointense lesion, with asymmetry of the gland.

A diagnosis of inappropriate TSH secretion probably caused by a TSH-producing pituitary microadenoma was established and the patient was started on gradually increasing doses of bromocriptine (up to 10 mg/d). After 2 mo of medication, he was clinically and biochemically (T3 190 ng/dL, T4 12 ng/dL, free T4 1.3 ng/dL, TSH 1.7 mU/L) euthyroid (see Fig. 2). Two months later he returned to the clinic with symptoms and signs of hyperthyroidism, and testing showed free hyperthyroxinemia with a normal TSH (see Fig. 2). Octreotide 100 mg TID subcutaneously was instituted with resolution of his symptoms and improvement of his free T4 level (see Fig. 2). A few weeks later, he underwent transsphenoidal surgery with resection of a 4-mm adenoma that immunostained strongly for TSH-β and FSH-β, weakly for GH and LH-β, and negative for ACTH and PRL. Postoperatively, his TFTs returned to normal and he became asymptomatic off all medications. Three years after surgery, the patient remains clinically euthyroid with normal TFTs and potassium levels.

Discussion

This case is an example of inappropriate TSH secretion, i.e., a situation whereby free hyperthyroxinemia occurs in the presence of a nonsuppressed TSH. In the differential diagnosis of this situation, it first is important to document that the thyroid hormone elevation is real and not caused by an elevated TBG, be it congenital or acquired (estrogen therapy, pregnancy, hepatitis), a condition frequently referred to as "euthyroid hyperthyroxinemia" *(1,2)*. People with euthyroid hyperthyroxinemia are clinically euthyroid and have normal TSH and free T4 values. Thus, this is an indication for the measurement of free thyroid hormone concentrations, which can presently be accomplished by commercially available, two-step immunoassays, that separate a fraction of the free T4 pool from the binding proteins before the T4 assay is performed *(2)*.

The differential diagnosis of true inappropriate TSH secretion includes selective pituitary resistance to thyroid hormones and TSH-secreting pituitary tumors (thyrotropinomas) *(3)*. Whereas in the former condition some of the feedback regulatory mechanisms are preserved, in the latter, a situation of autonomous TSH secretion prevails *(3)*. In the syndrome of selective pituitary resistance to thyroid hormone, TSH can be further stimulated with TRH administration and suppressed upon ingestion of thyroid hormone *(4)*. In contrast, in TSH-secreting adenomas, the TSH level should not be modified by the administration of either TRH or T3 *(5,6)*. The results of dynamic testing in these circumstances should be interpreted with caution, however, as up to 30% of TSH-producing adenomas respond to both TRH stimulation and T3 suppression *(6)*. Another biochemical characteristic that aids in the differentiation of these two conditions is the measurement of α-subunit *(3,6)*. Because of abnormal protein processing mechanisms, TSH-secreting adenomas produce an excess of α-subunit *(6)*. In the case described, the α-subunit was measured indirectly, separating the patient's serum using molecular exclusion chromatography and determining the proportion of TSH immunoreactivity that elutes in the fraction that corresponds to the α-subunit. α-subunit levels can also be measured directly in serum by specific immunoassays.

Patients with TSH-secreting pituitary adenomas usually present with symptoms and signs of thyrotoxicosis and a diffuse goiter *(3,6)*. Depending on the size and invasiveness of the tumor, these patients may have visual field defects and significant headaches *(3,6)*. Most thyrotropinomas are macroadenomas and may be accompanied by clinical and biochemical evidence of other pituitary hormone deficiencies *(6)*. Although the clinical features of hyperthyroidism are indistinguishable from those of Graves' disease, patients with TSH-secreting adenomas do not have any of the extrathyroidal manifestations of autoimmune thyroid disease such as exophthalmos or pretibial myxedema. Unilateral exophthalmos as a result of tumor invasion of the orbit has been reported, but thyroid acropachy has not been found *(7)*.

The case described in this chapter presented with thyrotoxicosis and well-documented episodes of hypokalemic paralysis. Thyrotoxic, hypokalemic periodic paralysis is a condition that occurs predominantly in Oriental and Latin-American male patients with hyperthyroid Graves' disease *(8,9)*. Although there are a few reports of hypokalemic paralysis developing in patients with toxic multinodular goiter, there is only one other reported case occurring in the setting of central hyperthyroidism *(10)*.

The treatment of choice of thyrotropinomas is transsphenoidal surgery *(11)*. Many patients with this condition had previously undergone thyroid ablation with radioidine *(3,6)*. This is obviously inappropriate and has been associated with a higher incidence of macroadenoma and tumor invasiveness *(3)*. The patient described in this chapter had a small microadenoma without chiasm compression, and therefore medical therapy was initially attempted. His initial response to bromocriptine was quite good, although it did not last long. His hyperthyroidism was then controlled, albeit incompletely, with octreotide until he underwent successful transsphenoidal removal of the microadenoma. TSH-secreting tumors respond to dopamine agonists rather poorly *(6,12,13)*, whereas they respond relatively well to somatostatin analogs both in terms of control of hyperthyroidism and tumor-size reduction *(6,13,14)*.

TSH-producing adenomas usually synthesize other hormones as well, most commonly, PRL and GH, and more rarely, FSH β-subunit *(6)*. The microadenoma in this patient was a chromophobic tumor that strongly immunostained for TSH-β and FSH-β, and was moderately positive for GH and LH-β. In most cases, the production of these other hormones is not accompanied by the corresponding clinical syndrome, because the peptides are either defective or simply not secreted. Interestingly, positive TSH immunostaining without clinical evidence of hyperthyroidism can be found in many clinically nonfunctioning pituitary adenomas *(15,16)*.

REFERENCES

1. Bartalena L. Recent achievements in studies on thyroid hormone binding proteins. Endocr Rev 1990;11: 47-63.
2. Klee GG, Hay ID. Biochemical testing of thyroid function. Endocrinol Metab Clin North Am 1997;26: 763-775.
3. McDermott MT, Ridgway CE. Central hyperthyroidism. Endocrinol Metab Clin North Am 1998;27: 187-203.
4. Refetoff S. Clinical and genetic aspects of resistance to thyroid hormone. The Endocrinologist 1992;2: 261-271.
5. Wynne AG, Gharib H, Scheithauer BW, et al. Hyperthyrodism due to inappropriate secretion of thyrotropin in 10 patients. Am J Med 1992:92:15-24.
6. Beck-Peccoz P, Brucker-Davis F, Persani L, et al. Thyrotropin-secreting pituitary tumors. Endocr Rev 1996;17:610-633.
7. Yovos JG, Falko JM, O'Dorisio TM, et al. Thyrotoxicosis and a thyrotropin secreting pituitary tumor causing unilateral exophtalmos. J Clin Endocrinol Metab 1981;53:338-342.
8. Ober KP. Thyrotoxic periodic paralysis in the United States. Report of 7 cases and review of the literature. Medicine 1992;71:109-120.
9. Nellen H, Mercado M, Villanueva S, et al. Thyrotoxic periodic paralysis in Mexican Mestizo patients: a clinical, biochemical and HLA-serological study. Arch Med Res1999;30:74-76.
10. Kiso Y, Yoshida K, Kaise K. A case of thyrotropin (TSH) secreting tumor complicated by periodic paralysis. Jpn J Med 1990;29:399-404.
11. McCutcheon IE, Weintraub BD, Oldfield EH. Surgical treatment of thyrotropin secreting pituitary adenomas. J Neurosurg 1990;73:674-683.
12. Smallridge RC. Thyrotropin-secreting pituitary tumors. Endocrinol Metab Clin North Am 1987;16: 765-792.
13. Shomali ME, Katznelson L. Medical therapy for gonadotroph and thyrotroph tumors. Endocrinol Metab Clin North Am 1999;28:223-240.
14. Comi RJ, Gesundheit N, Murray L, et al. Response of thyrotropin-secreting pituitary adenomas to a long-acting somatostatin analogue. N Engl J Med 1987;317:12-17.
15. Black PM, Hsu DW, Klibanski A. Hormone production in clinically non-functioning pituitary adenomas. J Neurosurg 1987;66:244-250.
16. Heshmati HM, Turpin G, Kujas M. The immunocytochemical heterogeneity of silent pituitary adenomas. Acta Endocrinol 1988;118:533-537.
17. Zuñiga S, Mendoza V, Felix-Espinosa I, et al. A plurihormonal TSH-secreting pituitary microadenoma: report of a case with an atypical clinical presentation and transient response to bromocriptine therapy. Endocr Pathol 1997;8:81-86.

CASE #4: 39-YR-OLD MAN
WITH A PITUITARY INCIDENTALOMA

Case Description

A 39-yr-old man presented to his physician because of facial herpes zoster and a related Bell's palsy. An MRI of the brain was normal except for the finding of an incidental pituitary adenoma arising out of the sella with a size of $1.2 \times 1.5 \times 1.2$ cm. He was referred directly to a neurosurgeon who found that his PRL was 28.1 ng/mL, his FSH was 5.5 mIU/mL, and his LH was 2.2 mIU/mL. He was scheduled for transsphenoidal resection of his apparently nonfunctioning adenoma. At surgery, when his nasopharynx was sprayed with a topical anesthetic prior to intubation, he had an anaphylactic reaction and suffered a cardiac arrest with a myocardial infarction. He subsequently had an uneventful recovery and was rescheduled 6 mo later for surgery.

However, he wished a second opinion and was seen by us. His endocrine review of systems was indeed negative, including normal sexual function. On examination, he was a well-appearing man with a weight of 213 lbs, a height of 69", and a BP of 138/86 mmHg. He had a partial paralysis of the left VII cranial nerve. There was mild abdominal obesity and mild facial plethora but no true facial rounding and no increase in the dorsal or supraclavicular fat pads. Hand and foot sizes appeared normal. Testes were of normal size and consistency. Testing showed a free T4 of 1.2 ng/dL (0.7-1.5), a morning cortisol of 22 µg/dL, a cortisol after overnight dexamethasone suppression of 2 µg/dL, an IGF-1 that was normal at 218 ng/dL, a testosterone of 352 ng/dL, and a PRL of 23.8 ng/dL. A PRL measurement after a dilution of 1:100 with saline was approximately the same.

We repeated the MRI scan, now 6 mo after the first, and compared them side-by-side. There was no change in tumor size and there was a clear 2–3-mm space between the tumor and the optic chiasm. We have advised the patient to have repeat scans now at yearly intervals and only have surgery if there is a clear increase in tumor size. He has seen his neurosurgeon again who wishes to operate now, as the chances of cure are greater now than later, when the tumor gets bigger.

Discussion

This patient presents with a rather common clinical dilemma, what to do with the patient with a pituitary "incidentaloma." As radiologic techniques have become more refined, we are now finding the clinical correlate of the observation that about 11% of pituitaries examined at autopsy harbor pituitary adenomas that were not suspected during life (1), although a number of other lesions can also be found (see Table 3). A similar frequency of incidentalomas is found when pituitary views are done in subjects having MRI scans for other reasons (2,3). In these series of autopsies and scans of normal subjects, virtually all the adenomas were microadenomas (1). However, in five series of patients with incidentalomas that have been reported (4–8), 94 of 152 patients had macroadenomas, such as this patient had.

This patient was evaluated for both hormone under- and oversecretion, finding neither to be present. Is this a worthwhile effort? In several series of patients with clinically nonfunctioning adenomas (CNFAs) who were undergoing surgery, hypopituitarism was present in about 50% (9–12). Furthermore, 52 of the 94 patients with macroadenomas that were incidentalomas mentioned earlier had pituitary function testing and 9 were reported as having hypopituitarism (4–8). Testing can be somewhat abbreviated, as clinical suspicion is generally low, consisting of measurement of free T4, testosterone, and AM cortisol levels. Should the cortisol have been borderline, e.g., 8–15 µg/dL, then further testing with metyrapone, hypoglycemia, or low-dose (1 µg) ACTH would have been done. He also had a quick screen for oversecretion with measurement of PRL, IGF-1, and an AM cortisol after overnight 1 mg dexamethasone suppression. The worth of such measurements in an asymptomatic patient has been questioned (13) but the tests are relatively inexpensive compared to repeated scans and/or surgery and the yield is not that low. One of the 18 incidentaloma patients studied by Reincke et al. (4) turned out to have a GH-secreting adenoma and in another similar series 8/67 patients had prolactinomas. Furthermore, in a recent series of 32 patients with CNFAs operated for a variety of reasons,

Table 3
Lesions of the Sella Turcica and Parasellar Areas

Pituitary Adenomas	Cell Rest Tumors
PRL-secreting	Craniopharyngioma
GH-secreting	Rathke's cleft cyst
ACTH-secreting	Epidermoid (cholesteatoma)
Gonadotropin-secreting	Chordoma
TSH-secreting	Lipoma
Nonsecreting	Colloid cyst
Primitive germ-cell tumors	Gliomas
Germinoma	Optic glioma
Dermoid	Oligodendroglioma
Teratoma	Ependymoma
Atypical teratoma (dysgerminoma)	Microglioma
Infundibuloma	
Astrocytoma	Metastatic cancer
Benign lesions	
Meningioma	Vascular aneurysms
Enchondroma	
Hypothalamic hamartomas	
Gangliocytomas	
Myoblastomas	
Granulomatous, infectious, inflammatory	Miscellaneous
Abscess, bacterial and fungal	Arachnoid cyst
Tuberculosis	Empty sella syndrome
Sarcoidosis	Mucocele (sphenoid)
Giant cell granuloma	
Lymphocytic hypophysitis	
Lymphocytic infundibulohypophysitis	
Histiocytosis X (eosinophilic granuloma)	
Echinococcal cyst	

Reprinted with permission from ref. *(1)*.

immunohistochemistry showed that three were silent lactotroph adenomas and one was a silent corticotroph adenoma *(14)*. It is not clear whether patients with "silent" somato-troph and corticotroph adenomas with minimal clinical evidence of hormone oversecretion are free from the increased risk for the more subtle cardiovascular, bone, oncological, and possibly other adverse effects we usually associate with such tumors. Because of these reasons, GH- and ACTH-secreting tumors with even minimal evidence of over-secretion should probably be resected. Tumors causing hypopituitarism should also be resected, as up to 40–50% of such patients can expect return of at least some pituitary function postoperatively *(9,15)*.

The patient was mildly hyperprolactinemic. But the level of hyperprolactinemia is more indicative of stalk dysfunction with the tumor impairing the ability of dopamine to reach the pituitary via the portal vessels rather than resulting from secretion by the tumor *(16–18)*. However, when two-site immunoradiometric assays (IRMA) or chemiluminometric (ICMA) assays are used, patients with very high PRL levels may appear to have PRL levels that are normal or only moderately elevated, i.e., on the order of 30–200 ng/

mL, because of the "hook effect" *(19,20)*. Thus, all patients with macroadenomas should have their PRL run undiluted and also at 1:100 dilution to be sure the lesion is not a prolactinoma. If this patient's hyperprolactinemia had been causing symptoms, these could easily be treated with a dopamine agonist.

However, this patient, as well as many others with incidental CNFAs did not have hypopituitarism or evidence of oversecretion and his mild hyperprolactinemia was causing no symptoms or hypogonadism. Is surgery indicated? In the five series already cited *(4–8)*, of 58 patients with microadenomas followed for 2.7–8.0 yr, there was tumor enlargement in only two patients. However, in these same series *(4–8)* of 94 patients with macroadenomas, 19 experienced tumor enlargement and in four of these 19, the enlargement was caused by sudden hemorrhage into the tumor. Thus, this patient only has about a 20% risk of tumor enlargement. Because of this and the fact that transsphenoidal surgery is not without complications *(21)*, we felt comfortable repeating his scans an intervals, with the idea that surgery could be deferred and only done if there was evidence of tumor enlargement. His history of anaphylaxis with cardiac arrest at the time of his prior transsphenoidal surgery clearly influenced our advice to him.

REFERENCES

1. Molitch ME. Pituitary incidentalomas. Endocrinol Metab Clin North Am 1997;26:725–740.
2. Chong BW, Kucharczyk AW, Singer W, et al. Pituitary gland MR: a comparative study of healthy volunteers and patients with microadenomas. Am J Neuroradiol 1994;15: 675–679.
3. Hall WA, Luciano MG, Doppman JL, et al. Pituitary magnetic resonance imaging in normal human volunteers: occult adenomas in the general population. Ann Intern Med 1994;120:817–820.
4. Reincke M, Allolio B, Saeger W, et al. The 'incidentaloma' of the pituitary gland. Is neurosurgery required? JAMA 1990;263:2772–2776.
5. Donovan LE, Corenblum B. The natural history of the pituitary incidentaloma. Arch Intern Med 1995; 153:181–183.
6. Nishizawa S, Ohta S, Yokoyama T, Uemura K. Therapeutic strategy for incidentally found pituitary tumors ("pituitary incidentalomas"). Neurosurgery 1998;43:1344–1350.
7. Feldkamp J, Santen R, Harms E, et al. Incidentally discovered pituitary lesions: high frequency of macroadenomas and hormone-secreting adenomas—results of a prospective study. Clin Endocrinol 1999;51:109–113.
8. Eguchi K, Migita K, Arita K, et al. Natural course and management of incidentally found pituitary lesions. Program of the 6th Int Pituitary Congress, Long Beach, CA, 1999, p. 99.
9. Arafah AM. Reversible hypopituitarism in patients with large nonfunctioning pituitary adenomas. J Clin Endocrinol Metab 1986;62:1173–1179.
10. Ebersold MJ, Quast LM, Laws ER, Scheithauer B, Randall RV. Long-term results in transsphenoidal removal of nonfunctioning pituitary adenomas. J Neurosurg 1986;64:713–719.
11. Comtois R, Beauregard H, Somma M, et al. The clinical and endocrine outcome to transsphenoidal microsurgery of nonsecreting pituitary adenomas. Cancer 1991;68:860–866.
12. Tominaga A, Uozumi T, Arita K, et al. Anterior pituitary function in patients with nonfunctioning pituitary adenoma: results of longitudinal follow-up. Endocrine J 1995;42:421–427.
13. King JT Jr, Justice AC, Aron DC. Management of incidental pituitary microadenomas: a cost-effectiveness analysis. J Clin Endocrinol Metab 1997;82:3625–3632.
14. Lillehei KO, Kirschman DL, Kleinschmidt-DeMasters B, Ridgway EC. Reassessment of the role of radiation therapy in the treatment of endocrine-inactive pituitary macroadenomas.Neurosurgery 1998; 43:432–439.
15. Webb SM, Rigla M, Wagner A, Oliver B, Bartumeus F. Recovery of hypopituitarism after neurosurgical treatment of pituitary adenomas. J Clin Endocrinol Metab 1999;84:3696–3700.
16. Molitch ME, Reichlin S. Hypothalamic hyperprolactinemia: neuroendocrine regulation of prolactin secretion in patients with lesions of the hypothalamus and pituitary stalk. In: Macleod RM, Thorner MO, Scapagnini U, eds. Prolactin. Basic and Clinical Correlates. Proc IVth Int Congr Prolactin. Liviana, Padova, Italy, 1985, pp. 709–719.

17. Bevan JS, Burke CW, Esiri MM, Adams CBT. Misinterpretation of prolactin levels leading to management errors in patients with sellar enlargement. Am J Med 1987;82:29–32.
18. Kruse A, Astrup J, Gyldensted C, Cold GE. Hyperprolactinaemia in patients with pituitary adenomas. The pituitary stalk compression syndrome. Br J Neurosurg 1995;9:453–457.
19. St-Jean E, Blain F, Comtois R. High prolactin levels may be missed by immunoradiometric assay in patients with macroprolactinomas. Clin Endocrinol 1996;44:305–309.
20. Barkan A, Chandler WF. Giant pituitary prolactinoma with falsely low serum prolactin: the pitfall of the "high-dose hook effect": case report. Neurosurgery 1998:9;13–15.
21. Ciric I, Ragin A, Baumgartner C, Pierce D. Complications of transsphenoidal surgery: results of a national survey, review of the literature and personal experience. Neurosurgery 197;40:225–237.

2

Hypopituitarism

Baha M. Arafah, MD and Mona P. Nasrallah, MD

CONTENTS

CASE #1: SARCOIDOSIS

Case Description

A 44-yr-old African-American woman presented with a 7-yr history of amenorrhea, tiredness, unexplained fatigue, weakness, dry skin, and thinning of the hair. She remained healthy until age 37, when she developed oligomenorrhea and thinning of axillary and pubic hair, with loss of hair over the parietal area. Serum thyroid-stimulating hormone (TSH) levels done on two separate occasions were reported to be "normal." Three years before her presentation, and at the age of 41, she was admitted to a hospital with headaches, lethargy, and nausea. The diagnosis of obstructive hydrocephalus was made. She had an emergency ventriculostomy, followed by a right-sided V-P shunt, which she continues to have. Work-up at that time included a lumbar puncture (WBC = 6/mL, glucose = 64 mg/dL, protein = 17 mg/dL, VDRL = nonreactive) and a MRI of brain without contrast, which revealed an empty sella and postoperative changes. Other findings during that admission included hyponatremia (Na = 122 mmol/L), normocytic anemia, and leukopenia (WBC = 2500/µL, Hct = 33 %). A bone marrow biopsy revealed noncaseating granulomas. The diagnoses of collagen vascular disease, not otherwise specified and the syndrome of inappropriate antidiuretic hormone (SIADH) were made. She was discharged home on oral sodium supplements (NaCl, 2 g/d), fluid restriction, and phenobarbital for seizure prophylaxis. The latter was discontinued because of increasing lethargy.

She remained chronically unwell, with exacerbating illnesses requiring several hospitalizations. Six months prior to this evaluation, she was admitted to the hospital for abdominal pain, nausea, vomiting, and weight loss of 15 lbs. Ultrasound of the gall bladder and liver enzymes were normal. At that time, morning serum cortisol levels were measured on two occasions and were in the "low-normal range" of 6 to 8 µg/dL.

From: *Contemporary Endocrinology: Challenging Cases in Endocrinology*
Edited by: M. E. Molitch © Humana Press Inc., Totowa, NJ

An outpatient endocrine consult was requested in view of the following thyroid function studies done at that time: a serum TSH of 0.94 mU/L, a total thyroxine level of 4.1 µg/dL (normal 5–11) and a calculated free thyroxine index of 4.0 (normal 5–11). Additional complaints included several years of history of dyspareunia and lack of libido.

In the clinic, she appeared tired and fatigued. Her exam was notable for a blood pressure of 90/70, a heart rate of 75/min, and a weight of 122 lbs. (baseline approximately 140). The thyroid was barely palpable. The skin was dry and there was sparse axillary and pubic hair. She had normal eye motility, full visual fields, and normal fundi. Her neurologic exam was remarkable for significant delay in the relaxation phase of the deep tendon reflexes.

Based on the past medical history and available clinical biochemical and pathological data, the diagnosis of hypopituitarism secondary to neurosarcoidosis was entertained. Additional studies were performed to assess pituitary function and confirm the etiology of hypopituitarism. Studies included the following serum levels: total thyroxine of 2.1 µg/dL, a free thyroxine index of 3 (normal 5–11), prolactin of 39 µg/L, an FSH of 1.1 IU/L, an LH of 0.9 IU/L, an estradiol of <10 ng/L, a total testosterone of 11 ng/dL, an AM cortisol of 5.5 µg/dL, a total calcium of 8.8 mg/dL, an albumin of 3.8 gm/dL, a Na^+ of 132 mmol/L, a K^+ of 4.2 mmol/L, and a normal ACE level.

A lumbar puncture revealed the following cerebrospinal fluid (CSF) data: WBC = 26/mL (70% lymphocytes and 15% monocytes, RBC = 0/mL, protein of 270 mg/dL, a glucose of 20 mg/dL, and negative stains and growth for bacteria, myobacteria, or fungi). Urinalysis showed a specific gravity of 1.015. Pulmonary function tests and chest X-ray were unremarkable. The electrocardiogram was reported as low voltage with sinus bradycardia. MRI of the pituitary with contrast showed meningeal enhancement in the region of the optic chiasm and a normal-appearing pituitary stalk. Neuroophthalmologic evaluation revealed granulomas in the tarsal conjunctiva but no uveitis.

Dynamic studies of pituitary hormone secretion were done, as shown in the Fig. 1. Briefly, they showed an elevated serum prolactin level on multiple occasions, associated with partial hypopituitarism, with loss of gonadal, thyroidal, and adrenal functions. Antidiuretic hormone (ADH) secretion was considered to be normal. The pattern of response to the administration of hypothalamic releasing hormones was consistent with deficiency of hypothalamic releasing hormones. Thus, despite the presence of clinical hypothyroidism and peripheral hypothyroxinemia, serum TSH levels were inappropriately in the "normal" range and increased further after thyrotropin-releasing hormone (TRH) was administered. The pattern of response to GnRH administration was similar and consistent with partial deficiency of the latter hypothalamic releasing factor. The patient had partial adrenocorticotropic hormone (ACTH) deficiency as evidenced by the subnormal rise in serum cortisol following insulin-induced hypoglycemia (nadir glucose of 22 mg/dL). The cortisol response to cortrosyn in this patient was considered "normal." Such discordance in cortisol responses is seen in 40–50% of patients with ACTH deficiency, particularly when the latter is partial.

The diagnosis of neurosarcoidosis and hypothalamic hypopituitarism was made and the patient was started on prednisone therapy (40 mg/d) as well as physiologic thyroid hormone replacement. Two weeks later, she felt like 'she was given a new life'. Premarin and provera were subsequently added with further improvement in her well being.

She did relatively well over the years, requiring careful monitoring. Seven years after the diagnosis was made, she developed cervical and brachial plexus neuritis, and was given high-dose steroids. As a result of steroid therapy, she had hypertension, weight

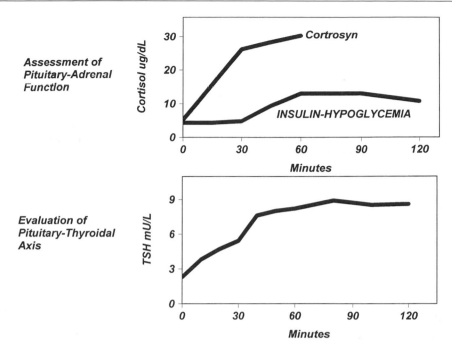

Fig. 1. Dynamic testing of pituitary function in a patient with hypopituitarism is shown. The upper graph shows evaluation of pituitary–adrenal function using cortrosyn stimulation test (250 μg, IV) and insulin-induced hypoglycemia (nadir glucose of 22 mg/dL). The lower panel of the graph shows the response to TRH administration in a patient with clinical and biochemical (low thyroxine) features of hypothyroidism.

gain, and developed cataracts and avascular necrosis of the hip, requiring total hip replacement. Currently, she is 54 yr old, doing very well with minimal neurologic sequale. She is an active housewife and a baby sitter. She continues to be on prednisone (7.5 mg/d), thyroxine, and premarin as hormone replacement. Although she was documented to have GH deficiency, she declined physiologic replacement therapy.

Discussion

This case illustrates many of the difficulties and problems encountered in establishing the diagnosis of hypopituitarism and in defining its etiology. The long duration of symptoms and their "nonspecific nature" clearly contributed to the delay in diagnosis. The patient had signs and symptoms of, at least, partial hypopituitarism 7 yr before her presentation. In addition, she had histologic findings 3 yr before presentation that were consistent with systemic sarcoidosis. At that time, she had anemia, hyponatremia, and noncaseating granulomas on bone marrow biopsy. She also had clinical features suggestive of adrenal insufficiency (tiredness, fatigue, hypotension, hyponatremia, loss of axillary and pubic hair) as well as hypogonadism (amenorrhea and dyspareunia).

Repeated assessment of thyroid function using TSH as a marker expectedly revealed normal values. The original thyroid function tests done a few months before endocrine evaluation were interpreted to be consistent with euthyroid-sick syndrome. It was not until the clinical and biochemical data were looked at together, that the diagnosis of hypopituitarism was entertained.

Sarcoidosis is a multisystem granulomatous disorder of unknown etiology *(1)*. Its prevalence varies from 5–50/100,000 depending on the population studied. In the United States, there is a 3.8-fold increased risk among African-Americans, with a slight female preponderance. The peak incidence of sarcoidosis is in the fourth decade of life. There seems to be a threefold higher incidence of family history of sarcoidosis among African-Americans. It is interesting to note that the patient's mother and sister had the disease. In these respects, our patient's presentation and background were typical.

Despite extensive epidemiological studies, there is incomplete understanding of the etiology of this disease. Both a genetic/immunologic predisposition and an environmental trigger seem involved in the pathogenesis. The hallmark of the disease is the presence of noncaseating granulomas. The clinical manifestations range in severity and in spectrum, depending on the specific organs involved. Whereas some symptoms can also be related to the products of granulomas such as vitamin D and the resulting hypercalcemia *(1)*, others are related to tissue and organ destruction such as the case with pulmonary manifestations. The following organ systems *(1)* are involved in sarcoidosis: pulmonary (90%), ocular (20%), dermatological (20%), reticuloendothelial (20%), gastrointestinal, salivary and hepatic (20%), musculoskeletal (10%), cardiac (5%), and nervous system (5%).

In the CNS, sarcoidosis has a predilection to the base of the skull and manifests clinically as cranial neuropathy (most commonly optic and facial nerves), lymphocytic meningitis, hydrocephalus (obstructive and nonobstructive), hypothalamic dysfunction, and hypopituitarism *(2–5)*. The patient under discussion has most of these manifestations.

The diagnosis of sarcoidosis in general is established based on three criteria: a) the recognition of the characteristic clinical findings; b) histologic evidence of noncaseating granulomas; and c) ruling out other causes of granulomas, particularly tuberculosis *(1)*. In the case of CNS involvement, the search for extraneurological manifestations should be undertaken, as these are present in 90% of patients and are easier to biopsy *(2,3)*. Lumbar puncture and gadolinium-enhanced MRI of brain are useful adjuncts in the diagnosis, especially in the absence of apparent systemic pathology *(2,3)*. CSF abnormalities are present in 80% of cases and most commonly include an elevated protein level and increased lymphocytes. MRI abnormalities are also detected frequently. The most specific finding for hypothalamic involvement is pituitary stalk thickening and leptomeningeal enhancement in the optic chiasm area. The latter helps to differentiate neurosarcoidosis from hypothalamic disease resulting from other causes such as multiple sclerosis and lymphocytic hypophysitis *(2,3)*. Products of granulomas such as ACE levels and IL-2 are nonspecific and depend on disease activity *(2,3)*. However, the finding of an elevated ACE level in the CSF fluid is indicative of active neurosarcoidosis.

The cause of hypopituitarism in neurosarcoidosis was demonstrated to be hypothalamic insufficiency by dynamic endocrine testing *(5)*. The general principles of testing outlined in earlier studies remain the mainstay of the diagnosis, and were applied to our patient. As shown in Fig. 1, the administration of TRH to our patient with clinical hypothyroidism resulted in a delayed and sustained release of TSH that is typically described in patients with tertiary or hypothalamic hypothyroidism. The latter pattern of response is also seen in patients with pituitary stalk section or compression. It is not surprising to note that such patients just as ours had mild hyperprolactinemia. Other dynamic studies using other stimulatory hypothalamic factors or hormones such as CRH and GnRH (performed on our patient, but not shown) can demonstrate the similar phenomena. In the study by Stuart et al., 6 out of 10 patients with neurosarcoidosis had a normal LH rise (greater than three- to six-fold basal) following GnRH infusion, and a lack of response after clomiphene citrate was observed in all 10 patients *(5)*.

After establishing the diagnosis, management of patients with sarcoidosis requires comprehensive and meticulous care. Attention to the details of specific organ involvement and management of problems arising from the disease itself (e.g., hypopituitarism, anemia), or as a complication of therapy (e.g., ulcer, weight gain, osteoporosis, fluid retention, and so on), represent some of the challenges encountered. Patients with neurosarcoidosis are often managed by multiple specialists with variable areas of interests and expertise, who should regularly interact and communicate with each other.

Even with steroid therapy, recovery of hypothalamic function is extremely unusual and, therefore, hypopituitarism necessitates permanent hormone replacement. Physiologic steroid replacement is roughly the equivalent of 5 mg prednisone per day. Most patients with neurosarcoidosis receive therapeutic doses of prednisone, and may therefore exhibit relative adrenal insufficiency at physiologic doses. Management of hypothyroidism is these patients is similar to that of patients with hypopituitarism, regardless of its etiology and relies primarily on oral thyroxine. Sex hormone replacement is crucial because of the high risk for osteoporosis. Similarly, GH therapy may be beneficial, but was refused by our patient. Diabetes insipidus, when present, is usually central and would respond well to oral or intranasal DDAVP. However, occasionally it may be partially nephrogenic when hypercalcemia is a complicating feature.

Chronic steroid therapy requires as much monitoring as hypopituitarism itself. Our patient developed cataracts, avascular necrosis of the hip, hypertension, and kidney stones. She is on prophylactic therapy for peptic ulcer disease.

REFERENCES

1. Newman LS, Rose CS, Maier LA. Sarcoidosis. N Engl J Med 1997;336:1224–1234.
2. Zajicek JP, Scolding NJ, Foster O, Rovaris M, Evanson J, Moseley IF, Scadding JW, Thopson EJ, Chamoun V, Miller DH, McDonald WI, Mitchell D. Central nervous system sarcoidosis. Diagnosis and management. QJM 1999;92:103–117.
3. Lower EE, Broderick JP, Brott TG, Baughman RP. Diagnosis and management of neurological sarcoidosis. Arch Intern Med 1997;157:1864–1868.
4. Bullman C, Faust M, Hoffmann A, Heppner C, Jockenhovel F, Muller-Wieland D, Krone W. Five cases with central diabetes insipidus and hypogonadism as first presentation of neurosarcoidosis. Eur J Endocrinol 2000;142:365–372.
5. Stuart CA, Neelon FA, Lebovitz HE. Hypothalamic insufficiency. The cause of hypopituitarism in sarcoidosis. Ann Intern Med 1978;88:589–594.

CASE #2: HYPOPHYSITIS

Case Presentation

A 25-yr-old woman was referred to our institution for evaluation of increasing fatigue, tiredness, sleepiness, decreased appetite, nausea, and a 5-kg weight loss over a 3-mo period. The patient noted gradual loss of libido, a decrease in axillary and pubic hair over the 2 mo preceding her evaluation. Six months before her visit, she underwent an eventful vaginal delivery after a full-term uncomplicated pregnancy. Menses resumed several weeks postpartum and remained regular since. The patient did not breastfeed her infant and she was treated briefly with bromocriptine. The patient denied having headaches or visual symptoms. Her past medical history was otherwise unremarkable. The family

Table 1
Pituitary Hormone Response to Dynamic Testing

Dynamic test	At Presentation		38 Months After Biopsy	
	Baseline level	Peak	Baseline peak	Level
Insulin-Induced Hypoglycemia*				
GH (µg/L)	2	8.9	0.1	6.9
ACTH (ng/L)	<3	3.1	<3	<3
Cortisol (µg/dL)	0.5	1.1	0.5	0.6
TRH Stimulation Test				
TSH (mU/L)	1.2	8.2	1.7	9.9
Prolactin (µg/L)	2.1	1.9	1.3	1.4
GnRH- Stimulation Test				
FSH (IU/L)	3.5	11.8	4.9	12
LH (IU/L)	4.6	23.5	6.7	33

*Nadir glucose of 25 mg/dL

history revealed a mother with Grave's disease and a maternal aunt with systemic lupus erythematosus (SLE).

On physical examination, pertinent findings included a recumbent blood pressure of 116/74 mmHg, which decreased to 100/60 upon assuming upright posture. She appeared tired, exhausted, and pale. The skin was not dry and the thyroid was not enlarged. Axillary and pubic hair were diminished. There was no increased pigmentation over mucous membranes or the skin. Eye exam revealed normal extraocular movement, pupillary reactions, visual fields, and fundi. Deep tendon reflexes were normal.

Initial laboratory data revealed the following: Na^+:127 mmol/L; K^+: 4.0 mmol/L; Cl^-:101 mmol/L; HCO_3^-: 28 mmol/L; BUN: 23 mg/dL, and a creatinine of 0.6 mg/dL. The hematocrit was 33% and the WBC was 3800/µL.

Initial endocrine data included the following: Am cortisol of 0.6 µg/dL, which increased to 3.5 µg/dL after IV cortrosyn (250 µg), a morning plasma ACTH level of <3 ng/L (10–52), DHEA-S of 5 µg/dL (50–400), free thyroxine of 0.8 ng/dL (0.6–1.5), a TSH of 1.7 mU/L, a prolactin of 2.0 µg/L, an FSH of 10 mU/L, an LH of 11 mU/L, an estradiol of 65 ng/L, a total testosterone of 15 ng/dL (10–70), and a free testosterone of 0.2 ng/dL (0.2–7).

A magnetic resonance imaging scan (MRI) of the sella turcica showed an enhancing sellar mass that extended into the suprasellar area, and was close to, but not in contact with the optic chiasm or the cavernous sinus.

The diagnosis of adrenal insufficiency was clinically suspected and biochemically confirmed. The patient was started on physiologic hydrocortisone replacement therapy (20 mg daily, in three divided doses), with prompt clinical improvement in symptoms. The treatment was discontinued for 2 d a week later when pituitary dynamic studies were performed. The results are illustrated in Table 1. Briefly, FSH and LH responses to GnRH were normal. Similarly, serum TSH increased normally after TRH administration. In contrast, baseline serum prolactin levels were low and did not increase after stimulation with TRH. Plasma cortisol and ACTH levels were low or undetectable and failed to increase after insulin-induced hypoglycemia (Nadir glucose level of 25 mg/dL). In contrast, serum GH levels increased appropriately after insulin-induced hypoglycemia.

Because of the unusual nature of mass, its proximity to the optic chiasm, and the endocrine data, biopsy of the mass was recommended. A transsphenoidal biopsy of the sellar mass showed findings consistent with lymphocytic hypophysitis, with scattered normal pituitary cells. Multiple sections throughout the specimen were immunostained and showed cells staining positive for prolactin, TSH, FSH, LH, GH, but not for corticotropin. The lymphocyte population consisted of a mixture of B and T cells. The B-cell population was composed of a polyclonal mixture of cell types by immunohistochemical staining for immunoglobulin heavy and light chains.

Postoperatively, corticotropin deficiency persisted and physiologic hydrocortisone replacement therapy was continued. A repeat MRI scan of the sella performed 6 mo after the biopsy showed no interval changes in the appearance of the pituitary mass. A MRI done 38 mo after the biopsy showed spontaneous resolution of the pituitary mass. Shortly thereafter, pituitary dynamic studies were repeated and were unchanged (see Table 1). Ten months later (i.e., 4 yr after initial presentation, she developed signs and symptoms of primary hypothyroidism). She was found to have a goiter, an elevated serum TSH level, as well as a positive antithyroid peroxidase antibody. Treatment with thyroxine reversed all symptoms of hypothyroidism. Currently, she continues to do well, 6 yr after the diagnosis of hypophysitis was made. She continues to have normal menses while receiving chronic physiologic hydrocortisone and thyroxine replacement.

Discussion

The current case has many of the features that have been reported in most cases of hypophysitis, particularly the temporal relationship to pregnancy. The pattern of pituitary hormone losses (ACTH and prolactin) with sparing of the gonadotropins is also typical of hypophysitis. The presence of a family history of autoimmune diseases and the subsequent development of such a disease (Hashimoto's thyroiditis) in our patient are consistent features of patients with adenohypophysitis (1–3).

Lymphocytic hypophysitis is one of the recently appreciated entities that can cause a pituitary mass and hypopituitarism. It is an inflammatory process, likely to be autoimmune in nature that involves the pituitary gland. Even though the inflammatory process is diffuse, corticotrophs appear to be the most susceptible, whereas gonadotrophs are the least affected by the inflammatory process. Thus, in patients with hypophysitis, ACTH deficiency is the most commonly impaired axis, whereas gonadal function is often normal (1–3). Lactotrophs are often affected by the inflammatory process, as reflected by the fact that serum prolactin levels are low in approximately one-half of the patients (1,2). A variant of this disease entity involves predominantly the posterior lobe of the pituitary and/or the stalk and, as expected, results in diabetes insipidus (4). Most patients with hypophysitis or their relatives have other autoimmune illnesses such as Grave's disease, Hashimoto's thyroiditis, vitiligo, lupus, and inflammatory arthritis (1,2).

A few of the reported cases have been noted to have serum antibodies against pituitary tissue as well as other autoantibodies (1,2). The latter finding in addition to the described histologic changes suggest that the disease is autoimmune in nature. In a study of sera from patients with biopsy proven lymphocytic hypophysitis, Crock (5) found that 70% had antibody to a 79-Kd cytosolic protein. Antibodies to the same antigen were seen in some patients with Addison's disease suggesting that the antigen is not restricted to the pituitary (5).

Precise diagnosis of this entity can only be made by biopsy. Definitive data on the long-term natural history of the disease are sparse. This case and a few others reported in the literature indicate that such patients can have spontaneous regression of the inflammatory process *(1–3)*. The natural course of the disease as constructed by the various presentations and manifestations suggest progressive fibrosis and loss of pituitary cells after an initial episode of edema, inflammation, and associated mass lesion. Depending on the stage of the disease at the time of diagnosis, patients may present with a large pituitary mass lesion as a result of the inflammatory process or with an atrophic and fibrotic gland. Although lymphocytic adenohypophysitis has been described in men and women of all age groups, the typical patient is a young woman presenting during pregnancy or within 1–2 yr after delivery. Despite the well-recognized tendency of gonadotropin secretion in these patients to be spared, subsequent fertility was not well appreciated. A few reports have indicated that such patients can get pregnant after the first episode of hypophysitis without unusual complications *(3)*.

The diagnosis is often difficult without a biopsy because of the variable mode of presentation and the lack of a serologic marker for the disease *(1,2,6)*. A few clues to the diagnosis include presentation during or within 2 yr after pregnancy in a woman who has other autoimmune diseases. The pattern of pituitary hormone deficit can also be very helpful in suspecting the diagnosis. ACTH and prolactin deficiencies associated with normal gonadotropin secretion are very likely to be caused by hypophysitis because impairment of pituitary-gonadal function is one of the earliest manifestation of hypopituitarism caused by mass lesions or vascular necrosis. Surgery is sometimes necessary at the time of first presentation especially in patients with mass lesions compressing the optic apparatus. When the clinical presentation, radiological and endocrine manifestation are all consistent with the diagnosis, tissue diagnosis may not be essential as long as the patient is followed closely. Although some advocate high-dose glucocorticoid therapy, there are no data to support efficacy of such treatment *(6)*. Hormone replacement therapy is the main form of treatment and should thoroughly address individual needs.

REFERENCES

1. Patel MC, Guneratne N, Haq N, West TET, Weetman AP, Clayton RN. Peripartum hypopituitarism and lymphocytic hypophysitis. QJM 1995;88:571–580.
2. Thodou E, Asa SL, Kontogeorgos G, Kovacs K, Horvath E, Ezzat S. Clinical case seminar: lymphocytic hypophysitis; clinicopathological findings. J Clin Endocrinol Metab 1995;80:2302–2311.
3. Gagneja H, Arafah B, Taylor HC. Histologically proven hypophysitis: spontaneous resolution and subsequent pregnancy. Mayo Clin Proc 1999;74:150–154.
4. Imura H, Nakao K, Shimatsu A, et al. Lymphocytic infundibulo-neurohypophysitis as a cause of central diabetes insipidus. N Engl J Med 1993;329:683–689.
5. Crock PA. Cytosolic autoantigens in lymphocytic hypophysitis. J Clin Endocrinol Metab 1998;83:609–618.
6. Feigenbaum SL, Martin MC, Wilson CB, Jaffe RB. Lymphocytic adenohypophysitis: a pituitary mass lesion occurring in pregnancy; proposal for medical treatment. Am J Obstet Gynecol 1991;164:1549–1555.

CASE #3: PITUITARY APOPLEXY

Case Presentation

A 46-yr-old man presented to the emergency room of a community hospital with a 6-h history of a sudden, severe, frontal headache that awakened him from sleep. He denied having similar episodes or frequent headaches. Evaluation by the emergency room physician was reported to have shown a temperature of 38.1°C, a blood pressure of 150/80, and a pulse of 99/min. He was described to have tenderness over the frontal and maxillary sinuses. His neck was supple and the remainder of his physical exam was reported to be unremarkable. He was discharged home on antibiotics and decongestants for presumed acute sinusitis. He returned to the same emergency room the next morning with persistent headaches and new onset of diplopia. He reported that he was unable to take the antibiotics he was previously prescribed because of nausea and vomiting. Evaluation by the emergency room physician showed a temperature of 39.4°C, a blood pressure of 120/68 and a pulse of 110/min. He was suspected by the emergency room physician to have meningitis and was transferred to our institution for further management.

On arrival to our institution, the patient appeared ill, but was alert and oriented, complaining of headaches, diplopia, and photophobia. He reported to have been previously healthy except for diminished libido and potency, for which he was prescribed Viagra® for 1 yr. He denied having chronic headaches or visual symptoms. On examination, the patient was slightly overweight with normal features. His vital signs were similar to those obtained at the emergency room. He had ptosis of the right eye, right abducen palsy, as well as bitemporal hemianopsia. Fundoscopic exam showed normal venous pulsation and mild, bilateral temporal disk pallor. The patient had minimal tenderness over maxillary and frontal sinuses, whereas his neck showed minimal stiffness. He was noted to have a slight bilateral gynecomastia, without a nipple discharge. The rest of the physical exam was negative.

After blood samples were drawn, iv fluids were administered. The patient had a non-contrast CT scan in the emergency department that showed a 2-cm hyperintense sellar mass with suprasellar extension. Following iv contrast, the mass became more intense. The endocrine team was consulted when the presumptive diagnosis of pituitary tumor apoplexy was made. Intravenous hydrocortisone (100 mg) was administered, a lumbar puncture was done followed by wide spectrum antibiotic therapy. The patient was admitted to the neurological intensive care unit for monitoring. Studies on the CSF specimens showed 15 WBC/mL, mostly lymphocytes, a normal glucose of 79 mg/dL, and an elevated protein concentration to 220 mg/dL. Cultures done on a CSF specimen showed no bacterial growth.

Pertinent laboratory studies done on arrival showed normal values for electrolytes, calcium, BUN, and creatinine. Total WBC was 15,500/µL with 75% neutrophils, 5% bands, 5% basophils, and 10% lymphocytes. Endocrine studies on blood samples drawn before therapeutic intervention showed the following: a serum cortisol of 6.5 µg/dL, a plasma ACTH of 13 ng/L, a free T4 of 1.1 ng/dL (0.6–2.0), a serum TSH of 1.9 mU/L (0.5–5.0), a free testosterone of 1 ng/dL (2.5–10), an FSH level of 0.7 mU/L (2–10), an LH level of 0.2 mU/L (2–10), and a prolactin of 2 µg/L (4–18).

In the intensive care unit, the patient was monitored and continued on hydrocortisone (25 mg IV, every 6 h), iv fluids and iv antibiotics. Clinical improvement was noted within a few hours of admission such that he became afebrile and noted some relief from the headaches. On repeated examinations, the third and sixth nerve-palsies were noted to persist. Twenty-four hours after admission to the ICU, the patient had transsphenoidal decompression of the necrotic tumor. Immunostaining of the resected tissue was limited because of the extensive necrosis. However, available viable tumor tissue showed a few prolactin-staining cells. Twenty-four hours after surgery, hydrocortisone therapy was discontinued while the patient continued to be clinically monitored. Resolution of the headaches and improvement of eye motility were noted within 24 h of surgery. Plasma ACTH and cortisol levels measured >36 h after hydrocortisone therapy was discontinued were appropriately elevated (55 ng/L, 33 µg/dL, respectively), indicating normal pituitary–adrenal function.

The patient continued to do well postoperatively and was discharged home on the fourth postoperative day only on pseudoephedrine for congestion. At the time of discharge, he had normal eye motility and visual fields. When tested 4 wk after discharge, his pituitary function was considered normal, including a free testosterone of 6.9 ng/dL (2.5–10), an AM cortisol of 27 µg/dL and a serum prolactin of 4.5 µg/L. A MRI scan done 6 mo after surgery showed no residual tumor. The patient continued to do well with normal pituitary function and no recurrence of the tumor, 7 yr after surgery.

Discussion

This case illustrates many of the issues and difficulties encountered in the management of patients with pituitary tumor apoplexy. Although the patient had a 1-yr history of symptoms suggestive of hypogonadism, the pituitary adenoma was previously undiagnosed and apoplexy was the first manifestation of the tumor. This is seen in approximately 50% of patients with pituitary tumor apoplexy *(1–3)*. It is likely that the patient had a prolactin secreting pituitary adenoma although this could not be documented with certainty. The low serum prolactin level seen at presentation does not necessarily argue against the latter diagnosis. It is well known that serum prolactin levels decrease precipitously in patients with prolactinomas, after complete adenomectomy *(4)*, or after hemorrhagic infarction *(5)*, as was the case in this patient.

Pituitary tumor apoplexy represents a rare clinical syndrome usually resulting from hemorrhagic infarction of an existing large adenoma. Although many precipitating factors are known, most episodes occur spontaneously as was the case in this patient. Pituitary tumor apoplexy is a clinical, rather than a pathological diagnosis. The term should be used only when signs of compression of perisellar structures or meningeal irritation occur after hemorrhagic infarction of an adenoma *(1)*.

As illustrated by the current case, the diagnosis of pituitary tumor apoplexy can be difficult and is frequently missed because, in addition to its relative rarity, the existence of an adenoma is not often suspected at the time of ictus. The clinical manifestations at the time of presentation consist of neurological and endocrinological signs and symptoms *(1)*. The pathophysiology of the clinical manifestations of pituitary tumor apoplexy can be divided into any combination of the following mechanisms:

1. Hemorrhagic infarction of the tumor leading to sudden increases in intrasellar pressure. The latter results in compression of the normal pituitary tissue as well as its vascular blood supply, leading to hypopituitarism, particularly acute adrenal insufficiency. In addition, the increased intrasellar pressure contributes to the development of headaches which is described as sudden in onset, severe and persistent in nature and bifrontal or occipital in location.
2. Sudden increase in intrasellar contents leading to increased pressure on adjacent vascular and neural structures, laterally, superiorly, and inferiorly.
   a. Laterally, increased pressure leads to damage to cavernous sinus neural structures e.g. cranial nerves III, IV, V, and VI. The patient under discussion has both third and sixth nerve palsies that explain his clinical symptoms.

b. Superiorly, increased pressure will lead to compression of the optic apparatus that can present clinically as decreased visual acuity as well as visual field deficit as was demonstrated in our patient.

c. Inferiorly, increased pressure can lead to CSF leak. The patient under discussion did not have any evidence for a CSF leak.

3. Leakage of blood or necrotic tissue into the subarachnoid space; leading to signs and symptoms of chemical meningitis. The patient under discussion had a clinical picture consistent with meningeal irritation, photophobia and fever associated with negative bacterial cultures, a finding quite characteristic of patients with tumor apoplexy.

The diagnosis of pituitary tumor apoplexy can, at times, be difficult as it may mimic a number of other intracranial illnesses (1). The two most important diseases that should be considered are aneurysmal subarachnoid hemorrhage and bacterial meningitis. Imaging studies are helpful in differentiating these illnesses.

Hypopituitarism often contributes to the morbidity and mortality of pituitary tumor apoplexy. Impaired secretion of all anterior pituitary hormones may be seen after pituitary tumor apoplexy. The most clinically important deficit is that of ACTH because it leads to acute glucocorticoid insufficiency at a time of severe physical stress. In that respect, the patient under discussion had what appeared to be a "normal " serum cortisol at a time when he was extremely stressed. Thus, he was presumed to have partial ACTH deficiency even though his serum levels were in the so-called "normal range." The vast majority of patients present with at least partial hypopituitarism (1,2). It is important to point out that many patients would be expected to have hypopituitarism even before the apoplectic episode, because practically all have large tumors (1,2). Our patient had clinical and biochemical features consistent with central hypogonadism at the time of presentation. It was not clear whether the hypogonadism in this patient was caused by a presumed long-standing hyperprolactinemia (not documented) or whether it was a component of the state of hypopituitarism. Even though GH secretion was not tested at presentation, it is more than likely that the patient had GH deficiency.

Management schemes for pituitary tumor apoplexy should address systemic, neurological, and endocrinological abnormalities. Patients presenting with clinical symptoms consistent with apoplexy require immediate medical attention, thorough clinical evaluation and continuous monitoring. Some of the most important interventions that must be urgently addressed in a patient with suspected pituitary tumor apoplexy are corticosteroid replacement and vigorous supportive measures to ensure hemodynamic stability (1).

Once the diagnosis of pituitary tumor apoplexy is clinically suspected, routine blood studies as well as additional blood samples should be drawn for subsequent determination of all pituitary hormone levels. Urgent imaging studies such as CT or MRI scan should be obtained to confirm the diagnosis. Glucocorticoid deficiency, seen in the vast majority of patients, results in significant morbidity, if left untreated. As was demonstrated in our patient, once glucocorticoids are administered, clinical improvement is invariably noted and hemodynamic stability is easier to maintain. The glucocorticoids are administered in supraphysiological doses to serve not only as replacement for endogenous hormone deficiency, but also to help control the effects of swelling on parasellar structures. We recommend either 100 mg hydrocortisone administered intravenously every 6 h or 4–6 mg dexamethasone administered intravenously every 6 h as the initial choice of steroid therapy.

Documentation of any visual field defect is important and should be obtained if the clinical condition permits. Analysis of CSF fluid is usually not necessary, unless the diagnosis of meningitis can not be safely excluded on clinical grounds. When the patient's physiological status is stabilized, the decision regarding the best method for reversing or preventing further neurological compromise should be considered. Several reports have documented that spontaneous neurological recovery is possible despite unilateral ophthalmoplegia and partial visual field defects. Thus, nonoperative, conservative medical management of patients with pituitary tumor apoplexy has been recommended by some (1–3,6). Even though improvement in neurological symptoms may be seen in patients treated conservatively, worsening of pituitary function is usually seen in such patients.

Because some patients may deteriorate rapidly (1–3,6) and the effects of continued compression on neural structures and endocrine function may be deleterious, we believe that urgent decompression should be undertaken by an experienced neurosurgeon, unless there are strong contraindications to surgical intervention. In view of the low morbidity and mortality associated with transsphenoidal surgical decompression, this approach is routinely used for the vast majority of patients.

Conservative medical therapy is a reasonable alternative option, particularly in areas that lack expertise in this type of surgery. Similarly, patients who are poor surgical candidates and those who have strong contraindications for surgical intervention are treated conservatively. This would involve supportive therapy, continued use of supraphysiologic doses of glucocorticoids for several weeks and hormone replacement. Improvement in neurologic symptoms is often seen in the majority of patients treated conservatively and at times to a similar degree to that seen in surgically treated patients. The role of conservative, medical therapy in the immediate management of patients with this disorder, was recently investigated in a recent study by Maccagnan et al. (6). The authors conducted a nonrandomized study on patients presenting with apoplexy and treated them all with dexamethasone. Patients who failed to improve after 1 wk of dexamethasone were surgically treated. The authors found that patients treated conservatively had a similar neurologic and neuroophthalmologic improvement when compared to surgically treated patients. However, it is obvious from the design of the study that surgically treated patients had more severe symptoms at presentation. Despite that limitation, it is clear that conservative therapy can be used in selected patients with minimal symptoms and those who improve dramatically after glucocorticoid administration.

Surgical decompression does not always result in complete resection of these infarcted macroadenomas, and routine postoperative radiological and endocrinological assessment is mandatory. Depending on the type of tumor, additional forms of therapy can be employed to control residual tumor growth.

Impairment in pituitary function may be reversed, in some patients, after surgery. Therefore, patients undergoing surgery are routinely monitored in the intensive care unit for several days after transsphenoidal decompression. We recommend that all patients should be continued on glucocorticoid therapy until the second postoperative day, at which time the dosage can be tapered or stopped abruptly. Once steroids are discontinued, serum cortisol levels are measured twice a day, and the patient is carefully monitored for any signs or symptoms of glucocorticoid deficiency (1). As demonstrated by the patient under discussion, those with an intact pituitary-adrenal axis postoperatively will have high or high-normal serum cortisol levels, and several levels should be >15 µg/dL. Patients with equivocal (<10 µg/dL) or low (<5 µg/dL) levels should be restarted on physiologic glucocorticoid therapy, particularly if they had symptoms. These patients can be tested later for further delineation of pituitary-adrenal function. In the authors' experience, most patients have high-normal serum cortisol levels within 24–36 h after discontinuing glucocorticoid therapy. As an alternative approach to rapid discontinuation of glucocorticoid therapy, steroids may be tapered slowly over several weeks, and then the patient's pituitary-adrenal axis should be tested. Although both approaches are reasonable, we favor the former method because it avoids the confounding effects of longer steroid therapy on evaluating the remaining pituitary function as well as the unnecessary use of medication with potential side effects.

The remainder of pituitary function should be assessed a few weeks after the episode. In our patient, this was done 4 wk after surgery and showed normalization of adrenal and gonadal functions. Growth hormone deficiency is the most commonly observed abnormality in patients with pituitary macroadenomas with or without apoplexy *(1,7)*. Current evidence indicates that physiologic replacement with GH is clinically beneficial.

REFERENCES

1. Arafah BM, Ybarra J, Tarr RW, Madhun ZT, Selman WR. Pituitary tumor apoplexy: pathophysiology, clinical manifestations and management. J Intensive Care Med 1997;12:123–134.
2. Ebersold MJ, Laws ER Jr, Scheithauer BW, et al. Pituitary apoplexy treated by transsphenoidal surgery; a clinicopathological and immunocytochemical study. J Neurosurg 1983;58:315–320.
3. Reid RL, Quigley ME, Yen SSC. Pituitary apoplexy, a review. Arch Neurol 1985;42:712–719.
4. Arafah BM, Brodkey JS, Pearson OH. Gradual recovery of lactotroph responsiveness to dynamic stimulation following surgical removal of prolactinomas: long-term follow-up studies. Metabolism 1986;35:905–912.
5. Arafah BM, Taylor HC, Salazar R, Saadi H, Selman WR. Apoplexy of a pituitary adenoma after dynamic testing with gonadotropin-releasing hormone. Am J Med 1989;87:103–105.
6. Maccagnan P, Macedo CLD, Kayath MJ, et al. Conservative management of pituitary apoplexy: a prospective study. J Clin Endocrinol Metab 1995;80:2190–2197.
7. Arafah BM. Reversible hypopituitarism in patients with large nonfunctioning pituitary adenomas. J Clin Endocrinol Metab 1986;62:1173–1179.

CASE #4: METASTASIS TO PITUITARY

Case Presentation

A 55-yr-old man presented to the neurology service with, a 2-d history of diplopia and headaches. Diplopia occurred primarily while the patient was looking sideways, although it was also reported on looking up. He had been unable to drive because of the new symptoms. The headaches came on gradually and were predominantly frontal and throbbing in nature. He had been previously healthy until approximately 2–3 mo prior to admission when he noted progressive tiredness and fatigue for no apparent reason. On further questioning, he also complained about diminished libido and potency for 2–3 mo prior to the onset of fatigue. He was reported by his wife to be more cold intolerant and to have started snoring only a few weeks before his presentation. His appetite has diminished, although the weight has not changed significantly. Two weeks prior to the hospital admission, the patient noted increasing thirst, polyuria, and nocturia of 4–6 times every night. At that time, he saw his primary physician who noted that a random glucose level was 195 mg/dL, whereas the urinalysis was unremarkable. The patient was told to have "borderline diabetes" and was advised to decrease carbohydrate and calorie intake. His symptoms persisted despite strict adherence to the latter recommendations.

The past medical history was significant for an episode of hemoptysis, 8 mo prior to admission and was otherwise unremarkable. The latter episode resolved spontaneously and the patient did not pursue further medical care. The patient was involved in an automobile accident 1 yr before the current presentation and apparently lost consciousness for several hours because of a concussion. A CT scan of the head (with and without contrast) then was reported to be negative. The patient had a 45 pack/year history of cigarette smoking and drinks only socially. The family history was remarkable for a father who had type 2 diabetes mellitus, as well as hypertension.

On physical exam, the patient appeared well nourished, yet fatigued while the left eye was covered with a patch to avoid diplopia. Vital signs were unremarkable as was the skin exam. He had mild ptosis of the left eye, left abducens nerve palsy, and an 8 mm minimally reactive left pupil. He also had upper-outer quadrianopsia in the left eye and normal fundi. There was no gynecomastia and the genital exam was normal. Except for a delayed relaxation phase of deep tendon reflexes, the rest of the exam was negative.

Initial laboratory studies revealed the following values; Na^+: 147 mmol/L, K^+: 4.8 mmol/L, Cl^-: 95 mmol/L, $HCO3^-$; 21 mmol/L, BUN:64 mg/dL, Creatinine: 1.8 mg/dL, total Ca: 12.9 mg/dL, albumin 4.5 gm/dL, total protein 8.5 gm/dL, alkaline phosphatase 289 IU/L with normal AST and ALT, urine specific gravity of 1.002 with negative dip stick for protein and glucose. A chest X-ray showed a 3-cm mass in the right upper lobe of the lung. A bone scan showed multiple areas of increased activity in the spine as well as the right femur. A CT scan of the head and a subsequent MRI scan demonstrated an enhancing, large suprasellar mass invading the left cavernous sinus and compressing the optic chiasm as well as the optic tracts. The sella turcica was not grossly enlarged. Review of the CT scan done 1 yr ago when the patient had a concussion confirmed the negative study, particularly in the suprasellar region.

Endocrine evaluation included the following: A free thyroxine of 0.45 ng/dL (0.6–2.0), a TSH level of 1.4 mU/L, a serum prolactin level of 43 µg/L, an AM cortisol of 1.9 µg/dL, a plasma ACTH of 11 ng/L, a total testosterone of 55 ng/dL (300–1000), a free testosterone of 0.7 ng/dL (2.5–10), an LH of 0.7 IU/L, and an FSH of 1.2 IU/L. Plasma PTH level was 5 ng/L (10–55), whereas that of PTH-rP was 18 pmol/L (normal : <5).

The patient was given iv saline and dexamethasone (6 mg every 6 h) and phenytoin for seizure prophylaxis. Oral thyroxine was started and then subcutaneous insulin was added 2 d later when glycemic control worsened. Slight clinical improvement was noted a few days later. Cranial irradiation was initiated after biopsy of the lung mass confirmed lung malignancy. The patient refused further treatment of the lung cancer and died within 2 mo of diagnosis. Postmortem examination confirmed the diagnosis of metastatic lung cancer to the bone, liver, as well as the suprasellar region.

Discussion

Although this was an unusually complicated clinical history, the diagnosis was not difficult to make on admission. The patient presented with third and sixth cranial nerve palsies as a result of tumor invasion into the cavernous sinus. In addition, the patient had headaches, perhaps as a result of rapid increase in the size of the suprasellar mass. From an endocrine standpoint, the patient also had clinical history suggestive of hypopituitarism, diabetes mellitus, as well as partial diabetes insipidus. Diabetes insipidus appears to be both central (partial loss of ADH secretion) as well as nephrogenic (secondary to hypercalcemia). The increased serum calcium level in this patient, was predominantly humoral in nature resulting from secretion of PTH-rP by the lung cancer, although osseous metastasis could have been an additional contributing factor. Biopsy of the lung mass confirmed the diagnosis of lung cancer. Thus, the patient presented with a newly discovered suprasellar mass associated with clinical and biochemical evidence for hypopituitarism and diabetes insipidus. The mass was relatively fast growing, as it was not noted on a previous CT scan done 1 yr earlier for a different reason. The findings of abnormal uptake in the bones associated with the increased alkaline phosphatase and otherwise normal liver function tests clearly suggest metastatic cancer. In view of the convincing nature of the clinical history as well as the biochemical findings, a biopsy of the suprasellar mass was not attempted. The presence of a relatively large suprasellar mass associated with normal-size sella suggest a rapidly expanding mass, rather than a benign, slowly growing tumor.

The clinical setting in this patient was somewhat typical of metastatic disease to the pituitary and suprasellar region (1–6). The rapid onset of symptoms and the associated ocular dysmotility at presentation favored the diagnosis of metastatic cancer rather than a pituitary adenoma. The large size of the suprasellar mass, particularly because it was not detected a year earlier, provided further support for the presumptive diagnosis (4). In this patient with osseous metastasis with a strong clinical history consistent with the diagnosis, biopsy of the sellar lesion is not necessary. Biopsy may be necessary if there were doubts about the diagnosis or if the patient had no known primary cancer (1–6).

Breast, prostate, lung, and gastrointestinal malignancies are the most common primary tumors that are documented to have metastasis to the pituitary and parasellar region. Of the malignancies that metastasize to the pituitary, breast cancer appears to be the most common, accounting for approximately 50%, while lung (20%), GI (5–10%) and prostate (5–10%), and others representing the rest. It is estimated that up to 9% of patients with metastatic breast cancer have pituitary and/or perisellar involvements (1–6). Other areas of distant metastasis are often recognized before pituitary involvement can be demonstrated.

Metastasis to the pituitary fossa is often not limited to the anterior lobe, as it commonly involves the posterior lobe of the pituitary and the hypothalamus. Consequently, diabetes insipidus is diagnosed in 35–70% of these patients (1–6). In contrast, diabetes insipidus is seen in <5% of patients with pituitary adenomas or other benign growths in the region. In fact, the most common cause of diabetes insipidus in patients with adenomas and even those with benign growths in the perisellar region is secondary to surgical procedures. Furthermore, and for the same reason, the hypopituitarism seen in patients with metastatic cancer is associated with mild hyperprolactinemia. Similarly, patients with metastatic tumors to the pituitary often (40–50%) present with cranial nerve palsies as a result of invasion of the cavernous sinuses (1–6). A mass lesion is often, but not always, seen in such patients, especially those with lymphoproliferative diseases. In patients with pituitary/perisellar metastasis, the bony sella turcica is often eroded, although its size is usually normal despite the presence of an intrasellar or suprasellar mass lesion (1,3,4).

Overall management of patients with metastasis depends to some degree on the type of malignancy and extent of metastasis. Immediate management involves the use of large doses of glucocorticoids (usually dexamethasone) and initiating external irradiation. In addition, thyroxine replacement therapy should be initiated whenever the diagnosis of hypothyroidism is confirmed. Oral or intranasal DDAVP are the mainstay in the management of diabetes insipidus, once confirmed. Other hormone replacement therapy (sex steroids, GH) is not warranted until the overall prognosis is appreciated. Most patients with metastatic cancer to the pituitary die within 3–6 mo *(1–6)*.

Despite some of the distinctive features, it is, at times, difficult to differentiate metastatic cancer to the pituitary from benign pituitary adenomas. Features that would favor the diagnosis of metastatic tumor rather than an adenoma include: rapid onset of symptoms and progression over a short period of time, known history of a malignancy, cranial nerve palsies, and the presence of diabetes insipidus. As discussed earlier, diabetes insipidus is very unusual in patients with pituitary adenomas who have not had surgery. Thus, even in patients with no known malignancies, metastatic cancer should be seriously considered in the differential diagnosis of a pituitary mass, particularly in those presenting with diabetes insipidus or ocular nerve palsies. Repeat imaging studies over several weeks often shows progression of metastatic cancer.

REFERENCES

1. Morita A, Meyer FB, Laws ER Jr. Symptomatic pituitary metastases. J Neurosurg 1998;89:69–73.
2. Aaberg TM, Kay M, Sternau L. Metastatic tumors to the pituitary. Am J Ophth 1995;119:779–785.
3. Teears RJ, Silverman EM. Clinicopathologic review of 88 cases of carcinoma metastatic to the pituitary gland. Cancer 1975;36:216–220.
4. Max MB, Deck DF, Rottenberg DA. Pituitary metastasis: Incidence in cancer patients and clinical differentiation from pituitary adenoma. Neurology 1981;31:998–1002.
5. Kovacs K. Metastatic cancer of the pituitary gland. Oncology 1973;27:533–542.
6. Allen EM, Kannan SR, Powell A. Infundibular metastasis and panhypopituitarism. J Natl Med Assoc 1988;81;325–330.

3

Posterior Pituitary

Disorders of Water Metabolism

Lisa L. Wong, MD *and Joseph G. Verbalis,* MD

CONTENTS

CASE #1: CHRONIC HYPONATREMIA UNRESPONSIVE TO DEMECLOCYCLINE, MINERALOCORTICOID, AND GLUCOCORTICOID THERAPY

Case Description

A 74-yr-old male first presented in 1990 for evaluation of recurrent syncope. He had six episodes of syncope since 1979, and these were usually associated with stressful events, recent alcohol intake, or rapid standing. Neurologic evaluation, including electroencephalogram (EEG) and head computed tomography (CT), were unrevealing, and he was diagnosed with vasovagal syncope. Subsequent cardiac evaluation with Holter monitoring and tilt table testing also supported a diagnosis of vasovagal syncope. At his initial presentation in 1990, he was found to have serum sodium = 130 mEq/L, potassium = 4.1 mEq/L, blood urea nitrogen = 13 mg/dL, and serum creatinine = 1.1 mg/dL. On review of his past medical records, it was apparent that his hyponatremia was long-standing, with serum sodium concentrations ranging from 128–134 mEq/L over the past 20 yr. He was on no medications. Further evaluation revealed a random urine osmolality of 717 mOsm/kg H$_2$O and a urine sodium of 71 mEq/L when his serum sodium was 130 mEq/L. He had normal thyroid function and a normal cosyntropin stimulation with a baseline cortisol level of 12.3 µg/dL and post-adrenocorticotropic hormone (ACTH) cortisols of 28.5 µg/dL at 30 min and 33.6 µg/dL at 60 min. In addition, he had a supine

From: *Contemporary Endocrinology: Challenging Cases in Endocrinology*
Edited by: M. E. Molitch © Humana Press Inc., Totowa, NJ

plasma renin activity (PRA) of 0.3 ng/mL/h (normal 0.2–2.3) and aldosterone of 36 ng/dL (normal <16), and an upright PRA of 0.3 ng/mL/h (normal 1.3–4.0) and aldosterone of 57 ng/dL (normal 3–19). His 24-h urine aldosterone was 8.6 µg/TV and 24-h urine sodium was 197 mEq/TV. He had a normal chest CT scan. An abdominal CT scan demonstrated a 4.5-cm left renal cyst and normal adrenal glands.

In 1995, he was started on fludrocortisone 0.1 mg daily for a presumptive diagnosis of hypoaldosteronism, but his serum sodium did not improve. However, he did feel somewhat stronger with less frequent syncopal episodes. In 1996, he was found to have an inappropriate plasma arginine vasopressin (AVP) level of 1.9 pg/mL with a concurrent serum osmolality of 265 mOsm/kg H_2O. He was started on demeclocycline 150 mg bid for a diagnosis of SIADH, but still did not have any improvement in his serum sodium concentration. He subsequently self-discontinued both the fludrocortisone and demeclo-cycline, and noted no change in his symptoms. In March 1999, he was hospitalized for another syncopal episode at which time his serum sodium was 131 mEq/L with a normal serum potassium level. He was restarted on demeclocycline and fludrocortisone 0.1 mg daily. By May 1999, the demeclocycline was increased to 300 mg tid and hydrocortisone 10 mg daily was added for presumed adrenal insufficiency.

In June 1999, he presented for a second opinion regarding his persistent hyponatremia (serum sodium ranging from 129–131 mEq/L). He denied weight loss, salt craving, nausea, emesis, polyuria, or polydipsia. His fluid intake was approximately 2.5 L/d. Past medical history was notable for hypertension and obstructive sleep apnea. His medications included fludrocotisone 0.1 mg daily, hydrocortisone 10 mg daily, demeclocycline 300 mg tid, labetalol 100 mg qd, and hydralazine 25 mg tid. Physical examination revealed a blood pressure of 148/66 mmHg and a pulse of 76 beats/min with no orthostatic changes. The skin had no hyperpigmentation or vitiligo, cardiopulmonary examination was normal, and there was no edema. Based on his history, exam, and laboratory data, he was pre-sumptively diagnosed with the reset osmostat variant of SIADH. His hydrocortisone was discontinued and demeclocycline gradually tapered off. Over the following three months, his serum sodium remained in the range from 128–132 mEq/L on only fludrocortisone 0.1 mg daily.

He was then admitted for a standard water load test. The patient ingested 1514 mL (20 mL/kg) of water over 30 min. Urine was collected hourly thereafter for 4 h for determinations of volume and osmolality. The results are shown in Table 1. It should be apparent that the entire water load was promptly excreted within 2 h, with a maximally dilute urine of 70 mOsm/kg H_2O. Consequently, this was interpreted as a normal response, except for the plasma sodium and osmolality levels. By 4 h, his plasma osmolality was 272 mOsm/kg H_2O and his serum sodium was 127 mEq/L, virtually identical to his starting values.

Discussion

Normally, plasma osmolality is maintained within narrow limits by osmotically regulated AVP secretion and thirst. Despite large variations of water intake, the osmolality of body fluids in a healthy individual is maintained within a relatively narrow range (275–295 mOsm/kg H_2O). This constancy is achieved through osmoreceptors located in the anterior hypothalamus. In 1947, Verney first introduced the term "osmoreceptors" to describe a collection of osmotically sensitive receptive elements that could influence the release of AVP from the posterior pituitary gland (1). Both the thirst osmoreceptors and

Table 1
Water Loading Test

Time (h)	Urine volume (mL)	Urine osmolality (mOsm/kg H_2O)	Serum osmolality (mOsm/kg H_2O)	Plasma AVP (pg/mL)	Serum sodium (mEq/L)
0		545	270	2.6	127
1	580	70			
2	1205	70	268	0.6	125
3	180	248			
4	200	361	272	2.0	127
Total	2165				

the osmoreceptors that regulate vasopressin secretion are located in or around the organum vasculosum of the lamina terminalis and the anterior wall of the third ventricle. Whether the thirst osmoreceptors are actually different cells than the vasopressin osmoreceptors has not been determined.

The most sensitive stimulus for AVP release is an increase in plasma osmolality. There are individual variations in the osmotic threshold, or set-point, for AVP release, probably reflecting variations in the sensitivity of individual osmoreceptor cells. At all plasma osmolalities below the set-point, plasma AVP is suppressed to low or undetectable levels. Above this set-point, secretion of the hormone increases rapidly in direct proportion to the increasing plasma osmolality. Therefore, with plasma hypoosomolality, AVP is suppressed and urine osmolality should be maximally dilute, and with plasma hyperosmolality, AVP levels rise and allow for maximal antidiuresis. In general, the osmotic threshold for thirst is usually set approximately 5–10 mOsm/kg H_2O above that for AVP release. This has the effect of allowing the kidney to regulate body water homeostasis in response to small changes in plasma osmolality, although thirst is only activated by larger and more threatening perturbations.

The patient presented in this case was incorrectly diagnosed with hypoaldosteronism and adrenal insufficiency, probably on the basis of his syncopal episodes, even though he never had documented orthostatic changes suggesting hypovolemia. In fact, his hyponatremia met all of the classic criteria of Schwartz and Bartter (2) for a diagnosis of the syndrome of inappropriate antidiuretic hormone secretion (SIADH): he had hypoosmolar hyponatremia; he had an inappropriately concentrated urine despite the presence of plasma hypotonicity; he was clinically euvolemic and this was supported by a high urinary sodium concentration; and his thyroid, adrenal, and renal function were normal. However, there are several different patterns of AVP secretion in patients with SIADH (3). Most interesting among these is the reset osmostat pattern, in which AVP is secreted appropriately to relative increases in plasma osmolality, but starting at an abnormally low threshold for secretion. The distinguishing characteristic of the patient with the reset osmostat variant of SIADH is the ability to excrete free water. Most patients with SIADH will fail to maximally suppress AVP when plasma osmolality falls below the normal osmotic threshold for AVP secretion, and as a result will demonstrate a marked impairment in their ability to excrete an orally administered water load. In contrast, a patient with a reset osmostat will be able to excrete a water load normally once the plasma osmolality falls below their threshold for AVP secretion, but this threshold will be lower than that of normal subjects.

The hallmark of the reset osmostat variant of SIADH is that the patient regulates his or her plasma osmolality appropriately around a reduced set-point *(4,5)*. There is a downward resetting of the level of plasma osmolality at which osmoreceptors control AVP secretion. AVP is normally responsive to osmotic influences, but the osmotic threshold or set-point for AVP release is subnormal. Thus, water retention occurs above the reset osmostat level although plasma osmolality is still below normal ranges. Nonetheless, AVP secretion can be suppressed and maximal urinary dilution and free water excretion can occur if plasma osmolality is decreased to sufficiently low levels. In some cases, the entire osmoregulatory system is reset, with the osmotic threshold for thirst also reduced. Resetting of the AVP osmostat is a relatively common variant of SIADH, occurring in 15–20% of studied cases *(3)*, and has been found in association with a variety of diseases, such as tuberculosis *(5,6)*, malnutrition *(5)*, gastric cancer *(7)*, and encephalitis *(8)*. This variant is also seen in early pregnancy and occasionally in otherwise healthy subjects *(9,10)*, such as the patient presented here.

Michelis et al. described the first well-documented case of downward resetting of the osmostat in 1974 *(4)*. In 1976, DeFronzo et al. studied four patients with stable hyponatremia who regulated their serum osmolality at hypotonic levels and had normal urinary diluting capacity *(5)*. These patients were euvolemic and hypoosmolar and had normal responses to a standard water load. Three had advanced pulmonary tuberculosis, and one had severe malnutrition with alcoholic abuse. Treatment of the underlying disease resulted in correction of the hyponatremia in three patients. Besides fulfilling the criteria for SIADH, patients with a reset osmostat must demonstrate normal diluting capacity, which is defined as the ability to excrete more than 80% of a standard water load within 4 h and to decrease their urine osmolality to or less than 100 mOsm/kg H_2O.

The mechanism underlying the reset osmostat variant of SIADH is still unclear. Resetting of the osmotic threshold for AVP secretion has been well described with volume depletion, and also has been shown to occur in various edema-forming states, presumably as a result of decreases in effective arterial blood volume. However, most patients with a reset osmostat are clinically euvolemic. It has been suggested that chronic hypoosmolality itself may reset the intracellular threshold for osmoreceptor firing, but studies in animals have not supported a major role for this mechanism since chronic hyponatremia does not appear to significantly alter the osmotic threshold for AVP secretion *(11)*. Perhaps the best-known physiological example of a reset osmostat for AVP secretion is the hypoosmolality and hyponatremia that occurs during pregnancy. Despite intensive studies over many years to identify potential hormonal factors that might be responsible for this resetting, a single factor has not yet been identified *(12)*, though recent studies have indicated that the placental hormone relaxin causes a stimulation of AVP and oxytocin secretion that closely resembles the reset osmostat pattern of AVP secretion *(13,14)*. Perhaps the most perplexing aspect of the reset osmostat pattern is its occurrence in patients with tumors, which suggests that some of these cases represent tumor-stimulated pituitary AVP secretion rather than paraneoplastic AVP secretion *(3,7,15)*.

The hyponatremia of the reset osmostat variant of SIADH is characteristically asymptomatic and fairly stable. In general, serum sodium levels are only mildly or moderately decreased. In this case, unequivocal symptomatic hyponatremia had never been documented. Although the patient had frequent episodes of vasovagal syncope, there is no indication that this was related to his hyponatremia, since he had been hyponatremic for a long time and his syncope was only intermittent. Furthermore, despite a very liberal fluid intake, he had never been shown to decrease his serum sodium below 127 mEq/L. This patient's hyponatremia was therefore chronic, mild, and well-tolerated. Neither the demeclocycline nor fludrocortisone impacted significantly on his serum sodium level, because he would simply drink fluids to defend his new osmotic thresholds for thirst and AVP secretion. In contrast, most patients with SIADH are able to normalize serum sodium levels on demeclocycline by producing nephrogenic diabetes insipidus, and patients with aldosterone deficiency should normalize serum sodium levels with mineralocorticoid replacement to prevent urinary sodium wasting.

In this case, AVP is being secreted abnormally at low levels of serum sodium and plasma osmolality, but it is secreted in a normal fashion relative to changes in plasma osmolality. At some point of serum sodium and plasma osmolality, the AVP levels can in fact be suppressed to near zero, allowing normal free water excretion. Based on the water-load results, this patient's threshold for AVP secretion is probably set around a serum sodium of 125 mEq/L, because he was able to excrete a maximally dilute urine normally at this level; his threshold for thirst is probably set a bit higher at 128–130 mEq/L, because this is what his resting sodium level is most of the time. This accounts for his stability over several decades. His ability to normally dilute his urine once he falls below his reset set-point has protected him from experiencing more serious and symptomatic degrees of hyponatremia. In general, no specific therapy is required for the patient with a reset osmostat, and we do not advise treatment of such patients other than avoiding excessive amounts of water intake over short periods of time, when they may overwhelm their urinary diluting capacity and drop to lower, and more dangerous, levels of hyponatremia.

REFERENCES

1. Verney EB. The antidiuretic hormone and the factors which determine its release. Proc Roy Soc Lon Ser B 1947;135:68.
2. Bartter FC, Schwartz WB. The syndrome of inappropriate secretion of antidiuretic hormone. Am J Med 1967;42:790–806.
3. Zerbe R, Stropes L, Robertson G. Vasopressin function in the syndrome of inappropriate antidiuresis. Annu Rev Med 1980;31:315–327.
4. Michelis MF, Fusco RD, Bragdon RW, Davis BB. Reset of osmoreceptors in association with normovolemic hyponatremia. Am J Med Sci 1974;267:267–273.
5. DeFronzo RA, Goldberg M, Agus ZS. Normal diluting capacity in hyponatremic patients. Reset osmostat or a variant of the syndrome of inappropriate antidiuretic hormone secretion. Ann Intern Med 1976;84: 538–542.
6. Hill AR, Uribarri J, Mann J, Berl T. Altered water metabolism in tuberculosis: role of vasopressin. Am J Med 1990;88:357–364.
7. Wall BM, Crofton JT, Share L, Cooke CR. Chronic hyponatremia due to resetting of the osmostat in a patient with gastric carcinoma. Am J Med 1992;93:223–343.
8. Howe JG, Penney MD, Currie S, Morgan D. Thirst, resetting of the osmostat, and water intoxication following encephalitis. Ann Neurol 1983;13:201–204.
9. Lipschutz JH, Arieff AI. Reset osmostat in a healthy patient. Ann Intern Med 1994;120:574–576.
10. Assadi FK, Agrawal R, Jocher C, John EG, Rosenthal IM. Hyponatremia secondary to reset osmostat. J Pediatr 1986;108:262–264.
11. Verbalis JG, Dohanics J. Vasopressin and oxytocin secretion in chronically hypoosmolar rats. Am J Physiol 1991;261:R1028–R1038.
12. Lindheimer MD, Davidson JM. Osmoregulation, the secretion of arginine vasopressin and its metabolism during pregnancy. Eur J Endocrinol 1995;132:133–143.

13. Weisinger RS, Burns P, Eddie LW, et al. Relaxin alters the plasma osmolality-arginine vasopressin relationship in the rat. J Endocrinol 1993;137:505–510.
14. Wilson BC, Summerlee AJ. Effects of exogenous relaxin on oxytocin and vasopressin release and the intramammary pressure response to central hyperosmotic challenge. J Endocrinol 1994;141:75–80.
15. Robertson GL, Aycinena P, Zerbe RL. Neurogenic disorders of osmoregulation. Am J Med 1982;72;339–353.

CASE #2: HYPONATREMIA AND HYPOTENSION FROM SIADH AND RENAL SALT WASTING

Case Description

A 65-yr-old man was diagnosed with small cell lung cancer in 1983 and subsequently underwent chemotherapy and radiation of the thorax. In 1984, he also received prophylactic whole brain irradiation consisting of 30 Gy (3000 rad) in 10 fractions. For 5 yr prior to the current presentation, he was noted to have persistent hyponatremia. He was given a diagnosis of SIADH and treated alternately with demeclocycline and fluid restriction. During this time, he also had recurrent episodes of orthostatic hypotension, frequently requiring hospitalization. Because urine sodium levels were always high during these episodes, he was felt to have renal salt wasting and was treated with NaCl administration.

He was hospitalized again in July 1999 with hypotension and hyponatremia. Review of systems was significant for pallor, loss of libido, and impotence since 1983. His only medication was NaCl tablets. On physical examination, he had markedly hypopigmented and finely wrinkled skin, pale areolae, absence of axillary hair, and small testes. He was afebrile. His supine pulse and blood pressure were 90 bpm and 129/70 mmHg. Upon sitting, his pulse rose to 100 bpm and blood pressure fell to 104/64 mmHg.

Laboratory evaluation included serum sodium = 123 mEq/L, potassium = 3.9 mEq/L, blood urea nitrogen (BUN) = 11 mg/dL, creatinine = 1.0 mg/dL, plasma osmolality = 264 mOsm/kg H_2O, urine osmolality = 254 mOsm/kg H_2O, urine sodium = 100 mEq/L, hemoglobin = 10.3 g/dL, and hematocrit = 30%. His FT4 level was 0.5 ng/dL (normal range, 0.7–2.8 ng/dL) and TSH = 1.76 µIU/mL. An cosyntropin stimulation test revealed a baseline cortisol level of 6.2 µg/dL with a 30-min post-ACTH cortisol level of 17.8 µg/dL. His PRL level was 20.9 ng/mL (2.6–13.1 ng/mL), free testosterone <0.2 pg/mL (10.8–24.6 pg/mL), and IGF-1 = 26.5 ng/mL (71–290 ng/mL).

Based on his physical exam and laboratory evaluation, a presumptive diagnosis of panhypopituitarism was made. He was placed on a twice-maintenance dose of hydrocortisone (40 mg qAM and 20 mg qPM), and his hypotension and hyponatremia resolved within 48 h. He was discharged on maintenance hydrocortisone (20 mg qAM and 10 mg qPM), levothyroxine, and a few weeks later he was started on testosterone replacement.

An MRI with gadolinium enhancement was consistent with an empty sella syndrome (see Fig. 1). Subsequent dynamic pituitary function testing with 400 µg of TRH showed a basal TSH of 0.51 µIU/mL, 15' = 0.42 µIU/mL, and 30' = 0.26 µIU/mL. Stimulation testing with 100 µg of gonadotropin-releasing hormone (GnRH) showed a basal follicle stimuating hormone (FSH) of 0.7 mIU/mL (normal range 1.27–19.26 mIU/mL), 15' = 0.6 mIU/mL and 30' = 0.8 mIU/mL. Basal LH was 0.44 mIU/mL (normal range 1.24–8.62 mIU/mL), 15' = 0.76 mIU/mL, and 30' = 0.34 mIU/mL.

Over the course of the next 7 mo, the patient dramatically improved on full hormone replacement therapy. He noted increased energy level, strength, and libido. His blood pressure remained stable. He developed increased facial and body hair, and his marked

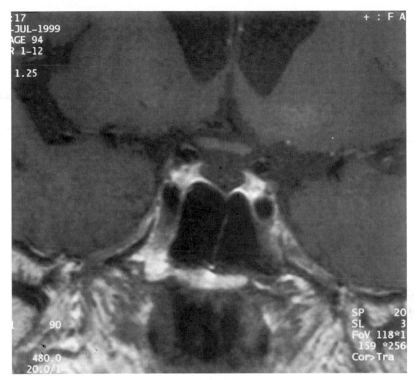

Fig. 1. Coronal section through the pituitary from a T1-weighted MR image following intravenous gadolinium administration demonstrates an absence of pituitary tissue in the sella turcica characteristic of the empty sella syndrome.

pallor improved. His serum sodium has remained in the normal range (137–139 mmol/L). His free testosterone level was 11.3 pg/mL (7.0–24.5) on testosterone enanthate injections. Thyroid function tests showed a free T4 = 1.13 and thyroid-stimulating hormone (TSH) = 0.014 on 0.1 mg of levothyroxine daily. His prolactin level has remained elevated at 50.3 ng/mL (2.6–13.1 ng/mL). He has declined a trial of growth hormone replacement therapy at this time.

Discussion

This case illustrates the importance of defining the underlying cause of hyponatremia before assuming that all such cases represent the SIADH. Hyponatremia is a well-known manifestation of primary adrenal insufficiency. Among 264 reported cases of primary adrenal insufficiency, 88% demonstrated hyponatremia. Less frequently, hyponatremia develops in patients with secondary adrenal insufficiency, e.g., in 28% of 47 reported cases of isolated ACTH deficiency *(1)*. Although hyponatremia may develop in either primary or secondary adrenal insufficiency, the mechanisms for hyponatremia clearly differ in each case. Patients with Addison's disease have a solute depletion hyponatremia. Destruction of the zona glomerulosa renders these patients mineralocorticoid deficient. The lack of aldosterone results in renal salt wasting at the distal tubule. The negative external sodium balance produces a decreased absolute extracellular fluid volume. Thus, Addisonian patients clinically present with vascular collapse. They are hypotensive and dehydrated because of volume contraction.

In contrast, patients with secondary adrenal insufficiency have a dilutional hyponatremia. Hyponatremia is not because of a lack of mineralocorticoid effect and renal sodium wasting, but rather because of an inability to excrete water normally. These patients have normal mineralocorticoid levels because aldosterone regulation still occurs via the renin-angiotensin system. They do not present with hyperkalemia because aldosterone levels are normal. Unlike the hyperpigmented Addisonian patient, the patient with secondary adrenal insufficiency appears hypopigmented, because ACTH is absent, rather than increased as in primary adrenal insufficiency. In this case, it was possible to differentiate primary from secondary adrenal insufficiency by the patient's lack of hyperpigmentation and hyperkalemia. Nonetheless, patients with glucocorticoid deficiency often present with hyponatremia because of free water retention owing to inappropriately increased vasopressin levels.

Just as hyponatremia occurs less often in patients with secondary adrenal insufficiency compared to those with primary adrenal insufficiency, so does hypotension occur less frequently in those with secondary adrenal insufficiency. When hypotension does occur, it is usually less severe than the hypotension in an Addisonian patient. Because patients with secondary adrenal insufficiency are not mineralocorticoid deficient, their hypotension is not a reflection of dehydration. With normal aldosterone levels, these patients are not prone to salt and volume depletion. Instead, their hypotension reflects a decreased vascular sensitivity to pressors. Hypocortisolism leads to decreased peripheral vascular adrenergic tone by decreasing vascular sensitivity to norepinephrine and angiotensin II *(2)*.

Besides hyponatremia and hypotension, patients with secondary adrenal insufficiency can also exhibit high urine sodium levels. This patient's urine sodium was 100 mEq/L. In caring for a patient who presents with hypotension and hyponatremia, the physician may be easily misled to believe that a high urine sodium level must represent renal salt wasting in this setting. However, in this case, the high urine sodium level simply reflected an appropriate natriuretic response by the kidney to a mild volume expansion from free water retention. Thus, one cannot assume that a patient with orthostatic hypotension, hyponatremia, and a high urine sodium must have renal salt wasting. All these findings might actually be attributable to glucocorticoid deficiency with secondary free water retention.

Animal and human studies have repeatedly documented that glucocorticoid deficiency results in an inability to excrete a water load *(3,4)*. Ikkos et al. studied 24 patients after hypophysectomy and found that they could not excrete a water load 4 wk postoperatively *(5)*. A defect in water excretion is detectable in almost all patients with panhypopituitarism. Normally, hyperosmolality stimulates vasopressin secretion in the supraoptic and paraventricular nuclei of the hypothalamus. There are also several nonosmotic stimuli for vasopressin that include hypotension, nausea, hypoglycemia, and hypoxia. Glucocorticoid deficiency represents another nonosmotic stimulus for vasopressin secretion. Oelkers demonstrated this nicely in a study of five women with hypopituitarism presenting with severe symptomatic hyponatremia *(6)*. In these patients, plasma vasopressin levels were inappropriately high in relation to plasma osmolality. After several months of hydrocortisone therapy, their hyponatremia resolved, and a normal relation of plasma vasopressin to plasma osmolality was reestablished. In patients with secondary adrenal insufficiency, short-term glucocorticoid administration is often associated with prompt restoration of normal kidney diluting ability and a water diuresis. A trial of glucocorticoid therapy was diagnostically helpful in this case, because the ACTH stimulation test resulted in a near normal response with a peak cortisol level of 17.8 µg/dL. Nonetheless, the patient's rapid correction of his hyponatremia and hypotension with just a twice-maintenance dose of hydrocortisone strongly supported the diagnosis of secondary adrenal insufficiency.

As early as 1949, increased vasopressin was suggested as a factor in impaired ability to excrete a water load in adrenal insufficiency. In 1967, Ahmed et al. found increased plasma vasopressin levels in untreated patients with hypopituitarism (7). Within 3 h after the administration of glucocorticoids, vasopressin levels decreased to within or slightly above the range for normal controls, who were similarly dehydrated. Vasopressin levels were increased in the absence of steroids and returned toward normal in their presence.

Increased vasopressin levels during cortisol deficiency have been well documented and this is currently well accepted (3,4,7). However, there had been an ongoing debate regarding the presence of a vasopressin-independent mechanism for hyponatremia in hypocortisolism. Linas et al. studied mineralocorticoid replaced adrenalectomized Brattleboro rats with central diabetes insipidus following a water load (8). They found no defect in water excretion after 24 h of glucocorticoid deficiency, but after 14 d there was a significant impairment in water excretion. This suggested a vasopressin-independent factor causing abnormal water excretion after 14 d in these animals. The authors hypothesized that decreased cardiac output and renal blood flow resulted in decreased distal fluid delivery, which might account for the defect in water excretion.

Patients with secondary adrenal insufficiency develop hyponatremia because of an inability to excrete free water, which is most likely a consequence of both inappropriately high vasopressin levels and possible direct renal effects. Glucocorticoids can increase free water excretion by suppressing the release of vasopressin from the magnocellular neurons of the neurohypophysis; in this case, glucocorticoid deficiency might result in a loss of tonic inhibition of vasopressin secretion at the level of the hypothalamus. Alternatively, because vasopressin is cosecreted with corticotropin releasing hormone (CRH) from the hypothalamic paraventricular nucleus to stimulate ACTH secretion, perhaps the lack of suppression of vasopressin by hypoosmolality represents a loss of normal feedback inhibition of these parvocellular neurons by cortisol. In addition, as noted earlier, there may also be a direct renal effect of glucocorticoid deficiency that impairs free water clearance by decreasing glomerular filtration rate (GFR) and volume delivered to the distal tubule.

This case is instructive not only from the standpoint of secondary adrenal insufficiency presenting with hyponatremia and hypotension, but also that of panhypopituitarism presenting after prophylactic whole brain irradiation. Early reports suggested that the normal pituitary gland was relatively radioresistant (9). However, in 1966 Tan et al. reported the first case of radiation induced pituitary dwarfism (10). Since then, deficiencies of all anterior pituitary hormones have been documented after radiotherapy when the hypothalamus and pituitary are included in the treatment field (11,12). This has been best demonstrated in patients receiving radiotherapy for pituitary tumors (13,14), nasopharyngeal carcinoma (15,16), and primary brain tumors (17,18).

Radiation can damage the pituitary gland directly or damage the hypothalamus or pituitary stalk, leading to a defect in delivery of hypothalamic releasing factors to the pituitary. The hypothalamus appears to be more radiosensitive than the pituitary and is more commonly the site of damage, particularly following lower doses, e.g., <40 Gy irradiation (19,20). However, at higher doses, there is evidence for both hypothalamic and anterior pituitary damage.

Deficiencies of all anterior pituitary hormones occur, but prolactin is the only hormone that tends to be secreted at supranormal levels after cranial irradiation, again reflecting hypothalamic damage, because disruption of hypothalamic dopaminergic inhibition of prolactin secretion by the pituitary lactotrophs results in hyperprolactinemia. Mild increases in prolactin are particularly common after cranial irradiation with doses exceeding 50 Gy (17,19). In this case, our patient had persistent mild hyperprolactinemia supporting probable radiation-induced hypothalamic damage.

There is evidence that the severity of radiation-induced tissue damage is correlated with time after radiation, leading to a characteristic delay in the onset of radiation-induced neuroendocrine dysfunction (20–22). Consequently, all patients treated with pituitary radiation should be monitored regularly for early detection of pituitary gland failure.

In our review of the literature, there has been no other reported case of radiation-induced hypopituitarism in a patient who received cranial irradiation for whole brain prophylaxis. A conventional dose for prophylactic whole brain irradiation in patients with small cell lung cancer is approximately 36 Gy in 20–25 fractions. A total dose of 36 Gy may actually be less toxic than a total dose of 30 Gy if delivered in more fractions. Perhaps one reason there has been no other case report of hypopituitarism occurring after prophylactic cranial irradiation is because this patient received more toxic levels of radiation. Another equally plausible reason is that given the prognosis of small cell carcinoma, these patients usually do not survive long enough for hypopituitarism to become manifest.

Although hypopituitarism secondary to pituitary irradiation and hyponatremia as a presenting manifestation of hypopituitarism are both well recognized (23), it is noteworthy that this patient went undiagnosed for many years. This can be ascribed to many reasons:

1. A general lack of appreciation of the clinical manifestations of hypopituitarism in adults;
2. A continuing misconception that hyponatremia is only seen with primary adrenal insufficiency as a result of renal salt-wasting from aldosterone deficiency;
3. A previous diagnosis of small cell carcinoma of the lung, which is commonly associated with SIADH and led to this incorrect diagnosis in this case;
4. The presence of orthostatic hypotension in combination with hyponatremia and a high urine sodium concentration, which was incorrectly interpreted as being indicative of renal salt wasting. Treatment with NaCl tablets was ineffective at abolishing the orthostatic hypotension and correcting the hyponatremia, and the patient was unable to comply with a strict fluid restriction because of exacerbation of his orthostatic symptoms. However, the orthostasis in this patient was, in fact, because of cortisol insufficiency, rather than volume depletion. He had a dilutional hyponatremia due to water retention with an appropriate natriuresis for the degree of water retention present.

This case therefore emphasizes that it is essential to consider secondary adrenal insufficiency, as well as primary adrenal insufficiency, in the differential diagnosis of unexplained hyponatremia.

REFERENCES

1. Stacpoole PW, Interlandi JW, Nicholson WE, et al. Isolated ACTH deficiency: a heterogeneous disorder. Clinical review and report of four new cases. Medicine 1982;61:13–24.
2. Ishikawa S, Schrier, RW. Vascular effects of arginine vasopressin, angiotensin II, and norepinephrine in adrenal insufficiency. Am J Physiol 1984;246:H104–H113.
3. Mandell IN, DeFronzo, RA, Robertson GL, et al. Role of plasma arginine vasopressin in the impaired water diuresis of isolated glucocorticoid deficiency in the rat. Kidney Int 1980;17:186–195.

4. Boykin J, DeTorrente A, Erickson A, et al. Role of plasma vasopressin in impaired water excretion of glucocorticoid deficiency. J Clin Invest 1978;62:738–744.

5. Ikkos D, Luft R, Olivecrona, H. Hypophysectomy in man: effect on water excretion during the first two postoperative months. J Clin Endocrinol Metab 1954;15:553–567.

6. Oelkers W. Hyponatremia and inappropriate secretion of vasopressin (antidiuretic hormone) in patients with hypopituitarism. N Engl J Med 1989;321:492–496.

7. Ahmed A, George BC, Gonzalex-Auvert C, et al. Increased plasma arginine vasopressin in clinical adrenocortical insufficiency and its inhibition by glucosteroids. J Clin Invest 1967;45:111–123.

8. Linas SL, Berl T, Robertson GL, et al. Role of vasopressin in the impaired water excretion of glucocorticoid deficiency. Kidney Int 1980;18:58–67.

9. Tobias CA, Lawrence JH, Born JL, et al. Pituitary irradiation with high-energy proton beams: preliminary report. Cancer Res 1958;18:121–134.

10. Tan BC, Kunaratnam N. Hypopituitary dwarfism following radiotherapy for nasopharyngeal carcinoma. Clin Radiol 1966;17:302–304.

11. Chen MS, Lin FJ, Huang, MJ, et al. Prospective hormone study of hypothalamic-pituitary function in patients with nasopharyngeal carcinoma after high dose irradiation. Jpn J Clin Oncol 1989;19:265–270.

12. Lam KS, Tse VK, Wang C, et al. Early effects of cranial irradiation on hypothalamic-pituitary function. J Clin Endocrinol Metab 1987:64:418–424.

13. Snyder PJ, Fowble B F, Schatz NJ, et al. Hypopituitarism following radiation therapy of pituitary adenomas. Am J Med 1986;81:457–462.

14. Littley MD, Shalet SM, Beardwell, CG, et al. Hypopituitarism following external radiotherapy for pituitary tumours in adults. Q J Med 1989;70:145–160.

15. Lam KS, Tse VKC, Wang C, et al. Effects of cranial irradiation on hypothalamic-pituitary function—a five year long study in patients with nasopharyngeal carcinoma. Q J Med 1991:78:165–176.

16. Samaan NA, Schultz PN, Yang KP, et al. Endocrine complications after radiotherapy for tumors of the head and neck. J Lab Clin Med 1987;109:364–372.

17. Constine LS, Woolf PD, Cann D, et al. Hypothalamic-pituitary dysfunction after radiation for brain tumors. N Engl J Med 1993;328:87–94.

18. Arlt W, Hove U, Muller B, et al. Frequent and frequently overlooked: treatment-induced endocrine dysfunction in adult long-term survivors of primary brain tumors. Neurology 1997;49:498–506.

19. Sklar CA, and Constine LS. Chronic neuroendocrinological sequelae of radiation therapy. Int J Rad Onc Biol Phys 1995;31:1113–1121.

20. Littley MD, Shalet SM, Beardwell CG, et al. Radiation-induced hypopituitarism is dose-dependent. Clin Endocrinol 1989;31:363–373.

21. Clayton, PE, Shalet SM. Dose dependency of time of onset of radiation-induced growth hormone deficiency. J Pediatr 1991;118:226–228.

22. Duffner PK, Cohen ME, Voorhess ML, et al. Long-term effects of cranial irradiation on endocrine function in children with brain tumors. A prospective study. Cancer 1985;56:2189–2193.

23. Bethune JE, Nelson DH. Hyponatremia in hypopituitarism. N Engl J Med 1965;272:771–776.

CASE #3: POLYURIA AND POLYDIPSIA
IN A YOUNG WOMAN WITH AN ENHANCING INFUNDIBULAR MASS

Case Description

A previously well 18-yr-old female suddenly developed polyuria and polydipsia 6 mo after an uncomplicated spontaneous vaginal delivery of her first child. She complained of nocturia every 2 h and excessive thirst with ice-water craving. Six months later, she was diagnosed with central diabetes insipidus. Her urine volume was 9 L/d. Urinary and plasma osmolality were 62 and 300 mOsm/kg H_2O, respectively, during *ad libitum* water intake. Following overnight water deprivation, her serum sodium was 153 mEq/L, potassium 4.7 mEq/L, and plasma arginine vasopressin level was <1.0 pg/ml. Treatment with desmopressin (dDAVP) 10 µg intranasally twice a day resulted in marked improvement of her symptoms.

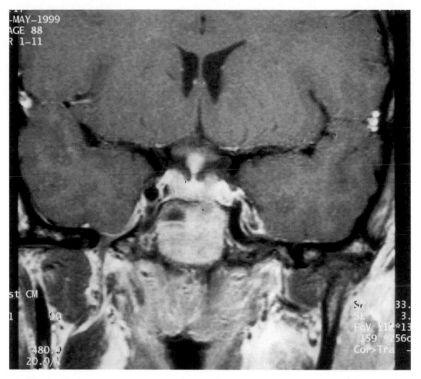

Fig. 2. Coronal section through the pituitary from a T1-weighted MR image following intravenous gadolinium administration demonstrates an enhancing infundibular mass measuring 7 mm in width. The optic chiasm, hypothalamus, and pituitary gland all appear to be normal.

She had normal menstrual cycles postpartum while on oral contraceptives. However, after discontinuing her oral contraceptives, her menses did not return. In addition, although she only breastfed for 1 mo, she noted persistent galactorrhea afterward. Her prolactin level was elevated to 28.5 ng/mL, and she was started on bromocriptine soon after the initiation of dDAVP. She had some improvement of her galactorrhea, but amenorrhea persisted. She also noted a 40-lb weight gain over 1 yr, despite a decreased appetite. Her only other complaint was episodic hot flashes.

Chest X-ray and serum angiotensin converting enzyme concentration were both normal. Lumbar puncture with cerebrospinal fluid (CSF) analysis was also normal. A magnetic resonance imaging (MRI) of the brain after 5 mo of dDAVP therapy disclosed a nodular enlargement of the pituitary infundibulum measuring $7 \times 6 \times 7$ mm, which enhanced homogenously with gadolinium (see Fig. 2). A repeat MRI 2 mo later revealed persistent enlargement of the infundibular mass, but with a suggestion of a slight decrease in the size of the lesion.

She presented to our institution for a second opinion after 6 mo of treatment with dDAVP and bromocriptine. On physical examination her blood pressure was 100/64 mmHg, pulse was 100 bpm and regular. She was obese with a BMI of 38.4 kg/m^2. Neuroophthalmologic evaluation was normal. The rest of her exam was unremarkable except for bilateral expressible galactorrhea.

Laboratory evaluation revealed a FT4 = 0.85 ng/dL (normal range, 0.80–1.50 ng/dL) and TSH = 0.95 μU/mL. Her estradiol level was 9 pg/mL, FSH = 4.3 mIU/mL, and LH = 3.5 mIU/mL. Her prolactin level was 1.2 ng/mL (2.6–13.1 ng/mL) on bromocriptine.

Subsequent dynamic pituitary function testing with 400 μg of TRH revealed a basal TSH of 1.06 μU/mL, 15' = 9.20 μU/mL, 30' = 9.98 μU/mL, 60' = 6.76 μU/mL, and 90' = 4.36 μU/mL. Stimulation testing with 100 μg of GnRH showed a basal FSH of 0.5 mIU/ mL, 30' = 4.7 mIU/mL and 60' = 7.0 mIU/mL. Basal LH was <0.2 mIU/mL, 30' = 5.41 mIU/mL and 60' = 4.84 mIU/mL. Insulin-induced hypoglycemia testing revealed adequate plasma cortisol response, but impaired growth hormone response. She had a baseline cortisol of 13.3 μg/dL, 45' = 16.6 μg/dL, 60' = 19.8 μg/dL, and 90' = 14.2 μg/dL. Basal GH was <0.1 ng/mL, 30' = 0.1 ng/mL, and 60' = 0.2 ng/mL.

Based upon her clinical presentation, a presumptive diagnosis of lymphocytic infundibuloneurohypophysitis was made. She was continued on a dopamine agonist and dDAVP, and was restarted on an oral contraceptive. Neither surgery nor corticosteroid therapy was recommended at the time of the initial evaluation. Instead, continued observation and close follow-up was suggested.

Discussion

In neurogenic diabetes insipidus, a deficiency of osmoregulated vasopressin secretion can result from a variety of acquired and familial diseases. Destructive lesions of the hypothalamus and pituitary stalk are often caused by brain tumors or head trauma. Rarely, the disease may result from infiltration of the infundibulum by histiocytosis X, granulomatous diseases (e.g., tuberculosis, sarcoidosis) or lymphoma. However, approximately 30–50% of cases of acquired diabetes insipidus are idiopathic, and it has been proposed that many of these may be a consequence of an autoimmune process.

Lymphocytic infundibuloneurohypophysitis (LIN) is a rare disorder characterized by central diabetes insipidus (CDI) caused by a chronic inflammatory infiltrate confined to the neurohypophysial system. Its pathogenesis is poorly understood, but it is thought to be the result of an autoimmune response to neurohypophysial antigens. The case presented illustrates several important points about the diagnosis and treatment of LIN. Before beginning a discussion of LIN, it is helpful to review the distinguishing features of a related pituitary disorder, lymphocytic hypophysitis, which affects the adenohypophysis via an autoimmune process.

Lymphocytic hypophysitis (LH) is a rare autoimmune disease that was first described in 1962. It classically presents as an intrasellar mass in females during late pregnancy or in the postpartum period. Patients often initially present with symptoms of mass effect, i.e., visual symptoms or headaches. They then progress to develop partial or complete hypopituitarism. Isolated ACTH deficiency or combined corticotropin and thyrotropin deficiencies can occur despite normal gonadotropin function. The pathophysiology is characterized by destruction of the anterior pituitary gland by infiltration with lymphocytes (mainly T cells) and plasma cells. Subsequently, the pituitary tissue is replaced by fibrosis. An autoimmune pathogenesis for the disease is well established. Cases of concurrent lymphocytic thyroiditis, adrenalitis, atrophic gastritis, and pernicious anemia have been reported *(1)*.

Management is controversial, but a conservative approach without surgical intervention is generally recommended unless there are signs of optic nerve compression or increased intracranial pressure. It is unresolved whether corticosteroid therapy influences the natural course of the disease, because some patients demonstrate spontaneous remission without any therapy.

LH and LIN both result from a chronic inflammatory infiltrate, but the lesion in LH occurs in the anterior pituitary gland, whereas the lesion in LIN is restricted to the hypothalamic neurohypophysial system. Imura et al. first proposed the pathological entity of lymphocytic infundibuloneurohypophysitis in 1993 (2). However, two autopsy cases described the underlying pathophysiology prior to this report. In 1970, a woman with CDI was found to have infiltration of lymphocytes and plasma cells as well as fibrosis confined to the neurohypophysis at autopsy (3). In 1989, an autopsy of a man with CDI revealed that he had chronic lymphocytic inflammation limited to the infundibulum, pituitary stalk, and posterior lobe of the pituitary gland. In addition, there was bilateral neuronal loss in the supraoptic and paraventricular nuclei (4).

To date, there are only 18 reported cases of histologically proven LIN in the literature (2,5–9). Within this limited series, there is an apparent female preponderance of the disorder, and most patients present with the sudden or gradual onset of central diabetes insipidus. The MRI often discloses an infundibular mass or enlargement of the neurohypophysial system reflecting the destruction of the neurohypophysis by infiltration with lymphocytes (mainly T cells) and plasma cells. Most lesions spontaneously regress by MRI over time as the inflammatory infiltrate is replaced by fibrosis and subsequent atrophy of the neurohypophysis occurs. The anterior pituitary is typically not involved except for an impaired GH response to insulin-induced hypoglycemia, which has been reported in some cases (2,5). Imura et al. postulated that there might be a derangement in the regulation of growth hormone releasing hormone (GHRH) secretion in some cases, either at the level of the the hypothalamus or the median eminence (2).

A case of postpartum LIN was described by Van Havenbergh et al. (9). A woman presented with central DI and a thickened pituitary stalk by MRI 6 mo postpartum. She had a remarkably similar presentation to this case. She also had persistent galactorrhea with moderate hyperprolactinemia and a subnormal response of GH to insulin-induced hypoglycemia. She underwent biopsy of the stalk lesion, which showed a lymphocytic infiltrate predominated by T cells. Four months after biopsy, the MRI showed marked decrease in thickening of pituitary stalk and infundibulum. If our patient indeed has LIN, we would similarly predict that her future MRIs will likewise demonstrate shrinkage of the infundibular lesion over time as a result of decreased inflammation.

Like LH, an autoimmune pathogenesis for LIN seems likely, but has not been as well defined. Few patients have concurrent autoimmune diseases. However, Watanabe et al. documented a case of central diabetes insipidus caused by nonspecific chronic inflammation of the hypothalamus and found the presence of HLA class I antigen A2 and HLA class II antigen DR4, which are associated with a variety of autoimmune diseases (10). The female preponderance and T-lymphocyte predominant chronic inflammation of LIN, as well as these two cases occurring in the postpartum period also imply an autoimmune pathogenesis. More direct evidence in support of an autoimmune pathogenesis has been the detection of antibodies against specific neurohypophyseal antigens in many patients with idiopathic DI presumed to be secondary to LIN (11,12).

Although a definite diagnosis of LIN can only be made by biopsy and pathologic examination of the infundibulum, a presumptive diagnosis can be made clinically. The differential diagnosis of CDI caused by a mass lesion in posterior lobe of pituitary or pituitary stalk includes Langerhans cell histiocytosis (LCH), sarcoidosis, tuberculosis, germinoma, and hypothalamic and optic gliomas. A recent retrospective study of CDI in children indicated that 24% of cases were caused by intracranial tumors, 16% to Langerhans' histiocytosis, 6% were familial, and 54% were idiopathic *(13)*. Granulomatous infiltrative diseases like sarcoidosis and LCH usually involve other organ systems, and anterior pituitary function is often impaired in LCH. Germinomas usually occur in children, and hypopituitarism is generally present in early stages. It is important to perform lumbar puncture to help exclude sarcoidosis, as well as germinoma. Because the clinical course over time may be the distinguishing feature of LIN versus these other disorders, close observation with frequent neuroimaging is indispensable.

In general, patients with LIN do not have progression or remission of their disease. No cases of spontaneous recovery from complete DI have been reported, though a recent report has suggested that dDAVP therapy may have ameliorated partial DI in patients with positive neurohypophysial antibodies *(14)*. Patients generally require lifelong administration of dDAVP and have a good long-term prognosis on HRT. Although this appears to be a self-limited inflammatory process, surgical intervention should be avoided in typical cases of LIN. Most documented cases of histologically proven LIN underwent biopsy to exclude a tumor. The decision of whether or not to biopsy an enhancing lesion of the infundibulum and pituitary stalk is difficult. We believe biopsy is unnecessary in most cases of presumed LIN and recommend close observation with frequent follow-up including neuroimaging at 6-mo intervals. Progressive increase in the size of the lesion is an indication to perform a biopsy, because involution generally occurs with LIN as the inflammatory process subsides. Corticosteroid therapy has been suggested, but there are no data to support the efficacy of such treatment. In this case, because the patient presented to us 1.5 yr after she first developed polyuria and polydipsia, corticosteroid therapy would not be of likely benefit. Corticosteroid treatment might be better attempted during the phase of acute inflammation in early LIN, but there are no studies to date that demonstrate that corticosteroids alter the natural course of the disease.

Although we consider LH and LIN distinct entities, i.e., LH is confined to the adenohypophysis and spares the neurohypophysis while LIN is confined to the neurohypophysis, a few cases of DI presenting in patients with histologically diagnosed LH have been reported *(15)*. Hashimoto et al. found 20 of 124 patients with LH who developed DI before treatment *(16)*. In some cases, neuroimaging studies revealed a thickened pituitary stalk, and in a few cases, chronic lymphocytic infiltration was found in both the adenohypophysis and infundibuloneurohypophysis. Ahmed described two cases presenting with hypopituitarism and DI with histological findings of pituitary necrosis involving the adenohypophysis, neurohypophysis and hypothalamus, which he termed necrotizing infundibular hypophysitis *(17)*. It is not known whether this disorder is a separate entity from LH and LIN or if it represents an extreme within a spectrum of presentations of a single autoimmune disorder.

It is possible that the intrasellar mass in the anterior pituitary of LH could compress the hypothalamus, thereby inhibiting synthesis of vasopressin. However, MRI of the cases of LH with DI suggest that such compression is unlikely *(18)*. Another explanation is that the inflammatory process of LH may extend into the pituitary stalk and/or neurohypophysis, destroying the hypothalamic pathways which transport vasopressin to the posterior pituitary. Finally, a variant of LH might exist in which there is a coexistence of LH and LIN. It is unclear whether the inflammatory lesions of LIN and LH are explained by the same pathogenetic process. Although both LH and LIN are likely caused by similar autoimmune processes, the antigens involved are probably distinct.

Thus, it is also imperative to carefully evaluate the anterior pituitary function of a patient who presents with CDI secondary to LIN, or any other inflammatory process involving the infundibulum and pituitary stalk. Our patient demonstrated an impaired growth hormone response to insulin-induced hypoglycemia, hypogonadotropic hypogonadism and possible early central hypothyroidism on baseline laboratory testing. Dynamic pituitary testing revealed functioning gonadotrophs, thyrotrophs, and corticotrophs in the anterior pituitary, which responded appropriately to hypothalamic releasing hormone stimulation. However, the inflammatory infiltrate and fibrosis in the area of the pituitary stalk likely impaired delivery of endogenous hypothalamic releasing hormones to the anterior pituitary. This would also explain the patient's mild hyperprolactinemia as secondary to decreased delivery of hypothalamic dopamine to the lactotrophs. Although the etiology of her weight gain in uncertain, it might be ascribed to a destruction of the basal hypothalamus by the inflammatory process in the infundibulum, an area known contain leptin receptors and to be important for coordination of hypothalamic systems regulating body weight homeostasis *(19)*.

In summary, as many as half of all cases of acquired central DI are idiopathic, and many of these may be caused by LIN, which is characterized by a lymphocytic infiltration of the neurohypophysial system with subsequent enlargement of the infundibulum and pituitary stalk by MRI. Patients with LIN require long-term dDAVP replacement and close follow-up to rule out other causes of infundibular enlargement. Patients with LIN tend to have a benign course without progression of the disease into other areas. Evaluation of anterior pituitary function is important to identify adenohypophyseal deficits due to LH that may occur concurrently with LIN, or as a result of impaired delivery of releasing hormones to the pituitary from the presence of an inflammatory mass in the area of the median eminence and pituitary stalk.

REFERENCES

1. Cosman F, Post KD, Holub DA, et al. Lymphocytic hypophysitis. Report of 3 new cases and review of the literature. Medicine 1989;68:240–256.
2. Imura H, Nakao K, Shimatsu A, et al. Lymphocytic infundibuloneurohypophysitis as a cause of central diabetes insipidus. N Engl J Med 1993;329:683–689.
3. Saito T, Yoshida S, Nako K, et al. Chronic hypernatremia associated with inflammation of the neurohypophysis. J Clin Endocrinol Metab 1970;31:391–396.
4. Kojima H, Nojima T, Nagashima K, et al. Diabetes insipidus caused by lymphocytic infundibuloneurohypophysitis. Arch Pathol Lab Med 1989;113:1399–1401.
5. Hoshimaru M, et al. Central diabetes insipidus resulting from a nonneoplastic tiny mass lesion localized in the neurohypophyseal system. Surg Neurol 1992;38:1–6.
6. Atkins D, Sanford R, Thomas B, et al. Infundibuloneurohypophysitis in children. A report of 2 cases. Pediatr Neurosurg 1999;30:267–271.
7. Kamel N, Ilgin SD, Corapcioglu D, et al. Lymphocytic infundibuloneurohypophysitis presenting as diabetes insipidus in a man. J Endocrinol Invest 1998;21:537–540.
8. Tsujii S, Takeuchi J, Koh M, et al. A candidate case for lymphocytic infundibulo-neurohypophysis mimicking a neurohypophysial tumor. Intern Med 1997;36:293–297.
9. Van Havenbergh T, Robberecht W, Wilms G, et al. Lymphocytic infundibulohypophysitis presenting in the postpartum period: case report. Surg Neurol 1996;46(3):280–284.
10. Watanabe A, Ishii R, Hirano K, et al. Central diabetes insipidus caused by nonspecific chronic inflammation of the hypothalamus: case report. Surg Neurol 1994;42:70–73.

11. Scherbaum WA. Autoimmune hypothalamic diabetes insipidus ("autoimmune hypothalamitis"). Prog Brain Res 1992;93:283–292.
12. De Bellis A, Bizzarro A, Amoresano PV, et al. Detection of vasopressin cell antibodies in some patients with autoimmune endocrine diseases without overt diabetes insipidus. Clin Endocrinol 1994;40:173–177.
13. Maghnie M, Cosi, G, Genovese E, et al. Central diabetes insipidus in children and young adults. N Engl J Med 2000;343:998–1007.
14. De Bellis A, Colao A, Di Salle F, et al. A longitudinal study of vasopressin cell antibodies, posterior pituitary function, and magnetic resonance imaging evaluations in subclinical autoimmune central diabetes insipidus. J Clin Endocrinol Metab 1999;84:3047–3051.
15. Nishioka H, Ito H, Toshiaki S, et al. Two cases of lymphocytic hypophysitis presenting with diabetes insipidus: a variant of lymphocytic infundibulo-neurohypophysitis. Surg Neurol 1996;46:285–290.
16. Hashimoto K, Tako T, Makino S. Lymphocytic adenohypophysitis and lymphocytic infundibuloneurohypophysitis. Endocr J 1997;44:1–10.
17. Ahmed SR, Aiello DP, Page R, et al. Necrotizing infundibulo-hypophysitis: a unique syndrome of diabetes insipidus and hypopituitarism. J Clin Endocrinol Metab1993;76:1499–1504.
18. Imura H. Some new aspects in etiologies and diagnosis of neurogenic diabetes insipidus. In: Saito T, Yoshida S, eds. Neurohypophysis: Recent Progress of Vasopressin and Oxytocin Research. Elsevier Science BV, Amsterdam, 1995, pp. 15–20.
19. Schwartz MW, Woods WC, Porte D, et al. Central nervous system control of food intake. Nature 2000; 404:661–671.

4

Hyperthyroidism

David S. Cooper, MD

CASE #1: TSH-SECRETING PITUITARY ADENOMA

Case Description

A 54-yr-old African-American woman was seen at an urgent care facility because of the recent development of palpitations. When examined, she was noted to have a pulse of 100 bpm. Her thyroid was normal in size, and the rest of the physical examination was normal. Thyroid function tests were as follows: T4 14 μg/dL, T3RU 43% (25–35), thyroid-stimulating hormone (TSH) 1.6 mU/L. These results were interpreted as indicating that the patient was euthyroid, and she was started on a β-blocker for symptomatic relief. However, one of the physicians in the urgent care center felt that the thyroid function tests were somewhat inconsistent, and called for further advice.

Two weeks later, the patient presented for an evaluation. Since starting on atenolol 50 mg twice daily, her palpitations had resolved. She denied nervousness, tremor, hyperdefecation, insomnia, weakness, shortness of breath, chest pain, or symptoms of ophthalmopathy. She had not noticed anterior neck discomfort, dysphagia, hoarseness, or neck swelling. She also denied headaches, visual changes, or a personal or family history of thyroid disease.

Her past history was unremarkable except for mild hypertension, controlled with a diuretic. There was no family history of thyroid or autoimmune disease. She was taking no medications other than the diuretic and the atenolol. She was 1 yr postmenopausal and had not taken hormonal replacement therapy (HRT).

On physical exam, pulse 80/min, BP 140/85 mmHg, wt 200 lbs. There was no proptosis and extraocular movements were full. The thyroid gland was twofold enlarged, firm, and symmetrical. No nodules were appreciated, and a bruit was not audible. The trachea

From: *Contemporary Endocrinology: Challenging Cases in Endocrinology*
Edited by: M. E. Molitch © Humana Press Inc., Totowa, NJ

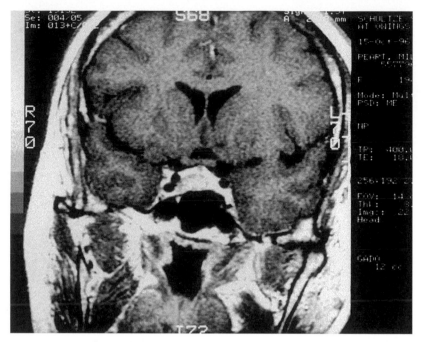

Fig. 1. Coronal section of a pituitary MRI showing an 11 mm pituitary tumor.

was in the midline and there was no cervical lymphadenopathy. The lungs, heart, abdomen, and extremities were unremarkable. There was no tremor and the skin was warm and dry.

Repeat laboratory testing of thyroid function was as follows: fT4 1.9 ng/dL (n:0.8–1.5), T3 265 ng/dL, TSH 1.6 mU/L. A 24-h radioiodine uptake was elevated at 42% (normal 10–30%). Other tests that were done included: estradiol 4 pg/mL, LH 26 mIU/L (postmenopausal 40–103), follicle stimulating hormone (FSH) 43 mIU/L (postmenopausal 34–96), prolactin 7.8 ng/mL, α subunit 1.5 ng/mL (n:<1.0; <3.6 for postmenopausal women), insulin-like growth factor (IGF)-1 269 ng/mL (90–360), morning cortisol 17 μg/dL. Sex hormone binding globulin (SHBG) was 91 nmol/L (n:20–106). A T4 binding panel, which is an electrophoretic analysis of the distribution of radiolabeled thyroxine among serum proteins, was normal. A magnetic resonance imaging (MRI) of the pituitary revealed an 11-mm pituitary microadenoma, which was close to, but did not impinge on the optic chiasm (see Fig. 1). A formal visual field examination was normal. The patient was started on Methimazole (Tapazole) 20 mg/d. One month later, her thyroid function tests were as follows: fT4 1.5 ng/mL, T3 131 ng/mL, TSH 4.6 mU/L. She was referred for neurosurgical evaluation, and underwent transsphenoidal hypophysectomy shortly thereafter. She recovered uneventfully from surgery, and had normal thyroid function off antithyroid drugs. Postoperative testing of the pituitary-adrenal axis showed normal adrenal function. Two years after surgery, on estrogen replacement therapy T4 was 11.4 mcg/dL, T3RU 23% (28–40), FTI 2.7 (1.6–3.7), thyroid stimulating hormone (TSH) 1.1 mU/L.

Discussion

This case illustrates a "classic" case of hyperthyroidism caused by a TSH-secreting pituitary tumor (TSHoma). TSHomas are rare, with a prevalence of about 1 in 1 million, but seem to be recognized with increasing frequency because of improved TSH assays. TSHomas can occur at any age and affect women and men equally *(1,2)*. By the time they are discovered, as in this case, 90% of TSHomas are macroadenomas. Approximately 30% of TSHomas are mixed tumors, with the most common situation being cosecretion with either growth hormone or prolactin. There was no evidence for cosecretion of either hormone in this case. The TSH molecules secreted by the tumor may have variable glycosylation, giving rise to variations in the biologic activity of the TSH. This may account for the lack of correlation between the level of TSH in the blood and the degree of hyperthyroidism.

This patient was typical, in that she presented with symptoms and signs of hyperthyroidism, which were quite mild. There is usually a goiter present, but the findings characteristic of Graves' disease (orbitopathy, dermopathy) are not seen. Features of a pituitary mass lesion (headache, visual field abnormalities) may occur in a minority of patients, and were not observed in this patient. Acromegaly is present in about 15% of cases, and amenorrhea/galactorrhea in about 10% *(1)*. Hypopituitarism, especially hypogonadism, may also be a presenting feature. In this patient, FSH and luteinizing hormone (LH) were appropriately elevated for her postmenopausal status.

In TSHomas, there is an increased or inappropriate level of TSH in the face of elevated thyroid hormone levels. Thyroid hormone resistance (THR) is the main entity that needs to be excluded in the differential diagnosis, since both conditions give rise to similar biochemical profiles. Although there is usually a positive family history of thyroid functional abnormalities in THR, which is an autosomal dominant condition, further diagnostic testing is almost always required. The TSH levels in patients with TSH-secreting tumors usually are not responsive to TRH or T3 administration, while TSH levels in patients with THR remain responsive. Interestingly, in the present case, the serum TSH level increased to 4.6 mU/L from 1.6 mU/L when her thyroid hormone levels were normalized with antithyroid medication.

Biochemical markers of thyroid hormone action, such as SHBG are elevated in TSHoma patients, but not in THR patents. In this case, the SHBG level was normal, albeit at the upper limit of the normal range. The measurement serum α subunit is one of the most helpful tests in differentiating TSHomas from THR. Most TSHomas oversecrete alpha subunit, while the α subunit is secreted in an equimolar manner with TSH in THR. This leads to an α subunit/TSH ratio >1 in the serum of TSHoma patients. This ratio may be calculated using the following formula:

$$[\alpha \text{ subunit (ng/mL)/TSH mU/L}] \times 10$$

It should be stressed that this ratio is not valid in postmenopausal women, as was the case here, or in men with primary hypogonadism, because they will have high serum α concentrations resulting from high serum gonadotropin levels. Of course, pituitary MRI will show a mass lesion in >95% of TSHoma patients, and should be normal in THR.

Another potential source of confusion may arise in euthyroid patients with familial dysalbuminemic hyperthyroxinemia (FDH). For reasons that are unclear, some FDH patients will have not only an elevated total T4, but also an elevated free T4 in some free T4 assays. Thus, a patient with FDH may present with symptoms suggesting hyperthyroidism (e.g., nervousness) and have high total T4 and free T4 levels and a normal, but seemingly inappropriate serum TSH level. Such patients will not have a goiter and the radioiodine uptake is normal. FDH can be ruled out by obtaining a free T4 by equilibrium dialysis and by performance of electrophoretic T4 binding studies, as was the case in this patient.

The treatment of TSHomas is transsphenoidal surgery. The chances of cure increase with smaller tumor size and absence of cavernous sinus invasion; overall, about 35% of patients can be cured surgically. Patients should be prepared for surgery with antithyroid drugs and/or β adrenergic blocking drugs. The criteria for "cure" are: euthyroidism with a normal serum TSH and no residual tumor on MRI (3,4).

For patients with residual tumor, radiation therapy should be considered. Octreotide in doses of 50–100 mcg bid or tid will normalize the serum TSH in most patients (5), but there may be escape from the effects of the drug in about 10% of cases (6). Long-acting somatostatin analogs have also been used effectively in TSHomas (7). Treatment with radioiodine or surgery to ablate the thyroid should be avoided if at all possible, since hypothyroidism could cause tumor growth.

REFERENCES

1. Beck-Peccoz P, Brucker-Davis F, Persani L, Smallridge RC, Weintraub BD. Thyrotropin-secreting pituitary tumors. Endocr Rev 1996;17:610–638.
2. Smallridge RC. Thyrotropin-secreting pituitary tumors. Endocrinol Metab Clin North Am 1987;16:765–792.
3. Losa M, Giovanelli M, Persani L, Mortini P, Faglia G, Beck-Peccoz P. Criteria of cure and follow-up of central hyperthyroidism due to thyrotropin-secreting pituitary adenomas. J Clin Endocrinol Metab 1996; 81:3084–3090.
4. Brucker-Davis F, Oldfield EH, Skarulis MC, Doppman JL, Weintraub BD. Thyrotropin-secreting pituitary tumors: diagnostic criteria, thyroid hormone sensitivity, and treatment outcome in 25 patients followed at the National Institutes of Health. J Clin Endocrinol Metab 1999;84:476–486.
5. Comi RJ, Gesundheit N, Murray L, Gorden P, Weintraub BD. Response of thyrotropin-secreting pituitary adenomas to a long-acting somatostatin analogue. N Engl J Med 1987;317:12–17.
6. Chanson P, Weintraub BD, Harris AG. Octreotide therapy for thyroid-stimulating hormone-secreting pituitary adenomas. A follow-up of 52 patients. Ann Intern Med 1993;119:236–240.
7. Gancel A, Vuillermet P, Legrand A, Catus F, Thomas F, Kuhn JM. Effects of a slow-release formulation of the new somatostatin analogue lanreotide in TSH-secreting pituitary adenomas. Clin Endocrinol (Oxf) 1994;40:421–428.

CASE #2: AMIODARONE-INDUCED HYPERTHYROIDISM AND ANTITHYROID DRUG-RELATED AGRANULOCYTOSIS

Case Description

An 80-yr-old man with a past history of myocardial infarction (MI) and ventricular arrhythmias presented to his internist with a 1 mo history of weight loss (approximately 15 lbs.) and weakness. He had been treated with amiodarone 200 mg bid for approximately 24 mo. Thyroid function tests had been normal 6 mo earlier, but now showed a suppressed serum TSH of <0.02 mU/L. In consultation with his cardiologist, it was felt not appropriate to discontinue the amiodarone, and the patient was referred for endocrinologic evaluation. Aside from the weight loss and weakness, there were no other hyperthyroid symptoms. His past history was unremarkable except for the MI. There was no family history of thyroid disease or autoimmune disease. His other medications included atenolol, atorvastatin, and ranitidine.

On physical examination, the patient was thin, but otherwise well appearing. His pulse was 60/min, BP 120/70 mmHg, weight 126 lbs. There was no proptosis and extraocular movements were full. The thyroid gland was not palpable, and no nodules were appreciated. The trachea was in the midline and there was no cervical lymphadenopathy. The lungs, heart, abdomen, and extremities were unremarkable. There was no tremor, and the skin was warm and dry.

Thyroid function tests were as follows: fT4 3.0 ng/dL, T3 190 ng/dL, TSH <0.02 mU/L. An interleukin 6 (IL-6) level was drawn, which returned 2 wk later within normal limits. A continuous flow Doppler ultrasound study was ordered, but the patient only received a conventional thyroid ultrasound: it showed a normal-sized gland with scattered 3–4 mm nodules in both lobes.

The patient was thought to have probable amiodarone-induced thyroiditis. He was started on prednisone 40 mg/d as a single daily dose. One week later, he noted no improvement in his symptoms, and repeat thyroid function tests were unchanged (fT4 2.8 ng/dL, T3 277 ng/dL). For this reason, Tapazole 40 mg/d was added to the regimen. One week later, thyroid function testing was unchanged, with fT4 2.9 ng/dL, T3 282 ng/dL. The prednisone and methimazole were continued. Two weeks later, the patient developed severe shortness of breath and was hospitalized with a diagnosis of congestive heart failure. Three days after admission, he developed a fever to 103°F with shaking chills. A chest X-ray showed a hazy infiltrate in the right lower lung field. Blood cultures were drawn, and subsequently grew *Strep. pneumoniae*. Broad spectrum antibiotics were started. A complete blood count (CBC), which had been normal on admission, revealed a white blood count (WBC) of 3000/mm^3 with 10% granulocytes. The methimazole was discontinued, but the WBC and granulocyte count continued to fall. Two days later, the WBC was 100/mm^3 with 0% granulocytes. A bone marrow examination revealed severe depletion of myelocytic precursors. A hematologist recommended therapy with recombinant G-CSF, which was started at a dose of 300 mcg/d. Two days later, the patient became unresponsive and had a respiratory arrest. He was intubated and transferred to the ICU. An MRI of the brain revealed an intracerebellar hemorrhage. Over the course of the next week, the granulocyte count rose gradually, and the patient defervesced. On prednisone therapy, his thyroid function became normal. However, he remained comatose and respirator-dependent for the next 2 wk. Life support was withdrawn at the urging of his family, and he died shortly thereafter.

Discussion

AMIODARONE-INDUCED THYROTOXICOSIS

The antiarrhythmic drug amiodarone is 37% iodine by weight: therefore, a daily 400-mg amiodarone dose would yield over 100 mg of inorganic iodine after deiodination. In addition to the potential effects of this large iodine load on thyroid function, the intact drug is a potent inhibitor of peripheral T4 to T3 conversion. Therefore, even in euthyroid subjects taking the drug, serum T4 and free T4 levels may be high-normal or even elevated and serum T3 levels are usually low-normal. The serum TSH may be slightly elevated early on in the treatment course *(1)*, but should be normal after 6 mo of treatment *(1)*.

The prevalence of amiodarone-induced thyrotoxicosis (AIT) in the United States is in the range of 2–4% of patients who take the drug *(2,3)*. The prevalence is much higher in areas of the world that are marginally iodine-deficient *(4)*. Most experts recognize two distinct forms of AIT, termed Type 1 and Type 2. Type 1 AIT is really a form of iodine-induced hyperthyroidism (also termed Jod–Basedow), which classically occurs in patients with an underlying multinodular goiter or subclinical Graves' disease. Type 2 AIT develops in individuals with normal thyroid glands, and is thought to represent a thyroiditis owing to a direct, toxic effect of the drug on thyroid follicular epithelial cells *(5)*.

Distinguishing between the two forms of AIT is crucial, as treatment is very different. Unfortunately, it may be difficult to tell the two forms of AIT apart, but some clinical and biochemical clues may be of help *(6)*. For unclear reasons, Type 1 AIT usually develops after a patient has been on the drug for over 2 years, while Type 2 disease develops after an average of 1–2 yr of treatment *(7)*. Patients with Type 1 disease usually have a palpably abnormal multinodular thyroid gland, and patients with Type 2 disease have no palpable thyroid abnormalities. Although a thyroiditis exists histopathologically in Type 2 AIT *(8)*, it is usually painless, but rare cases can mimic subacute thyroiditis with thyroidal pain. The literature suggests that Type 1 AIT patients have normal or high 24 h radioiodine uptake (RAIU) values in the face of high circulating iodine levels, whereas Type 2 patients invariably will have low values *(9)*. However, in the experience of many American thyroidologists, the RAIU is low (<2%) in both types. Serum IL-6 levels have been advocated to discriminate between the two types, because this inflammatory cytokine would be expected to be elevated in Type 2 AIT but not in Type 1 AIT *(10)*. However, in the author's experience and that of others *(11)*, the IL-6 may be normal in unequivocal cases of Type 2 AIT. Doppler flow ultrasound is another potentially valuable test, which reveals increased flow in Type 1 AIT, but normal or decreased flow in Type 2 due to the thyroidal inflammation *(12)*.

In the case presented above, the patient had been on the drug for about 2 yr, which does not really help in the differential diagnosis of AIT. His presenting complaints of weight loss and weakness are typical of elderly thyrotoxic patients; patients on amiodarone do not usually have palpitations or tachycardia because the drug has β-blocking effects. The fact that the thyroid gland was not palpable strongly suggested the diagnosis of Type 2 AIT. The thyroid function tests were typical of hyperthyroid patients taking amiodarone, with T4 predominance or "T4 toxicosis" owing to the inhibitory effects of amiodarone on 5'deiodinase *(13)*. Prior studies have suggested that thyroid function tests are similar in the two forms of the disease *(6)*, and it should be stressed that some patients with AIT may even have normal serum T3 levels *(14)*. The patient's IL-6 levels were normal, but as noted earlier, this does not rule out Type 2 AIT. The patient did not have a Doppler study of the thyroid.

Clinically, the patient was thought to have Type 2 AIT, and for that reason he was started on prednisone therapy. It would have been preferable to have stopped the amiodarone, but there have been cases reported in whom the thyroiditis resolved even though the amiodarone was continued *(15)*. Usually, there is a rapid and very gratifying response to prednisone in Type 2 AIT *(9)*. In the present case, when there was no such response, methimazole was added because the possibility of Type 1 disease could not be ruled out. Some authors have recommended a combination of glucocorticoids and antithyroid drugs in cases in which the diagnosis is uncertain *(16)*. Perchlorate may also be effective in Type 1 AIT as an inhibitor of thyroidal iodine uptake, and lithium has been reported to be a useful adjunct in patients that appear to have either Type 1 or Type 2 AIT *(17)*. In some patients in whom there is a poor response to pharmacologic therapy, and whose cardiac status is tenuous because of unremitting thyrotoxicosis, surgery is the only other option *(18)*. In the patient under discussion, his thyroid function tests remained elevated on prednisone and methimazole for unclear reasons, and surgery might have been a consideration had he not developed the severe problems that ultimately proved fatal.

ANTITHYROID DRUG-INDUCED AGRANULOCYTOSIS

As events unfolded, the patient developed a granulocytosis, one of the most feared complications of antithyroid drug therapy. Studies have shown a dose-related increase in the frequency of methimazole related complications *(19)*, and the elderly may be more susceptible *(19)*. Agranulocytosis may develop slowly *(20)*, making routine monitoring of the WBC reasonable, but in most cases, like this one, the problem develops precipitously.

In a review of 13 cases of antithyroid drug-induced agranulocytosis from a single institution, it was found that the most common infections were acute pharyngitis, acute tonsillitis, and pneumonia *(21)*. In 168 cases of drug-induced agranulocytosis, the overall mortality rate was 16%; older age, marrow hypoplasia, and shock were significant risk factors for mortality in univariate analysis, but in multivariate analysis, only preexisting renal dysfunction and bacteremia were significant predictors of death *(22)*. In the present case, sepsis may have been exacerbated by the concomitant administration of prednisone for presumed Type 2 AIT.

Although G-CSF has been used widely in the treatment of drug-induced agranulocytosis, and has been thought to decrease recovery time and mortality *(23)*, a recent randomized trial of G-CSF in antithyroid drug-induced agranulocytosis showed no apparent benefit *(24)*. However, there may be of benefit in a subset of patients with less severe degrees of myelocytic hypoplasia. There is no apparent benefit of glucocorticoid therapy in patients with antithyroid drug-related agranulocytosis *(25)*.

This patient had a cascade of drug-related side effects that ultimately led to his death. Unfortunately, the elderly are the most likely to receive amiodarone because of underlying cardiovascular disease, and when thyrotoxicosis develops, are more vulnerable to severe cardiac consequences. The elderly are also at higher risk for the development of complications of glucocorticoids and antithyroid drug-induced agranulocytosis as noted above. His death was clearly related to his development of agranulocytosis, even though the proximal cause was a cerebrovascular event.

REFERENCES

1. Burger, A, Dinichert, D, Nicod, P, Jenny, M, Lemarchand-Beraud, T, Vallotton, MB. Effect of amiodarone on serum triiodothyronine, reverse triiodothyronine, thyroxin, and thyrotropin: A drug influencing peripheral metabolism of thyroid hormones. J Clin Invest 1976;58:255–259.
2. Nademanee K, Singh BN, Callahan B, Hendrickson JA, Hershman JM. Amiodarone, thyroid hormone indexes, and altered thyroid function: long-term serial effects in patients with cardiac arrhythmias. Am J Cardiol 1986;58:981–986.
3. Harjai KJ, Licata AA. Effects of amiodarone on thyroid function. Ann Intern Med 1997;126:63–73.
4. Martino E, Safran M, Aghini-Lombardi F, Rajatanavin R, Lenziardi M, Fay M, Pacchiarotti A, Aronin N, Macchia E, Haffajee C. Environmental iodine intake and thyroid dysfunction during chronic amiodarone therapy. Ann Intern Med 1984;101:28–34.
5. Chiovato L, Martino E, Tonacchera M, Santini F, Lapi P, Mammoli C, Braverman LE, Pinchera A. Studies on the in vitro cytotoxic effect of amiodarone. Endocrinology 1994;134:2277–2282.
6. Bartalena L, Brogioni S, Grasso L, Bogazzi F, Burelli A, Martino E. Treatment of amiodarone-induced thyrotoxicosis, a difficult challenge: results of a prospective study. J Clin Endocrinol Metab 1996;81: 2930–2933.

7. Trip MD, Wiersinga W, Plomp TA. Incidence, predictability, and pathogenesis of amiodarone-induced thyrotoxicosis and hypothyroidism. Am J Med 1991;91:507–511.

8. Brennan MD, van Heerden JA, Carney JA. Amiodarone-associated thyrotoxicosis (AAT): experience with surgical management. Surgery 1987;102:1062–1067.

9. Martino E, Bartalena L, Mariotti S, Aghini-Lombardi F, Ceccarelli C, Lippi F, Piga M, Loviselli A, Braverman L, Safran M. Radioactive iodine thyroid uptake in patients with amiodarone-iodine-induced thyroid dysfunction. Acta Endocrinol (Copenh) 1988;119:167–173.

10. Bartalena L, Grasso L, Brogioni S, Aghini-Lombardi F, Braverman LE, Martino E. Serum interleukin-6 in amiodarone-induced thyrotoxicosis. J Clin Endocrinol Metab 1994;78:423–427.

11. Bauters C, D'Herbomez M, Nocaudie M, Decoulx M, Marchandise X, Wemeau JL. Interleukin-6 and thyroid radioactive iodine uptake in patients with amiodarone-induced thyrotoxicosis. J Endocrinol Invest 1999;22:94 (abstract).

12. Bogazzi F, Bartalena L, Brogioni S, Mazzeo S, Vitti P, Burelli A, Bartolozzi C, Martino E. Color flow doppler sonography rapidly differentiates type I and type II amiodarone-induced thyrotoxicosis. Thyroid 1997;7:541–545.

13. Rao RH, McCready VR, Spathis GS. Iodine kinetic studies during amiodarone treatment. J Clin Endocrinol Metab 1986;62:563–568.

14. Harjai KJ, Licata AA. Amiodarone-Induced Hyperthyroidism. PACE 1996;19:1548–1554

15. Roti E, Minelli R, Gardini E, Bianconi L, Braverman LE. Thyrotoxicosis followed by hypothyroidism in patients treated with amiodarone. A possible consequence of a destructive process in the thyroid. Arch Intern Med 1993;153:886–892.

16. Seminara S, Daniels G. Amiodarone and the thyroid. Endoc Pract 1998;4:48–57.

17. Dickstein G, Shechner C, Adawi F, Kaplan J, Baron E, Ish-Shalom S. Lithium treatment in amiodarone-induced thyrotoxicosis. Am J Med 1997;102:454–458.

18. Mulligan, DC, McHenry, CR, Kinney, W, Esselstyn, CB. Amiodarone-induced thyrotoxicosis: clinical presentation and expanded indications for thyroidectomy. Surgery 1993;114:1114–1119.

19. Cooper DS, Goldminz D, Levin AA, et al. Agranulocytosis associated with antithyroid drugs. Ann Intern Med 1983;98:26–29.

20. Tajiri J, Noguchi S, Murakami T, Murakami N. Antithyroid drug-induced agranulocytosis: the usefulness of routine white blood cell count monitoring. Arch Int Med 1990;150:621–624.

21. Sheng WH, Hung CC, Chen YC, Fang CT, Hsieh SM, Chang SC, Hsieh WC. Antithyroid-drug-induced agranulocytosis and infectious complications. Q J Med 1999;92:455–461.

22. Julia A, Olona M, Bueno J, et al. Drug-induced agranulocytosis: prognostic factors in a series of 168 episodes. Br J Haematol 1991;79:366–371.

23. Somogyi A, Rosta A, Lang I, Werling K. Treatment of drug-induced bone marrow suppression with recombinant human granulocyte/monocyte colony stimulating factor. Adverse Drug Reac Toxicol Rev 1996;15:119–124.

24. Fukata S, Kuma K, Sugawara M. Granulocyte colony-stimulating factor (G-CSF) does not improve recovery from antithyroid drug-induced agranulocytosis: a prospective study. Thyroid 1999;9:29–31.

25. Tamai H, Mukuta T, Matsubayashi S, et al. Treatment of methimazole-induced recombinant human granulocyte colony-stimulating factor (rhG-CSF). J Clin Endocrinol Metab 1993;77:1356–1360.

CASE #3: A TEENAGER WITH SEVERE HYPERTHYROIDISM DUE TO GRAVES' DISEASE

Case Description

A 14-yr-old girl developed typical symptoms of Graves' disease, including heat intolerance, weight loss, insomnia, and declining school performance. When seen by her pediatrician, she was noted to be tachycardic, with a stare, mild proptosis, and a large goiter. Thyroid function tests were consistent with thyrotoxicosis, and she was started on methimazole 10 mg tid and atenolol 50 mg/d. After 2 wk of therapy, she developed a diffuse pruritic rash, and was switched to PTU 100 tid. Over the next 6 mo, her thyroid function tests improved, but did not normalize, and she was referred to a pediatric endocrinologist for further evaluation. He determined that she was taking her medication faithfully, and increased the PTU dose to 200 mg tid. On this dose, the free T4 became normal, but the serum T3 remained elevated, and she was referred for consideration of radioiodine therapy.

At the time she was seen, at age 15, she continued to have heat intolerance, occasional palpitations, and nervousness. She had been amenorrheic for 6 mo. Her schoolwork had deteriorated to the point that she was required to enroll in summer school in order to be promoted into the tenth grade. She had no ophthalmologic complaints. Her family history was significant for a mother and maternal aunt who had had Graves' disease, and who had both been treated with radioiodine. Her past history was unremarkable except for a recent shoulder injury that had required placement of pins in the scapula.

On physical examination, pulse was 100/bpm, BP 130/60 mmHg, weight 176 lbs, height 65 inches. There was mild periorbital edema and mild bilateral proptosis with Hertel measurements of 21 mm OU. Extraocular movements were full. The thyroid was three-fold enlarged (60 g), and was firm, symmetrical, and smooth. No bruit was heard. There was a large pyramidal lobe present. The lungs were clear and the cardiac exam was normal except for a hyperdynamic precordium. The abdomen was benign. A fine tremor was present, and the skin was warm and moist. The reflexes were brisk. There was no evidence of dermopathy.

Thyroid function tests that had been done the week before were as follows: fT4 0.3 ng/dL, T3 650 ng/dL, TSH <0.02 mU/L. A pregnancy test was negative.

A lengthy discussion was held with the patient and her mother. Surgery was suggested as a reasonable option, but neither the patient nor her mother was so inclined, and they elected to proceed directly to radioiodine therapy. PTU was discontinued for 3 d, and a 24-h radioiodine uptake was 65%. She received 15 mCi ^{131}I, PTU was not restarted, and atenolol 50 mg once or twice a day was continued. After 3 mo, she was feeling generally well with β blockade, but she was still hyperthyroid, with the following thyroid function tests: fT4 3.5 ng/dL, T3 445 ng/dL, TSH <0.02 mU/L.

At this time, her orthopedic surgeon told the patient that the pins in her shoulder needed to be removed, a procedure requiring general anesthesia. Because of her abnormal thyroid status, surgery was delayed. PTU was restarted to prepare her for shoulder surgery. Two weeks later, the patient developed malaise, right upper quadrant pain, and dark urine. She was seen by her pediatrician, who noted her to be jaundiced and to have an enlarged tender liver. Liver function tests revealed a serum bilirubin of 12 mg/dL and transaminase levels that were 20-fold above normal. Serum ammonia levels and clotting times were normal, and serologic tests for hepatitis A, B, and C were negative. PTU was discontinued and liver function tests gradually normalized over the course of the next 3 wk.

The patient was started on SSKI 2 drops three times a day and atenolol 50 mg bid. Her serum levels of fT4 and T3 declined to 2.3 ng/dL and 225 ng/dL, respectively, and she underwent shoulder surgery uneventfully. The SSKI was continued, but after 6 wk, thyroid function returned to baseline elevations and the medication was stopped. Two months later, she was still hyperthyroid, with fT4 2.4 ng/dL and T3 550 ng/dL. The thyroid was still two–threefold enlarged and firm. There was continuing mild ophthalmopathy, which had not progressed, and she was treated with a second 20 mCi dose of radioiodine without glucocorticoid coverage. Six weeks later, fT4 was 0.6 ng/dL and T3 was 115 ng/dL, but after an additional 6 wk, fT4 rose to 2.1 ng/dL, and T3 was 350 ng/dL. She remained persistently hyperthyroid for the next 6 mo. A third dose of radioiodine (20 mCi) was administered, and the patient developed hypothyroidism 2 mo later. When last seen, she was doing well in school and had normal thyroid function taking thyroxine 0.125 mg daily.

Discussion

This case illustrates a number of issues surrounding the management of Graves' disease, especially in adolescents and young adults. Although many have typical symptoms and signs, a decline in school performance may be one of the most remarkable and disturbing manifestations. Other behavioral problems, such as anger, emotional lability, and antisocial activity may be attributed to "normal teenage behavior."

In a survey of members of the American Thyroid Association, radioiodine was the preferred method of therapy by a wide margin for Graves' disease in middle-aged or older persons, but antithyroid drugs were favored as initial therapy in young adults *(1)*. Unfortunately, antithyroid drug therapy often needs to be abandoned for a variety of reasons, including poor compliance and toxicity in patients in this age group *(2)*. Methimazole is an ideal drug in children and adolescents because of once-a-day dosing, thereby improving compliance *(3)*. Owing to her drug reaction (a rash), PTU was prescribed instead, to which she responded poorly. It is likely that she was taking the medication faithfully, because her fT4 level was subnormal, in the face of a remarkable elevation in serum T3. Such discordance between the serum T4 (or fT4) concentration and the serum T3 have been noted by others *(4)*, and stresses the need for monitoring serum T3 levels when following patients while they are on antithyroid medications.

Radioiodine is becoming increasingly acceptable as a form of therapy for Graves' disease in children and adolescents *(5)*. About 20% of individuals with Graves' disease fail to respond to a first dose of radioiodine *(6)*. Patients with very large glands are most likely to fail, and there is some evidence that high circulating titers of thyroid stimulating immunoglobulins also predict a worse outcome *(7)*. There is also accumulating evidence that PTU exposure prior to radioiodine treatment may increase the failure rate, by conferring a radioprotective effect upon the thyroid; interestingly, this phenomenon does not seem to occur in patients receiving methimazole therapy *(8)*. The reasons for this difference are unknown, since the two drugs are thought to have similar mechanisms of action.

There has been much controversy about the relationship between the method of treatment of Graves' disease and possible worsening of preexisting ophthalmopathy. Several prospective controlled trials *(9,10)* have rather convincingly shown that radioiodine therapy may worsen Graves' eye disease, especially if there is moderate to severe eye disease before therapy. Other factors that seem to be important in predicting whether worsening of eye problems will occur postradioiodine therapy include high serum T3 levels *(7)*, smoking *(11)*, and perhaps the development of unrecognized and untreated hypothyroidism following the radioiodine *(12)*. Previous studies have also demonstrated that glucocorticoid therapy (e.g., prednisone 40–60 mg/d with tapering over 2–3 mo) started at the time of radioiodine administration will prevent any potential worsening in virtually all cases *(8,13)*. In this case, only mild eye problems were present, and it was felt that the potential complications of glucocorticoid therapy outweighed any possible benefits. Fortunately, there was no apparent effect of radioiodine therapy on her eye disease.

The need for surgery that would necessitate general anesthesia became an issue in this patient who remained thyrotoxic after radioiodine therapy. Surgery and a variety of other stresses (infection, childbirth, trauma), are known to be precipitants of thyroid storm, although the risks are probably very low. Although several studies have shown that the outcomes after surgery in hypothyroid patients who are operated upon are no different from age and operation-matched controls, published data do not exist for hyperthyroidism. Therefore, it makes sense to attempt to normalize thyroid function, especially for an elective procedure.

Unfortunately, the patient developed a rare, but potentially fatal hepatotoxic reaction to PTU, even though she had previously taken it without toxicity. This illustrates the important point that major antithyroid drug reactions can occur on restarting therapy after a prior benign exposure to the drug. There are numerous case reports of PTU-induced hepatitis in the literature, summarized in a recent review *(14)*. The frequency is unknown, and although rare, patients should always be reminded about this rare side effect.

The use of SSKI to try to restore normal thyroid function prior to her shoulder surgery was based on studies showing that iodine has blocks hormone secretion, and has transient effects on hormone synthesis *(15)*. In patients previously treated with radioiodine, the inhibition of hormone synthesis is more dramatic and long lasting *(16)*, and patients can quickly become hypothyroid if not monitored carefully. In the present case, however, the effects were only partial and relatively short-lived. Had she not had the hepatotoxic reaction to PTU, the iodinated oral cholecystographic agents sodium ipodate (Oragraffin) or sodium iopanoate (Telepaque) might have been tried in this circumstance. Both are potent inhibitors of T4 to T3 conversion and also serve as a source of iodine *(17)*. There are no controlled trials that demonstrate the efficacy of these agents in this context, but many thyroid experts routinely use them in patients who require rapid restoration of normal thyroid function. Recently, it was announced that Oragraffin was being withdrawn from the market.

After her second dose of radioiodine, the patient developed transient hypothyroidism. This occurs in up to 90% of patients 2–4 mo after therapy *(18)*. The fact that the thyroid is still palpable or enlarged is a useful clinical clue that the hypothyroidism is likely to be transient *(19)*. After her third radioiodine dose, the patient finally became hypothyroid. One wonders with the benefit of hindsight whether she would have been better off if she had had surgery at the very beginning of her illness, 2 yr previously. Although surgery is not a favored treatment in this country, it is more routine in other parts of the world, especially in children. In a recently reported prospective trial from Sweden, in which patients with Graves' disease were randomized to receive antithyroid drugs, radioiodine, or surgery, patient satisfaction with their treatment, and patient fears of possible complications of treatment were not different for the three treatment arms *(20)*.

REFERENCES

1. Solomon B, Glinoer D, Lagasse R, Wartofsky L. Current trends in the management of Graves' disease. J Clin Endocrinol Metab 1990;70:1518–1524.
2. Hamburger JI. Management of hyperthyroidism in children and adolescents. J Clin Endocrinol Metab 1985;60:1019–1024.
3. Nicholas WC, Fischer RG, Stevenson RA, Bass JD. Single daily dose of methimazole compared to every 8 hours of propylthiouracil in the treatment of hyperthyroidism. South Med J 1995;88:973–976.
4. Chen JJ, Ladenson PW. Discordant hypothyroxinemia and hypertriiodothyroninemia in treated patients with hyperthyroid Graves' disease. J Clin Endocrinol Metab 1986;63:102–106.
5. Rivkees SA, Sklar C, Freemark M. The management of Graves' disease in children, with special emphasis on radioiodine treatment. J Clin Endocrinol Metab 1998;83:3767–3776.
6. Holm LE, Lundell G, Dahlqvist I, Israelsson A. Cure rate after 131I therapy for hyperthyroidism. Acta Radiol Oncol 1981;20:161–166.

7. Chiovato L, Fiore E, Vitti P, et al. Outcome of thyroid function in Graves' patients treated with radio-iodine: role of thyroid-stimulating and thyrotropin-blocking antibodies and of radioiodine-induced thyroid damage. J Clin Endocrinol Metab 1998;83:40–46.

8. Imseis RE, VanMiddlesworth L, Massie JD, Bush AJ, VanMiddlesworth NR. Pretreatment with propyl-thiouracil but not methimazole reduces the therapeutic efficacy of Iodine-131 in hyperthyroidism. J Clin Endocrinol Metab 1998;83:685–687.

9. Tallstedt L, Lundell G, Torring O, et al. Occurrence of ophthalmopathy after treatment for Graves' hyper-thyroidism. N Engl J Med 1992;326:1733–1738.

10. Bartalena L, Marcocci C, Bogazzi F, et al. Relation between therapy for hyperthyroidism and the course of Graves' ophthalmopathy. N Engl J Med 1998;338:73–78.

11. Bartalena L, Marcocci C, Tanda ML, et al. Cigarette smoking and treatment outcomes in Graves ophthal-mopathy. Ann Int Med 1998;129:632–635.

12. Tallstedt L, Lundell G, Blomgren H, Bring J. Does early administration of thyroxine reduce the devel-opment of Graves' ophthalmopathy after radioiodine treatment? Eur J Endocrinol 1994;130:494–497.

13. Bartalena L, Marcocci C, Bogazzi F, et al. Use of corticosteroids to prevent progression of Graves' oph-thalmopathy after radioiodine therapy for hyperthyroidism. N Engl J Med 1989;321:1349–1352.

14. Cooper DS. The side-effects of antithyroid drugs. The Endocrinologist 1999;9:457–467.

15. Schimmel M, Utiger RD. Acute effect of inorganic iodide after 131I therapy for hyperthyroidism. Clin Endocrinol 1977;6:329–332.

16. Ross DS, Daniels GH, DeStefano P, et al. Use of adjunctive potassium iodide after radioactive iodine (131I) treatment of Graves' hyperthyroidism. J Clin Endocrinol Metab 1983;57:250–253.

17. Braga M, Cooper DS. Oral cholecystographic agents and the thyroid. J Clin Endocrinol Metab 2001; 86:2354–2359.

18. Gomez N, Gomez JM, Ortiz A, et al. Transient hypothyroidism after Iodine-131 therapy for Graves' disease. J Nucl Med 1995;36:1539–542.

19. Sawers JSA, Toft AD, Irvine WJ, Brown NS, Seth J. Transient hypothyroidism after iodine-131 treat-ment of thyrotoxicosis. J Clin Endocrinol Metab 1980;50:226–229.

20. Torring O, Tallstedt L, Wallin G, et al. Graves' hyperthyroidism: treatment with antithyroid drugs, sur-gery, or radioiodine-a prospective randomized study. J Clin Endocrinol Metab 1996;81:2986–2993.

CASE #4: THYROID STORM

Case Description

A 25-yr-old woman presented to her physician two yr previously with weight loss, palpitations, and tremulousness. She was diagnosed with hyperthyroidism due to Graves' disease and started on therapy with an antithyroid drug. Because of a variety of circum-stances, including an inability to afford the medication, she became increasingly symp-tomatic. Over the next two yr, she lost approximately 40–50 lbs, and developed significant proximal muscle weakness. When referred to the Endocrine Clinic, she was severely debilitated. The patient had no other medical problems. There was a positive family his-tory of thyroid disease; her mother had had "an overactive thyroid" treated surgically many years earlier. She smoked two packs of cigarettes daily and was unemployed.

On physical exam, pulse was 130/bpm, BP 150/60 mmHg, weight 110 lbs, height 67 inches. The patient was emaciated and had severe temporal muscle wasting. There was a stare, lid lag, and mild bilateral proptosis. Extraocular movements were full. The thy-roid gland was twofold enlarged, firm, smooth, and symmetrical, with a palpable pyramidal lobe. There was no bruit or thrill over the gland. The lungs were clear and the precordium was hyperdynamic with a Grade 2/6 systolic ejection murmur at the left sternal border. The abdomen was scaphoid, but otherwise unremarkable. There was a fine tremor, the skin was warm and moist, and reflexes were brisk.

Thyroid function tests were as follows: fT4 5.1 ng/dL, T3 650 ng/dL, TSH <0.02 mU/L. Various options for therapy were discussed with the patient. Radioiodine was recommended, but the patient had a strong desire to have surgery. Accordingly, she was started on methimazole 40 mg/d and atenolol 50 mg bid in preparation for thyroidectomy. Four weeks later, she had gained 15 lbs, and was symptomatically much improved. Her thyroid function tests were as follows: fT4 2.5 ng/dL, T3 250 ng/dL. Methimazole was continued and the patient returned for follow up 4 wk later. She was now asymptomatic. The thyroid was still twofold enlarged, but there were no other manifestations of thyrotoxicosis. Thyroid function tests were repeated and were as follows: fT4 1.8 ng/dL T3 195 ng/dL. The patient was informed that she was now ready for surgery; surgical consultation was arranged, and surgery was scheduled two weeks hence. Six days before surgery, the surgeon's office contacted the patient by phone and instructed her not to take aspirin before surgery. She misconstrued the message, and discontinued both the methimazole and atenolol, as well as the SSKI that had been prescribed by the surgeon 5 d earlier to decrease vascularity of the gland. The morning of surgery she arrived in the preoperative area with tremor and palpitations. On physical examination, pulse 110 bpm, and the skin was warm and moist. The patient was cleared for surgery and underwent bilateral near total thyroidectomy without incident.

While in the recovery room, she became more tachycardic and was treated with 5 mg of intravenous propranolol, which reduced the heart rate from 140 bpm to 95 bpm. Her blood pressure and temperature were normal, and she was transferred to the surgical floor. Several hours later, her pulse was noted to be 120 bpm, her temperature increased to 100°F, and she became agitated and anxious. She remained oriented to person, place, and time. She was treated with another intravenous dose of propranolol and started on atenolol 150 mg orally every 12 h. Thyroid function tests that had been drawn that morning prior to surgery returned showing the following: fT4 3.0 ng/dL, T3 350 ng/dL. Six hours later she had a pulse of 90 bpm, a normal temperature, and she was less hyperkinetic. Atenolol was continued and she continued to improve over the next 12 h. She was discharged from the hospital on the second postoperative day on atenolol 50 mg/d for 2 d, and she was started on thyroxine 10 d later when she became biochemically hypothyroid (fT4 0.4 T3 50 ng/dL TSH <0.02).

Discussion

This patient illustrates several important points. Patients frequently ask what would "happen" to them if their hyperthyroidism were left untreated. In addition to the risk of atrial arrhythmias (21) and osteoporosis (22), a clinical outcome similar to what was seen in this patient on presentation is seen all too frequently. Graves' disease usually does not spontaneously remit, although there are certainly patients who have what appear to be spontaneous remissions.

The indications for surgery in Graves' disease include:

1. The presence of a large goiter;
2. Allergy to or noncomplicance with antithyroid drugs in children in whom radioiodine may not be considered to be appropriate;
3. The presence of a malignant or suspicious nodule within the gland;
4. Patient preference, usually based on an emotional reaction to the idea of radioiodine. Such was the case in this patient, based on her mother's having had uneventful surgery.

Preparation for surgery traditionally means rendering the patient euthyroid with antithyroid drugs. Because this may take as long as 12 wk to accomplish, some experts have recommended more rapid preparation with β blocking agents with or without potassium iodide for 2–3 wk. Generally speaking, these latter preparative methods have permitted safe surgery, although there is a higher frequency of postoperative fever and tachycardia in patients prepared in this manner (23). In patients requiring more rapid preparation, another strategy uses a combination of glucocorticoids, β-blockers, and sodium ipodate, permitting surgery to be done safely in 5 d (24).

In addition to measures designed to normalize thyroid function, some surgeons prefer to add SSKI 10 d prior to surgery to decrease blood flow to the gland. Although there is evidence that iodine does decrease thyroid vascularity, one study showed that blood loss during surgery was similar in patients who were and were not prepared with iodine (25). The major long-term complications of surgery are recurrent laryngeal nerve damage and hypoparathyroidism, and these are less frequent in experienced hands (26). Recurrent hyperthyroidism develops in 5–15% of patients, often many years after the initial surgery (27).

Thyroid storm is a decompensated state of severe thyrotoxicosis, and the syndrome generally includes fever, tachycardia or tachyarrhythmia, and altered mental status as primary manifestations. Burch and Wartofsky have attempted to formulate a set of diagnostic criteria for thyroid storm using a scoring system (28), but this idea has not gained wide acceptance. Most studies have not found differences in thyroid function tests between hyperthyroid patients with and without thyroid storm, although a higher level of free T4 has been noted by some authors (29). In the patient under discussion, thyroid function rapidly deteriorated when methimazole was discontinued, which is not unexpected. In a recent study, serum free T4 and T3 rose by 39% and 70%, respectively, within days of stopping methimazole therapy (30). The simultaneous discontinuation of atenolol probably made the patient even more vulnerable to a decompensated state (perhaps thyroid "squall" rather than "thyroid storm" would best describe this case).

The polypharmaceutical treatment of thyroid storm is designed to block thyroid hormone synthesis (antithyroid drugs), thyroid hormone release (iodine), T4 to T3 conversion (propranolol, steroids, oral cholecystographic agents), and thyroid hormone action at the tissue level (β-blocking drugs). In the present case, the patient was status post-thyroidectomy, so antithyroid agents and iodine would have no therapeutic role. Therapy with an oral cholecystographic agent was considered in this patient to block T4 to T3 conversion (31), but it was felt that her problem would quickly resolve owing to endogenous clearance of thyroid hormone. Therefore, β blockade was the only specific therapy used, and the patient recovered uneventfully, if somewhat memorably, from the surgery.

REFERENCES

1. Kahaly GJ, Nieswandt J, Mohr-Kahaly S. Cardiac risks of hyperthyroidism in the elderly. Thyroid 1998; 8:1165–1169.
2. Jodar E, Munoz-Torres M, Escobar-Jimenez F, Quesada-Charneco M, Lund del Castillo JD. Bone loss in hyperthyroid patients and in former hyperthyroid patients controlled on medical therapy: influence of aetiology and menopause. Clin Endocrinol 1997;47:279–285.
3. Feely J, Crooks J, Forrest AL, et al. Propranolol in the surgical treatment of hyperthyroidism, including severely thyrotoxic patients. Br J Surg 1981;68:865–869.
4. Baeza A, Aguayo M, Barria M, Pineda G. Rapid preoperative preparation in hyperthyroidism. Clin Endocrinol 1991;35:439–442.

5. Coyle PJ, Mitchell JE. Thyroidectomy: is Lugol's iodine necessary? Ann R Coll Surg Engl 1982;64: 334–345.
6. Sosa JA, Bowman HM, Tielsch JM, Powe NR, Gordon TA, Udelsman R. The importance of surgeon experience for clinical and economic outcomes from thyroidectomy. Ann Surg 1998;228:320–330.
7. Sugino K, Mimura T, Ozaki O, et al. Management of recurrent hyperthyroidism in patients with Graves' disease treated by subtotal thyroidectomy. J Endocrinol Invest 1995;18:415–419.
8. Burch HB, Wartofsky L. Life-threatening thyrotoxicosis. Endocrinol Metab Clin North Am 1993;22: 263–277.
9. Brooks MH, Waldstein SS. Free thyroxine concentrations in thyroid storm. Ann Intern Med 1980;93:694–697.
10. Andrade VL, Gross JL, Maia AL. Effect of methimazole pretreatment on serum thyroid hormone levels after radioactive treatment in Graves' hyperthyroidism. J Clin Endocrinol Metab 1999;84:4012–4016.
11. Roti E, Robuschi G, Gardini E, et al. Comparison of methimazole, methimazole and sodium ipodate, and methimazole and saturated solution of potassium iodide in the early treatment of hyperthyroid Graves' disease. Clin Endocrinol 1988;28:305–314.

5

Hypothyroidism and Thyroiditis

Donald A. Meier, MD
and Michael M. Kaplan, MD

CONTENTS

CASE #1: RECURRENT PAINFUL HASHIMOTO'S THYROIDITIS

Case Description

Case 1 presented to us in 1982, at age 67, after taking levothyroxine (T4) for 10 yr. Her thyroid was nontender, quite firm, and diffusely enlarged, with an estimated size of 50 g. Her antithyroid microsomal antibody titer was 1:1 600,000 and her antithyroglobulin antibody level was 50 radioimmunoassay (RIA) units*. On a T4 dose of 150 µg daily, her serum thyrotropin [thyroid stimulating hormone (TSH)] level was 3.5 mU/L (normal 0.5–5.2). The presumed diagnosis was chronic lymphocytic (Hashimoto's) thyroiditis. T4 was continued. In 1987, because her thyroid size had not decreased, she had a fine-needle aspiration biopsy (FNAB), that produced only a few groups of oxyphilic follicular cells (Hürthle cells), consistent with Hashimoto's thyroiditis, but insufficient for a definite diagnosis. Her goiter was stable until May 1995, when she reported 2 wk of severe anterior neck pain that radiated to her ears and jaw. Thyroid size was still about 50 g, the erythrocyte sedimentation rate (ESR) was 76 mm/h (normal up to 18) and the white blood cell count (WBC) was normal. Another FNAB produced adequate numbers of cohesive groups of benign follicular cells, many of which were Hürthle cells, mixed with a polymorphous

---

*The reference ranges for laboratory tests cited in these cases reports are as follows (unless stated otherwise in the text for individual values): free thyroxine (free T4) 0.6–2.2 ng/dL, free thyroxine index (FTI) 1.4–4.0 index units, total serum triiodo-thyronine (T3) 80–220 ng/dL, thyrotropin (TSH) 0.5–5.2 mU/L, antithyroglobulin antibody up to eight RIA units, antithyroid microsomal antibody titer up to 1:100, 24 h thyroidal radioiodine uptake 10–35%, erythrocyte sedimentation rate (ESR) up to18 mm/h. Thyroid size was estimated by palpation and the upper limit of normal size was considered to be 20 g.

From: *Contemporary Endocrinology: Challenging Cases in Endocrinology*
Edited by: M. E. Molitch © Humana Press Inc., Totowa, NJ

Table 1
Sequence of Painful Episodes for Case 1

Date	Intensity of pain	Duration of pain	Thyroid size	Treatment
May 95	severe	3–4 wk	50 g	acetaminophen + T4
June–Sep. 95	mild, intermittent		35 g	T4
Sep. 96	no pain		35 g	
Dec. 96	moderate	2–3 wk	50 g	acetaminophen + T4
Apr. 97	no pain		35 g	T4
Nov. 97	severe	3–4 wk	50 g	acetaminophen + T4
1998–Jan. 99	3 more moderately painful episodes			T4, acetaminophen as needed
Apr. 99	severe	3–4 wk	60 g	acetaminophen
early Aug. 99	severe	1 week	50 g	corticosteroids + T4
mid Aug. 99	severe	1 week	50 g	corticosteroids + T4
Sep. 99	no pain		50 g	external radiation + T4
Feb. 00	no pain		30 g	T4
Sep. 00	no pain		25 g	T4

lymphocytic population, and occasional connective tissue fragments. This was typical for the fibrous variant of Hashimoto's thyroiditis, and with no evidence of subacute thyroiditis or lymphoma.

Her subsequent course is summarized in Table 1. The neck pain subsided and thyroid size decreased spontaneously, but mild pain recurred intermittently over the next 4 mo. Neurologic and dental evaluations were unremarkable. Computed tomography (CT) of the neck showed only a diffuse goiter. Between December 1996 and January 1999, she had five episodes of anterior neck pain and thyroid enlargement, each lasting several weeks. Because she had diabetes and a history of gastritis, corticosteroids were avoided, and she was treated with acetaminophen and T4. In April 1999, she had yet another painful episode and her thyroid size was now about 60 g. T4 was discontinued to determine if she had enough intrinsic thyroid function to allow treatment with radioiodine, but 6 wk later, when her free T4 was <0.2 ng/dL and her TSH was >45 mU/L, her 24-h thyroidal radioiodine uptake was only 1.7%. Thus, radioiodine therapy was not feasible, but her neck pain cleared in the interim. Oral T4 was resumed.

On August 3, 1999, severe neck pain recurred, now radiating to the shoulders and chest as well as the jaw and ears. The neck pain responded in 24 h to oral methylprednisolone, which was tapered and discontinued over 6 d. Another FNAB produced a mixed cellular harvest of benign follicular cells, Hürthle cells, background lymphocytes, and. irregularly circumscribed bands of sclerotic stroma (see Fig. 1). The diagnosis again was fibrous variant of Hashimoto's thyroiditis without evidence for granulomatous thyroiditis. Two weeks later, when another episode of severe pain occurred, she was treated with prednisone, 20 mg tid for 5 d, which was then tapered and discontinued over nine additional days. Again, the pain cleared within 2 d, but she had marked hyperglycemia. Definitive therapy was necessary, but the patient, now age 84, did not want surgery. She therefore received 1000 cGy of external beam radiation therapy in four fractions, in October 1999. In December 1999, her thyroid was nontender and about 30 g in size. Only minor painful episodes subsequently occurred through September 2000, when her thyroid gland was about 25 g. She was very gratified with the results of the radiation therapy.

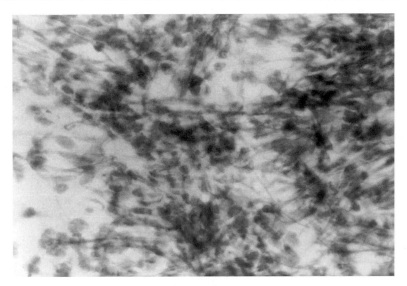

Fig. 1. There are cohesive groups of benign thyroidal follicular cells: occasional groups of Hürthle cells and scattered background lymphocytes. In addition to the mixed cellular harvest, there are irregularly circumscribed bands of sclerotic stroma.

Discussion

Classically, Hashimoto's thyroiditis causes a firm, diffuse, painless goiter. The clinical spectrum includes euthyroid goiter, subclinical hypothyroidism, overt hypothyroidism, and severe myxedema. The size of the goiter may range from near normal to very large, with little correlation between thyroid size and function. Histopathologically there are varying degrees of lymphocytic infiltration, mainly by T cells, as well as the presence of lymphoid follicular centers, predominantly B cells *(1)*. This process can be focal, leading to mild palpable nodularity. In some severe cases, the thyroid may be normal sized or enlarged, but with the normal thyroid tissue replaced by small follicles, scant colloid, and extensive infiltrates of lymphocytes, plasma cells, macrophages, and scattered giant cells *(2)*. In other severe cases, sometimes termed chronic atrophic thyroiditis, the thyroid is small and markedly hypofunctional, containing predominantly connective tissue, with only scattered thyroid follicular cells, small groups of lymphocytes, and plasma cells *(2)*.

The etiology of Hashimoto's thyroiditis is autoimmune. Beside the lymphocytic infiltration of the thyroid, autoantibodies to thyroglobulin or thyroid peroxidase are usually present in the serum. Antibodies to the sodium/iodide symporter and blocking TSH-receptor antibodies are occasionally present, also. The incidence of Hashimoto's thyroiditis has been reported to be 0.3–1.5 cases per 1000 persons per year *(3)*, and it is much more common in females than males. The onset is most common in the 30–50 age group, but occurs at all ages including childhood. It is often familial. Hashimoto's thyroiditis is associated with other autoimmune endocrine and rheumatologic syndromes. In the polyglandular syndrome type 2, Hashimoto's thyroiditis coexisits with insulin-dependent diabetes mellitus, Addison's disease, premature ovarian failure, and pituitary failure. Myasthenia gravis, celiac disease, pernicious anemia, alopecia areata, and serositis can also occur. The associated rheumatologic disorders include rheumatoid arthritis, systemic lupus erythematosus, Sjögren's syndrome, systemic sclerosis, and temporal arteritis. Chronic active hepatitis, biliary cirrhosis, and celiac disease are also statistically associated with Hashimoto's thyroiditis.

It was long thought that once patients with Hashimoto's thyroiditis became hypothyroid, lifelong T4 replacement was necessary. However, it is now appreciated that there is a spectrum of autoimmune thyroid disease, with Graves' hyperthyroidism—caused by stimulating TSH-receptor antibodies—at one end and Hashimoto's thyroiditis at the other end. Over several years, some hypothyroid patients treated with T4 need smaller replacement doses and may become euthyroid or, occasionally, overtly hyperthyroid. This is discussed more fully in our last case.

Painful Hashimoto's thyroiditis is rare. Zimmerman et al. identified eight patients from the Mayo Clinic with Hashimoto's thyroiditis who presented with neck pain and a tender goiter, diffuse in seven patients, and with unilateral enlargement and tenderness in one (4). Painful episodes lasted from 10 d to 9 mo. One patient had three episodes of recurrent neck pain over 5 yr. All had histopathologic confirmation of Hashimoto's thyroiditis, with pathologic changes no different from the usual nonpainful Hashimoto's thyroiditis. Five had normal thyroid function. The 24-h radioiodine thyroid uptake was low in only one of seven patients in whom it was measured. All eight were treated with thyroid hormone. Of the five patients also treated with corticosteroids, three had pain relief but experienced recurrence of pain after the steroid dosage was decreased. Of the four patients treated with aspirin, one had complete relief of pain, two had no relief, and one had pain relief after 3 mo of aspirin therapy, but 4 yr later had recurrent pain. Two patients required surgery to relieve their thyroid tenderness. Therapeutic suggestions were high dose aspirin along with suppressive doses of T4, and consideration of thyroidectomy if there is no relief of pain in 6 mo.

Shigemasa et al. reported eight patients with chronic thyroiditis who presented with painful tender thyroid glands (5). All had histologic verification of Hashimoto's thyroiditis by cutting needle biopsy. There were varying degrees of lymphocytic infiltration and fibrosis. Seven patients had radioiodine uptakes; in six, the uptake was low associated with transient thyrotoxicosis. The duration of pain in all cases was less than 1 mo, but one patient had a previous similar episode. Although the initial presentation resembled subacute thyroiditis (SAT), six patients developed sustained hypothyroidism and needle biopsy showed no changes of granulomatous thyroiditis.

Our patient differed from other reported cases of painful Hashimoto's thyroiditis (4,5) in that she did not develop pain until 13 yr after the onset of Hashimoto's thyroiditis. The cause of the pain in painful Hashimoto's thyroiditis is not known. One possibility is stretching of the thyroid capsule. Another possibility is release of cytokines or activation of cytotoxic immune cells, causing acute destruction of thyroid parenchyma. These mechanisms are presumably involved in other painful thyroid conditions, the most common of which are hemorrhage into a thyroid nodule and subacute thyroiditis. In our patient, the size of the thyroid gland did vary, and stretching of the thyroid capsule is plausible, but unprovable. Some of the other conditions associated with pain originating in the thyroid gland or the surrounding structures are listed in Table 2 and discussed later.

For the rare patient with painful Hashimoto's thyroiditis unresponsive to antiinflammatory analgesics, thyroidectomy is definitive. External irradiation has occasionally been used for cases of severely painful granulomatous subacute thyroiditis (6). It is effective in many cases, but there is concern about the potential neoplastic effects of low-level radiation to the thyroid gland. We are not aware of other cases of painful Hashimoto's

Table 2
Causes of Pain Originating in or Near the Thyroid Gland

Condition	Frequency of pain
Thyroid diseases	
hemorrhage into, or infarction of, a thyroid nodule	common
subacute (deQuervain's) thyroiditis	very common
thyroid cancer	occasional
lymphoma originating in the thyroid	occasional
Graves' disease	very rare
Hashimoto's thyroiditis	rare
Amiodarone-induced thyrotoxicosis	occasional
infective thyroiditis or infected thyroglossal duct cyst	almost always
infiltrative diseases such as amyloidosis or sarcoidosis	variable
Nonthyroid diseasess	
anterior neck abcess	
carotodynia	
neck muscle tension or spasm	
sialitis or salivary duct obstruction	
tracheitis or tracheal hypersensitivity	
lymphadenopathy	
pneumocystis carinii infection	

thyroiditis treated with radiation therapy. Based on this patient, external radiation would seem to be a useful alternative for patients who have increased surgical risks or are unwilling to have surgery.

REFERENCES

1. LiVolsi VA. Pathology of thyroid diseases. In: Braverman LE, Utiger RD, eds. Werner and Ingbar's The Thyroid, 8th ed. Lippincott Williams & Wilkins, Philadelphia, PA, 2000, pp. 490–491.
2. LiVolsi VA. The pathology of autoimmune thyroid disease: a review. Thyroid 1994;4:333–339.
3. DeGroot LJ, Larsen PR, Hennemann G. Hashimoto's thyroiditis. In: DeGroot LJ, Larsen PR, Hennemann G, eds. The Thyroid and Its Diseases, 6th ed., Churchill Livingstone, New York, 1996, pp. 309–310.
4. Zimmerman RS, Brennan MD, McConahey WM, et al. Hashimoto's thyroiditis, an uncommon cause of painful thyroid unresponsiveness to corticosteroid therapy. Ann Intern Med 1986;104:355–357.
5. Shigemasa C, Ueta Y, Mitani Y, et al. Chronic thyroiditis with painful tender thyroid enlargement and transient thyrotoxicosis. J Clin Endocrinol Metab 1990;70:385–390.
6. Volpe R. Subacute thyroiditis. In: Burrow GN, Oppenheimer JH, Volpe R, eds. Thyroid Function and Disease. Saunders, Philadelphia, PA, 1990, p. 188.

CASE #2: LOCALIZED THYROID PAIN

Case Description

Case 2 is a 19-yr-old man who presented to us with 10 d of marked anterior neck pain and swelling. Two days earlier, he had been started on 60 mg of prednisone daily, which had improved the pain and reduced the neck swelling. Examination showed a 4-cm firm, tender mass in the lower right thyroid lobe and isthmus, which was hypofunctional by pertechnetate scintiscanning (see Fig. 2). Free T4 and TSH levels were normal, the erythrocyte sedimentation rate (ESR) was elevated at 32 mm/h, and the leukocyte count was elevated at 14,800 with 84% neutrophils. FNAB with 22- and 25-gauge needles was quite

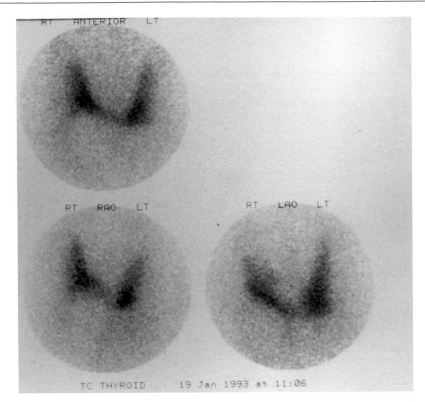

Fig. 2. Technetium-99m pertechnetate scan showing the large hypofunctional mass that seems to arise from the lower right thyroid lobe and isthmus. There is a faint suggestion of a rim of activity surrounding the mass. The projections are anterior, right anterior oblique (RAO) and left anterior oblique (LAO).

painful and produced only a scanty, nondiagnostic cellular sample. A tentative diagnosis of localized SAT was made. The patient was instructed to taper his prednisone over a week. After stopping it, he was virtually pain free and had resumed normal activities. One month later, the patient still felt well and thyroid function remained normal. The mass was 3 cm, and was hard but not at all tender. A repeat FNAB was diagnostic of Hodgkin's disease (see Fig. 3). CT images showed a 7 × 5-cm superior mediastinal mass, which probably extended up into the right thyroid lobe, but the possibility of a separate thyroid mass could not be excluded.

Discussion

This man's initial findings strongly suggested classic, painful subacute, or deQuervain's thyroiditis (SAT). SAT is generally felt to have a viral etiology. Patients with SAT experience neck pain and thyroid tenderness. The pain may involve the whole gland, one lobe, or part of one lobe. If the pain is initially unilateral, it will usually spread to the other lobe in days to weeks. There are often some prodromal symptoms of muscle aching and fatigue, and there may be a preceding upper respiratory infection. On examination, the thyroid is typically extremely tender and mildly to moderately enlarged. Usually the enlargement is diffuse, but it may be unilateral or nodular and is firm to hard in consistency. Corticosteroids are very effective in relieving symptoms of SAT, often within 24 h. Microscopi-

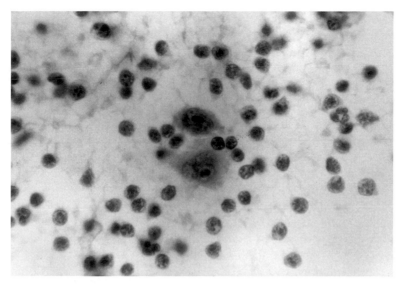

Fig. 3. There is a lymphocytic cellular background including immature and mature cells. Scattered among the lymphocytes are many multinucleated cells with large vesicular nuclei and prominent nucleoli. There are occasional binucleated cells consistent with Reed–Sternberg cells. No thyroid material is evident.

cally there are varying degrees follicular cell destruction, extravasation of colloid, and infiltration of lymphocytes and histiocytes, which congregate around colloid and coalesce into giant cells. In later stages, there is variable fibrosis and areas of follicular regeneration so that after recovery the thyroid appears normal except for minimal residual fibrosis *(1)*.

The intense inflammation of SAT can cause discharge of preformed thyroid hormone into the circulation, resulting in high serum T4 and T3 levels and low TSH levels. The damage to the follicular cells impairs iodine transport, causing low radioiodine and pertechnetate uptakes. Thyroid scintiscans generally show very patchy or no tracer uptake, although in localized disease there can be visualization of uninvolved areas if the serum TSH is not too low. There can be a changing pattern on scintiscan as the inflammation progresses from one lobe to the other and as recovery occurs in the two lobes at different time intervals *(2)*. If corticosteroids are employed and the pain and swelling do not resolve within 72 h, SAT is likely not the etiology. However, as our case illustrates, and as we have seen in other cases of lymphoma, prompt relief of thyroid pain by corticosteroid treatment can occur in conditions other than SAT.

Other etiologies for a painful thyroid are listed in Table 2. Acute suppurative thyroiditis may be difficult to distinguish from SAT by symptoms and physical examination, but is quite rare and readily identified when FNAB produces pus. Painful Hashimoto's thyroiditis can have a transient hyperthyroid phase *(3)*, as previously discussed, and may be indistinguishable from SAT except by needle biopsy. Painful Graves' disease has a normal or elevated radioiodine uptake *(4,5)*. In amyloidosis involving the thyroid, the radioiodine uptake is low, the ESR is high, and the response to glucocorticoids is dramatic, but there are features of systemic amyloidosis as well *(6)*. Pneumocystis carinii infection can be painful and involved areas have low tracer uptake (7), but the etiology may be suggested by the history, and the organism can be detected on FNAB specimens. Most malignant neoplasms of the thyroid are painless, but a few are painful, presumably because of rapid growth (8,9). The radioiodine uptake and thyroid scintiscan appearance will depend upon the extent of neoplastic involvement in the gland. Hemorrhage into a thyroid nodule also causes variable scintiscan findings, depending upon the extent of the bleeding and the functional properties of the nodule (10). FNAB is usually diagnostic for malignancy or hemorrhage.

Lymphoma accounts for only about 1–2% of thyroid malignancies. Most are B-cell lymphomas of the mucosal associated lymphoid tissue (MALT) type (11). Kossev and LiVolsi discuss the nature of these thyroid lymphomas and forthcoming changes in their classification and nomenclature (11). About 10–15% of thyroid lymphomas are painful (12). Primary Hodgkin's disease of the thyroid is exceedingly rare (11,13,14), and most cases involving the thyroid are secondary to mediastinal and/or cervical primary lesions (13,14). This was probably true for our patient.

If the initial presentation of a painful thyroid does not have the typical clinical findings of SAT, including a high ESR and and diffusely decreased tracer uptake on scintiscanning, FNAB should be performed to establish the diagnosis. This is especially true if the process is localized to a nodule or one lobe. If FNAB is inconclusive, more aggressive approaches to obtaining a tissue diagnosis can be considered, according to the physician's index of suspicion of the other possibilities.

REFERENCES

1. Lazarus JH. Silent thyroiditis and subacute thyroiditis. In: Braverman LE, Utiger RD, eds. Werner and Ingbar's The Thyroid, 7th ed. Lippincott–Raven, Philadelphia, PA, 1996, p. 584.
2. Hamburger JI, Kadian G, Rossin HW. Subacute thyroiditis evolution depicted by serial 131I scintigram. J Nucl Med 1965;6:560–565.
3. Shigemasa C, Ueta Y, Mitani Y, et al. Chronic thyroiditis with painful tender thyroid enlargement and transient thyrotoxicosis. J Clin Endocrinol Metab 1990;70:385–390.
4. Stanley JM, Najjar SS. Painful thyroid gland: an atypical presentation of Graves' disease. Clin Endocrinol 1992;27:468–469.
5. Fukata S, Matsuzuka, F, Hara T, et al. Rapidly progressive thyroid failure in Graves' disease after painful attack in the thyroid gland. Arch Intern Med 1987;107:118–119.
6. Ikenoue H, Okamura K, Kuroda T, et al. Thyroid amyloidosis with recurrent subacute thyroiditis-like syndrome. J Clin Endocrinol Metab 1988;67:41–45.
7. Drucker DJ, Bailey D, Rotstein L. Thyroiditis as the presenting manifestation of disseminated extrapulmonary pneumocystis carinii infection. J Clin Endocrinol Metab 1990;71:1663–1665.
8. Prakash R, Jayaram G, Singh RP. Follicular thyroid carcinoma masquerading as subacute thyroiditis. Australas Radiol 1991;35:174–177.
9. Watts NB, Sewell CW. Case report: carcinomatous involvement of the thyroid presenting as subacute thyroiditis. Am J Med Sci 1998;296:126–128.
10. Hamburger JI, Taylor CI. Transient thyrotoxicosis associated with acute hemorrhagic infarction of autonomously functioning thyroid nodules. Ann Intern Med 1979;91:406–409.
11. Kossev P, LiVolsi VA. Lymphoid lesion of the thyroid: review in light of the revised European-American lymphoma classification and upcoming World Health Organization classification. Thyroid 1999;9:1273–1280.
12. Hamburger JI, Miller JM, Kini SR. Lymphoma of the thyroid. Ann Int Med 1983;99:685–693.
13. Vailati A, Marcena C, Aristia L, et al. Primary Hodgkin's disease of the thyroid: report of a case and review of the literature. Haematologica 1991;76:69–71.
14. Granados R, Pinkus G, West P, et al. Hodgkin's disease presenting as an enlarged thyroid gland. Report of a case diagnosed by fine needle biopsy aspiration. Acta Cytol 1991;35:439–441.

CASES #3 AND 4: MALABSORPTION OF LEVOTHYROXINE

Case Descriptions

Case 3

A 49-yr-old female with primary hypothyroidism had been euthyroid for several years, taking 200 µg T4 daily, until March 2000, when her free T4 was normal at 1.6 ng/dL, but her TSH level was elevated at 33 mU/L. Questioning revealed that she had started ingesting two 330-mg calcium tablets with magnesium, chromium picolinate, vitamin E, and a "high potency" multivitamin tablet simultaneously with her T4. She was instructed to separate her daily T4 dose from her vitamin and mineral supplements by 4 h. Six weeks later, her free T4 was high-normal at 2.2 ng/dL and her TSH was 0.06 mU/L.

Case 4

A 45-yr-old female had a 3-yr history of hypothyroidism. For the past year she had taken 300 µg T4 tablets 6 d a week. She was intermittently fatigued and sometimes needed excessive sleep. She took no other medication. On examination, her height was 66 in and her weight was 198 lb. Her thyroid gland was small. Her serum free T4 was 1.7 ng/dL (normal 0.8–1.8) and her TSH was 4.0 mU/L, both normal. T4 was continued. One year later, she returned and was now ingesting her T4 tablets simultaneously with multiple supplements including St. John's wort, Kava-Kava, a "natural energy" tablet, vitamin B-12, vitamin E, and a multivitamin preparation. She reported that she took her thyroid tablets faithfully, 6 d a week as prescribed. Her tablets were inspected and they were the same brand tablets she was taking the year before. Her serum free T4 was normal at 1.3 ng/dL, but her TSH was elevated to 11.38 mU/L. She was instructed to take her T4 dose 4 h apart from her supplements. Nine weeks later, she had discontinued all of her tablets but the T4. Her free T4 was now 1.4 ng/dL and her TSH was normal at 0.5 mU/L.

Discussion

Oral T4 is approximately 60–90% absorbed, primarily in the small bowel. There is considerable intra- and intersubject variation *(1)*. Wenzel and Kirschsieper showed about a 15% increase in absorption when T4 was taken in the fasting state vs when it was taken with food *(2)*. However, we are not aware of studies of effects of concomitant food on T4 absorption from the T4 preparations currently used in the U.S. Other conditions that alter T4 replacement dose requirements are listed in Table 3. Patients over age 70 need smaller average T4 replacement doses *(3,4)*. Pregnancy can cause a 50–100% increase in T4 dosage depending upon the amount of residual functioning thyroid tissue present in the patient *(5)*. Patients with a variety of intestinal disorders such as regional enteritis, celiac disease, pancreatic diseases, and hepatic cirrhosis can have decreased absorption of T4. Hypothyroid patients with surgical short bowel syndromes may require three times the usual replacement T4 dose *(1)*. The subject of a recent case report was hypothyroid taking 500 µg of T4 daily, had no known cause for a high T4 requirements, did not respond when the 500-µg dose was administered under controlled conditions, but responded promptly to intravenous T4 *(6)*.

Many pharmacologic agents can alter a patient's response to orally ingested T4 (see Table 3). Some clearly decrease gastrointestinal absorption, including ferrous sulfate *(7)*, cholestyramine (and presumably colestipol) *(8)*, and sucralfate *(9)*. Sertraline, when given to hypothyroid patients stabilized on a T4 dose, can cause a TSH elevation *(10)*, by an

Table 3
Causes of Altered T4 Dose Requirements

Decreased requirement
  Aging
Increased requirement
  Pregnancy
  Drugs known to interfere with absorption
      ferrous sulfate
      cholestyramine (and probably colestipol)
      sodium polystyrene sulfonate
      calcium carbonate
      aluminum hydroxide
      sucralfate
      soy-based infant feeding formulas
  Drugs with unknown mechanism
      sertraline
      lovastatin (1 case report)
  Drugs that increase T4 clearance
      rifampin
      carbamazepine
      phenytoin
      phenobarbital
  Drugs that inhibit T4 to T3 conversion
      amiodarone
  Malabsorption
      high fiber diet
      intestinal diseases
          celiac disease
          inflammatory bowel diseases
          short bowel syndromes
          protein losing enteropathy
      pancreatic exocrine insufficiency
      hepatic cirrhosis

unknown mechanism. There are isolated cases of lovastatin *(11)*, sodium polystyrene sulfonate *(12)*, and aluminum hydroxide *(13)* causing increased T4 dose requirements, presumably by decreasing absorption. Patients who consume high fiber diets may need larger T4 replacement doses *(14)*, but the frequently used oral fiber supplements psyllium and polycarbophil do not appear to alter T4 absorption *(15)*. It has been long known that soy-based infant feeding formulas interfere with T4 absorption *(16)*. Currently, there are many soy-based dietary supplements on the market as sources of calcium or as remedies for menopausal symptoms; whether any of them alter T4 absorption is unknown.

A recently discovered absorption interaction between calcium carbonate and T4 is of considerable clinical significance because hypothyroidism is most prevalent in women over age 50, who are now appropriately urged to make sure they have an ample calcium intake to protect their bone mineral density. Schneyer *(17)* reported three thyroid cancer patients who had suppressed TSH values on T4, then began taking calcium carbonate simultaneously with their T4 in the morning. The TSH values rose to 7.31–13.3 mU/L, but became suppressed again when calcium carbonate was either discontinued or taken after lunch or dinner *(17)*. Another single case was recently reported *(18)*. Singh et al. studied 20 hypothyroid patients who had normal free T4 and TSH values on T4 replacement and were then given 1200 mg of elemental calcium as the carbonate, together with the patients' usual T4 dose, for 3 mo *(19)*. There was a slight but statistically significant decrease in the mean serum free T4 value from 1.3 ng/dL at baseline, to1.2 ng/dL during the calcium ingestion, and to 1.4 ng/dL after calcium discontinuation ($p < 0.001$). Mean TSH levels increased from 1.6 mU/L at baseline to 2.7 during the calcium ingestion, and decreased to 1.4 after calcium discontinuation ($p = 0.008$). Four of the 20 patients had TSH values above the normal range during the calcium period and would have required an increased T4 dose if they had continued to ingest their T4 simultaneously with the calcium carbonate. Case 3 exemplifies this problem, and illustrates that taking T4 and calcium 4 h apart is a satisfactory solution.

Case 4 was not taking calcium, but started taking a variety of herbal, vitamin, and mineral preparations. There was a dramatic change in the thyroid function studies when these agents were ingested with T4. We have seen this problem in other patients taking various combinations of multiple herbal supplements, but have not been able to identify the responsible agent(s). Several of the patients have taken ginseng, ginkgo, echinacea, or St. John's wort, but always with other supplements. Taking all such preparations more than 4 h apart from the T4 dose has consistently restored responsiveness to the T4 dose that was adequate before the supplements were started.

Our current recommendation is that patients already taking herbal and mineral supplements who need to start T4 treatment, or patients taking T4 who want to take such supplements, take T4 and the supplements at least 4 h apart. Because the interaction between calcium and T4 appears to be clinically significant in only about 20% of patients, it is probably not necessary for patients already taking both calcium and T4 to change their medication schedule.

REFERENCES

1. Choe W, Hays MT. Absorption of oral thyroxine. The Endocrinologist 1995;5:222–228.
2. Wenzel KW, Kirschsieper HE. Aspects of the absorption of oral l-thyroxine in normal man. Metabolism 1977;26;1–8.
3. Rosenbaum RL, Barzel US. Levothyroxine replacement dose for primary hypothyroidism decreases with age. Ann Intern Med 1982;96:53–55.
4. Swain CT, Herman T, Molitch ME, et al. Aging and the thyroid. Decreased requirement for thyroid hormone in older hypothyroid patients. Am J Med 1983;75:206–209.
5. Kaplan MM. Management of thyroxine therapy during pregnancy. Endocr Pract 1996;2:281–286.
6. Jauk B, Mikosch HJ, Gallowitsch E, et al. Case history. Unusual malabsorption of levothyroxine. Thyroid 2000;10:93–95.
7. Campbell NR, Hasinoff BB, Stalts H, et al. Ferrous sulfate reduces thyroxine efficiency in patients with hypothyroidism. Ann Intern Med 1991;117:1010–1013.
8. Harmon SM, Seifert CF. Levothyroxine-cholestyramine interaction reemphasized (letter). Ann Intern Med 1991;115:658–659.
9. Sherman SI, Tielens ET, Ladenson PW. Sucralfate causes malabsorption of l-thyroxine. Am J Med 1994;96:531–535.
10. McCowen MB, Garber JR, Spark R. Elevated serum thyrotropin in thyroxine-treated patients with hypothyroidism given sertraline (letter). N Engl J Med 1997;337:1010–1011.
11. Demke DM. Drug interaction between thyroxine and lovastatin (letter). N Engl J Med 1989;321:1341–1342.

12. McLean M, Kirkwood I, Epstein M, et al. Cation-exchange resin and inhibition of intestinal absorption of thyroxine. Lancet 1993;341:1286.
13. Liel Y, Sperber AD, Shany S, et al. Nonspecific intestinal adsorption of levothyroxine by aluminum hydroxide. Am J Med 1994;97:363–365.
14. Liel Y, Harman-Boehm I, Shany S. Evidence for a clinically important adverse effect of fiber-enriched diet on the bioavailability of levothyroxine in adult hypothyroid patients. J Clin Endocrinol Metab 1996;81:857–859.
15. Chiu AC, Sherman SI. Effects of pharmacological fiber supplements in levothyroxine absorption. Thyroid 1998;8:667– 671.
16. Pinchera A, MacGillivray MH, Crawford JD, et al. Thyroid refractoriness in an athyreotic cretin fed soybean formula. N Engl J Med 1965;273:83–87,
17. Schneyer C. Calcium carbonate and reduction of levothyroxine efficiency (letter). JAMA 1998;279:750.
18. Butner LE, Fulco PP, Feldman G. Calcium carbonate-induced hypothyroidism (letter). Ann Intern Med 2000;132:595.
19. Singh N, Singh PN, Hershman JM. Effect of calcium carbonate on the absorption of levothyroxine. JAMA 2000;283:2822–2825.

CASE #5: CHANGING AUTOIMMUNE THYROID DISEASE: HYPOTHYROIDISM IS NOT ALWAYS PERMANENT

Case Description

This woman presented in February 1982, at age 34, with marked fatigue, cold intolerance, a 15-lb weight gain in 6 mo, and muscle cramps. Her thyroid size was about 15 g, her skin was quite dry and coarse, and the relaxation phase of her deep tendon reflexes was prolonged. The free T4 index (FTI) was 0.6 index units (normal 1.4–4.0), the TSH was 56.6 mU/L, the antithyroglobulin antibody level was elevated at 42 RIA units, and the antithyroid microsomal antibody titer was elevated at 1:1600. She was started on 150 μg of T4 daily. In June, she was clinically improved with an FTI of 2.3 units, but her TSH was still high at 23.0 mU/L. The T4 dose was increased to 200 μg daily. In October 1982, the FTI was 3.6 U and the TSH was normal, 3.1 mU/L.

In November 1983, she reported feeling well and had lost 20 lb, but her FTI was elevated at 4.8 U and her thyroid gland was now about 25 g. The T4 dosage was reduced to 200 μg 6 d a week. She did not return until August 1984, when she reported palpitations and nervous feelings. She had lost 7 more pounds, and had a pulse of 100 bpm with a 30-g thyroid gland. Her FTI was up to 8.0 U. The T4 dosage was reduced to 100 μg daily, but 2 mo later, her FTI was still high at 7.6, and she had no TSH increase after thyrotropin-releasing hormone (TRH) infusion. T4 was discontinued. Two months later (December 1984) palpitations and nervousness persisted, her heart rate was 120, thyroid size was still 30 g, and there was bilateral proptosis. The FTI was 7.6, the total serum T3 was greatly elevated at 531 ng/dL, and there was no increase in serum TSH after TRH infusion. The 24-h radioiodine uptake was elevated at 41%. Her findings were now diagnostic of Graves' disease with hyperthyroidism, and she was treated definitively with radioactive iodine. Three months later, she was again hypothyroid, and has required T4 replacement therapy for the ensuing16 yr.

Discussion

The continuum of autoimmune thyroid disease extends from classic Graves' hyperthyroidism to hypothyroidism caused by Hashimoto's thyroiditis. There are intermediate forms of autoimmune thyroid disease in which patients have elements of both conditions simultaneously, or in which they move along the continuum over time.

Progression from hyperthyroidism to hypothyroidism is probably the most common change. It is now accepted that virtually all patients with Graves' disease have stimulating TSH-receptor autoantibodies that act as TSH-agonists, promoting thyroid follicular cell growth and function, like TSH *(1)*. Some hypothyroid patients have blocking or inhibitory TSH-receptor autoantibodies, but reported frequencies vary widely, from 0–75% *(2)*. Changes in levels of stimulatory or blocking TSH-receptor autoantibodies, or a shift from production of one type of TSH-receptor antibody to the other, would alter thyroid function, and evidence exists for these phenomena.

Of patients with Graves' disease whose hyperthyroidism goes into remission after treatment only with antithyroid drugs, as many as half become hypothyroid or have evidence of a subclinical impairment of thyroid function years later *(3,4)*. Tamai et al. *(5)* studied 26 patients with Graves' disease previously treated only with antithyroid drugs and who later developed hypothyroidism, Eight (31%) had TSH-blocking antibodies. Based on needle biopsy findings in nine patients, they estimated that TSH-blocking antibodies accounted for the hypothyroidism in about a third of the patients, and chronic autoimmune thyroiditis was responsible in the remaining two-thirds.

Some patients have hypothyroidism that resolves spontaneously. Takasu found TSH-blocking antibodies in 15 of 172 (9%) patients with Hashimoto's thyroiditis and 16 of 64 patients (25%) with chronic atrophic thyroiditis *(2)*. Of 21 patients whose blocking antibodies were identified before T4 treatment, 15 (71%) had disappearance of these antibodies after 3.5–8 yr of T4 therapy, and six of the latter 15 (40%) remained euthyroid after a mean follow-up of 2.1 yr. Rieu et al. found TSH-blocking antibodies in 22 (23%) of 96 hypothyroid goitrous patients with Hashimoto's thyroiditis *(6)*. After 1 yr of T4 treatment, TSH blocking antibody levels decreased in 11 patients, whose T4 medication was discontinued for 2 mo. The TSH blocking antibody levels increased, but not to pre-treatment levels, and none of the 11 patients remained euthyroid. Other series of hypothyroid patients with Hashimoto's thyroiditis, which excluded patients with reversible forms of hypothyroidism (subacute and silent thyroiditis, iodine deficiency and excess, drugs) have also found that some patients remain euthyroid after T4 treatment is discontinued *(7,8)*.

Although, in a relatively small percentage of patients with Hashimoto's thyroiditis, hypothyroidism is not permanent, there is no reliable way to identify such patients prospectively *(9)*. Disappearance of TSH blocking antibodies is only a rough guide, and measurement of these antibodies is not routinely available. The only reliable way to determine whether T4 replacement remains necessary is to discontinue it. Depending on the patient's age and general health this can be done all at once or in phases. Even if T4 withdrawal is initally successful, patients should be monitored indefinitely, because the chances of recurrent hypothyroidism are unknown.

The least common pattern of change in thyroid function, exemplified by Case 5, is from hypothyroidism to hyperthyroidism. Fatourechi and Gharib reported on six patients who developed hyperthyroidism of the Graves' type 2 to 20 yr after the diagnosis of hypothyroidism *(10)*. They found reports of only 39 other cases, but postulated that this phenomenon occurred more commonly than was recognized. We agree, and estimate that we see about one such patient a year in our practice. To identify this change, we recommend that patients taking T4 for hypothyroidism caused by Hashimoto's thyroiditis, and whose TSH values fall to levels below 0.1 mU/L, have an estimate of their serum free T4 levels, and, if there is still uncertainty, serum T3 levels, rather than having a decrease in their T4 dose based just on the TSH result.

REFERENCES

1. McIver B, Morris JC. The pathogenesis of Graves' disease. Endocrinol Metab Clin North Am 1998;27: 7–89.
2. Takasu N, Yamada T, Takusa M, et al. Disappearance of thyrotropin-blocking antibodies and spontaneous recovery from hypothyroidism in autoimmune thyroiditis. N Engl J Med 1992;326:513–518.
3. Wood LC, Ingbar SH. Hypothyroidism as a late sequela in patients with Graves' disease treated with antithyroid agents. J Clin Invest 1979;64:1429–1436.
4. Hirota Y, Tamai H, Hayashi Y, et al. Thyroid function and histology in forty-five patients with hyperthyroid Graves' disease in clinical remission more than ten years after thionamide drug treatment. J Clin Endocrinol Metab 1986;62:165–169.
5. Tamai H, Kasagi K, Takaichi Y, et al. Development of spontaneous hypothyroidism in patients with Graves' disease treated with antithyroid drugs: clinical, immunological, and histological findings in 26 patients. J Clin Endocrinol Metab 1989:69:49–53.
6. Rieu M, Richard A, Rosilio M, et al. Effects of thyroid status on thyroid autoimmunity expression in euthyroid and hypothyroid patients with Hashimoto's thyroiditis. Clin Endocrinol 1994;40:529–535.
7. Takasu N, Komiya I, Asawa T, et al. Test for recovery from hypothyroidism during thyroxine therapy in Hashimoto's thyroidits. Lancet 1990;336:1084–1086.
8. Comtois R, Faucher L, Lafleche L. Outcome of hypothyroidism caused by Hashimoto's thyroiditis. Arch Intern Med 1995;155:1404–1408.
9. Utiger RD. Vanishing hypothyroidism (editorial). N Engl J Med 1992;326:562–563.
10. Fatourechi V, Gharib H. Hyperthyroidism following hypothyroidism. Data on six cases. Arch Intern Med 1988;148:976–978.

6

Thyroid Cancer

Richard T. Kloos, MD
and Ernest L. Mazzaferri, MD, MACP

CONTENTS

CASE #1: CHILD WITH SCLEROSING PAPILLARY CANCER

Case Description

A 9-yr-old girl was referred to an endocrinologist in November 1995 after her pediatrician found a goiter. Her paternal grandmother and paternal uncle (who also had Down syndrome) both had thyroidectomies by age 20 yr for unknown reasons. The endocrinologist found the patient had high titers of antithyroid peroxidase antibodies, diagnosed Hashimoto's thyroiditis, and initiated thyroxine suppression therapy.

In January 1996 her mother noted a "swollen gland" in the left posterior neck and in July 1997 found another swelling in the patient's anterior neck. Thyroid ultrasound and ^{123}I scan showed a solid, cold, left thyroid nodule. Her endocrinologist found an enlarged thyroid, left cervical lymphadenopathy, and a firm nodular mass involving the right thyroid lobe. The preoperative chest X-ray showed a diffuse interstitial nodular pattern consistent with metastases. She was referred to surgery and underwent open biopsy of a slightly enlarged Delphian lymph node and the thyroid isthmus. The final pathology sections revealed metastatic papillary thyroid cancer (PTC) in the lymph node extending through its capsule into the soft tissues, and skeletal muscle infiltrated by PTC, and she underwent total thyroidectomy, bilateral node dissection, and thymectomy. Final histologic sections showed that the thyroid gland was totally replaced by diffuse sclerosing variant PTC with extrathyroidal extension, vascular invasion, and prominent lymphocytic infiltration that was bilaterally metastatic to 7 of 11 lymph nodes. She was referred to one of us (RT Kloos) for ^{131}I therapy who palpated residual bulky left posterior neck lymphadenopathy and she was returned to the surgeon for further lymph node resection,

From: *Contemporary Endocrinology: Challenging Cases in Endocrinology*
Edited by: M. E. Molitch © Humana Press Inc., Totowa, NJ

Table 1
Case 1 Laboratory Summary

Date	Time since initial surgery (mo)	Tg on T4 (ng/mL)	Tg off LT4 (ng/mL)	TSH (normal 0.32–5.0 mIU/mL)	Anti-Tg ATB (normal <120 IU/mL)	[131]I therapy dose (mCi)	[131]I therapy cumulative (mCi)
8-18-97	1		210	287.6	57,166	252	252
3-17-98	8		177	437	75,690	275	527
11-5-98	16		13	417.6	188,383		
12-11-98	17					303	830
6-30-99	23	10		5.1	84,985		
11-11-99	28	15		0.02	84,487		

which was done in August 1997 resecting three lymph nodes, all of which demonstrated metastatic PTC.

Shortly after surgery, she underwent serum thyroid-stimulating hormone (TSH) and thyroglobulin (Tg) measurements (see Table 1), hypothyroid whole body ^{131}I imaging, and ^{131}I dosimetry while on a low iodine diet, which revealed bilateral cervical and diffuse pulmonary metastases. Her blood dosimetry estimate indicated that 276 mCi of ^{131}I would reach the 200 rad limit, and accordingly, she was treated with 252 mCi of [131]I. Immediately thereafter she was given prophylactic antiemetic therapy, sucked hard lemon candies for salivary gland stimulation, and took in abundant fluids, experiencing minimal emesis. Posttherapy imaging revealed ^{131}I uptake in cervical lymph nodes, the superior mediastinum and diffusely in both lungs. Her therapy was complicated by parotid swelling from subacute pseudoobstruction, and chronically by xerostomia treated with over-the-counter dry mouth products (Biothene®).

In March 1998, 7 mo after her initial ^{131}I therapy, her chest X-ray showed a slightly decreased size and number of tiny nodular metastases. Her whole body hypothyroid ^{131}I diagnostic imaging showed reduced activity in the lung metastases and neck, which was reduced to only one focus, and uptake in the left parietal skull caused by hair contamination. Based on her previous dosimetry and persistent, albeit reduced, pulmonary uptake, she was treated with 275 mCi of [131]I. Posttherapy imaging showed no change except for two additional neck foci not seen on the pretherapy images.

In November 1998, she had a negative hypothyroid diagnostic scan, a Tg of 13 ng/mL off thyroxine (in the presence of antithyroglobulin antibodies), and an unchanged chest X-ray. In December 1998, hypothyroid dosimetry estimated a limiting blood dose of 200 rads from 335 mCi ^{131}I, and she was thus treated with 303 mCi [131]I. Her posttherapy scan revealed a single focus in the neck, bilateral mediastinum, and no lung uptake. Since then, additional ^{131}I therapy has been withheld pending disease progression, because her Tg did not significantly fall with her last ^{131}I treatment.

Discussion

This is an unusual case of childhood thyroid cancer presenting as a diffuse goiter. Thyroid cancer is very uncommon in children: only about 1% of all thyroid cancers are diagnosed before age 10 yr, or less than 200 cases in 1999 (1). Most are PTCs presenting as a palpable thyroid nodule or enlarged cervical lymph node.

The most likely cause of diffuse goiter in a child of this age is Hashimoto's disease, although other less-common causes are euthyroid Graves' disease or congenital goiter. Ordinarily, fine-needle aspiration biopsy (FNAB) is not recommended for diffuse goiter unless there is a compelling reason to suspect malignancy (2). Few patients with diffuse goiters have clinically important thyroid cancer, although microscopic occult PTC (incidental thyroid cancer) is fairly common in diffusely enlarged thyroid glands that have been partially resected for benign disease, and such cancers are clinically indolent lesions requiring no further therapy (3). Although diffuse goiter is often treated with thyroxine sup-pression of TSH, there is debate about its efficacy (4,5). In one prospective, placebo-con-trolled study, treatment of small (approximately 50 g) sporadic nontoxic goiters with TSH-suppressive doses of thyroxine resulted in a mean decrease of thyroid volume of 25% after 9 mo of treatment, which occurred in 70% of treated patients compared with none in the controls; however, the goiters returned to their pretreatment size when thyroxine was discontinued (6). All of the patients in this study had a FNAB showing benign goiter. Thyroid hormone suppression of goiter should not be used in lieu of FNAB as a diagnostic test for thyroid carcinoma (2). The main clue to the diagnosis of thyroid cancer in this patient was the rapidly growing lymph node metastases.

Death from thyroid cancer is rare in young patients: in national studies, only about 0.1% of thyroid cancer deaths occurred before age 20 yr, which amounts to about 51 of 5139 deaths from thyroid cancer between 1988 and 1992 recorded in the database (7). Typically, survival rates are very favorable in children, although their tumors are usually more advanced at the time of diagnosis, with more local and distant metastases than those of adults (8,9). Thyroid cancer recurrence rates, however, are much higher in children than in adults, averaging about 40% in patients whose thyroid cancer is diagnosed during the first two decades of life compared with 20% in adults (10,11). Moreover, their rate of pulmonary metastases is more than 20% in some series, almost twice those in adults (9,10,12). Prognosis for long-term survival in children is nonetheless excellent, except for those under age 10 who have very high thyroid cancer mortality rates (8,11,13). This may be the main reason that survival rates are lower among children with thyroid cancer than those of normal children (14).

The patient under discussion has diffuse sclerosing PTC, which is an uncommon variant found in approximately 5% of spontaneously occurring papillary carcinomas and in approx-imately 10% of children in Chernobyl with radiation-induced PTC (15,16). It is often initially confused with Hashimoto's disease and is typically accompanied by elevated serum antithyroid antibodies. The diagnosis usually becomes apparent when a patient with diffuse goiter develops palpable lymph node metastases or the gland undergoes rapid or asymmetrical growth. This is typically a bilateral tumor that presents as a goiter with extensive squamous metaplasia, sclerosis, and many psammoma bodies and abun-dant lymphatic invasion involving the entire thyroid gland. Almost all have lymph node metastases and about 25% have lung metastases at the time of diagnosis (15,17). Although metastases are more frequent than usual, there is some disagreement about whether long-term prognosis is worse than that of typical PTC, mainly because it commonly afflicts young patients who ordinarily have an extended life expectancy even with lung metas-tases (15,17).

This patient's prognosis was predictably poor, both in terms of recurrence and cancer mortality, at the time the diagnosis. Her tumor was infiltrating the thyroid gland capsule, was bilaterally metastatic to cervical lymph nodes, and was associated with mediastinal lymph nodes and lung metastases, all of which portend a poor outcome *(10)*. Tumor growing through the capsule of a lymph node is as serious a prognostic sign as is tumor invading the thyroid capsule *(18)*.

Lymph node metastases are found in almost half of adults and more than 80% of children at the time of diagnosis; whereas even more patients—up to 85% in some studies—have microscopic nodal metastases found on more detailed histologic study *(19,20)*. The number and size of lymph node metastases increase as the primary tumor size increases *(12)*. When the isthmus or both lobes are involved with tumor, nodal metastases are often bilateral or extend into the mediastinum, and in other cases, tumor penetrates the lymph node capsule and invades the soft tissues, which are all poor prognostic signs and were found in this patient *(21,22)*.

Less than 5% of adults with PTC have distant metastases at the time of diagnosis and another 5% develop them over the next two or three decades *(12)*; however, about twice this many children have distant metastases at the time of diagnosis and even more occur during follow-up. For example, in our series, 8% of children under age 10 yr had distant metastases at the time their thyroid cancer was diagnosed and eventually 33% developed them compared with only 2.5% of adults who had distant metastases at the time of diagnosis, and about 10% who developed them over the course of their disease *(10)*.

The lung is the most common site of distant metastases and its involvement the most usual cause of death from PTC. In a review of 1231 patients with distant metastases, 49% were in the lung alone and another 15% were in lung and bone, 25% were in bone alone, and 12% were in the central nervous system or in multiple organs *(12)*. Lung metastases may be large and discrete or may have a "snowflake" appearance from diffuse lymphangitic spread and may concentrate sufficient ^{131}I to be detected on whole-body scan. Others are not seen on the chest X-ray but only become visible on ^{131}I whole body scans, sometimes only after the administration of a therapeutic dose of [131]I *(23)*. Prognosis for children with lung metastases is better than that for adults, but once they become visible on X-ray, most patients eventually die of their disease, albeit decades later in the case of children. Respiratory insufficiency is the most common specific fatal condition, and accounts for almost half the deaths caused by thyroid cancer *(24)*.

In this patient with a poor prognosis at the time of initial diagnosis, the first several operations failed to completely remove the cervical component of her tumor burden. In our experience, this occurs when surgeons are not very experienced in the treatment of thyroid cancer. This has been documented in a large study from Maryland *(25)*. Surgery is always more effective in debulking large tumor masses than is ^{131}I or X-ray therapy. Hence, the referral back to surgery for this patient when residual palpable lymph nodes were appreciated.

This patient has anti-Tg antibody in her serum, which is found in up to 20% of patients with thyroid cancer (it is about half this in the general population) and almost always invalidates the serum Tg result *(26)*. Most Tg measurements are now done by immunometric assays in which the presence of anti-Tg antibodies usually falsely lowers the serum Tg level. The high serum Tg levels in this patient despite these antibodies simply reflect the extensive nature of her disease and the last serum Tg of 15 ng/mL is likely spuriously low. Serum Tg can be detected by a newly introduced Tg mRNA method, which can reliably detect serum Tg mRNA concentrations in patients with circulating antithyroglobulin antibodies *(27)*.

Although this patient's pulmonary metastases were evident on her X-ray, some patients, especially children and young adults, have lung metastases with high serum Tg levels, negative chest X-rays and no lung uptake on the diagnostic ^{131}I whole body scans. The lung metastases are typically seen on the posttherapeutic scan after 100 or 200 mCi of ^{131}I and are found in about 20% of patients with serum Tg levels above about 15 ng/mL during thyroid hormone withdrawal in whom chest X-rays and diagnostic ^{131}I whole body scans are negative *(23)*.

This patient was treated with very large doses of ^{131}I based on upper bound limits set by blood dosimetry. This approach establishes an upper limit on the amount of ^{131}I that can be given safely, which is generally considered to be 200 rad to the whole blood from a single dose *(28)*. Nonetheless, nonthyroidal tissues are exposed to high radiation doses, which is especially true of the parotid glands, colon and gonads. After the therapeutic dose of ^{131}I is administered, oral fluid intake should be large to increase urine output and avoid bladder radiation injury. Also, the patient should suck on lemon drops to stimulate salivary flow to minimize the risk of radiation-induced sialadenitis. Amifostine may protect the salivary glands, but its use has been limited *(29)*. Constipation routinely caused by hypothyroidism should be treated with cathartics to reduce colon and gonadal radiation. Gonadal injury is a greater problem in men than women, but can occur in women treated with ^{131}I near menopause. Emesis is a particularly serious problem in children being treated with ^{131}I and should be anticipated and treated with antiemetic drugs.

Ordinarily, repeat ^{131}I doses are administered at about yearly intervals, although ^{131}I can be given more frequently if the clinical situation warrants. The interval between treatments should be long enough to permit full recovery of the bone marrow, which nearly always shows some effects, albeit usually mild, from ^{131}I therapy. The risk of serious complications rises with cumulative doses of ^{131}I that exceed about 800 mCi in adults and 500 mCi in children. Bone marrow damage and induction of other tumors are the most serious late problems of ^{131}I therapy. Large doses of ^{131}I (usually >1000 mCi) can cause a small but significant excess of deaths from bladder cancer and leukemia *(30)*. Bladder cancer tends to occur most often in those with relatively little ^{131}I uptake in the neck or metastases. In a report from Germany, 80% of 35 thyroid carcinoma patients treated with ^{131}I had bone marrow abnormalities, including three with acute myeloid leukemia *(31)*. Patients with abnormalities of erythrocytes, platelets, and granulocytes had received very high ^{131}I cumulative doses, all >1000 mCi *(31)*. In 13 large series comprising a total of 2753 patients with thyroid carcinoma, 14 cases of leukemia were detected *(32)*. The resulting prevalence of about 0.5% is higher than expected in the general population. Acute myeloid leukemia, the type associated with ^{131}I therapy, usually has occurred within 10 yr of treatment. Leukemia was less likely when ^{131}I was given annually rather than every few months, and when total blood doses per administration was less than 200 rad *(32)*. Despite this report, the lifetime risk of leukemia is so small (<0.33%) that it does not outweigh the benefit of radioiodine therapy *(33)*. The absolute risk of life lost because of recurrent thyroid carcinoma exceeds that from leukemia by fourfold to 40-fold, depending upon the age at which the patient is treated *(33)*. When lower total cumulative ^{131}I doses (600 to 800 mCi, 22000 to 29600 MBq) are given at widely spaced intervals (12 mo), long-term effects on the bone marrow are minimal *(34)* and few cases of leukemia occur. Pulmonary fibrosis occurs rarely in patients with diffuse pulmonary metastases treated with ^{131}I *(35)*. It can be avoided by using smaller than usual doses (e.g., 75 mCi, 2775 MBq) of ^{131}I when diagnostic scans show high uptake in the lungs. These were the considerations in with-holding further ^{131}I therapy in the patient under discussion since her tumor did not appear to be further responding to treatment.

Thyroid hormone therapy significantly reduces recurrence and cancer-specific mortal-ity rates *(10,36)*. The levothyroxine dosage needed to maintain serum TSH levels in the euthyroid range is greater among thyroid cancer patients (2.11 µg/kg/d) than among those with primary hypothyroidism caused by nonmalignant disease (1.62 µg/kg/d) *(37)*. How-ever, the degree of TSH suppression required for this benefit is debated. One study found that patients who had undergone total thyroid ablation for thyroid carcinoma required 2.7 ± 0.4 (SD) µg/kg/d of thyroxine to achieve an undetectable basal serum TSH level that did not increase after TRH administration *(38)*. A French study found that a con-stantly suppressed TSH (<0.05 µU/mL) was associated with a longer relapse-free survi-val than when serum TSH levels were always 1 µU/mL or greater, and that the degree of TSH suppression was an independent predictor of recurrence *(39)*. One potential conse-quence of TSH suppression is loss of bone mineral density even in children *(40)*. Con-versely, a prospective U.S. study of 617 patients in the National Thyroid Cancer Treatment Cooperative Study found that disease stage, patient age, and ^{131}I therapy independently predicted disease progression, but that the degree of TSH suppression did not *(41)*.

Thyroxine therapy is resumed ~24 h after ^{131}I therapy, but it may take up to 2 mo for serum TSH concentrations to fall to normal or below when suppression doses of thyrox-ine are given *(42)*. In our experience, the dose of thyroxine may be doubled in selected patients for the first week to shorten this interval without adverse consequences.

REFERENCES

1. Landis SH, Murray T, Bolden S, Wingo PA. Cancer statistics, 1998. CA 1998;48:6–30.
2. Mazzaferri EL. Management of a solitary thyroid nodule. N Engl J Med 1993;328:553–559.
3. Moosa M, Mazzaferri EL. Occult thyroid carcinoma. Cancer J 1997;10:180–188.
4. Gharib H, Mazzaferri EL. Thyroxine suppressive therapy in patients with nodular thyroid disease. Ann Intern Med 1998;128:386–394.
5. Csako G, Byrd D, Wesley RA, et al. Assessing the effects of thyroid suppression on benign solitary thyroid nodules. A model for using quantitative research synthesis. Medicine (Baltimore, MD) 2000;79: 9–26.
6. Berghout A, Wiersinga WM, Drexhage HA, Smits NJ, Touber JL. Comparison of placebo with L-thy-roxine alone or with carbimazole for treatment of sporadic non-toxic goitre. Lancet 1990;336:193–197.
7. Kosary CL, Ries LAG, Miller BA, Hankey BF, Harras A, Edwards BK. SEER Cancer Statistic Review, 1973–1992: Tables and Graphs. Bethesda, MD: National Cancer Institute. NIH Pub. No. 96-2789, 1995.
8. Dottorini ME, Vignati A, Mazzucchelli L, Lomuscio G, Colombo L. Differentiated thyroid carcinoma in children and adolescents: A 37-year experience in 85 patients. J Nucl Med 1997;38:669–675.
9. Samuel AM, Rajashekharrao B, Shah DH. Pulmonary metastases in children and adolescents with well-differentiated thyroid cancer. J Nucl Med 1998;39:1531–1536.
10. Mazzaferri EL, Jhiang SM. Long-term impact of initial surgical and medical therapy on papillary and follicular thyroid cancer. Am J Med 1994;97:418–428.
11. Hung W. Well-differentiated thyroid carcinomas in children and adolescents: a review. Endocrinologist 1994;4:117–126.
12. Mazzaferri EL. Thyroid carcinoma: papillary and follicular. In: Mazzaferri EL, Samaan N, eds. Endocrine Tumors. Blackwell Scientific, Cambridge, MA, 1993, pp. 278–333.
13. Harach HR, Williams ED. Childhood thyroid cancer in England and Wales. Br J Cancer 1995;72:777–783.
14. Schlumberger M, De Vathaire F, Travagli JP, et al. Differentiated thyroid carcinoma in childhood: long term follow-up of 72 patients. J Clin Endocrinol Metab 1987;65:1088–1094.
15. LiVolsi VA. Unusual variants of papillary thyroid carcinoma. In: Mazzaferri EL, Kreisberg RA, Bar RS, eds. Advances in Endocrinology and Metabolism. Mosby-Year Book, St. Louis, MO, 1995, pp. 39–54.

16. Nikiforov Y, Gnepp DR. Pediatric thyroid cancer after the Chernobyl disaster: pathomorphologic study of 84 cases (1991–1992) from the Republic of Belarus. Cancer 1994;74:748–766.

17. Ain KB. Papillary thyroid carcinoma etiology, assessment, and therapy. Endocrinol Metabol Clin North Am 1995;24:711–760.

18. Yamashita H, Noguchi S, Murakami N, et al. Extracapsular invasion of lymph node metastasis—A good indicator of disease recurrence and poor prognosis in patients with thyroid microcarcinoma. Cancer 1999;86:842–849.

19. Noguchi M, Yamada H, Ohta N, et al. Regional lymph node metastases in well-differentiated thyroid carcinoma. Int Surg 1987;72:100–103.

20. Sugino K, Ito K Jr, Ozaki O, Mimura T, Iwasaki H, Ito K. Papillary microcarcinoma of the thyroid. J Endocrinol Invest 1998;21:445–448.

21. Yamashita H, Noguchi S, Murakami N, Kawamoto H, Watanabe S. Extracapsular invasion of lymph node metastasis is an indicator of distant metastasis and poor prognosis in patients with thyroid papillay carcinoma. Cancer 1997;80:2268–2272.

22. Mazzaferri EL, Young RL, Oertel JE, Kemmerer WT, Page CP. Papillary thyroid carcinoma: the impact of therapy in 576 patients. Medicine (Baltimore, MD) 1977;56:171–196.

23. Schlumberger M, Mancusi F, Baudin E, Pacini F. 131-I Therapy for elevated thyroglobulin levels. Thyroid 1997;7:273–276.

24. Kitamura Y, Shimizu K, Nagahama M, et al. Immediate causes of death in thyroid carcinoma: clinico-pathological analysis of 161 fatal cases. J Clin Endocrinol Metab 1999; 84:4043–4049.

25. Sosa JA, Bowman HM, Tielsch JM, Powe NR, Gordon TA, Udelsman R. The importance of surgeon experience for clinical and economic outcomes from thyroidectomy. Ann Surg 1998;228:320–328.

26. Spencer CA, Takeuchi M, Kazarosyan M, et al. Serum thyroglobulin autoantibodies: prevalence, influence on serum thyroglobulin measurement, and prognostic significance in patients with differentiated thyroid carcinoma. J Clin Endocrinol Metab 1998;83:1121–1127.

27. Ringel M, Ladenson P, Levine MA. Molecular diagnosis of residual and recurrent thyroid cancer by amplification of thyroglobulin messenger ribonucleic acid in peripheral blood. J Clin Endocrinol Metab 1998;83:4435–4442.

28. Benua RS, Cicale NR, Sonenberg M, et. al. The relation of radioiodine dosimetry to results and complications in the treatment of metastatic thyroid cancer. AJR 1962;87:171–178.

29. Bohuslavizki KH, Klutmann S, Brenner W, Mester J, Henze E, Clausen M. Salivary gland protection by amifostine in high-dose radioiodine treatment: results of a double-blind placebo-controlled study. J Clin Oncol 1998;16:3542–3549.

30. Edmonds CJ, Smith T. The long-term hazards of the treatment of thyroid cancer with radioiodine. Br J Radiol 1986;59:45–51.

31. Gunter HH, Schober O, Schwarzrock R, Hundeshagen H. Hematologic long-term modifications after radio-iodine therapy in carcinoma of the thyroid gland. II. Modifications of the bone marrow including leukemia. Strahlentherapie und Onkologie 1986;163:475–485.

32. Maxon H III, Smith HS. Radioiodine-131 in the diagnosis and treatment of metastatic well differentiated thyroid cancer. Endocrinol Metabol Clin North Am 1990;19:685–718.

33. Wong JB, Kaplan MM, Meyer KB, Pauker SG. Ablative radioactive iodine therapy for apparently localized thyroid carcinoma. A decision analytic perspective. Endocrinol Metabol Clin North Am 1990; 19:741–760.

34. Van Nostrand D, Neutze J, Atkins F. Side effects of "rational dose" iodine-131 therapy for metastatic well-differentiated thyroid carcinoma. J Nucl Med 1986;27:1519–1527.

35. Brown AP, Greening WP, McCready VR, Shaw HJ, Harmer CL. Radioiodine treatment of metastatic thyroid carcinoma: the Royal Marsden Hospital experience. Br J Radiol 1984;57:323–327.

36. Mazzaferri EL. Thyroid remnant ^{131}I ablation for papillary and follicular thyroid carcinoma. Thyroid 1997;7:265–271.

37. Burmeister LA, Goumaz MO, Mariash CN, Oppenheimer JH. Levothyroxine dose requirements for thyrotropin suppression in the treatment of differentiated thyroid cancer. J Clin Endocrinol Metab 1992; 75:344–350.

38. Bartalena L, Martino E, Pacchiarotti A, et al. Factors affecting suppression of endogenous thyrotropin secretion by thyroxine treatment: retrospective analysis in athyreotic and goitrous patients. J Clin Endocrinol Metab 1987;64:849–855.

39. Pujol P, Daures JP, Nsakala N, Baldet L, Bringer J, Jaffiol C. Degree of thyrotropin suppression as a prognostic determinant in differentiated thyroid cancer. J Clin Endocrinol Metab 1996;81:4318–4323.

40. Radetti G, Castellan C, Tatò L, Platter K, Gentili L, Adami S. Bone mineral density in children and adolescent females treated with high doses of L-thyroxine. Horm Res 1993;39:127–131.
41. Cooper DS, Specker B, Ho M, et al. Thyrotropin suppression and disease progression in patients with differentiated thyroid cancer: results from the National Thyroid Cancer Treatment Cooperative Registry. Thyroid 1999;8:737–744.
42. Maini CL, Sciuto R, Tofani A. TSH suppression by octreotide in differentiated thyroid carcinoma. Clin Endocrinol 1994;40:335–339.

CASE #2: GRAVES' DISEASE AND PAPILLARY CANCER

Case Description

In March 1997, a 41-yr-old white woman presented with a recent onset of hoarseness and the history of a "knot in her neck." She had heat intolerance and weight loss despite a normal appetite, and fatigue and muscle weakness. Her mother had undergone a thyroid lobectomy in the past for a thyroid "mass." On examination she was clinically thyrotoxic, showing resting tachycardia, fine tremor, stare, lid lag, and a diffusely enlarged thyroid with increased fullness in the left lobe that seemed adherent to surrounding tissues. Her serum free T4 was 3.6 ng/dL (normal 0.8–2.4) and TSH was undetectable. A thyroid scan showed a diffusely enlarged gland with uniform uptake of radioiodine except for a cold area in the left lower lobe. Thyroid ultrasound revealed a 2.7-cm echogenic solid mass with an internal 1-cm hypoechoic area in the left lobe. Her chest X-ray was normal. FNA revealed PTC and she was referred to surgery after control of her thyrotoxicosis with methimazole.

At time of surgery done in June 1997 the normal thyroid tissue planes were obliterated and the left thyroid lobe was adherent to the surrounding muscles and soft tissues. Gross tumor, which was invading the thyroid capsule and encasing the left recurrent laryngeal nerve, was identified as PTC by frozen section. She underwent total thyroidectomy with sacrifice of the left recurrent laryngeal nerve without neck node dissection. Final sections showed a multifocal tumor, the largest focus of which was 3.5 cm, with vascular invasion and extension through the thyroid capsule.

In July 1997, her Tg was 1,490 ng/mL after thyroid hormone withdrawal (see Table 2) and she received 150 mCi of ^{131}I without diagnostic imaging. The posttherapy scan demonstrated uptake in the thyroid bed and suprasternal notch areas.

In June 1998, when she received 206 mCi of ^{131}I because of a rising thyroglobulin, her posttherapy imaging revealing only uptake in the suprasternal notch area.

By January 1999, her neck MRI was negative but noncalcified pulmonary nodules ranging from 2 to 8 mm were seen on chest X-ray.

After being treated with 300 mCi ^{131}I in March 1999, without dosimetry or pretherapy imaging, her posttherapy imaging demonstrated suprasternal notch, left thyroid bed, and slight bilateral diffuse pulmonary uptake.

In June 1999, when her care was transferred to one of us (RTK), her thyroid stimulating immunoglobulin (TSI) was 22% (normal 0–9). In September, her chest X-ray demonstrated progression of the lung nodules, the largest of which was 9 mm. In December, she underwent hypothyroid whole body imaging and dosimetry after therapy with retinoic acid (Accutane, 1.3 mg/kg in divided doses twice daily) and lithium to promote ^{131}I uptake and retention. A diagnostic whole-body scan was negative despite her elevated Tg. Dosimetry studies indicated an upper limit of 200 rads to blood would be delivered by

Table 2
Case 2 Laboratory Summary

Date	Months since thyroidectomy	Tg on LT4 (ng/mL)	Tg off LT4 (ng/mL)	TSH (normal 0.32–5.0 mU/mL)	I-131 Rx
6-20-97	0 (post-op)	3727.5		—	
7-29-97	1		1490	—	150 mCi
10-2-97	4	370		—	
4-2-98	10	601		—	
6-9-98	12			60.38	206 mCi
7-20-98	13	183		0.13	
1-28-99	19	1050		—	
3-22-99	21			65.07	300 mCi
6-17-99	24	457		<0.04	
9-16-99	27	1055		<0.04	
12-15-99	30		6090	36.7	298 mCi
3-14-00	33	1535			
7-17-00	37	11600		<0.04	

290 mCi ^{131}I and she was treated with 298 mCi of [131]I. A posttherapy scan 1 wk later was similar to the one done in March 1999, showing little uptake in the pulmonary metastases. A follow-up chest X-ray done March 2000 showed slight progression of pulmonary metastases compared to September 1999.

Discussion

This patient had Graves' disease and PTC. At the time of diagnosis the thyroid tumor was grossly invasive and probably metastatic to the lungs, despite the normal chest X-ray and diagnostic ^{131}I whole body scans. Symptoms or signs that are highly suspicious of cancer include rapid tumor growth, a very firm nodule, fixation to adjacent structures, vocal-cord paralysis and enlarged regional lymph nodes *(1)*. According to one study, when two or more of these highly suspicious symptoms or signs were present there is nearly a 100% likelihood of malignancy *(2)*. Although this patient did not undergo direct laryngoscopy to document vocal cord paralysis, she undoubtedly had it, which in itself is nearly diagnostic of thyroid cancer.

Extrathyroidal extension of tumor has a particularly poor prognosis. Symptoms and signs of invasion that this patient experienced (hoarseness and fixation of tumor to surrounding structures) forecast a difficult tumor resection, as was the case in this patient whose laryngeal nerve was sacrificed to remove bulky gross tumor. In our study, the likelihood of distant metastases was threefold higher in patients with local tumor invasion than in those without it (21% and 7%) *(3)*. Likewise, cancer-specific mortality rates were, respectively, with and without tumor invasion, 15% and 3% at 5 yr and 18% and 5% at 10 yr follow-up *(3)*.

The presence of Graves' disease raises important questions about the diagnosis of a thyroid nodule and the virulence of thyroid cancers that occur in such cases. Although the prevalence of thyroid carcinoma in Graves' disease has been examined over many years, the issue still remains controversial *(5,6)*. This is because most of the studies are confounded by ascertainment biases of one sort or another. More recent studies generally have found the overall incidence of thyroid carcinoma to be close to about 5% among patients undergoing surgery for Graves' disease *(7–11)*. Whether this is higher than expected incidence remains problematic because there is not a good control group with which to compare these frequency figures.

In retrospective surgical series many of the neoplasms found in patients with Graves' disease are small incidentally discovered PTCs *(9–11)*. Whether a nodule is palpable preoperatively is an important point. In one large study, the risk of malignancy in patients with a palpable cold nodule was 45.8% *(12)*. In another large study, 34% of 315 patients with Graves' disease had thyroid nodules 8 mm or larger in diameter detected by ultrasonography, but fine-needle aspiration biopsy revealed carcinoma in only one *(13)*.

The benchmark Cooperative Thyrotoxicosis Therapy Follow-up Study of Dobyns et al. *(14)* gathered data from 36,050 patients treated for hyperthyroidism between 1946 and 1968 at 26 medical centers. Thyroid nodules were palpable in 15.8% of the 31,190 patients with Graves' disease, giving an incidence at least two-fold that expected in the general population during that period. At first glance, the prevalence of thyroid carcinoma in this study appears low—only 86 carcinomas were found in the entire group—but 700 patients had thyroid nodules that had not been biopsied or excised. Moreover, the prevalence of carcinoma may have been as much as twice that in the general population at that time *(5)*. Like other studies, many thyroid carcinomas were occult (<5 mm) but its incidence in palpable nodules was over twice that found in patients with diffuse goiters, although an equal proportion (about 35%) of each group had undergone surgery.

Thus, the evidence from a number of studies suggests that the prevalence of thyroid carcinoma in patients undergoing surgery for Graves' disease is about 5% and that the frequency of thyroid cancer in palpable thyroid nodules may be as high as twice this rate. Clearly, alternative etiologies for such nodules are more frequent than thyroid carcinoma. One retrospective study of 468 Graves' disease patients, who were almost all treated with ^{131}I or antithyroid drugs in an ambulatory setting, found that almost 13% had thyroid nodules. Of these 5.8% were solitary hypofunctional nodules, 4.5% were multiple nodules and 4% were autonomous nodules and 1.7% were patchy Graves' disease.

The clinical implications of these data are as follows: thyroid nodules in patients with Graves' disease are more common than usual and should intensify the concern about coexisting thyroid malignancy even more than usual. The workup must include FNA although the cytology may demonstrate atypia if the patient has been treated with ^{131}I, and this may be severe enough to be mistaken for a malignancy. If doubt remains after the FNA, the patient requires thyroid surgery.

Almost all papillary and follicular carcinomas express TSH receptor mRNA at varying levels, and the sodium-iodine symporter (NIS) at levels usually lower than those found in normal thyroid tissues *(15–18)*. The TSH receptors and NIS in papillary and follicular carcinoma are often functional, responding to native and recombinant human TSH stimulation by concentrating ^{131}I in malignant follicular cells and releasing thyroglobulin (Tg) from them *(19)*. This response is important for diagnostic follow-up and therapy. Equally important is the inhibition of growth and Tg release by TSH suppression *(20)*. However, in high-risk papillary and follicular tumors that do not concentrate[131]I, low expression of TSH receptors are found more commonly *(21)*. Similarly, noniodine avid carcinomas may not express NIS (see Case 3).

The interaction of Graves' disease and thyroid cancer is also controversial. The notion that Graves' disease may stimulate growth of thyroid cancer comes from the long held idea that TSH is the most important factor promoting the growth of normal and neoplastic thyroid tissues. However, several arguments are at odds with this concept. For example, most current evidence suggests that TSH suppression is not effective in shrinking the majority of benign thyroid nodules *(22)*. And more to the point, a recent review *(23)* of the role of TSH in the growth of benign and malignant thyroid tumors concluded that TSH is but one of many factors that promote pathological thyroid growth and, even more relevant, that thyroid tumors may well evolve in the absence of TSH stimulation.

Molecular studies also show that oncogenes play a major role in the development of thyroid carcinoma and may also influence growth of a tumor. The RET/PTC oncogene, a rearranged form of the RET protooncogene, is associated with human PTCs in man *(24)* and causes PTC in a transgenic mouse model with targeted expression of RET/PTC1 in the thyroid gland *(25)*. Thus, there are powerful factors other than, or in addition to, TSH that direct the growth patterns of thyroid carcinoma. This fits with the concept proposed by Derwahl et al. *(23)* that TSH-dependent signaling is but one link in a complex network of interacting signals that regulates thyroid growth.

There is nonetheless substantial evidence that TSH-stimulation of thyroid neoplastic tissue promotes tumor growth and function. There are important functional similarities between TSH and TSH-receptor-stimulating antibodies (TRAb) of Graves' disease. Like TSH, TRAb occupies thyrotropin membrane receptors on normal thyroid cells and activates thyroid adenylate cyclase, causing normal thyroid tissue to become hyperplastic and hyperfunctional. Serum TRAb from patients with Graves' disease and thyroid carcinoma increases cAMP in human follicular thyroid carcinoma cells in vitro and enhances DNA production in cultured rat thyroid follicular cells *(18)*. The cAMP-signaling cascade is highly active in some benign toxic thyroid adenomas and in some hyperfunctioning thyroid nodules of multinodular goiters as the result of activating mutations in the TSH receptor or the $G_s\alpha$ gene. These mutations, which represent an initial step in the pathogenesis of some toxic adenomas, have been found in a few thyroid carcinomas *(26–28)*. When they are present, the mutations would be more likely to manifest as thyroid cancers that retain unusual differentiated function and may account for the rare cases of thyrotoxicosis caused by hyperfunctioning differentiated thyroid carcinomas that masquerade as an autonomously hyperfunctioning thyroid nodule *(29)* or cause thyrotoxicosis when widely metastatic. One case report *(30)* described a 48-yr-old man who presented with signs of thyrotoxicosis for 1 yr owing to severe Graves' disease associated with a nodular goiter and elevated levels of TRAb. Thyroid cancer metastatic to his lungs was diagnosed preoperatively. After total thyroidectomy, his thyrotoxicosis persisted with suppressed serum TSH levels, showing the functional nature of his lung metastases in response to TRAb.

Thus, considerable evidence supports the notion that TSH stimulates both the trapping function of iodide, the release of thyroglobulin and the growth of some thyroid carcinomas, forming the basis for the wide use of TSH suppressive doses of T4 in treating this disease and the idea that some differentiated thyroid carcinomas associated with Graves' disease may be more aggressive than usual.

Our patient developed metastases that failed to concentrate ^{131}I despite the presence of TRAb. This is similar to the case of a 49-yr-old woman who nine years after undergoing thyroidectomy and ablative treatment with 100 mCi ^{131}I for follicular carcinoma that

resulted in negative total body ^{131}I scans and negative Tg measurements, developed Graves'
disease and concurrent pulmonary metastases that did not respond to ^{131}I therapy *(31)*.

When this occurs, there are few strategies that improve ^{131}I uptake. Once it is clear that
the patient has not received large doses of iodine in food or drugs, which can be excluded
with urinary iodine measurements, then only a few options remain. Lithium therapy
increases the accumulation of ^{131}I in thyroid cancer lesions, prolongs its retention and
augments the therapeutic radiation dose from ^{131}I *(32)*. Given at a dosage of 400–800 mg
daily (10 mg/kg) for 7 d, it increases ^{131}I uptake in metastatic lesions while only slightly
increasing uptake in normal tissue *(33)*. Thus, it is not necessary to perform ^{131}I kinetic
studies in patients on lithium unless large therapeutic radioiodine doses are planned
which would be expected to approach established safety limits. The response of metastatic well-differentiated thyroid carcinoma to ^{131}I therapy is related to the amount of
radiation delivered to the tumor, which must receive more than 8000 cGy to ensure its
complete destruction *(34)*. The largest fractional change in effective half-life with lithium
occurs in lesions with a biological half-life of less than 3 d *(32)*. Thus, lithium is most
beneficial in the tumors that are less likely to respond to ^{131}I therapy. In our patient,
unfortunately this did not occur.

Likewise, retinoic acid (Accutane) has been used in patients with thyroid cancers that
fail to concentrate ^{131}I or concentrate it poorly. This drug, which partly redifferentiates
follicular thyroid carcinoma in vitro, may benefit a few patients. In one study, retinoic
acid given orally (1.18 ± 0.37 mg/kg) for at least 2 mo induced significant ^{131}I uptake in
two of 12 patients with differentiated carcinoma untreatable by other modalities *(35)*.
This response was associated with a rise in serum Tg concentration, suggesting tumor
redifferentiation. However, its beneficial effects have not been widely reproduced by
others. Potential adverse consequences of retinoic acid therapy include severe birth
defects, liver function test abnormalities, and hypertriglyceridemia.

Our patient unfortunately had a poor response to these strategies. Only about 50% to
80% of differentiated thyroid carcinomas and their metastases, and up to about one-third
of Hürthle cell carcinomas concentrate ^{131}I *(36–40)*. Iodine avidity is associated with
better tumor differentiation, younger patient age (90% if age <40 yr compared to 56%
for age >40 years), and smaller tumor deposits *(39)*. Radioiodine uptake is seen in 95%
of patients with pulmonary metastases and a normal chest X-ray, 88% of those with
micronodular disease, and 37% of those with macronodular disease *(39)*. Patients with
distant metastases that concentrate radioiodine have 10-yr survival rates of 57% compared with 8% for noniodine avid distant metastases *(39)*. The majority of patients who
die of thyroid cancer do so as the result of pulmonary metastases. One large study clearly
shows how patients die of thyroid cancer *(41)*. Most suffer a pulmonary death, either from
respiratory failure caused by pulmonary metastases or suffocation from tumor in the
airway. The authors of this study make the important observation that two thirds of the
patients who had airway stenosis (almost half of whom had differentiated thyroid cancer)
without tracheostomy died of asphyxia, however, since 1986 when tracheostomy was
done in almost all patients with airway stenosis, only one patient with distal tracheal
stenosis has died of airway obstruction.

As antithyroid drug therapy in Graves' disease may decrease TRAb *(4)*, it may be
reasonable (but unproven) in this patient given her tumor's aggressive course and the fact
that no conventional therapy has been effective. Consideration should also be given to
therapeutic trials.

REFERENCES

1. Mazzaferri EL. Management of a solitary thyroid nodule. N Engl J Med 1993;328:553–559.
2. Hamming JF, Goslings BM, vanSteenis GJ, Claasen H, Hermans J, Velde JH. The value of fine-needle aspiration biopsy in patients with nodular thyroid disease divided into groups of suspicion of malignant neoplasms on clinical grounds. Arch Intern Med 1990;150:113–116.
3. Mazzaferri EL, Jhiang SM. Long-term impact of initial surgical and medical therapy on papillary and follicular thyroid cancer. Am J Med 1994;97:418–428.
4. Takasu N, Akamine H, Komiya I, Yamada T. Simple and reliable method for predicting the remission of Graves' disease: Revised triiodothyronine-suppression test, indexed by serum thyroxine. J Endocrinol Invest 1995;18:288–294.
5. Mazzaferri EL. Thyroid cancer and Graves' disease. J Clin Endocrinol Metab 1990;70:826–829.
6. Mazzaferri EL. Thyroid cancer and Graves' disease: the controversy ten years later. Endo Pract 2000;6: 221–225.
7. Vaiana R, Cappelli C, Perini P, et al. Hyperthyroidism and concurrent thyroid cancer. Tumori 1999;85: 247–252.
8. Kraimps JL, Bouin-Pineau MH, Marechaud R, Barbier J. (Basedow's disease and thyroid nodules. A common association). Ann Chir 1998;52:449–451.
9. Vini L, Hyer S, Pratt B, Harmer C. Good prognosis in thyroid cancer found incidentally at surgery for thyrotoxicosis. Postgrad Med J 1999;75:169–170.
10. Chao TC, Lin JD, Jeng LB, Chen MF. Thyroid cancer with concurrent hyperthyroidism. Arch Surg 1999;134:130–134.
11. Oertli D, Harder F, Oberholzer M, Staub JJ. Hyperthyroidism and concurrent thyroid cancer—coincidence or association? Schweiz Med Wochenschr 1998;128:1910–1914.
12. Belfiore A, Garofalo MR, Giuffrida D, et al. Increased aggressiveness of thyroid cancer in patients with Graves' disease. J Clin Endocrinol Metab 1990;70:830–835.
13. Cantalamessa L, Baldini M, Orsatti A, Meroni L, Amodei V, Castagnone D. Thyroid nodules in Graves disease and the risk of thyroid carcinoma. Arch Intern Med 1999;159:1705–1708.
14. Dobyns BM, Sheline GE, Workman JB, Tompkins EA, McConahey WM, Becker DV. Malignant and benign neoplasm of the thyroid in patients treated for hyperthyroidism: a report of the Cooperative Thyrotoxicosis Therapy Follow-up Study. J Clin Endocrinol Metab 1974;38:976–998.
15. Caillou B, Troalen F, Baudin E, et al. Na$^+$/I$^-$ symporter distribution in human thyroid tissues: an immunohistochemical study. J Clin Endocrinol Metab 1998;83:4102–4106.
16. Jhiang SM, Cho JY, Ryu K-Y, et al. An immunohistochemical study of Na+/I- symporter in human thyroid tissues and salivary gland tissues. Endocrinology 1998;139:4416–4419.
17. Ryu K-Y, Senokozlieff ME, Smanik PA, et al. Development of an RT-cPCR method to quantitate the expression levels of human Na+/I- symporter (hNIS). Thyroid 1999;9:405–409.
18. Filetti S, Belfiore A, Amir SM, et al. The role of thyroid-stimulating antibodies of Graves' disease in differentiated thyroid cancer. N Engl J Med 1988;318:753–779.
19. Haugen BR, Pacini F, Reiners C, et al. A comparison of recombinant human thyrotropin and thyroid hormone withdrawal for the detection of thyroid remnant or cancer. J Clin Endocrinol Metab 1999;84: 3877–3885.
20. Pujol P, Daures JP, Nsakala N, Baldet L, Bringer J, Jaffiol C. Degree of thyrotropin suppression as a prognostic determinant in differentiated thyroid cancer. J Clin Endocrinol Metab 1996;81:4318–4323.
21. Tanaka K, Inoue H, Miki H, et al. Relationship between prognostic score and thyrotropin receptor (TSH-R) in papillary thyroid carcinoma: immunohistochemical detection of TSH-R. Br J Cancer 1997; 76:594–599.
22. Gharib H, Mazzaferri EL. Thyroxine suppressive therapy in patients with nodular thyroid disease. Ann Intern Med 1998;128:386–394.
23. Derwahl M, Broecker M, Kraiem Z. Thyrotropin may not be the dominant growth factor in benign and malignant thyroid tumors. J Clin Endocrinol Metab 1999;84:829–834.
24. Jhiang SM, Mazzaferri EL. The ret/PTC oncogene in papillary thyroid carcinoma. J Lab Clin Med 1994; 123:331–337.
25. Jhiang SM, Cho JY, Furminger TL, et al. Thyroid carcinomas in RET/PTC transgenic mice. Recent Results Cancer Res 1999;154:265–270.
26. Russo D, Arturi F, Schlumberger M, et al. Activating mutations of the TSH receptor in differentiated thyroid carcinomas. Oncogene 1995;11:1907–1911.

27. Russo D, Tumino S, Arturi F, et al. Detection of an activating mutation of the thyrotropin receptor in a case of an autonomously hyperfunctioning thyroid insular carcinoma. J Clin Endocrinol Metab 1997; 82:735–738.
28. Spambalg D, Sharifi N, Elisei R, Gross JL, Medeiros-Neto G, Fagin JA. Structural studies of the thyrotropin receptor and $G_s\alpha$ in human thyroid cancers: low prevalence of mutations predicts infrequent involvement in malignant transformation. J Clin Endocrinol Metab 1996;81:3898–3901.
29. Appetecchia M, Ducci M. Hyperfunctioning differentiated thyroid carcinoma. J Endocrinol Invest 1998;21:189–192.
30. Le Pommelet C, Denizot A, Costagliola S, et al. Graves' disease caused by metastatic thyroid cancer. Presse Med 1996;25:671–673.
31. Katz SB, Garcia AJ, Niepomniszcze H. Development of Graves' disease nine years after total thyroidectomy due to follicular carcinoma of the thyroid. Thyroid 1997;7:909–911.
32. Koong SS, Reynolds JC, Movius EG, et al. Lithium as a potential adjuvant to ^{131}I therapy of metastatic, well differentiated thyroid carcinoma. J Clin Endocrinol Metab 1999;84:912–916.
33. Pons F, Carrio I, Estorch M, Ginjuame M, Pons J, Milian R. Lithium as an adjuvant of iodine-131 uptake when treating patients with well-differentiated thyroid carcinoma. Clin Nucl Med 1987;8:644–647.
34. Maxon HR, Thomas SR, Hertzberg VS, et al. Relation between effective radiation dose and outcome of radioiodine therapy for thyroid cancer. N Engl J Med 1983;309:937–941.
35. Grünwald F, Menzel C, Bender H, et al. Redifferentiation therapy-induced radioiodine uptake in thyroid cancer. J Nucl Med 1998;39:903–1906.
36. Simpson WJ, Panzarella T, Carruthers JS, Gospodarowicz MK, Sutcliffe SB. Papillary and follicular thyroid cancer: impact of treatment in 1578 patients. Int J Radiat Oncol Biol Phys 1988;14:1063–1075.
37. Samaan NA, Schultz PN, Haynie TP, Ordonez NG. Pulmonary metastasis of differentiated thyroid carcinoma: treatment results in 101 patients. J Clin Endocrinol Metab 1985;60:376–380.
38. Ruegemer JJ, Hay ID, Bergstralh EJ, Ryan JJ, Offord KP, Gorman CA. Distant metastases in differentiated thyroid carcinoma: a multivariate analysis of prognostic variables. J Clin Endocrinol Metab 1988; 67:501–558.
39. Schlumberger M, Challeton C, De Vathaire F, et al. Radioactive iodine treatment and external radiotherapy for lung and bone metastases from thyroid carcinoma. J Nucl Med 1996;37:598–605.
40. Franceschi M, Kusic Z, Franceschi D, Lukinac L, Roncevic S. Thyroglobulin determination, neck ultrasonography and iodine-131 whole-body scintigraphy in differentiated thyroid carcinoma. J Nucl Med 1996;37:446–451.
41. Kitamura Y, Shimizu K, Nagahama M, et al. Immediate causes of death in thyroid carcinoma: clinicopathological analysis of 161 fatal cases. J Clin Endocrinol Metab 1999; 84:4043–4049.

CASE #3: PERSISTENT PAPILLARY CANCER

Case Description

A 45-yr-old woman who had been treated for primary hypothyroidism from age 29 noted a thyroid mass in August 1994 that was cold by ^{123}I scan and yielded indeterminate cytology by fine-needle aspiration (FNA) biopsy. At surgery done shortly after the FNA, frozen section biopsy revealed PTC and total thyroidectomy was performed. The final histologic sections showed this to be a multifocal bilateral PTC, the largest focus of which was 1.8 cm in the left lobe amidst a background of severe Hashimoto's thyroiditis.

She was treated with 29 mCi of ^{131}I in October 1994 when her thyroglobulin (Tg) was 73 ng/mL (Table 3) and her ^{131}I whole body scan (WBS) at 48 h showed an uptake of 0.4% in a thyroglossal duct remnant and bilateral thyroid bed. Fourteen months later, because of a persistent elevation in serum Tg and a nearly identical uptake and WBS, she was treated with 150 mCi of [131]I. Ten-day posttherapy images demonstrated no uptake in the left thyroid bed, suggesting thyroid stunning or rapid turnover of radioiodine.

In March 1996, 18 mo after her initial surgery, her Tg remained elevated and neck ultrasound was negative but neck MR imaging revealed nonpalpable lymph nodes maxi-

Table 3
Case 3 Laboratory Summary

Date	Months since thyroidectomy	Tg on LT4 (ng/mL)	Tg off LT4 (ng/mL)	TSH (normal 0.32–5.0 mU/mL)	Therapy
10-17-94	1		73	81.6	29 mCi
4-4-95	7	14.9		0.11	
10-10-95	13	21.1		0.08	
12-14-95	15		85.8	71.2	150 mCi
3-26-96	18	26.6		0.05	
7-8-96	22		339.7	96.2	203 mCi
1-14-97	28	33.7		<0.04	
7-1-97	34		275	44.9	203 mCi
11-6-97	38	23.1		0.06	
4-21-98	43	32.4		0.05	
8-6-98	47	27.6		0.05	
11-2-98	50	20.4		0.05	
1-25-99	52	12.3		0.05	
6-29-99	57	51		0.04	
7-28-99					Lymph node resection
10-21-99	61	15.1		0.16	
4-20-00	67	15.8		<0.04	
6-10-00	69				Lymph node resection
7-8-00	70	10.6		0.08	

mally measuring 1.6 cm in the left supraclavicular region and 1 cm anterior to the trachea. In July 1996 after a persistently elevated Tg and faint midline uptake (0.17%) of 4 mCi of ^{131}I were again demonstrated, she received 203 mCi of ^{131}I, which resulted in no abnormal uptake on the 12-d posttherapy scan.

In July 1997, because of persistent Tg elevation she was treated with another 203 mCi of ^{131}I, although both the diagnostic and posttherapy scans were negative. In August 1997, neck and chest CT and whole body ^{99m}Tc-sestamibi scans were negative.

In June 1999, 4 yr and 9 mo after her initial surgery, FNA of a palpable left supraclavicular lymph node was positive for PTC. Whole body F-18-flourodeoxyglucose-positron emission tomography (FDG-PET), done to rule out additional metastatic foci, demonstrated uptake only in the left supraclavicular region in the area of the biopsy (Fig. 1). One month later she underwent left modified neck dissection that yielded only 1 positive lymph node among the 27 that were resected. A histoculture of tumor from the lymph node demonstrated no in vitro uptake of ^{131}I in response to TSH stimulation despite adequate expression of TSH receptors and Tg, however, expression of sodium/iodine symporter (NIS) determined by RT-PCR was almost absent. In April 2000, neck ultrasonography was performed in response to the elevated postoperative Tg level that demonstrated a 1.1-cm-lymph node anterior to the trachea near the thyroid bed and just left of midline that was positive for PTC after ultrasound guided FNA. An adjacent 0.7 by 0.5 cm lymph node was also identified that was not biopsied given the high degree of

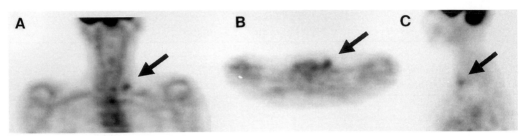

Fig. 1. FDG-PET scan coronal (**A**), transaxial (**B**), and sagittal (**C**) images from Case 3. Arrow indicates abnormal uptake in the left supraclavicular region.

suspicion of malignancy in the larger lymph node. In May 2000, she had neck and chest CT scans interpreted as negative and without change from August 1997. In June 2000, she underwent a central neck dissection that resected two metastatic lymph nodes with extranodal extension that corresponded to those seen on ultrasonography.

Discussion

This patient developed an aggressive, thyroid cancer that did not concentrate ^{131}I decades after she became hypothyroid as the result of chronic autoimmune thyroiditis. How the two diseases might be linked, however, is controversial. One large study (1) of surgical thyroid specimens found the prevalence of autoimmune thyroiditis among 626 Japanese, 330 white, and 90 African American patients was significantly higher among those with PTC than among patients with adenomatous goiter or follicular adenoma. Whether autoimmune thyroiditis is a predisposing factor for PTC or a response to the malignancy, nonetheless remains uncertain. Indeed, studies suggest that chronic thyroiditis has a favorable prognostic effect on PTC (2,3).

The diagnosis of PTC in this patient was not made on the initial FNA cytology, which was not examined at our institution. In most cases the diagnosis of PTC can be made by FNA cytology and usually is not confused with a follicular lesion (4). In contrast, Hürthle cell and follicular adenomas are typically difficult to differentiate from their malignant counterparts by FNA and by study of frozen tissue sections done at surgery. Large-needle aspiration biopsies and cutting-needle biopsies usually yield results similar to those of FNA but cause more serious complications (4). Thus, FNA cytology specimens showing sheets of normal or atypical follicular or Hürthle cells without an abundance of colloid in the background are often simply designated as follicular or Hürthle cell neoplasms, which poses a serious management predicament at the time of surgery (4,5–7). Ordinarily, ipsilateral lobectomy and isthmusectomy without frozen section study are advised for nodules yielding such cytology (8). Roughly three-fourths of these lesions are benign and the benign or malignant character of the tumor usually cannot be determined with certainty until the final histologic sections are available, and even then there may difficulty separating malignant and benign tumors (4). The patient under discussion, however, underwent frozen section in the setting of an indeterminate lesion that was diagnostic and allowed for a single procedure total thyroidectomy rather than requiring a subsequent completion thyroidectomy. However, as the patient was already hypothyroid and dependent of thyroid hormone therapy anyway, a total thyroidectomy without frozen section would have been reasonable as long as the risk of surgical complications was low.

Approximately 4–6 wk after surgery, most recommend serum TSH and Tg measurement and a 3–5 mCi diagnostic ^{131}I WBS after thyroid hormone withdrawal. However, there is concern that diagnostic doses of ^{131}I will reduce the subsequent uptake of ^{131}I given as treatment. This effect, referred to as "thyroid stunning," may be more pervasive than heretofore suspected. In one study, diagnostic ^{131}I doses as low as 3 mCi reduced the subsequent uptake of ^{131}I, particularly in thyroid remnants and cervical lymph nodes *(9)*. The effect became progressively greater with larger ^{131}I doses. Therapeutic ^{131}I uptake was not reduced by ^{123}I or 2 mCi ^{131}I scanning doses, but after 3, 5, and 10 mCi of ^{131}I it was reduced, respectively, 40%, 67%, and 89%. Serum Tg is high for about 2 wk after the administration of a 3–5 mCi scanning dose of ^{131}I, a finding often associated with incomplete ablation, perhaps reflecting the stunning effect on the thyroid remnants *(10)*. Unfortunately, the use of small ^{123}I doses (to minimize cost) or small doses of [131]I (2 mCi) that avoid the stunning effect are slightly less sensitive than larger scanning doses of ^{131}I in identifying thyroid remnants *(10,11)*. Although large scanning doses of ^{123}I in the range of 2 or 3 mCi may be more sensitive, they are generally regarded as too expensive for routine diagnostic scanning.

This patient's Tg level was strikingly elevated postoperatively, indicating that she had substantial residual disease that may have been best treated initially with a larger ablation dose of ^{131}I, despite her essentially negative ^{131}I WBS. Based upon her serum Tg of 73 ng/mL, her ^{131}I WBS showing only minimal uptake in the thyroid bed was most likely a false-negative study suggesting that her residual disease was already noniodine avid.

A study from France found that a 2–5 mCi diagnostic ^{131}I scan performed one year after thyroid ablation did not correlate with the results of Tg determination, but only confirmed the completeness of thyroid ablation *(12)*. If ^{131}I scans are negative and Tg is elevated (>10 ng/mL after thyroid hormone withdrawal or >5 ng/mL after recombinant human TSH), residual disease is likely. When the serum Tg concentration is higher than 40 ng/mL after thyroid hormone withdrawal and the diagnostic ^{131}I WBS is negative, up to 25% have occult lung metastases seen only on the posttherapy ^{131}I WBS *(13)*. The treatment of scan negative, thyroglobulin positive patients is controversial and challenging. The National Comprehensive Cancer Network guidelines for the treatment of thyroid cancer recognizes this controversy and supports radioiodine therapy or further evaluation with nonradioiodine imaging *(8)*. Rather than performing more diagnostic imaging studies other than perhaps neck ultrasonography to identify easily resectable disease, many clinicians first administer 100 to 200 mCi of ^{131}I when the serum Tg level is above 10 ng/mL after total or near-total thyroidectomy despite a negative diagnostic ^{131}I WBS *(14)*. The rationale is that radioiodine therapy is systemic and may be effective in reducing the mass of malignant tissue. The posttherapy scan may also localize the disease, which may assist in directing future diagnostic imaging studies, surgery, external beam radiation, or in supporting further ^{131}I therapy. An alternative to radioiodine therapy is to perform nonradioiodine imaging using various combinations of ultrasound, CT, MR, FDG-PET, thallium, sestamibi, tetrofosmin, and radiolabeled somatostatin analogs. In our experience, neck ultrasound and FDG-PET have the highest yield in this setting. Unfortunately, both strategies have limitations and uncommonly result in complete cure.

In this patient's case, the March 1996 neck ultrasound was negative. In retrospect, the March 1996 MR of the neck probably identified both of her sites of malignant lymph nodes more than 3 yr before they became palpable or were reimaged and biopsied; the nodes were not identified by CT or sestamibi imaging. This is unusual because cervical ultrasonography in experienced hands is typically much more sensitive for the identification of malignant cervical lymph nodes than is MR.

Throughout this patient's clinical course, her Tg level was elevated out of proportion to the ^{131}I uptake seen on both diagnostic and posttherapy ^{131}I scans because of the low expression of sodium-iodide symporters (NIS) in her tumor tissue. The recently cloned NIS *(15)* is the plasma membrane protein that mediates active iodide uptake into several tissues, including the thyroid and salivary glands and normal breast tissue *(16)*. Found heterogeneously expressed in the thyroid, NIS is clustered in the basal and lateral membranes of normal thyrocytes *(16)*. Activation of NIS, which is a key step in iodide transport from the circulation into the thyrocyte, occurs against an electrochemical gradient and requires energy, is coupled to the action of Na+/K+-ATPase and is stimulated by TSH, the main hormone regulating thyroid-specific functions. Increased NIS expression is found in autonomously hyperfunctioning thyroid adenomas and Graves' disease, and decreased levels of NIS protein and/or mRNA are observed in Hashimoto's disease, cold nodules, most differentiated thyroid cancers and cell lines derived from them *(16,17)*. Autoantibodies directed against NIS have been identified in autoimmune thyroid disease and blocking antibodies isolated from sera of patients with Hashimoto's disease inhibit NIS function in vitro *(18)*. NIS mRNA expression can be upregulated by retinoic acid in human thyroid carcinoma cell lines whereas retinoic acid treatment decreases NIS expression and function in differentiated rat thyroid FRTL-5 cells *(18)*. Low expression of NIS has serious diagnostic and therapeutic implications regarding radioiodine as is seen in this patient.

This patient underwent scanning with fluorine-18 fluorodeoxyglucose (FDG) positron emission tomography (PET), which should be considered in all patients with differentiated thyroid cancer in whom recurrence or metastases are suspected, particularly those with elevated Tg values and negative whole body ^{131}I scans.

A large multicenter European study evaluated the clinical significance of FDG-PET in 222 patients with differentiated thyroid carcinoma and compared the results with ^{131}I whole body scintigraphy (WBS) and [99m]Tc 2-methoxyisobutylisonitrile (MIBI) or thallium-201 chloride (Tl) scintigraphy *(19)*. The sensitivity of whole-body FDG-PET imaging was 75% for the whole patient group (*n* = 222) and 85% for those with negative ^{131}I scans (*n* = 166) compared to about 50% for WBS, MIBI, or Tl scans. The specificity of WBS was higher at 99%, however, compared with about 90% for FDG-PET and the other scans. In this study, FDG-PET and WBS in combination missed tumor in only 7% of the patients. Another study found FDG-PET to be superior to WBS and serum Tg measurement for detecting metastases to cervical lymph nodes and found FDG-PET helpful for determining the surgical management of these patients *(20)*.

Once distant metastases are discovered in patients with differentiated thyroid carcinoma, FDG-PET can identify high and low risk subsets. Poorly differentiated thyroid cancer lesions, which often lose the ability to concentrate ^{131}I, exhibit increased metabolic activity evidenced by enhanced glucose uptake seen on FDG-PET. One study of 124 patients with differentiated thyroid cancer, 14 of whom died during 41 mo of follow-up, found that the single strongest predictor of survival was the volume of FDG-avid disease *(21)*. The 3-yr survival of patients with FDG-positive tumor volumes of 125 mL or less was 96% compared with 18% in those with an FDG-positive tumor volume greater than 125 mL. All of 10 patients with distant metastases and negative PET scans remained alive and well during follow-up *(21)*.

This patient has persistent disease the location(s) of which is not yet certain. During follow-up an attempt will be made to identify the location of her persistent disease. About 85% of patients with differentiated thyroid cancer are free of disease within a year or 18 mo after initial surgery. The others have persistent disease, which in our experience can be eliminated in fewer than half the patients. In one study of patients with disease recurrence, almost one-third of patients died of their disease a median of 64 mo from diagnosis and initial therapy and about 10% were alive with persistent disease after a median follow-up of 9 yr *(22)*. Patients most likely to become disease-free had recurrences limited to cervical lymph nodes that concentrated ^{131}I without history of a locally invasive tumor. Patients most likely to die of their disease had noniodine avid disease with primary tumors demonstrating extrathyroidal or extranodal extension *(22)*. An aggressive imaging and surgical approach is reasonable if the patient has disease restricted to her neck and superior mediastinum that does not concentrate ^{131}I. Tumor mass is a predictor of outcome, and Tg level is correlated to tumor mass. It is thus not suprising that Tg levels correlate with prognosis *(23)*. For example, The 10-yr survival rate of patients with distant metastases is 80% when the Tg is 1–2 ng/mL on TSH suppressive therapy as opposed to 21% when the Tg is >100 ng/mL *(23)*.

REFERENCES

1. Okayasu I, Fujiwara M, Hara Y, Tanaka Y, Rose NR. Association of chronic lymphocytic thyroiditis and thyroid papillary carcinoma—A study of surgical cases among Japanese, and white and African Americans. Cancer 1995;76:2312–2318.
2. Kashima K, Yokoyama S, Noguchi S, et al. Chronic thyroiditis as a favorable prognostic factor in papillary thyroid carcinoma. Thyroid 1998;8:197–202.
3. Schäffler A, Palitzsch KD, Seiffarth C, et al. Coexistent thyroiditis is associated with lower tumour stage in thyroid carcinoma. Eur J Clin Invest 1998;28:838–844.
4. Mazzaferri EL. Management of a solitary thyroid nodule. N Engl J Med 1993;328:553–559.
5. Tielens ET, Sherman SI, Hruban RH, Ladenson PW. Follicular variant of papillary thyroid carcinoma: a clinicopathologic study. Cancer 1994;73:424–431.
6. Brennan MD, Bergstralh EJ, van Heerden JA, McConahey WM. Follicular thyroid cancer treated at the Mayo Clinic, 1946 through 1970: initial manifestations, pathologic findings, therapy, and outcome. Mayo Clin Proc 1991;66:11–22.
7. Emerick GT, Duh Q-Y, Siperstein AE, Burrow GN, Clark OH. Diagnosis, treatment, and outcome of follicular thyroid carcinoma. Cancer 1993;72:3287–3295.
8. Mazzaferri EL. NCCN thyroid carcinoma practice guidelines. Oncology 1999;13:391–442.
9. Park HM, Perkins OW, Edmondson JW, Schnute RB, Manatunga A. Influence of diagnostic radioiodines on the uptake of ablative dose of iodine-131. Thyroid 1994;4:49–54.
10. Muratet JP, Giraud P, Daver A, Minier JF, Gamelin E, Larra F. Predicting the efficacy of first iodine-131 treatment in differentiated thyroid carcinoma. J Nucl Med 1997;38:1362–1368.
11. Leger FA, Izembart M, Dagousset F, et al. Decreased uptake of therapeutic doses of iodine-131 after 185-MBq iodine-131 diagnostic imaging for thyroid remnants in differentiated thyroid carcinoma. Eur J Nucl Med 1998;25:242–246.
12. Cailleux AF, Baudin E, Travagli JP, Ricard M, Schlumberger M. Is diagnostic iodine-131 scanning useful after total thyroid ablation for differentiated thyroid cancer? J Clin Endocrinol Metab 2000;85: 175–178.
13. Schlumberger MJ. Diagnostic follow-up of well-differentiated thyroid carcinoma: historical perspective and current status. J Endocrinol Invest 1999; 22(Suppl 11):3–7.
14. Schlumberger M, Mancusi F, Baudin E, Pacini F. 131-I Therapy for elevated thyroglobulin levels. Thyroid 1997;7:273–276.
15. Smanik PA, Liu Q, Furminger TL, et al. Cloning of the human sodium iodide symporter. Biochem Biophys Res Commun 1996;226:339–345.

16. Jhiang SM, Cho JY, Ryu K-Y, et al. An immunohistochemical study of Na+/I- symporter in human thyroid tissues and salivary gland tissues. Endocrinology 1998;139:4416–4419.
17. Schmutzler C, Köhrle J. Implications of the molecular characterization of the sodium-iodide symporter (NIS). Exp Clin Endocrinol Diabetes 1998;106:S1–S10.
18. Castro MR, Bergert ER, Beito TG, McIver B, Goellner JR, Morris JC. Development of monoclonal antibodies against the human sodium iodide symporter: immunohistochemical characterization of this protein in thyroid cells. J Clin Endocrinol Metab 1999;84:2957–2962.
19. Gruenwald F, Kaelicke T, Feine U, et al. Fluorine-18 fluorodeoxyglucose positron emission tomography in thyroid cancer: results of a multicentre study. Eur J Nucl Med 1999;26:1547–1552.
20. Chung JK, So Y, Lee JS, et al. Value of FDG PET in papillary thyroid carcinoma with negative ^{131}I whole-body scan. J Nucl Med 1999;40:986–992.
21. Wang W, Larson SM, Fazzari M, et al. Prognostic value of [18F]fluorodeoxyglucose positron emission tomographic scanning in patients with thyroid cancer. J Clin Endocrinol Metab 2000;85:1107–1113.
22. Vassilopoulou-Sellin R, Schultz PN, Haynie TP. Clinical outcome of patients with papillary thyroid carcinoma who have recurrence after initial radioactive iodine therapy. Cancer 1996;78:493–501.
23. Schlumberger M, Challeton C, De Vathaire F, et al. Radioactive iodine treatment and external radiotherapy for lung and bone metastases from thyroid carcinoma. J Nucl Med 1996;37:598–605.

CASE #4: PAPILLARY CANCER
IN PATIENT WITH CHRONIC RENAL FAILURE

Case Description

A 43-yr-old man with chronic renal failure from autosomal dominant polycystic kidney disease developed a thyroid nodule diagnosed as PTC by FNA biopsy in July 1995. His preoperative thyroglobulin (Tg) and serum creatinine were elevated (see Table 4). He promptly underwent near total thyroidectomy for a multifocal PTC scattered throughout the gland, the largest of which was a 2.2 cm tumor in the isthmus that showed vascular invasion. Two lymph nodes were positive for cancer.

In September 1995, after a diagnostic hypothyroid whole body ^{131}I scan showed bilateral lateral neck uptake, he was treated with 182 mCi of ^{131}I and TSH-suppressive doses of thyroxine were begun. A computed tomography (CT) scan obtained several weeks after the radioiodine therapy demonstrated cervical lymph nodes as large as 1.5 cm bilaterally.

In February 1996, neck ultrasound showed a 2 cm right neck lymph node. A diagnostic hypothyroid whole body ^{131}I scan done 1 mo later demonstrated 1.2% uptake in the thyroid bed and bilateral uptake in the neck that was treated with 200 mCi [131]I. The posttherapy images demonstrated two foci of uptake in the left neck, one in the right neck and one in the superior mediastinum/suprasternal notch. Diffuse pulmonary metastases seen only on the posttherapy images, in retrospect, may have also been present on the 1995 posttherapy images. A few weeks after ^{131}I treatment a serum creatinine level done by his nephrologist had risen from 5.1 mg/dL to 6.2 mg/dL.

In January 1997, a whole body ^{131}I scan and dosimetry done at another institution demonstrated three foci of activity in the upper mediastinum and lower anterior neck, and diffuse pulmonary micrometastases. The patient was advised not to receive more than 60 mCi ^{131}I but therapy was not given.

In October 1997, after receiving IRB approval at our institution, he was treated in our medical center with 100 mCi of [131]I 24 h after being given rhTSH (Thyrogen®), 0.9 mg IM, on two consecutive days. A diagnostic ^{131}I whole body scan was not obtained, but posttreatment imaging showed less lung, left neck and midline uptake than had been seen

Table 4
Case 4 Laboratory Summary

Date	Months since thyroidectomy	Tg on LT4 (ng/mL)	Tg off LT4 of thyrogen stimulated (ng/mL)	TSH (normal 0.32–5.0 mU/mL)	Creatinine (normal 0.7–1.3 mg/dL)	I-131 Rx
6-21-95	Pre-operative	53.4			3.4	
9-8-95					4.6	182 mCi
10-31-95	3	12.4		0.19	4.1	
2-2-96	7	8.6		<0.04		
3-18-96	8		176	333	5.1	200 mCi
7-31-96	12	5.4		0.02		
1-21-97	18	6.7		0.05		
7-29-97	24	5.4		<0.04	6.5	
10-21-97	27	3.9		<0.04		
10-23-97	27		5.9	337.5	5.6	Thyrogen 100 mCi
5-17-98	34	3.3		—	7.3	
7-25-98	36	2.4		<0.04		
11-17-98	40	4.3		<0.04	7.3	
1-21-99	42		14.3	490.0		Thyrogen 100 mCi
4-27-99	45	4.3		0.01	7.7	
7-6-99	48	4.1		<0.04	Peritoneal dialysis begun	
12-28-99	53	4.2		<0.04		
2-7-00	55	5.2		<0.04	12.7	
2-16-00	55		27.8	743.6	10.4	Thyrogen 140 mCi
6-29-00	59	1.8		<0.04		

previously, and no uptake in the right neck. One month later, his neck and chest CT scans showed no evidence of tumor.

In January 1999, he was again treated with 106 mCi ^{131}I after rhTSH stimulation and his posttherapy images demonstrated one focus of uptake at the area of the suprasternal notch and less pulmonary uptake.

In February 2000, he underwent whole body and blood dosimetry under rhTSH stimulation followed by rhTSH-stimulated ^{131}I therapy (see Figs. 2 and 3). We did this by administering 0.9 mg of rhTSH IM on Monday and Tuesday at the same time performing nightly automated peritoneal dialysis. On Wednesday he received a 4-mCi-tracer dose of ^{131}I and underwent no dialysis for 24 h. On Thursday, he began manual peritoneal dialysis to minimize radiation contamination to his home equipment. Whole body and blood dosimetry data were collected daily through Friday and completed on the following Monday. Erroneously, blood for Tg (and TSH) measurements were not obtained on Friday. On Monday, he received a third injection of rhTSH after completing the dosimetry study and received a fourth injection on Tuesday. Dosimetry revealed 46% whole body retention at 48 h. Blood dosimetry (blood β plus whole body γ) revealed 1.52 rads/mCi yielding limits of 200 rad at 132 mCi and 300 rad at 197 mCi. Tuesday night he underwent

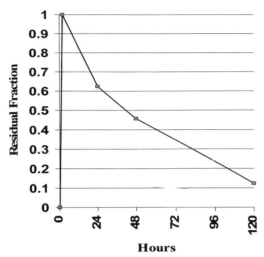

Fig. 2. Case 4 whole body ^{131}I retention as a function of time determined by serial whole body counts.

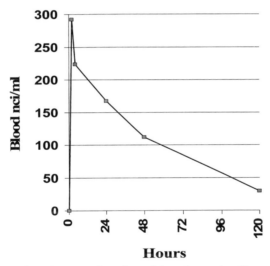

Fig. 3. Case 4 blood ^{131}I radioactivity as a function of time determined by serial whole blood counts.

automated nocturnal dialysis and then on Wednesday the laboratory studies shown in Table 4 were drawn and he was treated with 140 mCi of [131]I. After therapy, he underwent no dialysis until he resumed manual peritoneal dialysis on Thursday and continued until the following Tuesday when he resumed nocturnal automated peritoneal dialysis. Eight days after treatment, posttherapy imaging revealed faint suprasternal notch activity that had not changed from the previous study in January 1999, but less pulmonary activity. Following his last therapy, he developed chronic dry mouth.

Discussion

In retrospect, this patient had distant metastases at the time his PTC was diagnosed. Although the preoperative Tg of 53.4 ng/mL is high, it cannot be taken as *prima facie* evidence of distant metastases because there are two sources of Tg in the serum: normal thyroid tissue and well-differentiated thyroid cancer. The preoperative diagnosis of distant metastases cannot be made on the basis of serum Tg levels alone, even if they are higher than normal, because certain nonmalignant thyroid disorders such as thyroiditis raise them. The serum Tg level roughly correlates with the tumor mass, providing there is little or no normal thyroid tissue and the tumor synthesizes Tg, and antithyroglobulin antibodies are not present. These antibodies are found in up to 25% of patients with thyroid cancer, a rate almost threefold more common than in the general population (1). This is important because in the absence of antithyroglobulin antibodies, Tg measurements done after thyroid ablation provide the most sensitive means of detecting residual thyroid cancer.

Measuring serum Tg levels and performing whole-body ^{131}I imaging are the principal means of postoperatively assessing the patient's cancer status. Together, the two will detect recurrent or residual disease in most patients who have undergone total thyroid ablation. After the initial therapy is completed, serum Tg should be measured periodically and whole-body ^{131}I scanning should be done after thyroxine is discontinued or rhTSH is administered. A test for serum antithyroglobulin antibodies should be done in the sample obtained for serum Tg assay because these invalidate serum Tg measurements in most assays (1,2). Antithyroglobulin antibodies spuriously lower serum Tg levels in most immunometric assays (the more commonly used type) and raise Tg levels in most radioimmunoassays.

Although serum Tg can be measured when the patient is taking thyroxine, the measurement is more sensitive when thyroid hormone has been stopped or rhTSH is given to elevate the serum TSH (3,4). Under these circumstances, serum Tg has a lower false-negative rate than whole body ^{131}I scanning (3,4). In one study, the sensitivity of serum Tg was 50% before and 83% after thyroxine was discontinued (5). Detecting circulating Tg by a newly introduced Tg mRNA method is a more sensitive marker of residual thyroid tissue or cancer than measuring it by immunometric assay, particularly during thyroxine treatment or with circulating antithyroglobulin antibodies (6). However, this assay is not yet widely available.

In a comparative study, serum Tg and whole-body ^{131}I scanning results were concordant in only 44% of 233 patients who had undergone total thyroid ablation (7). Most with discordant studies had negative whole-body scans and positive serum Tg tests; only three had the opposite pattern. The test sensitivities were 96% for serum Tg and 48% for whole body ^{131}I scans. The few false-negative serum Tg tests occurred with small papillary carcinomas that had cervical or mediastinal lymph node metastases. In a study of serum Tg measurements in 180 patients who had undergone near-total or total thyroidectomy and ^{131}I ablation and were followed up to 18 years, 94% had Tg values less than 5 ng/mL and 98% had values less than 10 ng/mL during thyroxine therapy (8). The results of serum Tg and ^{131}I tests are complementary. Patients rarely have recurrent carcinoma after they have undergone near-total or total thyroidectomy and ^{131}I ablation and have a negative postablation scan and serum Tg values less than 2 ng/mL while receiving thyroid hormone and less than 3 ng/mL after it is discontinued (8). However, the sensitivity and specificity of various Tg assays vary widely in different laboratories, even with the use of a new international standard (CRM 457) (9).

We use a sensitive Tg immunometric assay with a detection limit of 0.5 ng/mL. A serum Tg above this level during thyroxine therapy in a patient who has undergone total or near-total thyroidectomy and ^{131}I ablation is a sign of persistent normal tissue or differentiated thyroid carcinoma, which is an indication for repeat scanning when there is no other evidence of disease. If serum Tg rises above 5–10 ng/mL after thyroid hormone is discontinued or rises above approximately 2.5 ng/mL after rhTSH is administered, normal or malignant thyroid tissue is usually present, even if the 2 to 4 mCi ^{131}I diagnostic scan is negative (i.e., <1% [131]I uptake) *(3,10,11)*. In this case, neck ultrasonography and/or CT or magnetic resonance imaging (MRI), and/or F-18-fluorodeoxyglucose-positron emission tomography (FDG-PET) should be considered to detect occult tumor that can be excised. However, if tumor is not found and the serum Tg is above 10 ng/mL, we give a therapeutic dose of [131]I—usually 100 to 150 mCi—and perform a posttreatment scan. In our experience, about 20% of such patients have lung metastases. Others use different cutoff values and a different dose of ^{131}I, but the Tg level to trigger treatment has been gradually coming down in recent years *(12)*. The patient under discussion had high enough serum Tg measurements at 3 and 7 mo after initial therapy, both while taking thyroxine and after its withdrawal (see Table 4), that distant metastases were almost certain to have been present, probably in the lung.

Treating this man's thyroid cancer was a particularly difficult problem, given the important interactions between chronic renal disease, hypothyroidism, and renal iodine clearance. His first two ^{131}I treatments were done after thyroid hormone withdrawal. During the second one in March 1996, his serum creatinine became so elevated after thyroid hormone withdrawal, as a consequence of the hypothyroidism-induced reduction in renal blood flow, that he and his attending nephrologist felt another such episode would cause permanent damage to his kidneys requiring chronic dialysis. For this reason, he was considered an appropriate candidate for rhTSH-stimulated ^{131}I treatment that does not reduce glomerular filtration rate (or radioiodine clearance) as does hypothyroidism. The FDA has approved recombinant TSH for diagnostic ^{131}I whole body scans and Tg measurement, but not for ^{131}I therapy because withdrawal may provide a more potent stimulus for uptake of therapeutic doses of ^{131}I by malignant thyroid tissue. The principal reason for this is that sustained TSH stimulation over weeks occurs after thyroid hormone withdrawal, but not with rhTSH, which typically has a serum half-life of 60 h following 0.9 mg IM. Also, with rhTSH there is no reduction in the renal clearance of iodine that hypothyroidism characteristically produces after thyroid hormone withdrawal, which enhances the whole-body retention and therapeutic effect of [131]I *(3)*.

The patient was treated with ^{131}I administered as large fixed doses and later was given ^{131}I doses calculated by dosimetry. His last dose of 140 mCi of radioiodine may be equivalent to 300–500 mCi therapy in a patient with normal renal function and a similar burden of disease. Of the three treatment methods available, the most widely used and simplest is to administer a fixed dose *(13)*. Most clinics use this method regardless of the percentage uptake of ^{131}I in the remnant or metastatic lesion. In the setting of normal renal function, lymph node metastases that are not large enough to excise are often treated with 100–175 mCi. Carcinoma extending through the thyroid capsule and invading the neck is often treated with 150–200 mCi, which will usually not induce radiation sickness or produce serious damage to other structures. Patients with distant metastases are often treated with 200 mCi of [131]I. Diffuse pulmonary metastases that concentrate 50% or more of the diagnostic dose of ^{131}I, which is very uncommon, may be treated with 75 mCi ^{131}I to avoid lung injury. Many believe that to eradicate a tumor it must concentrate at least 0.1% of the ^{131}I dose at 24 h. However, in some patients metastases detected only by high serum Tg concentrations can be treated effectively when uptake is much lower than 0.1% *(12)*. Translating these fixed radioiodine doses in the setting of normal renal function to that of various states of renal insufficiency is problematic.

A second approach is to use quantitative dosimetry methods to estimate tumor uptake and retention. Some favor this because radiation exposure from arbitrarily fixed doses of ^{131}I can vary substantially. Doses that will deliver 50,000 to 60,000 rads (500–600 Gy) to the residual normal tissue and 4000 to 5000 rads (40–50 Gy) to metastatic foci are likely to be effective. If the calculated dose is less than 3500 rads (35 Gy), it is unlikely that the cancer will respond to ^{131}I therapy *(14,15)*. To make these calculations, it is necessary to estimate tumor size, which is often difficult to do and impossible in patients with pulmonary metastases only visible with radioiodine imaging. Typically, lesions that receive only a few hundred rads from 150 to 200 mCi of ^{131}I should be considered for surgery, external radiation or medical therapy.

A third approach to radioiodine therapy is to administer a dose calculated to deliver a maximum of 200 rads (2 Gy) to the blood, keeping the whole-body retention less than 120 mCi at 48 h and the amount in the lungs less than 80 mCi (2960 MBq) when there is diffuse pulmonary uptake. The maximum administered dose is often kept at 300 mCi *(16)*. Large therapeutic doses, regardless of the method chosen to estimate or calculate them, deliver proportionally large radiation doses to the gonads, bone marrow, urinary bladder and colon, perhaps accounting for the observations that malignancies at these sites rise and gonadal dysfunction increases when large cumulative doses of ^{131}I are administered. About two-thirds of patients given 200 mCi or more develop mild radiation sickness characterized by headache, nausea and occasional vomiting, which begins about 4 h after ^{131}I administration and resolves in about 24 h, but almost never occurs with smaller doses although most children receiving ^{131}I develop these symptoms. Occasionally, patients have transient tongue pain or reduced taste *(14,15)*. In the months following high-dose radioiodine therapy, intermittent bouts of salivary pseudoobstruction may occur that typically resolve within about 1 yr. It is important that the patient be aware of this possibility to prevent unnecessary therapy for bacterial parotitis or salivary duct stones. More than a year after the last ^{131}I treatment, nearly half have reduced salivary gland function and some report recurrent conjunctivitis, but these are almost never serious problems.

Our patient was given rhTSH in preparation for his treatment with [131]I. Recombinant human TSH has been used to prepare some patients for ^{131}I therapy, especially those with hypopituitarism or other medical problems that blunt or abolish the normal rise of TSH in response to thyroid hormone withdrawal, or medical conditions that will be adversely affected by hypothyroidism. For example, Rudavsky and Freeman treated a patient with scan-negative, thyroglobulin-positive metastatic thyroid cancer using ^{131}I and rhTSH *(17)*. The patient had lung and bone metastases and was considered so desperately ill that rhTSH was used in lieu of thyroid hormone withdrawal. Their patient was given 0.9 mg rhTSH IM on 2 d and 515 mCi of ^{131}I was administered on the third day. A whole body scan obtained 1 wk later revealed uptake of ^{131}I in both lungs and in essentially all skeletal metastases. The bone pain ameliorated within two weeks and further improvement ensued over the next few months, permitting the patient to resume independent ambulation while his serum Tg fell from 7800 ng/mL to 1924 ng/mL on thyroid hormone therapy.

Our patient had a good response to [131]I. He had considerable uptake of radioisotope in his lungs on the earlier posttreatment scan (Fig. 4) but subsequently had a fall in his serum Tg levels and diminished uptake of isotope in his lungs (Fig. 5). Nonetheless, he has persistent disease.

Posttreatment ^{131}I scans are likely to yield the most important clinical information when pretreatment scans are negative and serum Tg levels are very high. In a study of 283

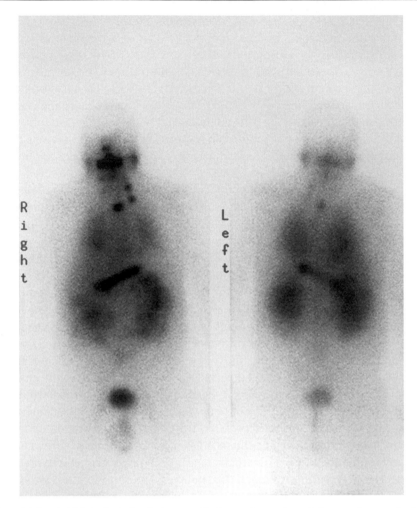

Fig. 4. Case 4 March 1996 whole body images (left panel anterior, right panel posterior) after 200 mCi of ^{131}I therapy with hypothyroid stimulation demonstrate two left neck foci consistent with metastatic lymph nodes, the superior mediastinum, and subtle uptake in the right neck. Bilateral diffuse lung uptake from pulmonary metastases is seen. Prominent bilateral renal activity is present consistent with enlarged polycystic kidneys. Diffuse hepatic radioiodine activity is best seen on the anterior image.

patients, over 6% had lung and bone metastases detected after treatment with 100 mCi ^{131}I that had been suspected on the basis of high serum Tg levels but had not been detected after 2 mCi scans *(18)*. In another study, all but one of 17 patients with elevated serum Tg levels and negative 5 mCi diagnostic scans showed ^{131}I uptake after 75 to 140 mCi ^{131}I; more than half had lung metastases *(19)*. Treating these lesions usually reduces the tumor burden, but complete tumor eradication may be difficult to achieve. The best prognosis— sometimes associated with apparent cure after ^{131}I therapy—is with lung metastases seen only on ^{131}I imaging (some are seen only on posttherapy imaging) and not by X-ray or computed tomography *(12,20)*. Among 23 patients treated with ^{131}I for diffuse pulmonary metastases detected only by ^{131}I imaging, 87% had no lung uptake on subsequent scans *(21)*. After ^{131}I therapy, serum Tg became undetectable and lung CT scans showed

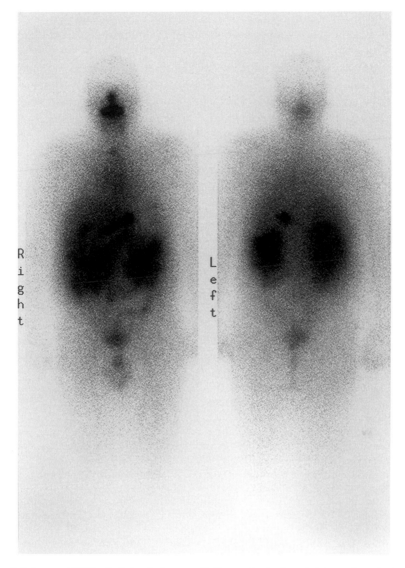

Fig. 5. Case 4 February 2000 whole body images (left panel anterior, right panel posterior) after 140 mCi of ^{131}I therapy with rhTSH stimulation demonstrate uptake in the superior mediastinum/suprasternal notch and faint bilateral diffuse lung uptake from pulmonary metastases. Prominent bilateral renal activity and diffuse hepatic uptake are again noted.

disappearance of the micronodules in almost half the patients, while lung biopsy showed no evidence of disease in two. Others also report a substantial fall in serum Tg levels after ^{131}I treatment of such patients *(22)*. In one study, patients considered free of disease after ^{131}I therapy survived three times longer than those with persistent disease *(23)*. In another study of 20 patients with pulmonary metastases, 65% had a complete response to ^{131}I therapy and there were no relapses after 4 to 32 yr *(24)*. Others report a reduction of metastatic disease in most patients but find that a complete remission of pulmonary metastases is uncommon *(25,26)*. Nonetheless, a partial response with reduction of metastatic disease is usually possible and patients generally have a good quality of life with no further disease progression and a low mortality rate. This is consistent with data that suggests that the tumor bulk of distant metastases is second only to patient age as a predictor of thyroid cancer mortality *(27)*.

Another problem encountered during our patient's whole-body ^{131}I scans was scan interpretation. His enlarged kidneys are seen quite well with radioiodine imaging (Figs. 4 and 5), which is a characteristic of this type of polycystic kidney disease and is a cause of a false-positive scan *(28)*. Furthermore, ^{131}I accumulated in his peritoneal dialysis fluid and was best seen on his 48 h diagnostic images (not shown). There are other important causes of false positive whole body ^{131}I scans. Body secretions, pathologic transudates and inflammation, nonspecific mediastinal uptake, or tumors of nonthyroidal origin may cause false-positive scans *(29)*. Misleading scans can be caused by physiologic secretion of ^{131}I from the nasopharynx, salivary and sweat glands, stomach, genitourinary tract, and from skin, hair, and clothing contamination with urine, sputum or tears. Pathologic pulmonary transudates and inflammation owing to cysts may also produce false positive scans, as may lung lesions caused by inflammatory disease. Diffuse physiologic hepatic ^{131}I uptake is seen after diagnostic and therapeutic doses of ^{131}I, which is the result of ^{131}I labeled thyroglobulin. The more ^{131}I uptake that appears in the residual thyroid or extrahepatic metastases, the more it appears in the liver. The frequency of hepatic uptake in the post-therapy scans is related to the dose of ^{131}I, ranging from 40% with a 30-mCi dose to 70% with 150–200 mCi of [131]I *(30)*. However, hepatic ^{131}I uptake without uptake in the thyroid bed or in extra-hepatic thyroid carcinoma may represent occult metastases *(30)*.

REFERENCES

1. Spencer CA, Takeuchi M, Kazarosyan M, et al. Serum thyroglobulin autoantibodies: prevalence, influence on serum thyroglobulin measurement, and prognostic significance in patients with differentiated thyroid carcinoma. J Clin Endocrinol Metab 1998;83:1121–1127.
2. Spencer CA. Recoveries cannot be used to authenticate thyroglobulin (Tg) measurements when sera contain Tg autoantibodies. Clin Chem 1996;42:661–663.
3. Haugen BR, Pacini F, Reiners C, et al. A comparison of recombinant human thyrotropin and thyroid hormone withdrawal for the detection of thyroid remnant or cancer. J Clin Endocrinol Metab 1999; 84:3877–3885.
4. Pacini F, Lari R, Mazzeo S, Grasso L, Taddei D, Pinchera A. Diagnostic value of a single serum thyroglobulin determination on and off thyroid suppressive therapy in the follow-up of patients with differentiated thyroid cancer. Clin Endocrinol 1985;23:405–411.
5. Muller-Gartner HW, Schneider C. Clinical evaluation of tumor characteristics predisposing serum thyroglobulin to be undetectable in patients with differentiated thyroid cancer. Cancer 1988;61:976–981.
6. Ringel M, Ladenson P, Levine MA. Molecular diagnosis of residual and recurrent thyroid cancer by amplification of thyroglobulin messenger ribonucleic acid in peripheral blood. J Clin Endocrinol Metab 1998;83:4435–4442.
7. Ronga G, Fiorentino A, Fragasso G, Fringuelli FM, Todino V. Complementary role of whole body scan and serum thyroglobulin determination in the follow-up of differentiated thyroid carcinoma. Ital J Surg Sci 1986;16:11–15.
8. Ozata M, Suzuki S, Miyamoto T, Liu RT, Fierro-Renoy F, DeGroot LJ. Serum thyroglobulin in the follow-up of patients with treated differentiated thyroid cancer. J Clin Endocrinol Metab 1994;79:98–105.
9. Spencer CA, Takeuchi M, Kazarosyan M. Current status and performance goals for serum thyroglobulin assays. Clin Chem 1996;42:164–173.
10. Schlumberger MJ. Medical progress—Papillary and follicular thyroid carcinoma. N Engl J Med 1998; 338:297–306.
11. Spencer CA, Wang CC. Thyroglobulin measurement—Techniques, clinical benefits, and pitfalls. Endocrinol Metabol Clin North Am 1995;24:841–863.

12. Schlumberger M, Mancusi F, Baudin E, Pacini F. 131-I Therapy for elevated thyroglobulin levels. Thyroid 1997;7:273–276.
13. Mazzaferri EL. Carcinoma of follicular epithelium: radioiodine and other treatment outcomes. In: Braverman LE, Utiger RD, eds. The Thyroid: A Fundamental and Clinical Text. Lippencott-Raven, Philadelphia, PA, 1996, pp. 922–945.
14. Brierley J, Maxon HR. Radioiodine and external radiation therapy. In: Fagin JA, ed. Thyroid Cancer. Kluwer Academic, Boston/Dordrecht London: 1998, pp. 285–317.
15. Maxon HR, Englaro EE, Thomas SR, et al. Radioiodine-131 therapy for well-differentiated thyroid cancer—a quantitative radiation dosimetric approach: outcome and validation in 85 patients. J Nucl Med 1992;33:1132–1136.
16. Benua RS, Cicale NR, Sonenberg M, et al. The relation of radioiodine dosimetry to results and complications in the treatment of metastatic thyroid cancer. AJR 1962;87:171–178.
17. Rudavsky AZ, Freeman LM. Treatment of scan-negative, thyroglobulin-positive metastatic thyroid cancer using radioiodine ^{131}I and recombinant human thyroid stimulating hormone. J Clin Endocrinol Metab 1997;82:11–14.
18. Schlumberger M, Tubiana M, De Vathaire F, et al. Long-term results of treatment of 283 patients with lung and bone metastases from differentiated thyroid carcinoma. J Clin Endocrinol Metab 1986;63:960–967.
19. Pacini F, Lippi F, Formica N, Elisei R, Anelli S, Ceccarelli C. Therapeutic doses of iodine-131 reveal undiagnosed metastases in thyroid cancer patients with detectable serum thyroglobulin levels. J Nucl Med 1987;28:1888–1891.
20. Casara D, Rubello D, Saladini G, et al. Different features of pulmonary metastases in differentiated thyroid cancer: Natural history and multivariate statistical analysis of prognostic variables. J Nucl Med 1993;34:1626–1631.
21. Schlumberger M, Arcangioli O, Piekarski JD, Tubiana M, Parmentier C. Detection and treatment of lung metastases of differentiated thyroid carcinoma in patients with normal chest X-rays. J Nucl Med 1988; 29:1790–1794.
22. Pineda JD, Lee T, Ain K, Reynolds J, Robbins J. Iodine-131 therapy for thyroid cancer patients with elevated thyroglobulin and negative diagnostic scan. J Clin Endocrinol Metab 1995;80:1488–1492.
23. Beierwaltes WH, Nishiyama RH, Thompson NW, Copp JE, Kubo A. Survival time and "cure" in papillary and follicular thyroid carcinoma with distant metastases: statistics following University of Michigan therapy. J Nucl Med 1982;23:561–568.
24. Brown AP, Greening WP, McCready VR, Shaw HJ, Harmer CL. Radioiodine treatment of metastatic thyroid carcinoma: the Royal Marsden Hospital experience. Br J Radiol 1984;57:323–327.
25. Samuel AM, Rajashekharrao B, Shah DH. Pulmonary metastases in children and adolescents with well-differentiated thyroid cancer. J Nucl Med 1998;39:1531–1536.
26. Sisson JC, Giordano TJ, Jamadar DA, et al. 131-I treatment of micronodular pulmonary metastases from papillary thyroid carcinoma. Cancer 1996;78:2184–2192.
27. Schlumberger M, Challeton C, De Vathaire F, et al. Radioactive iodine treatment and external radiotherapy for lung and bone metastases from thyroid carcinoma. J Nucl Med 1996;37:598–605.
28. Giuffrida D, Fornito MC, Pellegriti G, Regalbuto C, Vigneri G. False positive ^{131}I total body scan due to bilateral polycystic renal disease. J Endocrinol Invest 1997;20:342–344.
29. Greenler DP, Klein HA. The scope of false-positive iodine-131 images for thyroid carcinoma. Clin Nucl Med 1989;14:111–117.
30. Chung JK, Lee YJ, Jeong JM, et al. Clinical significance of hepatic visualization on iodine-131 whole-body scan in patients with thyroid carcinoma. J Nucl Med 1997;38:1191–1195.

CASE #5: POST-IRRADIATION INSULAR THYROID CANCER

Case Description

A 69-yr-old man with a history of external beam radiation therapy for acne as a teenager presented in July 1991 with superior vena cava syndrome thought owing to an enlarged thyroid. Although he could not date the onset of his symptoms precisely, his arm swelling seemed to have appeared over a few weeks. He underwent neck surgery at his local hospital where the surgeon found an invasive thyroid tumor that he considered

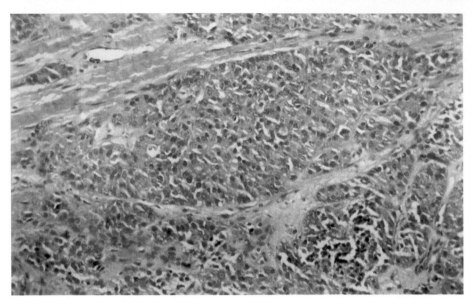

Fig. 6. A black and white photograph of an H & E stained slide from the initial tumor of Case 5 demonstrates a solid cluster of cells surrounded by fibrous tissue creating an island or "insular" architecture. (Image courtesy of Paul E. Wakely, M. D., Department of Pathology, The Ohio State University.)

unresectable and merely performed a wedge biopsy. The pathologists thought the tumor was an anaplastic thyroid carcinoma and he was referred to our medical center.

In August 1991, our initial examination disclosed a hoarse, but robust muscular man who had a large asymmetrical and very hard goiter that was adherent to surrounding tissues on the right. There was facial suffusion and edema, and dilatation of his neck veins and those of his right arm and thorax consistent with a superior vena cava syndrome. He had stridor with forced deep inspiration. Upon our review of the histologic sections (see Fig. 6) a diagnosis of insular thyroid carcinoma (ITC) was made, which prompted further surgical exploration at our institution.

At surgery a large invasive tumor was found that was difficult to separate from the neck tissues. The surgeon excised as much tumor as possible, including most of the right thyroid lobe, a large right supraclavicular mass and tumor that was enveloping, but not invading the trachea and the right carotid artery and subclavian vein. The procedure was completed with a modified right neck dissection and tracheostomy. Invasive tumor measuring 1 × 3 cm that could not be resected was left at the right pyriform sinus. The surgical specimen revealed a tumor that was completely occluding the excised right jugular vein lumen. Histologically, this was a multifocal ITC that was scattered throughout the thyroid gland, the largest focus of which was 2.3 cm.

From September through November 1991, he was treated with external beam radiation, receiving approximately 60 Gy to a wide field that included the neck and mediastinum extending to a few centimeters below the carina. At the same time, he was given doxorubicin 20 mg/m^2/week. Near the end of this course of therapy, he developed severe mucositis, neutropenia, and sepsis that required hospital admission. His thyroid laboratory studies are summarized in Table 5.

Table 5
Case 5 Laboratory Summary

Date	Months since thyroidectomy	Tg on LT4 (ng/mL)	New assay Tg on LT4 (ng/mL)	TSH (normal 0.32–5.0 mU/mL)
2-7-92	7	9.1		0.08
12-18-92	17	3.6		1.00
6-28-93	23	4.5		0.16
4-26-94	33	5.5		1.11
9-19-94	38	5.6		1.63
3-27-95	44	5.1	1.8	0.59
10-1-96	63		3.2	3.92
11-5-97	76		2.2	0.98
5-12-98	82		1.4	1.29
3-30-99	92		<0.5	0.06

His superior mediastinal syndrome resolved shortly after his initial therapy and he gradually recovered, gaining full strength and resuming his daily physical workouts, although his hoarseness persisted. In December 1991 and February 1992, neck CT imaging revealed a left thyroid lobe and soft tissue thickening in the right thyroid bed. In August 1994, a neck CT showed asymmetric soft tissue swelling in the region of his right pyriform sinus and permanent right vocal cord paralysis without change from July 1992. From August 1996 through June 1999, neck and upper mediastinal CT imaging continued to show right vocal cord paralysis and residual tissue in the left thyroid bed, but not in the pyriform sinus area. Serial chest CT imaging from December 1991 through October 1996 was negative for malignancy. A chest CT in May 1998 was essentially negative except for minimal pericardial thickening. During this time, the patient developed severe depression related to the death of his son and did not return for follow-up studies.

In January 2000, he developed symptoms of severe coronary artery disease necessitating three-vessel coronary artery bypass. At surgery, a rock hard "marble" sized mass was found overlying the aorta, which extended into the pericardium and surrounded the pulmonary artery out of the surgeon's reach. Biopsy of the unresectable tumor revealed carcinoma of undetermined origin on frozen section study. Final pathology showed this to be a poorly differentiated carcinoma, which demonstrated necrosis and many mitotic figures and which stained for cytokeratin, but not thyroglobulin, chromogranin, synaptophysin, polyclonal CEA, or calcitonin. Because the area of recurrent disease had been included in the previously irradiated field where he had received nearly maximal radiation, it was felt he would not benefit from additional radiotherapy. Because he was asymptomatic and the tumor was unlikely to respond to chemotherapy, no further treatment was offered at that time.

Discussion

This patient, who as a youngster had head and neck irradiation for acne, developed insular thyroid carcinoma (ITC) more than 50 yr later, which after about 9 yr degenerated into an anaplastic tumor. Ordinarily, PTC accounts for approximately 80% of all thyroid carcinomas in the U.S. (1,2), including more than 95% of the malignant tumors caused by thyroid irradiation *(3)*. Although most irradiation-induced tumors are typical PTCs, a variant of this tumor—diffuse sclerosis variant PTC—accounts for 10% of the malignant tumors found among the children of Chernobyl, a frequency over twice that in patients without prior irradiation *(4–6)*.

External radiation was widely used in the past to treat children with benign head and neck conditions. It is now well known that this caused thyroid carcinoma in a number of children, especially those exposed before the age of 15 yr, posing a major risk that becomes progressively larger with increasing doses of radiation between 0.10 Gy (10 rads) and 10 Gy (1000 rad) *(7)*. The incidence of thyroid carcinoma begins rising within 5 yr of exposure and continues unabated for 30 yr, after which it begins to decline *(7)*. It is slightly more likely to develop in females than males, but the difference is small, and is more likely to occur when there is a family history of thyroid carcinoma *(7)*. Nonetheless, only about 30% of irradiated patients develop palpable thyroid nodules, of which only about one third are malignant *(8)*. Typically, ITC does not occur after head and neck irradiation.

Our patient presented with an extremely aggressive thyroid tumor that initially was understandably mistaken for an anaplastic thyroid carcinoma (ATC) by his referring physicians. Differentiating ATC from other uncommon forms of thyroid cancer is extremely important and can be done with careful histological and immunohistologic study of the tumor. In addition, our patient's ITC appears to have evolved over time into ATC.

First described in 1984 by Carcangiu et al. *(9)*, ITC accounts for slightly less than 5% of all thyroid carcinomas *(10)*. Typically, the tumor shows solid clusters of cells with small follicles that resemble pancreatic islet cells but contain thyroglobulin *(11)*. Although often categorized as a variant of follicular carcinoma, some ITCs show papillary differentiation. Accordingly, some pathologists believe that ITC is derived from follicular epithelium but should be considered as a separate pathologic entity *(11)*. Point mutations found in some ITCs at codon 61 of the N-RAS gene also suggest that this tumor represents a *de novo* entity distinct from follicular carcinoma *(10)*.

ITCs are unusually large invasive tumors that often penetrate blood vessels and grow through the thyroid capsule. Although they can be diagnosed by FNA biopsy, the cytology is usually interpreted as "suspicious for follicular neoplasm" and ITC thus should be included in the differential diagnosis of such lesions *(12)*. Compared to PTC, ITC presents at an older age (54 vs 36 yr) with larger primary tumors (4.7 vs 2.5 cm) and fewer neck metastases (36% vs 50%) but more distant metastases (26% vs 2%), and has a worse 30-yr cancer-specific mortality rate (25% vs 8%) *(13)*. In a study of ITC and tall cell carcinoma (a highly virulent form of PTC), univariate analysis of disease-free interval showed that prognosis was determined by patient age, tumor size, extrathyroidal extension, and lymph node metastases *(14)*. However, patients with ITC had significantly worse outcomes than those with tall cell carcinoma. ITC can also occur in children in whom it is usually responsive to thyroidectomy and ^{131}I therapy, but may have an aggressive clinical course and may be fatal *(15,16)*. In older patients, ITC is less likely to concentrate [131]I *(15,17)*. However, this is not always the case. One patient, who presented with an autonomously functioning thyroid nodule that caused severe thyrotoxicosis, was found to have ITC metastatic to a cervical lymph node and both lungs *(18)*. The primary tumor and its metastases contained an activating mutation of the TSH receptor gene that accounted for its hyperfunction, and perhaps its aggressive behavior *(18)*.

ATC is an exceptionally invasive malignancy with extremely aggressive behavior and a poor prognosis. Mutations in the *p53* suppressor gene occur almost exclusively in poorly differentiated thyroid tumors and its prevalence is highest in ATC, suggesting that *p*53 inactivation may confer aggressive properties and further loss of differentiated function in these neoplasms. In the past, ATC accounted for approximately 5–10% of thyroid carcinomas *(19)*, but in recent years its incidence has been lower and now accounts for about 2% of all thyroid cancers in the U.S. *(2)*. In a review of 475 patients with this disease reported in six large studies, the mean age at the time of diagnosis was 65 yr with only a slight female predominance *(19)*. Almost all ATCs evolve from well-differentiated tumors *(19)*. Although an occasional case of anaplastic medullary thyroid carcinoma occurs, most arise from well-differentiated papillary or follicular thyroid carcinoma or occasionally from follicular adenomas *(19)*.

Typically both thyroid lobes are involved and the tumor is invasive and poorly demarcated from surrounding neck tissues. Histologically, ATCs exhibit three distinct morphologic patterns—spindle cell, giant cell, and squamoid features—often with frequent mitotic figures. The immunohistochemical proof of the follicular origin of ATC is staining with epithelial markers, the most useful of which is low-molecular-weight keratin (cytokeratin) expressed in up to 80% of cases, which our patient demonstrated *(20)*. Other markers may be detected, although as many as 30% of ATCs express no tumor markers *(21)*. Some stain for thyroglobulin, which is of little diagnostic value because its detection is so variable, ranging from none to 70% in different studies *(19)*. ATC usually contains little thyroglobulin and thus fails to raise the serum thyroglobulin very much or not at all, which happened in our patient as his tumor became more undifferentiated (see Table 5).

Almost two-thirds of patients with ATC present with a rapidly enlarging neck mass, often without preexisting goiter, and up to half have symptoms of tracheal compression and invasion, usually with dyspnea or stridor *(20)*. Symptoms often appear abruptly, being present for less than 3 mo in almost half the patients *(22)*. Rapid tumor growth often causes neck pain that may mimic subacute thyroiditis, probably caused by tumor necrosis and invasion of neck tissues. Hoarseness and cough, sometimes with hemoptysis, and systemic symptoms of fever or weight loss are often present. Although most patients have normal thyroid function, thyrotoxicosis rarely occurs, probably from rapid thyroid tissue necrosis releasing thyroid hormone *(19)*.

On examination, ATC is typically a stoney hard, poorly circumscribed mass that is fixed to surrounding structures. In one large study *(22)*, 60% of ATCs presented as a multinodular goiter and 38% presented as an apparently isolated thyroid nodule, whereas only 2% caused diffuse thyroid enlargement. The tumors are characteristically quite large and may be associated with palpable cervical lymph nodes. About 80% are larger than 5 cm and half are accompanied by palpably enlarged cervical lymph nodes; about one-third of the tumors cause vocal cord paralysis *(22)*. Stridor that occurs when the patient's neck is extended portends serious airway obstruction and should raise the question of elective tracheostomy to protect the airway. The tumor may cause a superior mediastinal syndrome with venous distention and edema of the face, arms, and neck. Thus at the time of his initial presentation, our patient had many clinical features of ATC caused by an extremely aggressive ICT.

At the time of diagnosis, only about one-third of patients with ATC have distant metastases, mostly to the lung, but about half the patients eventually developed them *(19,20,22)*. Metastases are typically large isolated lesions that do not concentrate [131]I.

Although a diagnosis of thyroid malignancy is almost always possible by FNA cytology, ATC may be difficult to distinguish from thyroid lymphoma, MTC and other forms of undifferentiated thyroid carcinoma such as ITC, or cancers metastatic to the thyroid gland. Nonetheless, the giant and spindle cell patterns of ATC usually predominate, sometimes with multinucleated giant cells, suggesting the correct diagnosis. Although MTC often shows a spindle cell population, it usually can be correctly identified by FNA cytology that may stain for amyloid or calcitonin (19). Non-Hodgkin's thyroid lymphoma can be identified by FNA, usually by its small cells, but open biopsy and histochemical staining may be necessary to differentiate it from ATC, especially when the lymphoma is composed of large cells. Poorly differentiated "insular" thyroid carcinoma may be mistaken for ATC, which occurred in our patient. Most cases of ATC diagnosed by FNA should have open biopsy with immunohistochemical staining to confirm the diagnosis.

ATC has a dismal prognosis. Typically, it cannot be completely resected because of its invasion into adjacent neck structures, causing death from the effects of local tumor invasion, particularly asphyxiation. In one large study (23), more than 50% of patients died from suffocation, whereas the others died of a combination of effects from the primary tumor and metastases. Median survival has been only 4–6 mo in most large series reported over the past two decades (19,22). This has not improved substantially in recent years. For example, a large study in 1961 reported that 61% of 119 patients with ATC died within 6 mo and 77% had died within a year of diagnosis (24). Almost 30 yr later, another large study of 121 patients with ATC reported a mean survival of 7 mo (20). This is why lymphomas, MTC, and other tumors such as insular carcinoma that resemble ATC—but typically are more responsive to therapy and have a substantially better prognosis—must be carefully identified by immunohistochemical studies.

It was apparent at the time of presentation that our patient had an aggressive thyroid malignancy with a poor prognosis. Men with thyroid carcinoma, especially those over age 60 yr at the time of diagnosis, have an especially poor prognosis. In our series of patients with differentiated thyroid carcinoma, 10-yr survival rate in patients over age 60 yr was 36% for men and 50% for women ($p < 0.03$) (25). Although our patient had ITC, based on his age, gender, clinical presentation, and tumor stage, therapy was approached as though this were an ATC, which typically is very resistant to any form of therapy and is rarely cured. Surgery, chemotherapy, or radiotherapy used separately generally has not been effective (26–28). The best survival rates are reported following combined surgery, external irradiation and chemotherapy (29).

Unlike surgery for differentiated thyroid carcinoma, less than total thyroidectomy with resection of the involved adjacent neck tissues and cervical lymph nodes should be done for ATC if possible, without resorting to radical surgery. In the large Mayo Clinic series (22), 41% of the patients had surgical resection—mostly total lobectomy with subtotal resection of the contralateral lobe—in an attempt to cure the patient. In the M. D. Anderson Hospital series (20), approximately 45% of the patients underwent total thyroidectomy. However, in neither series did the extent of surgery influence the survival rate. Total thyroidectomy and radical neck dissection results in an increased complication rate without conferring a clear advantage over a more conservative approach. When the tumor is resectable, an appropriately aggressive and safe surgical approach is to resect the tumor with wide margins of adjacent soft tissue on the involved side.

Airway management is an important facet of initial therapy. Our patient had a tracheostomy in place for almost 2 yr before we felt assured that he would not succumb from strangulation by local tumor, which may comprise the airway either by compression alone, displacement or infiltration with the malignancy, and less often as the result of neurogenic dysfunction. Management involves thyroid gland resection and decompression of the airway when there is compression or displacement alone, and tracheostomy when the airway is infiltrated with tumor. Many patients require tracheostomy during the course of their disease, mainly to relieve airway obstruction but also as a precautionary measure before initiating external radiation therapy. External irradiation may cause tumor edema that acutely exacerbates airway obstruction. More than half the patients in the Mayo Clinic series required tracheostomy at some time during the course of their disease *(22)*.

After treatment with surgery and conventional radiotherapy, less than 5% of patients with ATC survive 5 yr, although survivors who are disease-free at 2 yr may live for longer periods *(19)*. Because conventional external irradiation fails to eradicate local disease, larger radiation doses may be given at closer intervals, but the toxicity is very high, resulting in severe esophagitis and dysphagia, spinal cord necrosis, and death *(28,30)*.

There is no consensus on the selection of chemotherapeutic agents for patients with A:TC, mainly because this tumor is so resistant to chemotherapy. None provides clearly superior therapeutic efficacy, and the selection is often based as much upon the side-effect profiles of the drugs as potential efficacy. Doxorubicin is perhaps the most commonly used, administered either alone or in combination with other drugs. The usual doxorubicin dosage has been between 60–90 mg/m^2 body surface *(19)*. In one study *(31)*, the response rate (complete or partial remission) with this dose of doxorubicin used alone was almost 40% in 248 patients with advanced thyroid carcinoma of all types, but was only 22% for 77 patients with ATC *(31)*. Remission duration is relatively short, with a median period of 90 (range 33–560) d in the 20%–30% who respond to doxorubicin *(19)*. When there is a response to doxorubicin, pulmonary metastases respond to therapy most frequently, followed by bone metastases and local tumor growth; however, it may not control local disease *(19)*.

One regimen consisting of combination doxorubicin and hyperfractionated radiation therapy for anaplastic thyroid carcinoma has been shown to provide better results than either treatment given alone *(32)*. The protocol in this study consists of once weekly administration of low-dose doxorubicin (10 mg/m^2) and hyperfractionated radiation therapy carried out with a fractional dose of 160 cGy per treatment twice a day for 3 d per wk. The total tumor dose is nearly 6000 cGy delivered over about 40 d. Nine patients underwent this combination treatment and eight achieved complete tumor regression in the primary treated area; six remained free of neck disease until death or their last follow-up. The protocol was well tolerated with little morbidity. In 1987, the authors reported their results in 19 patients with ATC that were treated with the same protocol *(33)*. Complete tumor response was observed in 84% of the patients and local tumor control rate was 68% at two years. Median survival was 1 yr, but most patients eventually developed distant metastases and died from the disease.

This patient's low serum Tg levels portend a poor prognosis with degeneration of the ITC to ATC, which was found on the biopsy done in January 2000 that showed the tumor to be undifferentiated without intracellular thyroglobulin. His relatively asymptomatic state from the tumor despite its aggressive nature and the fact that no conventional therapy was available suggested that he should be entered into a therapeutic trial using a new class of drugs.

REFERENCES

1. Mazzaferri EL. Thyroid carcinoma: papillary and follicular. In: Mazzaferri EL, Samaan N, eds. Endocrine Tumors. Blackwell Scientific, Cambridge, MA, 1993, pp. 278–333.

2. Hundahl SA, Fleming ID, Fremgen AM, Menck HR. A National Cancer Data Base report on 53,856 cases of thyroid carcinoma treated in the US, 1985-1995. Cancer 1998;83:2638–2648.

3. Robbins J, Schneider AB. Radioiodine-induced thyroid cancer: studies in the aftermath of the accident at Chernobyl. Trends Endocrinol Metab 1998;9:87–94.

4. LiVolsi VA. Unusual variants of papillary thyroid carcinoma. In: Mazzaferri EL, Kreisberg RA, Bar RS, eds. Advances in Endocrinology and Metabolism. Mosby-Year Book, St. Louis, MO, 1995, pp. 39–54.

5. Nikiforov Y, Gnepp DR. Pediatric thyroid cancer after the Chernobyl disaster: Pathomorphologic study of 84 cases (1991-1992) from the Republic of Belarus. Cancer 1994;74:748–766.

6. Ain KB. Papillary thyroid carcinoma etiology, assessment, and therapy. Endocrinol Metabol Clin North Am 1995;24:711–760.

7. Ron E, Lubin JH, Shore RE, et al. Thyroid cancer after exposure to external radiation: A pooled analysis of seven studies. Radiat Res 1995;141:259–277.

8. Schneider AB, Shore Freedman E, Ryo UY, Bekerman C, Favus M, Pinsky S. Radiation-induced tumors of the head and neck following childhood irradiation. Prospective studies. Medicine (Baltimore) 1985; 64:1–15.

9. Carcangiu ML, Zampi G, Rosai J. Poorly differentiated ("insular") thyroid carcinoma. A reinterpretation of Langhans' "wuchernde Struma". Am J Surg Pathol 1984;8:655–668.

10. Pilotti S, Collini P, Mariani L, et al. Insular carcinoma—A distinct de novo entity among follicular carcinomas of the thyroid gland. Am J Surg Pathol 1997;21:1466–1473.

11. LiVolsi VA. Follicular lesions of the thyroid. In: LiVolsi VA, ed. Surgical Pathology of the Thyroid. W. B. Saunders, Philadelphia, PA, 1990, pp. 173–212.

12. Guiter GE, Auger M, Ali SZ, Allen EA, Zakowski MF. Cytopathology of insular carcinoma of the thyroid. Cancer 1999;87:196–202.

13. Burman KD, Ringel MD, Wartofsky L. Unusual types of thyroid neoplasms. Endocrinol Metabol Clin North Am 1996;25:49–68.

14. van den Brekel MW, Hekkenberg RJ, Asa SL, Tomlinson G, Rosen IB, Freeman JL. Prognostic features in tall cell papillary carcinoma and insular thyroid carcinoma. Laryngoscope 1997;107:254–259.

15. Hassoun AAK, Hay ID, Goellner JR, Zimmerman D. Insular thyroid carcinoma in adolescents—A potentially lethal endocrine malignancy. Cancer 1997;79:1044–1048.

16. Sanz J, Cerpa F, Dominguez M, et al. [Insular carcinoma of the thyroid]. Rev Med Chil 1999;127:329–331.

17. Marchesi M, Biffoni M, Biancari F, et al. Insular carcinoma of the thyroid. A report of 8 cases. Chir Ital 1998;50:73–75.

18. Russo D, Tumino S, Arturi F, et al. Detection of an activating mutation of the thyrotropin receptor in a case of an autonomously hyperfunctioning thyroid insular carcinoma. J Clin Endocrinol Metab 1997; 82:735–738.

19. Mazzaferri EL. Undifferentiated thyroid carcinoma and unusual thyroid malignancies. In: Mazzaferri EL, Samaan N, eds. Endocrine Tumors. Blackwell Scientific, Boston, MA, 1993, pp. 378–398.

20. Venkatesh YS, Ordonez NG, Schultz PN, Hickey RC, Goepfert H, Samaan NA. Anaplastic carcinoma of the thyroid. A clinicopathologic study of 121 cases. Cancer 1990;66:321–330.

21. LiVolsi VA, Brooks JJ, Arendash Durand B. Anaplastic thyroid tumors. Immunohistology. Am J Clin Pathol 1987;87:434–442.

22. Nel CJ, van Heerden JA, Goellner JR, et al. Anaplastic carcinoma of the thyroid: a clinicopathologic study of 82 cases. Mayo Clin Proc 1985;60:51–58.

23. Tallroth E, Wallin G, Lundell G, Lowhagen T, Einhorn J. Multimodality treatment in anaplastic giant cell thyroid carcinoma. Cancer 1987;60:1428–1431.

24. Woolner LB, Beahrs OH, Black BM, McConahey WM, Keating RF Jr. Classification and prognosis of thyroid carcinoma. Am J Surg 1961;102:354–387.

25. Mazzaferri EL, Jhiang SM. Long-term impact of initial surgical and medical therapy on papillary and follicular thyroid cancer. Am J Med 1994;97:418–428.

26. Lu WT, Lin JD, Huang HS, Chao T. Does surgery improve the survival of patients with advanced anaplastic thyroid carcinoma? Otolaryngol Head Neck Surg 1998;118:728–731.

27. Asakawa H, Kobayashi T, Komoike Y, et al. Chemosensitivity of anaplastic thyroid carcinoma and poorly differentiated thyroid carcinoma. Anticancer Res 1997;17:2757–2762.

28. Mitchell G, Huddart R, Harmer C. Phase II evaluation of high dose accelerated radiotherapy for anaplastic thyroid carcinoma. Radiother Oncol 1999;50:33–38.

29. Tennvall J, Lundell G, Hallquist A, et al. Combined doxorubicin, hyperfractionated radiotherapy, and surgery in anaplastic thyroid carcinoma: report on two protocols. Cancer 1994;74:1348–1354.
30. Simpson WJ. Anaplastic thyroid carcinoma: a new approach. Can J Surg 1980;23:25–27.
31. Ahuja S, Ernst H. Chemotherapy of thyroid carcinoma. J Endocrinol Invest 1987;10:303 310.
32. Kim JH, Leeper RD. Treatment of anaplastic giant and spindle cell carcinoma of the thyroid gland with combination Adriamycin and radiation therapy. A new approach. Cancer 1983; 52:954–957.
33. Kim JH, Leeper RD. Treatment of locally advanced thyroid carcinoma with combination doxorubicin and radiation therapy. Cancer 1987;60:2372–2375.

7

Cushing's Syndrome

James W. Findling, MD

CONTENTS

CASE #1: CUSHING'S DISEASE: DIFFICULTIES IN DIAGNOSIS

Case Description

A 38-yr-old woman was referred because of a 75-lb weight gain over the past 7 yr. She has noticed some increasing facial fullness and has had some problems with climbing stairs. She has had insomnia and nocturia for the past 3 yr and complains of some easy bruisability. She recently suffered a stress fracture in her right foot. She has maintained normal menstrual periods, but has had a decreased libido. She complains of emotional lability over the past 2 yr. She denied any history of diabetes, hypertension, or kidney stones.

Her past medical history is remarkable for a left oophorectomy 6 mo ago for a ruptured ovarian cyst. She has recently been receiving some counseling for depression. There is a family history of thyroid disease in her mother and diabetes in both maternal grandparents. She has had two pregnancies and two healthy children. There is no history of significant alcohol use and she does not smoke.

Examination showed a slightly cushingoid woman (see Fig. 1) with a BP of 130/90, pulse 88, height 63", weight 222 lbs. She had some mild facial rounding with very slight plethora. Her skin was not thin. She did have a slight increase in supraclavicular fullness as well as a dorsocervical fat pad. The thyroid examination was normal. She had good muscle strength and no peripheral edema.

Biochemical evaluation showed the following 24-h urine free cortisol (UFC) measurement obtained during a 3-mo period: 222 µg, 42 µg, 78 µg, and 54 µg (normal <50 µg/d). An overnight 1-mg dexamethasone suppression test yielded a serum cortisol of <1 µg/dL. An 11:00 PM salivary cortisol level was 5.3 nmol/L (0.4–3.6 nmol/L).

Computed tomography (CT) of the abdomen showed a 4-cm mass in the right adrenal gland and the left adrenal gland appeared normal. A cystic area of 2 cm was noted on the

From: *Contemporary Endocrinology: Challenging Cases in Endocrinology*
Edited by: M. E. Molitch © Humana Press Inc., Totowa, NJ

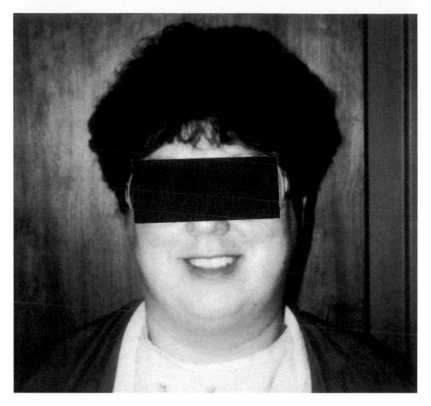

Fig. 1. A young woman with a 75-lb. weight gain over 7 yr.

right ovary. A CT scan of the pituitary gland showed a convexity of the pituitary gland but no discrete pituitary lesion was identified. Because of claustrophobia, the patient would not undergo an MRI of the pituitary.

The patient was referred for inferior petrosal sinus adrenocorticotropic hormone (ACTH) sampling. The results are outlined in Table 1. A left-sided pituitary corticotroph adenoma was suspected based on these results and she was referred to an experienced pituitary neurosurgeon.

At the academic medical center where she was referred, she was initially seen by an endocrinologist who did not believe she had spontaneous Cushing's syndrome. The patient was admitted to a clinical research center and underwent the 2-d low-dose dexamethasone suppression test (dexamethasone 0.5 mg every 6 h × 8 doses). On the second day of this test, the urine free cortisol and 17-hydroxycorticosteroids were undetectable. She was referred back to her private endocrinologist.

Another late-night salivary cortisol level was 4.9 nmol/L (0.3–3.6) and a dexamethasone corticotropin releasing hormone (CRH) test was performed. The results are shown in Table 1. After these studies, the pituitary neurosurgeon agreed to operate on this woman. Transsphenoidal surgery demonstrated a 2-mm left corticotroph microadenoma, which was successfully removed and was followed promptly by secondary adrenal insufficiency. Within 24 mo, her pituitary-adrenal axis recovered. Subsequent CT of the adrenals showed regression of the 4-cm adrenal nodule. The patient lost 60 lbs and is very pleased with her clinical outcome.

Table 1
Case 1

Inferior Petrosal Sinus Sampling
ACTH (pg/mL)

Time	Location		
	Rt IPS	*Lt IPS*	*P*
0	51	160	22
100 µg oCRH IV			
+2	73	406	30
+5	287	704	40

	Dexamethasone-CRH Test			
Time	[a]*0'*	*15'*	*30'*	*60'*
Cortisol (µg/dL)	1.1	1.9	3.2	2.9
ACTH (pg/mL)	8	19	19	22

[a]CRH 100 µg IV given after dexamethasone 0.5 mg orally every 6 h for 48 h.

Discussion

The diagnosis of Cushing's syndrome represents a very challenging problem for clinical endocrinologists, particularly when the degree of hypercortisolism is mild *(1)*. The differentiation of patients with true spontaneous Cushing's syndrome from the large number of patients with Cushing's phenotype may be very difficult. Clinicians are certainly familiar with the remarkable similarities between the metabolic syndrome X and Cushing's syndrome. Excessive and sustained cortisol secretion has long been associated with the entire spectrum of the metabolic syndrome X including obesity, insulin resistance, dyslipidemia, hypertension, and impaired glucose tolerance resulting in morbid sequelas of atherosclerosis and cardiovascular disease. Recognition of subclinical hypercortisolism in some patients with incidentally discovered adrenocortical tumors and the clinical improvement observed in these patients following adrenal surgery has increased the importance of discovering and treating even mild Cushing's syndrome *(2)*.

Clinical features that enhance the index of suspicion for endogenous hypercortisolism include the presence of facial rounding with plethora, increased supraclavicular fullness, proximal myopathy, cutaneous wasting (skin-fold thickness in the dorsum of the right hand <2 mm), osteoporosis, and neuropsychiatric problems. Although the patient described here did not have an established diagnosis of hypertension, elevated blood pressure is present in the majority of patients. Our patient had upper-body obesity, but did not appear grossly Cushingoid. She did have some mild plethora and increased supraclavicular fullness, as well as subjective (albeit no objective evidence) of weakness. She also had some neuropsychiatric issues (emotional lability, insomnia, decreased libido). Certainly, the constellation of clinical features in this patient mandated an evaluation for possible Cushing's syndrome.

The measurement of a 24-h UFC determination is considered the most useful diagnostic test in establishing the presence or absence of Cushing's syndrome. Introduction of high-performance liquid chromatography (HPLC) has provided the most specific means of measuring UFC. Normal subjects usually have UFC <50 µg/24 h with this technique. UFC determinations have been shown to have diagnostic sensitivity and specificity as high as 98–100% in some series (3); however, a recent study comparing UFC measured by HPLC with a competitive binding method for urine cortisol determination, showed that 7 of 29 patients with proven Cushing's syndrome had normal UFC with either method (4). This sobering observation creates considerable concern regarding the negative predictive value of urine cortisol measurements in the diagnosis of Cushing's syndrome. At least 10–15% of patients with Cushing's syndrome will have at least one of four 24-h UFCs within the normal range (5). The patient described here illustrates this point.

Low-dose dexamethasone suppression testing has been used as a diagnostic aid in the evaluation of patients with suspected Cushing's syndrome for four decades (6). Unfortunately, these tests have poor sensitivity and specificity. The case presented here amplifies this point. The classic 2-d low-dose dexamethasone suppression test (dexamethasone 0.5 mg orally every 6 h for 48 h with measurement of urine steroid) has been shown to have sensitivity of only 79%, specificity 74%, and diagnostic accuracy of 71% in patients with mild Cushing's syndrome (7). In addition, the overnight 1-mg dexamethasone suppression test has been shown to not be much better. Reported cutoff values for the suppression of serum cortisol in studies using contemporary immunoassay techniques range from 3.6–7.2 µg/dL (8). A recent extensive review assessing the utility of the overnight 1-mg dexamethasone suppression test in the diagnosis of Cushing's syndrome suggests that the dexamethasone-induced suppression of plasma cortisol to <1.8 µg/dL effectively excludes Cushing's syndrome (8). As it has become increasingly obvious that some patients with mild ACTH-dependent Cushing's syndrome demonstrate unusual sensitivity to dexamethasone suppression, this much lower criterion must be employed to provide adequate sensitivity for the test; however, the false-positive rate will almost certainly increase and thereby decrease the overall diagnostic utility of the test. A recent study (9) has shown that 13 of 73 patients (17.8%) with Cushing's syndrome suppressed serum cortisol to <5 µg/dL and that six of these patients actually had plasma cortisol levels <2 µg/dL following the overnight 1-mg dexamethasone suppression test. Obviously, the patient described here had exquisite glucocorticoid negative feedback and suppressed both plasma and urine cortisol to plasma urine steroids to very low levels following low-dose dexamethasone suppression testing. Needless to say, other clinical and biochemical features must be taken into consideration in establishing the presence or absence of Cushing's syndrome.

Patients with endogenous hypercortisolism of any etiology usually have a disrupted diurnal rhythm. Although morning cortisol levels in patients with Cushing's syndrome overlap those of normal subjects, increased cortisol secretion at or near the time of the nadir has been a consistent finding in patients with spontaneous Cushing's syndrome. Several studies have shown that late-night (11:00 PM–midnight) plasma cortisol determinations are useful in discriminating patients with Cushing's syndrome from those with Cushing's phenotype or pseudo-Cushing's states (e.g., depression, alcoholism, eating disorders) (10,11). Plasma cortisols >1.8 µg/dL while sleeping at midnight provides a diagnostic sensitivity of nearly 100% for Cushing's syndrome; however, this technique requires inpatient hospitalization for at least 48 h and is currently impractical as a screening test.

More recently, the determination of late-night salivary cortisol has been shown to be a simple and effective means of screening for possible Cushing's syndrome (12). Salivary cortisol concentration is highly correlated with free (biologically active) serum or plasma cortisol and is independent of the rate of saliva flow. Saliva can be easily collected in a commercially available collection device which involves chewing on cotton for 2 min. Elevations of salivary cortisol greater than the upper limit of the normal reference range (3.6 nmol/L) has been shown to yield a diagnostic sensitivity of 90–95%. In addition, late-night salivary cortisol has been shown to provide good discrimination between patients with proven Cushing's syndrome and patients referred with Cushing's phenotype. Our patient described here had modest but persistent elevations of 11:00 PM salivary cortisols consistent with her slightly elevated UFC determination. In our experience, the presence of elevations of UFC and 11:00 PM salivary cortisol yielded diagnostic specificity of essentially 100% for Cushing's syndrome. Similarly, normal UFC in combination with normal 11:00 PM salivary cortisol essentially exclude the diagnosis.

The endocrinologist who evaluated this patient prior to pituitary surgery relied on the low-dose dexamethasone suppression testing to exclude the diagnosis of Cushing's syndrome; however, the presence of mild but persistent elevations of UFC and salivary cortisol certainly seem to suggest the presence of mild Cushing's syndrome. The findings in the inferior petrosal sinus ACTH sampling are consistent with the diagnosis of Cushing's disease (pituitary ACTH-dependent Cushing's syndrome) only if the patient actually has spontaneous Cushing's syndrome. Obviously, normal subjects will have a pituitary ACTH gradient which surprisingly may often lateralize into either the left or right petrosal sinus *(13)*. In order to provide further diagnostic certainty, a dexamethasone-CRH test was performed.

This test has been designed to distinguish Cushing's syndrome from patients with pseudo-Cushing states (depression and alcoholism) as well as from normal subjects *(7, 14)*. The dexamethasone-CRH test takes advantage of the overt sensitivity of patients with Cushing's syndrome to both dexamethasone and CRH by combining these tests. Dexamethasone (0.5 mg every 6 h) is administered eight times starting with a dose at 12:00 PM and with the last dose at 6:00 AM prior to the dynamic studies. CRH (1 µg/kg) is administered intravenously at 8:00 AM. A plasma cortisol >1.4 µg/dL measured 15 min after the administration of CRH correctly identified patients with Cushing's syndrome. The major liability of this test is its cumbersomeness and the exquisite assay sensitivity needed for cortisol determinations. Most commercially available assays for cortisol do not provide the degree of sensitivity and specificity needed to interpret this test properly. Our group has seen at least four false-positive studies. In our experience, plasma ACTH response to this test is actually of greater diagnostic utility than the serum cortisol. Patients with Cushing's disease usually have plasma ACTH levels >15 pg/mL sometime during the test. Patients without Cushing's syndrome usually have plasma ACTH levels <10 pg/mL throughout the test. The dexamethasone-CRH test in our patient was abnormal by anyone's criterion.

Finally, our patient also had a large (4 cm) right adrenal nodule. At least 20% of patients with ACTH-dependent Cushing's syndrome may have unilateral or bilateral adrenal nodules that can, on occasion, be mistaken for an adrenal-dependent cortisol-producing neoplasm *(15)*. Now with the widespread availability of reliable, sensitive and specific plasma ACTH assays, the ACTH-dependency of these nodules should be easily established and diagnostic confusion avoided. As was the case in our patient, these nodules often regress following removal of the ACTH-secreting neoplasm.

REFERENCES

1. Findling JW, Raff H. Newer diagnostic techniques and problems in Cushing's disease. Endocrinol Metab Clin North Am 1999;28:191–210.
2. Reincke M, Nieke J, Kustin GP, et al. Preclinical Cushing's syndrome in adrenal incidentalomas: comparison with adrenal Cushing's syndrome. J Clin Endocrinol Metab 1992;75:826–832.
3. Huang CM, Zweig M. Evaluation of a radioimmunoassay of urinary cortisol with extraction. Clin Chem 1989;35:125,126.
4. Lin CL, Wu TJ, Machacek DA, Jiang NS, Kao PC. Urinary free cortisol and cortisone determined by high performance liquid chromatography in the diagnosis of Cushing's syndrome. J Clin Endocrinol Metab 1997;82:151–155.
5. Nieman LK, Cutler GB Jr. The sensitivity of the urine free cortisol measurement as a screening test for Cushing' syndrome. In: Program and Abstracts of the 72nd Ann Mtg Endocr Soc, June 1990, Atlanta, GA, p. 230.
6. Liddle GW. Tests of pituitary adrenal suppressibility in the diagnosis of Cushing's syndrome. J Clin Endocrinol Metab 1960;12:1539–1560.
7. Yanovski JA, Cutler GB Jr, Chrousos GP, et al. Corticotropin-releasing hormone stimulation following low-dose dexamethasone administration. JAMA 1993;269:2232–2238.
8. Wood PJ, Barth JH, Friedman DB, et al. Evidence for the low dose dexamethasone suppression to screen for Cushing's syndrome–recommendations for a protocol for biochemistry laboratories. Ann Clin Biochem 1997;34:222–229.
9. Findling JW, Shaker JL, Brickner RC, et al. Low-dose dexamethasone suppression testing cannot be used to exclude Cushing's syndrome. In: Programs and Abstracts of the 81st Ann Mtg Endocr Soc, June 1999, San Diego, CA, p. 90.
10. Papanicolaou DA, Yanovski JA, Cutler GB, et al. A single midnight cortisol measurement distinguishes Cushing's syndrome from pseudo-Cushing states. J Clin Endocrinol Metab 1998;83:1163–1167.
11. Newell-Price J, Trainer P, Perry L, et al. A single sleeping midnight cortisol has 100% sensitivity for the diagnosis of Cushing'' syndrome. Clin Endocrinol 1995;43:545–550.
12. Raff H, Raff JL, Findling JW. Late-night salivary cortisol as a screening test for Cushing's syndrome. J Clin Endocrinol Metab 1998;83:2681–2686.
13. Yanovski JA, Cutler GB Jr, Doppman JL, et al. The limited ability of inferior petrosal sinus sampling with corticotropin-releasing hormone to distinguish Cushing's disease from pseudo-Cushing states or normal physiology. J Clin Endocrinol Metab 1993;77:503–509.
14. Yanovski JA, Cutler GB Jr, Chrousos GP, Nieman LK. The dexamethasone-suppressed corticotropin-releasing hormone stimulation test differentiates mild Cushing's disease from normal physiology. J Clin Endocrinol Metab 1998;83:348–352.
15. Doppman JL, Miller DL, Dwyer AJ, et al. Macronodular adrenal hyperplasia in Cushing's disease. Radiology 1988;166:345–347.

CASE #2: ECTOPIC ACTH SYNDROME

Case Description

The patient is a 45-yr-old man referred to an endocrinologist because of rapid onset of severe hypertension and lower extremity edema. Severe weakness, fatigue, and a weight gain of 10–12 lbs developed over a 3 mo period of time. He was unable to perform his job as a maintenance worker. There had been some emotional lability.

His past medical history was remarkable for congenital absence of the left kidney. His family history was unknown as he was adopted. He had never smoked and rarely used alcohol.

Examination showed a mildly cushingoid man whose blood pressure was 142/98 mmHg, pulse 96, height 69-3/4", weight 191 lbs. There was some mild facial rounding but no real plethora. He did have a slight increase in supraclavicular fullness. There was no proptosis or abnormal eye findings. His thyroid gland was not enlarged. He had

Table 2
Case 2

| | Inferior Petrosal Sinus Sampling ACTH (pg/mL) | | |
| | *Location* | | |
Tme	*Rt IPS*	*Lt IPS*	*P*
0'	243	246	217
100 μg oCRH IV			
+2'	210	249	187
+5'	238	236	191

| Intravenous ACTH Sampling | |
Site	*Plasma ACTH (pg/mL)*
Arterial	63
Brachiocephalic Trunk (left)	132
R subclavian	87
Superior vena cava	77
R atrium	86
R pulmonary vein	84
Abd. vena cava	71

normal genitalia. He had significant proximal muscle weakness and he was unable to get out of the chair without assistance.

Initial laboratory studies showed a sodium of 143 mEq/L, potassium 2.4 mEq/L, chloride 98 mEq/L, bicarbonate 29 mEq/L. Random blood glucose was 132 mg/dL.

A basal 24-h UFC was 2200 μg/d and fell to 92 μg/d following the 2-d high-dose dexamethasone suppression test. A plasma ACTH level was 89 pg/mL (9–52). Pituitary CT was normal (MRI was precluded because of metal hardware in his left inner ear) and the patient was referred for pituitary neurosurgery.

Fortunately, the neurosurgeon referred this man for inferior petrosal sinus ACTH sampling. The results of the study are shown in Table 2. There was no evidence of pituitary ACTH gradient either before or after CRH administration. Somatostatin receptor scintigraphy (octreotide acetate) was normal. A chest CT did show a right lower lobe abnormality. Trimethoprim-sulfamethoxazole prophylaxis for *Pneumocystis carinii* was initiated and the patient underwent a right lower lobe lobectomy removing a noncaseating granuloma with no change in intraoperative ACTH and persistent hypercortisolism. A few days later, the patient underwent an intrathoracic venous sampling procedure. Remarkably, a significant increase in ACTH was found in the left brachiocephalic trunk (see Table 2). Repeat high-resolution CT scan through the anterior mediastinum did show an 8-mm mass. This lesion was removed by mediastinoscopy with immediate intraoperative decrease in ACTH and secondary adrenal insufficiency. The pathology report demonstrated a thymic carcinoid tumor with positive immunocytochemistry for ACTH.

The patient had complete clinical remission of Cushing's syndrome and secondary adrenal insufficiency persisted for 19 mo. Three years following surgery, the patient underwent further testing and was found to have a 24-h UFC of 9 μg/d and a plasma ACTH of

25 pg/mL. Five years following his initial presentation, the patient developed rapid onset again of generalized edema, hypertension, and weakness. A 24-h UFC was 3110 µg and a plasma ACTH was 1022 pg/mL. CT of the chest demonstrated a 2×1.2-cm soft-tissue mass in the anterior mediastinum just below the level of the previous surgical clips. Trimethoprim-sulfamethoxazole was started. A sternotomy was performed removing a well-differentiated 2-cm thymic carcinoid tumor. One small lymph node also demonstrated a small metastasis of 3 mm. Immunocytochemistry was strongly positive for ACTH. Postoperatively, hypercortisolism persisted (24-h UFC of 300 µg/d). The patient's postoperative course was complicated by intrathoracic hemorrhage following anticoagulation for a left subclavian vein thrombosis. After a protracted hospitalization and recovery from the venous thrombosis, the patient underwent laparoscopic bilateral adrenalectomy and clinical and biochemical resolution of his hypercortisolism. He is currently on maintenance glucocorticoid and mineralocorticoid support. The postoperative chromogranin A level is elevated at 15.5 ng/mL (1.6–5.6) and is serving as a potential tumor marker. The patient continues to have serial chest radiographs and CT imaging.

Discussion

This patient illustrates not only the great difficulty in distinguishing pituitary ACTH-dependent Cushing's syndrome from the occult ectopic ACTH syndrome, but also the problems frequently encountered in the discovery and treatment of patients with non-pituitary ACTH-dependent hypercortisolism. Distinguishing Cushing's disease from the occult ectopic ACTH syndrome with certainty requires a thoughtful and common sense approach. Cushing's disease is predominantly a disorder of women with most reported series showing a 6:1 female/male ratio. On the other hand, the ectopic ACTH syndrome is equally distributed between the sexes. As a rule, patients with Cushing's disease have, in retrospect, signs and symptoms of hypercortisolism developing over several years. In contrast, patients with ectopic ACTH-secreting neoplasms usually have the onset of signs and symptoms of hypercortisolism over a period of time of less than 1 yr. Furthermore, spontaneous hypokalemia and metabolic alkalosis is unusual in Cushing's disease (10% of patients), but is present in almost 50% of patients with the ectopic ACTH syndrome *(1)*. Therefore, the rapid onset of ACTH-dependent hypercortisolism with hypokalemia in our male patient must raise considerable concern regarding the possibility of a nonpituitary neoplasm regardless of the findings of any other tests.

The measurement of plasma ACTH is an important part of the evaluation *(2)*. Although plasma ACTH levels are generally higher in patients with the ectopic ACTH syndrome than those with Cushing's disease, there is overlap between these two disorders. Nonpituitary tumors may secrete many of the posttranslational peptides of proopiomelanocortin (POMC). Crosby et al. *(3)* have developed a two-site immunoradiometric assay for the measurement of ACTH precursors. This assay measures peptides containing POMC (31KD) or pro-ACTH (22KD). Although values are greater in patients with ectopic ACTH than those with Cushing's disease (see Fig. 2), we have still observed considerable overlap in these patient groups.

Traditionally, endocrinologists have used high-dose dexamethasone suppression testing to help distinguish pituitary from nonpituitary sources of ACTH hypersecretion. Unfortunately, the use of high-dose dexamethasone suppression testing in the differential diagnosis of ACTH-dependent Cushing's syndrome yields a diagnostic sensitivity,

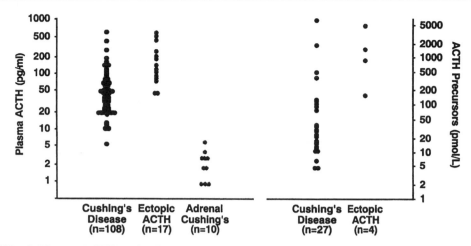

Fig. 2. Plasma ACTH and ACTH precursor levels in patients with Cushing's syndrome.

specificity, and accuracy of only 80% *(4)*. Several groups of investigators have attempted to improve the diagnostic accuracy of high-dose dexamethasone suppression testing by changing the diagnostic criterion. For example, Flack and coworkers *(5)* collected urine for 6 d with the first 2 d as controls. During the next 2 d, subjects were given 0.5 mg of dexamethasone every 6 h and during the last 2 d, 2 mg of dexamethasone every 6 h. Only the patients with Cushing's disease had >90% suppression of UFC and for 17-hydroxy-corticosteroids. This study demonstrated that the 50% cutoff value, which had been used in the past should be abandoned; however, the problem with using the strict 90% suppression cutoff was that it generated 30% misclassification of patients with Cushing's disease (false-negative results). Our patient suppressed basal elevations of UFC to 96% following the high-dose dexamethasone suppression test. This finding resulted in referral to a pituitary neurosurgeon in what could have been a surgical misadventure.

Our group has recently reported a series of patients with ectopic ACTH syndrome and Cushing's disease in whom high-dose dexamethasone suppression testing was performed by their referring endocrinologist *(6)*. In this series, 3 of 15 patients with ectopic ACTH syndrome had >90% suppression of high dose dexamethasone (see Fig. 3). There was really no difference in the characteristics of dexamethasone suppression testing in patients with Cushing's disease than those with the occult ectopic ACTH syndrome. Even more compelling is the finding that a logistic model of clinical variables was not only better than high-dose dexamethasone suppression testing, *per se*, but was not improved by the addition of high-dose dexamethasone suppression testing. For example, the combination of female gender, young age, long duration of symptoms, modest elevation of UFC, lack of hypokalemia, and a normal or only slightly elevated plasma ACTH showed a 98% sensitivity, 78% specificity, and 90% diagnostic accuracy for Cushing's disease. Surely, the continuation of high dose dexamethasone suppression testing in the differential diagnosis of ACTH-dependent Cushing's syndrome cannot be justified.

Fortunately, in our patient, common sense prevailed and more precise diagnostic studies were performed. Pituitary imaging with MRI is an important part of the evaluation of ACTH-dependent Cushing's syndrome. Rarely, patients with Cushing's disease may have a large corticotroph macroadenoma and further studies are not required. However, the

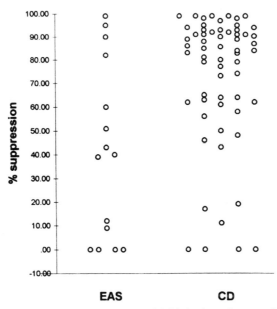

Fig. 3. Percent suppression of cortisol secretion with high-dose dexamethasone in patients with either Cushing's disease (CD) *n* = 61 or ectopic ACTH (EAS) *n* = 15.

majority of patients have either equivocal or normal findings. Because it is well appreciated that nearly 10% of normal subjects have pituitary MRI findings consistent with a small pituitary lesion *(7)*, the interpretation of any pituitary MRI patients with ACTH-dependent Cushing's syndrome must be interpreted cautiously. The normal pituitary CT in our patient offered no help in the differential diagnosis; even if the study has been consistent with a small lesion, the clinical presentation of this male patient demanded a more definitive diagnostic procedure.

The only reliable and accurate means of distinguishing pituitary from nonpituitary ACTH-dependent Cushing's syndrome is the use of bilateral simultaneous inferior petrosal sinus sampling (IPSS) with CRH stimulation. In experienced centers, the diagnostic accuracy of IPSS approaches 95–100% *(8,9)*. Nonetheless, the results from a recent large-scale retrospective multicenter study demonstrated that the overall sensitivity, specificity, accuracy of IPSS was only in the 80–90% range *(10)*. In addition, IPSS has been associated with morbid and even fatal complications including deep vein thrombosis, pulmonary emboli, and brainstem vascular damage *(11)*. In a recent series of 166 patients done in an experienced center *(12)*, IPSS was associated with only one episode of a transient neurologic event (VI nerve palsy), and there were no cases of pulmonary thromboembolism. IPSS is an invaluable resource in the differential diagnosis of many patients with ACTH-dependent Cushing's syndrome, but it must be performed in dedicated and experienced centers in order to provide accurate results with as little morbidity as possible.

The IPSS results in our patient were unequivocal. There was no evidence of pituitary ACTH-gradient either before or after CRH administration. As this patient illustrates, the search for the occult ectopic ACTH-secreting neoplasm may be difficult.

The ectopic ACTH syndrome is usually associated with neuroendocrine tumors. Small cell lung carcinoma is thought to represent such a neuroendocrine tumor and accounts for the majority of the cases with ectopic ACTH associated with a clinically apparent neo-plasm. On the other hand, bronchial carcinoid tumors represent the majority of cases with radiologically occult tumors (13). Medullary thyroid carcinoma, pancreatic islet cell neoplasia, pheochromocytoma, and carcinoid tumors of almost any other origin are also well recognized causes of ectopic ACTH production (1).

The majority of patients with occult ectopic ACTH are found to have small bronchial carcinoid tumors. Computed tomography of the chest and abdomen will be helpful in revealing potential sources of ectopic ACTH production. For example, islet cell tumors producing ACTH are always larger than 2 cm and usually have metastasized to liver by the time Cushing's syndrome appears. Medullary carcinoma of the thyroid may easily be detected by measurement of serum calcitonin and patients usually have extensive dis-ease by the time hypercortisolism is discovered. Pheochromocytoma may also be a source of ectopic ACTH and these tumors are always visible on CT imaging of the adrenal glands.

CT imaging of the chest identified a small lesion in the right lower lobe of our patient, which seemed to be the most obvious source of his ectopic ACTH. MRI of the chest has also been helpful in identifying central bronchial carcinoid tumors, which may be <1 cm in diameter and confused with normal pulmonary vasculature on CT scan. Our patient could not have an MR of the chest done because of metal hardware present in his inner ear for a hearing problem.

Unfortunately, a right lower lobectomy in our patient removed only a noncaseating granuloma with no decrease in plasma ACTH and persistence of hypercortisolism follow-ing the procedure. Our group has shown that a complete removal of ACTH-secreting bronchial carcinoid tumors can be detected intraoperatively by greater than 50% decrease in ACTH by 15 minutes. Modification of the ACTH immunochemiluminescent assay to 15-min incubation allows the documentation with successful tumor removal in the oper-ating room (14).

Although wide ranging venous sampling and bronchial lavage for ACTH are usually ineffective in detecting occult tumors, further investigation of our patient with sampling from pulmonary venous effluent discovered an increase in plasma ACTH in the left brachiocephalic (innominate) vein. High-resolution CT imaging showed a mediastinal mass of 8 mm. Primary thymic carcinoid tumors are also a potential source of ectopic ACTH production. Although some have suggested that thymic vein sampling may be a reliable technique for identifying ACTH-producing thymic carcinoid tumors, elevated levels of ACTH in thymic vein samples may reflect ACTH production by pulmonary bronchial carcinoid tumors, mediastinal metastasis, thymic carcinoid, or diffuse hyper-plasia in intrathymic neuroendocrine elements (15). Consequently, with no obvious tumor in the anterior mediastinum, it may not be consistent with a thymic lesion.

Thymic enlargement (pseudotumors of the thymus) has also been described in patients with ectopic ACTH syndrome following resolution of the hypercortisolism either medi-cally or with bilateral adrenalectomy. Tabarin et al. (16) has described five patients with the ectopic ACTH syndrome in whom a thymic mass was discovered 6–14 mo after remis-sion of hypercortisolism. Exploratory thoracotomy was performed in four cases and resulted in the removal of an enlarged, but normal thymus. The mechanism of this abnor-mality is thought to be thymic depletion resulting from hypercortisolism followed by (rebound) thymic hyperplasia when cortisol levels are decreased.

Because some ectopic ACTH-secreting neoplasms have somatostatin receptors, soma-tostatin receptor scintigraphy (SRS) has also been proposed as a means of localizing these ectopic ACTH-secreting tumors that are not found with conventional imaging. Recently, Tabarin et al. *(17)* reported this technique in 12 patients with the occult ectopic ACTH syndrome. Whole-body planar SRS using ^{111}In-pentetreotide was performed 19 times in these 12 patients. Five patients had negative SRS and conventional imaging studies and the source of ACTH secretion remains occult following several months of follow-up in four of these patients, whereas a 2-cm ileal carcinoid tumor with liver and micrometastasis was found at laparotomy in one patient 14 mo after presentation. SRS was positive in 4 of the 12 patients with a false positive in one patient with a follicular thyroid adenoma. SRS identified a 10-mm pancreatic tumor that became detectable using CT scanning 9 mo later in one patient and two mediastinal lymph nodes of 10 mm previously ignored by MRI in another patient. SRS had little influence on therapeutic options in these two patients in whom no final diagnosis could be made. Repetition of this imaging technique during follow-up of patients with previously negative scans was useless. In contrast, conventional imaging was positive in 6 to 12 patients. Sensitivity of SRS for the detection of bronchial carcinoids was lower than that of thin section CT scanning. Our patient had a negative somatostatin receptor scan.

The anterior mediastinal mass in our patient was discovered to be an ACTH-secreting thymic carcinoid and was successfully removed by mediastinoscopy. The patient had abrupt reduction in plasma ACTH levels and development of secondary adrenal insufficiency which persisted for several months following the surgery. Despite a prolonged clinical and biochemical remission, the patient presented 5 yr later with recurrent and prodigious hypercortisolism with a markedly elevated plasma ACTH. CT imaging again showed a mediastinal mass and removal of this recurrent thymic carcinoid tumor resulted in attenuation but not resolution of his hypercortisolism. Immunocytochemistry was positive for ACTH and the tumor was well differentiated.

Thymic neuroendocrine tumors are quite unusual and may have combined features ranging from well differentiated (carcinoid) to small cell carcinoma. Approximately 20% of patients with primary thymic neuroendocrine tumors have Cushing's syndrome. The variability in the spectrum of the differentiation of primary thymic tumors is relevant regarding prog-nosis. Patients with more poorly differentiated neuroendocrine features have a very poor prognosis. In a recent series of 11 cases of primary thymic neuroendocrine carcinoma (two patients had Cushing's syndrome), nine of the patients had died of their tumors between 1–4 yr after the diagnosis *(18)*. The persistence of Cushing's syndrome in our patient after the second operation suggests persistent micrometastasis. In retrospect, a sternotomy and complete removal of anterior mediastinal tumor lymph nodes should have been performed at the initial presentation. Similarly, a complete lobectomy and removal of regional lymph nodes should be performed in patients with bronchial carcinoid tumors rather than a more limited procedure in order to secure a better long-term outcome *(1)*.

The postoperative course in our patient was not a smooth one. Left subclavian vein thrombosis mandated anticoagulation, which then led to intrathoracic bleeding and the need for hemotransfusion. Cushing's syndrome is a hypercoagulable state and these patients are certainly at greater risk for many post-op complications *(19)*. Our patient was treated prophylactically with trimethoprim-sulfamethoxazole in order to prevent *Pneumocystis* pneumonia. It is well appreciated that patients with severe hypercortisolism—particularly with ectopic ACTH—have significant immunosuppression and are at risk for opportunistic infections. We have observed the development of *P. carinii* pneumonia in four patients with the ectopic ACTH syndrome following initiation of adrenostatic therapy. The recognition of *P. carinii* pneumonia during lowering of cortisol levels is a result of unmasking of the intense inflammation of the pneumonia, which has been suppressed by the hypercortisolism *(20)*. Because we have routinely used prophylaxis with trimethoprim- sulfamethoxazole, we have not observed any cases of *P.* pneumonia in 18 consecutive patients with the ectopic ACTH syndrome.

The persistence of hypercortisolism in this patient demanded definitive treatment. Medical therapy with adrenostatic agents such as ketoconazole, metyrapone, and aminoglutethimide may be beneficial on a short-term basis, but can rarely be used effectively for the long-term management of patients with significant hypercortisolism. Bilateral adrenalectomy serves as a definitive means of treating these patients. Now with the use of laparoscopic adrenalectomy, this procedure can be offered to patients with minimal morbidity and mortality and relatively short hospital stays *(21)*. It is important to recognize that the hypercortisolism is often a major cause of a patient's debilitating condition and that early surgical intervention may be indicated in order to gain prompt control of the hypercortisolism even when the patient seems desperately ill.

The prognosis of patients with the ectopic ACTH syndrome largely depends on the efficacy of therapies for the neoplasm. The mean survival of patients with ectopic ACTH resulting from small cell lung carcinoma can be measured in days *(22)*. Increased mortality in these patients may be related to the opportunistic infections and catabolic state associated with severe hypercortisolism. Certainly, the prognosis in our patient is guarded and vigilant imaging follow-up for residual carcinoid tumors in his mediastinum and chest is warranted on a long-term basis. The finding of a well-differentiated tumor provides a hopeful prognosis. Because adrenalectomy has been performed, ACTH can no longer be used as a reliable tumor marker. Because chromogranin A was elevated, this neuropeptide may serve as a reasonable barometer of tumor burden.

REFERENCES

1. Findling JW, Raff H. Ectopic ACTH. In: Mazzaferri EL, Samaan NA, eds., Endocrine Tumors. Cambridge, 1993, pp. 554–566.
2. Raff H, Findling JW. A new immunoradiometric assay for corticotropin evaluated in normal subjects and patients with Cushing's syndrome. Clin Chem 1989;35:596–600.
3. Crosby SR, Stuart MF, Ratcliffe JG, White A. Direct measurement of the precursors of adrenocorticotropin in human plasma by two-site immunoradiometric assay. J Clin Endocrinol Metab 1988;67:1271–1277.
4. Findling JW, Raff H. Newer diagnostic techniques and problems in Cushing's disease. Endocrinol Metab Clin North Am 1999;28:191–210.
5. Flack MR, Oldfield EH, Cutler GB Jr, et al. Urine free cortisol in the high-dose dexamethasone suppression test for the differential diagnosis of the Cushing syndrome. Ann Intern Med 1992;116:211–217.
6. Aron DC, Raff H, Findling JW. Effectiveness versus efficacy: the limited value in clinical practice of high dose dexamethasone suppression testing in the differential diagnosis of ACTH-dependent Cushing's syndrome. J Clin Endocrinol Metab 1997;82:1780–1785.
7. Hall WA, Luciano MG, Doppman JL, et al. Pituitary magnetic resonance imaging in normal volunteers: Occult adenomas in the general population. Ann Intern Med 1994;120:817–820.
8. Findling JW, Kehoe ME, Shaker JL, et al. Routine inferior petrosal sinus sampling in the differential diagnosis of adrenocorticotropin (ACTH)-dependent Cushing's syndrome: early recognition of the occult ectopic ACTH syndrome. J Clin Endocrinol Metab 1991;73:408–413.
9. Oldfield EH, Doppman JL, Nieman LK, et al. Petrosal sinus sampling with and without corticotropin-releasing hormone for the differential diagnosis of Cushing's syndrome. N Engl J Med 1991;325:897–905.

10. Invitti G, Giraldi FP, deMartin M, Cavagnini F. The Study Group of the Italian Society of Endocrinology on the Pathophysiology of the Hypothalamic-Pituitary-Adrenal Axis: Inferior petrosal sinus sampling in patients with Cushing's syndrome and contradicting responses to dynamic testing. Clin Endocrinol 1999;51:255–257.
11. Miller DL, Doppman JL, Peterman SB, et al. Neurologic complications of petrosal sinus sampling. Radiology 1992;185:143–147.
12. Lefournier V, Gatta B, Martinie M, et al. One transient neurological complication (sixth nerve palsy) in 166 consecutive inferior petrosal sinus samplings for the etiological diagnosis of Cushing's syndrome. J Clin Endocrinol Metab 1999:84:3401–3402.
13. Pass HI, Doppman JL, Nieman L, et al. Management of the ectopic ACTH syndrome due to thoracic carcinoids. Ann Thorac Surg 1990;50:52–57.
14. Raff H, Shaker JL, Siefert PE, Werner PH, Hazelrigg SR, Findling JW. Intraoperative measurement of adrenocorticotropin (ACTH) during removal of ACTH-secreting bronchial carcinoid tumors. J Clin Endocrinol Metab 1995;80:1036–1039.
15. Doppman JL, Pass HI, Nieman LK, et al. Corticotropin-secreting carcinoid tumors of the thymus: diagnostic unreliability of thymic venous sampling. Radiology 1992;184:71–74.
16. Tabarin A, Catargi B, Chausan P, et al. Pseudo-tumor of the thymus after correction of hypercortisolism in patients with ectopic ACTH syndrome: a report of five cases. Clin Endocrinol 1995;42:207–213.
17. Tabarin A, Valli N, Chanson P, et al. Usefulness of somatostatin receptor scintigraphy in patients with occult ectopic adrenocorticotropin. J Clin Endocrinol Metab 1999;84:1193–1202.
18. Noran CA, Suster S. Thymic neuroendocrine carcinomas with combined features ranging from well-differentiated (carcinoid) to small cell carcinoma. Am J Clin Pathol 2000;113:345–350.
19. Blevens, LS Jr, Clark RV, Owens DS. Thromboembolic complications after inferior petrosal sinus sampling in patients with Cushing's syndrome. Endocr Prac 1998;4:365–367.
20. Findling JW, Buggy BP, Segerson TP, Raff H. Pneumocystis carinii pneumonia complicating intermittent Cushing's syndrome. Wisc Med J 1986;85:23–25.
21. Weisnagel SJ, Gagner M, Beton G, Pomp A, Pharand D, Lacroix A. Laparoscopic adrenalectomy. The Endocrinologist 1996;6:169–178.
22. Dimopoulos NA, Fernandez JF, Samaan NA, Holoye PY, Vassilopou Lou-Sellin R. Paraneoplastic Cushing's syndrome as an adverse prognostic factor in patients who die early with small cell lung cancer. Cancer 1992;69:66–71.

CASE #3: CUSHING'S SYNDROME IN A CHILD

Case Description

The patient is an 11-yr-old female who has not grown in the past 18 mo despite an approximately 20-lb weight gain (see Fig. 4) associated with increasing facial rounding and plethora. She is prepubertal. There has been some evidence of breast development. She has noticed some increasing hair on her chest, back, and arms. Easy bruisability and emotional lability have been noted. She has no history of hypertension or diabetes. There is no family history of any endocrinopathy. She is not receiving any medications. She is a 6th-grade student maintaining excellent grades during the past year.

Examination showed a cushingoid-appearing 11-yr-old girl whose height was 130.7 cm (52") and weight 85 lbs. Her blood pressure was 104/70 mmHg, pulse 68 bpm. She had facial rounding with plethora and generalized obesity with increases in supraclavicular fullness. There were no abnormal eye findings and her thyroid gland was normal. She had good muscle strength and no peripheral edema.

Laboratory studies confirmed the presence of ACTH-dependent hypercortisolism. A 24-h urine free cortisol (UFC) was 205 µg/d (normal <30 µg/d) and morning serum cortisol 29 µg/dL decreased only to 22 µg/dL following overnight 1-mg dexamethasone suppression test. A pituitary MRI was unremarkable and a basal plasma ACTH was 54 pg/mL (normal: 9–52 pg/mL).

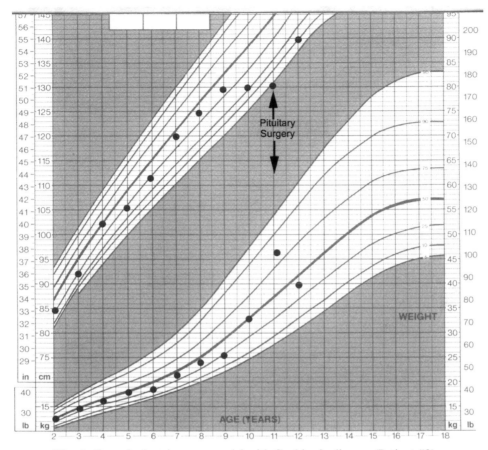

Fig. 4. Growth chart in a young girl with Cushing's disease (Patient #3).

In order to confirm the differential diagnosis of Cushing's syndrome in this girl, bilateral simultaneous inferior petrosal sinus ACTH sampling with CRH stimulation was performed. The results are shown in Table 3. There was an unequivocal pituitary ACTH gradient that lateralized before and after CRH administration into the right petrosal sinus. There was also an exaggerated peripheral ACTH response to CRH. These findings were consistent with a right-sided pituitary ACTH-secreting microadenoma and the patient was referred to an experienced pituitary neurosurgeon.

Transsphenoidal pituitary surgery was performed and complete exploration of the pituitary revealed no evidence of a microadenoma. Based on the results of the IPSS, a right hemi-hypophysectomy was performed. Despite the fact that no definite tumor was identified during surgery or even in the histological specimen submitted to the laboratory, the patient promptly developed secondary adrenal insufficiency, which persisted for 2 yr following surgery. The patient had a significant weight loss of 10 lbs and gained 8 cm in height within 6 mo of surgery. Menarche occurred 20 mo following surgery. She had normal thyroid and adrenal function, as well as normal menstrual cyclicity 6 yr following the procedure.

Table 3
Case 3

| | Inferior Petrosal Sinus Sampling ACTH (pg/ml) | | |
| | | Location | |
Time	Rt IPS	Lt IPS	P
0'	210	40	37
50 µg oCRII IV			
+2'	2326	141	53
+5'	3161	158	124

Discussion

Cushing's syndrome is rare in children. The hallmark of endogenous hypercortisolism in children is growth failure and weight gain. Some children whose illness starts before the first decade of life may present with premature sexual development, presumably caused by increased secretion of adrenal androgens. On the other hand, older children (13–14 yr of age) may be prepubertal possibly because of hypogonadism induced by the hypercortisolism. Bone age is actually consistent with chronological age in most patients, reflecting the combined effects of cortisol, which should have an inhibitory effect and adrenal androgens, which have a stimulatory effect on bone development. Mental changes are less common in children and their school performance is often excellent in contrast to the job performance of adults with Cushing's syndrome. Unlike adults, the female predominance in Cushing's disease is not as dramatic and spontaneous Cushing's syndrome occurs probably with equal frequency in boys and girls (1).

The differential diagnosis of Cushing's syndrome in children is similar to that of adults; however, ectopic ACTH may be less common, accounting for <5% of Cushing's syndrome in children. Primary adrenal disease is seen in approximately 10% of children with Cushing's and, like adults, pituitary ACTH-secreting tumors predominate (1).

The biochemical studies needed to secure the diagnosis of Cushing's syndrome in children are similar to those in adults. Determination of free cortisol in the urine over a 24-h period is felt to be the single best test. The normal range in children appears to be somewhat less than adults, the upper reference range usually being around 30 µg/24 h (usually 50 µg/24 h in adults). The overnight 1-mg dexamethasone suppression test has not been standardized in children. The 2-d, classic low-dose dexamethasone suppression test in children employs a dose of 20 µg/kg/d (2). One series showed that none of the children studied suppressed their free cortisol to <30 µg/d following low-dose dexamethasone for 2 d (2). In small children whose UFC determinations is difficult (if not impossible), late night (11:00 PM to midnight) salivary cortisols have been used with very good sensitivity and specificity.

Our patient had a typical presentation for Cushing's syndrome with mild hypercortisolism and very slight elevation of plasma ACTH. Despite a normal pituitary imaging study, the most likely cause of the Cushing's syndrome in this patient was a small pituitary ACTH-secreting microadenoma. The only reasonable way to secure this diagnosis was with inferior petrosal sinus sampling and IPSS provided evidence of a right-sided tumor.

Although IPSS is an extremely useful diagnostic aid for establishing the diagnosis of Cushing's disease, its use for the localization of pituitary microadenomas is more controversial. An intrapetrosal sinus ratio of 1.4 or greater has been suggested as being consistent with lateral localization of a microadenoma *(3)*. The clinical effectiveness of this procedure for lateralization appears to relate to the expertise and experience of the invasive radiologist *(4)*. Bilateral IPSS localizes the pituitary tumor in 85–90% of patients in our center; however, other series have reported rates ranging from 70–100%, with an average of about 75–80%. Booth et al. *(5)* have recently evaluated the ability of imaging and IPSS to localize an ACTH-secreting pituitary lesion in comparison with definitive histopathologic examination of the pituitary gland in patients with Cushing's disease. Lateralization of a pituitary tumor was identified in 31 of 32 patients in whom bilateral IPSS was achieved. Histological examination confirmed a corticotroph adenoma in 28 of these patients and corticotroph hyperplasia in the other two. One patient was found to have an ectopic sphenoid corticotroph adenoma. Accurate localization of the pituitary lesion was much better when based on IPSS results vs imaging studies (70% vs 49%, respectively). In eight patients with discrepant results, IPSS is more likely than pituitary imaging to reveal the final pathology (62% vs 13%, respectively). In nine patients with completely normal pituitary imaging, IPSS accurately localized the lesion in 89%.

Our patient certainly reflects the importance of IPSS in the localization of these tumors. Despite very careful intraoperative exploration, a microadenoma could not be located. Hemihypophysectomy in this young girl resulted in a very gratifying clinical remission manifested by secondary adrenal insufficiency and preservation of anterior pituitary function with development of menarche and a pubertal growth spurt. The histological absence of any corticotroph microadenoma is not unusual in patients cured from Cushing's disease *(6)*. The relatively high number of cases with negative histological findings who undergo remission following pituitary surgery suggest that these patients with Cushing's syndrome do not reflect a different etiologic group but the adenomatous tissue is lost during the process of surgical removal or pathologic examination. It certainly seems reasonable to offer hemihypophysectomy to patients who have unequivocal lateralization of their pituitary ACTH gradient, particularly if intraoperative findings are unremarkable.

The long-term outcome in children in adolescence after transsphenoidal surgery for Cushing's disease is favorable. Two large series of pituitary microsurgery for Cushing's disease in children has shown an initial remission rate of 83–95% *(7,8)*. Nonetheless, relapses may occur any time following successful surgery and long-term follow-up is necessary in these children. Devoe et al. *(9)* reported a recurrence rate of 27% 1–6 yr following successful surgical remission of Cushing's syndrome. Nonetheless, repeat transsphenoidal surgery in these patients resulted in remission in 6 of 8 patients. Although conventional radiation treatment, with or without concomitant mitotane treatment, can be offered as an alternative therapy, most experienced clinicians reserve such treatment to only those patients with more aggressive, invasive, and surgically unresectable tumors. As always, bilateral adrenalectomy may be necessary in some patients in whom pituitary surgery, radiation therapy, or medical treatment is unsuccessful.

REFERENCES

1. Leinung MC, Zimmerman D. Cushing's disease in children. Endocrinol Metab Clin North Am 1994;23: 629–639.

2. Streeten DH, Stevenson CT, Dalakos TG, et al. The diagnosis of hypercortisolism: biochemical criteria differentiating patients from lean and obese normal subjects and from females on oral contraceptives. J Clin Endocrinol Metab 1969;29:1191–1211.
3. Oldfield EH, Chrousos GP, Schulte HB, et al. Preoperative localization of ACTH-secreting pituitary microadenomas by bilateral and simultaneous inferior petrosal sinus sampling. N Engl J Med 1985;310: 100–103.
4. Findling JW. Inferior petrosal sinus sampling: pros and cons; when and where. J Endocrinol Invest 2000; 23:193–195.
5. Booth GL, Redelmeier DA, Grossman H, et al. Improved diagnostic accuracy of inferior petrosal sinus sampling over imaging for localizing pituitary pathology in patients with Cushing's disease. J Clin Endocrinol Metab 1998;83:2291–2295.
6. Semple PL, Vance ML, Findling J, Laws ER Jr. Transsphenoidal surgery for Cushing's disease: outcome in patients with a normal MRI scan. J Neurosurg 2000;46:553–559.
7. Styne DM, Grumbach MM, Kaplan SL, Wilson CB, Conte FA. Treatment of Cushing's disease in childhood and adolescence by transsphenoidal microadenomectomy. N Engl J Med 1984;310:889–893.
8. Magiakou MA, Nastorakas G, Oldfield EH, et al. Cushing's syndrome in children and adolescents: prevention, diagnosis, and therapy. N Engl J Med 1994;331:629–636.
9. Devoe DJ, Miller WL, Conte FA, et al. Long-term outcome in children and adolescents after transsphenoidal surgery for Cushing's disease. J Clin Endocrinol Metab 1997;82:3196–3202.

8

Adrenal Insufficiency and Adrenal Cancer

Erik K. Alexander, MD *and Robert Dluhy,* MD

CONTENTS

CASE #1: A RAPIDLY EXPANDING ADRENAL MASS

Case Description

A 43-yr-old male initially presented to his primary care physician with the complaint of 3 d of right-sided abdominal pain. The pain was dull, located diffusely in the right upper quadrant of his abdomen and flank, and at times penetrated to the back. He denied any relation of the pain to food intake. In addition, he denied any jaundice, nausea, vomiting, fevers, or chills. His exam was unremarkable with the exception of mild right upper quadrant abdominal pain with moderate palpation. His physician was concerned with the possibility of gall bladder pathology, and pursued an abdominal ultrasound of the right upper quadrant. The ultrasound revealed no evidence of biliary disease, but an incidental finding of a right adrenal mass, measuring approximately 2 cm, was noted (see Fig. 1). No further testing was performed, and the patient's pain resolved without therapy. Approximately 3 yr later, the patient again presented with pain located in his right upper abdomen, similar to his previous episode. An ultrasound of the biliary tract was performed, and revealed two gallstones, without signs of obstruction or inflammation. The incidental right adrenal nodule was again noted, and measured at 3 cm in size. Subsequently, an abdominal and pelvic computerized tomography (CT) scan was performed without contrast and revealed a 3.5-cm homogeneous right adrenal mass, rounded in configuration, with attenuation slightly less than the adjacent liver (20 Hounsfield units). No other masses or adenopathy were seen, and the contralateral adrenal gland was normal in appearance.

The patient was otherwise healthy except for borderline hypertension, with blood pressures averaging 140–150/85–90 mmHg. He denied paroxysmal headaches, sweating,

From: *Contemporary Endocrinology: Challenging Cases in Endocrinology*
Edited by: M. E. Molitch © Humana Press Inc., Totowa, NJ

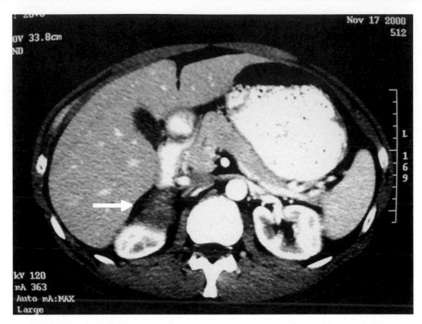

Fig. 1. CT scan of the abdomen revealing a 2 cm right adrenal mass.

or palpitations. In addition, he denied significant weight change, proximal weakness, acne, or striae. His physical exam was unremarkable, and he was noted to be noncushingoid. His abdomen was soft, without hepatosplenomegaly, and no masses could be appreciated. He would consistently note, however, vague tenderness in the right upper quadrant of his abdomen with deep palpation. Two separate 24-h urine collections were evaluated for excess catecholamine secretion, and were within normal limits. His serum electrolytes, including potassium, were normal.

Given the change in size of the adrenal mass on imaging, his physician was appropriately concerned, and pursued further radiologic evaluation by obtaining an abdominal magnetic resonance image (MRI). The study confirmed a 3.5-cm right adrenal nodule, occupying the anterior-most aspect of the gland. The mass did not completely replace the normal adrenal gland, and was, therefore, less likely to represent a malignant lesion. Gradient echo sequences showed no excess fat content in the lesion. It was recommended to the patient that CT scan-guided fine-needle aspiration biopsy (FNAB) be performed on the lesion to assess for malignancy. This procedure occurred uneventfully, and the results revealed adrenocortical cells with no evidence of a malignant process. With this information, the physician reassured the patient, and follow-up at regular intervals was suggested, or, if any change occurred in his clinical status.

The patient had an unrevealing course for the next year, but then again, had the occurrence of similar, but more intense, right-sided abdominal pain, that prompted a reevaluation. Repeat CT scanning of his abdomen and pelvis revealed a nonhomogeneous mass now measuring 5.5 cm, located superior to the right kidney. The remainder of the scan was normal. It was felt that the heterogeneity represented adrenal hemorrhage into the adrenal mass. His physical exam remained normal except for some vague tenderness in the right upper quadrant of his abdomen. Routine laboratory studies were normal.

He was then referred to another physician for further evaluation and possible treatment. A 24-h urine sample was collected, and revealed no sign of excess catecholamine excretion. Given the history of significant change in size of the adrenal lesion over time, as well as the change in appearance of the lesion on recent imaging, it was suggested that the patient undergo surgical excision. He tolerated the procedure well. The pathology was consistent with adrenal carcinoma, showing both capsular and lymphatic invasion.

The patient has subsequently had resolution of his abdominal pain, and follow-up CT scans have shown no signs of tumor recurrence over three years since his surgery.

Discussion

This case exemplifies many of the difficulties with initial evaluation and subsequent follow-up of incidentally discovered adrenal nodules. It is well documented that incidentally found, asymptomatic adrenal nodules (i.e., "incidentalomas") are quite prevalent, and increase in frequency as the population ages *(1–3)*. In the majority of cases, these lesions represent nonmalignant, nonhypersecreting, adrenocortical adenomas. However, it is clear that a small percentage of such lesions will secrete excessive amounts of adrenal hormones, or represent malignant disease (either primary adrenal carcinoma, or metastatic disease to the adrenal gland).

The patient presented at age 43 with new onset, vague, abdominal pain. His physicians were appropriately concerned with the possibility of gallbladder pathology, but imaging noted only an adrenal mass, and no other anatomic etiology for his complaints. As incidentally discovered adrenal nodules present with no associated local symptoms, an adrenal nodule associated with pain is not asymptomatic, and therefore cannot truly be viewed as an incidentaloma. Therefore, adrenal masses associated with pain should be aggressively investigated, as such lesions may represent more serious disorders.

On initial evaluation of an adrenal mass, the physician should consider possible hyperfunctionality by means of a thorough history and physical examination. Hypertension may be an important clue because many functioning adrenal masses are associated with elevated blood pressure. Biochemical testing should assess for possible overproduction of cortisol, aldosterone, or catecholamines. Although this patient received appropriate evaluation for excessive catecholamine production via a 24-h urine collection, no assessment of excess cortisol, androgen, or aldosterone was pursued. Generally, this would be accomplished with a 1-mg overnight dexamethasone suppression test or 24-h urine collection for free cortisol, and random serum aldosterone and renin levels. Mantero et al. studied 992 patients with adrenal incidentalomas over 1 cm in size, and found hyperfunctionality in 9.0% of their study population *(4)*. In this study, 5.2% of this population had Cushing's syndrome, 3.1% had pheochromocytomas, and 0.7% had primary hyperaldosteronism *(4)*. In addition, a recent study by Kudva et al. found that as many as 10% of all adrenal pheochromocytomas present as adrenal incidentalomas *(5)*. It is also important to note that a negative history or the lack of clinical findings do not rule out the possibility of overproduction of cortisol, catecholamines, aldosterone, or dehydroepiandosterone sulfate (DHEA-S). There is general agreement that hyperfunctionality of any adrenal lesion warrants surgical removal.

The patient was subsequently seen on an infrequent basis, and no further follow-up of his adrenal lesion was performed for 3 yr. This point is of utmost importance, as the second major predictor used to determine need for resection of an adrenal lesion is its size. Both size of the lesion at the time of diagnosis, and change in size over time, are very useful predictors of the probability of adrenal carcinoma. Although rare, the possibility of adrenal carcinoma increases with the size of the lesion at initial diagnosis. In addition, whereas the 5-yr survival for all patients with adrenocortical carcinoma is approximately 16%, the 5-yr survival for patients with limited disease is approximately 40%. This stresses the point that removal of such lesions prior to continued growth and invasion is crucial, as surgical resection at early stages is the most effective therapy.

The exact size of an adrenal incidentaloma at which to recommend surgical removal is controversial. Numerous studies have suggested size cutoffs ranging between 3–6 cm. The seminal recommendation for removal of lesions greater than 6 cm was made by Copeland et al. in 1983 (1). This study reported the prevalence of biochemically silent adrenocortical carcinomas was <1/250,000, and the prevalence of benign adenomas >6 cm, based on autopsy series, was about 1/4000. Using these data, it was noted that 60 operations on such patients would be needed to discover one adrenocortical carcinoma. These data, however, have been recently reevaluated by Herrera et al. (6) who suggest significantly different recommendations. Specifically, they note that it would take only three operations (not 60) to remove one carcinoma on patients with 6 cm incidental adrenal masses. Using 5 and 4 cm as cutoffs, they suggest it would require only 6 and 12 operations, respectively (6). One other important caveat is that radiologic determination of adrenal nodule size has been shown to significantly underestimate (about 80%) the actual size of the lesion when subsequently measured after resection. The current consensus suggests removal of an adrenal mass that is greater that 4–5 cm, or demonstrates significant increase in size on close follow-up (3–6 mo). The patient clearly did not meet criteria for surgical removal of his lesion based on size at the time of initial presentation (2 cm), but importantly, a CT scan was not performed to accurately determine the true size of the lesion or other radiographic features such as heterogeneity.

It is generally felt prudent to follow patients such as above with routine, periodic CT scan examinations. The exact interval needed has not been conclusively determined, in part, will be dictated by the age of the patient, suitability for surgery, and other risk/benefit assessments (7). Shorter intervals (every 3–6 mo) are recommended the first 1–2 yr following diagnosis, and in younger patients. If no evidence of growth is documented, it is then generally recommended to follow such lesions on a yearly or bi-yearly basis. This patient did not receive appropriate radiologic follow-up, which would likely have noted significant growth of the lesion.

Three years later, the patient was found to have a significant change in the size of his adrenal lesion, and his physicians were appropriately concerned. After finding no evidence for pheochromocytoma, they chose to pursue CT scan-guided biopsy of the lesion. This technique has proven useful in establishing the diagnosis of metastatic malignancies to the adrenal gland, but has no role in differentiating adrenocortical adenoma from an adrenocortical carcinoma. This patient underwent such a procedure, and the results revealed adrenocortical cells. The clinicians were falsely reassured by this finding. Pathological findings that differentiate adrenal adenoma from carcinoma cannot be determined from cytology and include capsular and vascular invasion in the surgical specimen. Thus, fine-needle or core biopsy of an adrenal mass has utility only in helping diagnose possible metastatic disease to the adrenal gland.

Recently, some attention has also been given to the use of adrenal iodocholesterol scintigraphy with [6-β-I131]iodomethyl-19-norcholesterol (NP-59). Some data had suggested that those lesions that took up NP-59 were usually benign *(3)*. However, recent studies have found that both the sensitivity and specificity of this test are poor, and it is not clinically useful.

Finally, in the evaluation of adrenal incidentalomas, the utility of DHEA-S measurement may be useful as well. Although not highly sensitive or specific, DHEA-S is a helpful marker if it is found to be very high, or subnormal *(4)*. When found to be elevated, it is supportive of the diagnosis of adrenal carcinoma. In contrary, when found to be suppressed, it is often supportive of cortisol-producing adrenal adenomas, as excess cortisol will suppress ACTH secretion and, as a result, androgen production from the normal adrenocortical tissue.

The patient subsequently was found to have a large, rapidly enlarging adrenal mass, which became heterogeneous in appearance. Although acute hemorrhage into a benign adrenocortical adenoma is possible, the heterogeneity of the lesion as described is also a more-common finding in adrenal carcinoma. The location within the adrenal gland, or the amount of unaffected gland seen radiographically have no diagnostic value. At the point of his referral to a tertiary center, there were now multiple, obvious reasons to recommend removal of his lesion. These reasons included size of the lesion (>4 cm), rapid growth of the lesion with a heterogeneous appearance, and symptoms (abdominal pain), which, in retrospect, were probably related to the mass.

In conclusion, diagnosis and follow-up of adrenal incidentalomas can be difficult, but should be primarily dictated by hyperfunctionality, and size (initially, and change over time) of the lesion.

REFERENCES

1. Copeland PM. The incidentally discovered adrenal mass. Ann Intern Med 1983;98:940–945.
2. Angeli A, Osella G, Ali A, Terzolo M. Adrenal incidentaloma: an overview of clinical and epidemiological data from the National Italian Study Group. Horm Res 1997;47:279–283.
3. Kloos RT, Gross MD, Francis IR, Korobkin M, Shapiro B, et al. Incidentally discovered adrenal masses. Endocr Rev 1995;16:460–484.
4. Mantero F, Masini AM, Opocher G, et al. Adrenal incidentaloma: an overview of hormonal data from the National Italian Study Group. Horm Res 1997;47:284–289.
5. Kudva YC, Young WF Jr, Thompson GB, Grant CS, van Heerden J. Adrenal Incidentaloma: An important component of the clinical presentation spectrum of benign sporadic adrenal pheochromocytoma. The Endocrinologist 1999;9:77–80.
6. Herrera MF, Grant CS, van Heerden JA, Sheedy, PF, Ilstrup DM. Incidentally discovered adrenal tumors: an instituitional perspective. Surgery 1991;110:1014–1021.
7. Barzon L, et al. Risk factors and long-term follow-up of adrenal incidentalomas. J Clin Endocrinol Metab 1999;84:520–526.

CASE #2: HYPERTENSION AND HYPOKALEMIA

Case Description

A 45-yr-old male presented for evaluation of hypertension. The patient first came to medical attention 30 yr ago when he was noted to be hypertensive at age 14. This was discovered in high school during a routine physical exam where he was found to have a blood pressure of approximately 190/95 mmHg. A physical exam was performed and no abnormalities were noted except for obesity (body mass index = 34 kg/m^2). An electrocardiogram (EKG), basic electrolytes (including potassium), creatinine, and urinalysis were also noted to be normal. A 24-h urine collection for catecholamine excretion was normal. His hypertension was attributed to obesity, and he was instructed to start a weight loss and exercise program; hydrochlorothiazide was started. At age 19, his blood pressure was 170/90 mmHg while on therapy. An intravenous pyelogram (IVP) and nephrogram was performed, but no renal abnormalities were identified. He had lost 25 lbs and his blood pressure was moderately improved; his medication was changed to propranolol. He continued on this medication for the next 15 yr with only moderate control of his hypertension (140–160/85–100 mmHg); he also complained of frequent headaches.

At age 40, he was seen by a new physician for worsening blood pressure control on propranolol treatment. His exam was notable for obesity, but no other abnormalities were identified. He was specifically noted not to be Cushingoid, and no abdominal bruits could be appreciated. However, he was found to be hypokalemic (3.0 mmol/L), and was started on potassium replacement (80 mmoL/d). His blood pressure was now noted to be 200/100 mmHg. He denied any excess licorice ingestion.

His past medical history was otherwise notable for peptic ulcer disease, spastic colitis, frequent headaches, and a transient (5 min) episode of left-sided weakness at age 20 that spontaneously resolved. His family history was notable for a maternal grandmother who had hypertension and died of a cerebral hemorrhage at age 66. His mother also had hypertension, as did eight maternal uncles and aunts (all diagnosed in adulthood). He has one brother, 5 yr younger, who had started treatment for hypertension at age 23.

Given the strong family history of hypertension, young age of onset, and appearance of hypokalemia, his physician pursued testing for secondary causes of his hypertension. Twenty-four-hour urine collections for catecholamine and cortisol excretion were normal. Random plasma aldosterone (PA) and plasma renin activity (PRA) levels revealed values of 37.1 ng/dL (normal = 3.0–35.0 ng/dL, normal salt diet) and <0.1 ng/mL/h (normal upright value = 0.4–8.8 ng/mL/h, normal salt diet), respectively. Given these data, a diagnosis of primary hyperaldosteronism was made. He was started on spironolactone 50 mg daily, but additionally required labetalol and losartan for blood pressure conrol. Later, his dose of spironolactone was increased to 200 mg daily. A CT scan with 5-mm slices of the adrenal glands showed no evidence of an adenoma, and was reported as normal. Given the patient's extensive family history of early-onset hypertension, it was thought he may suffer from glucocorticoid-remediable aldosteronism (GRA). However, a blood sample for the chimeric gene duplication characteristic of GRA was negative. He was, therefore, diagnosed with bilateral, idiopathic adrenal hyperplasia as a cause for primary hyperaldosteronism. The patient pursued a second opinion, and was referred to another physician who performed further testing.

To confirm the diagnosis of primary hyperaldosteronism, the patient was asked to undergo a saline suppression test (measurement of aldosterone following administration of two liters 0.9% normal saline over 4 h), which revealed failure of normal aldosterone suppression (aldosterone = 12.0 ng/dL; normal value <5.0 ng/dL). His blood pressure remained poorly controlled on spironolactone, losartan, labetalol, and hydrochlorothiazide. Potassium levels were within normal limits. A repeat CT scan with 1-mm slices revealed bilateral micronodular adrenal glands: two 4-mm nodules were seen in both the right and left adrenal glands, and a 6-mm nodule was seen in the right adrenal gland.

Given the history of early-onset hypertension, hypokalemia, and multiple small, sub-centimeter adrenal nodules seen radiographically, it was felt the exact cause of his hyper-

Table 1
Results of Right and Left Adrenal Vein
Sampling with Continuous ACTH Infusion

Time	Sampling location	Aldosterone (ng/dL)	Cortisol (mcg/dL)	Aldo/cortisol ratio
0 min	Infrarenal IVC	102	46.6	2.2
	Suprarenal IVC	24	22.4	1.1
	Lt Adrenal Vein	81	704	0.1
	Rt Adrenal Vein	2325	700	3.3
5 min	Lt Adrenal Vein	324	350	0.5
	Right Adrenal Vein	9740	560	17.4
10 min	Left Adrenal Vein	379	810	0.5
	Right Adrenal Vein	10430	560	18.6
15 min	Left Adrenal Vein	340	640	0.5
	Right Adrenal Vein	12897	620	20.8
20 min	Left Adrenal Vein	276	760	0.4
	Right Adrenal Vein	6390	480	13.3
30 min	Left Adrenal Vein	220	510	0.4
	Right Adrenal Vein	7717	520	14.8

aldosteronism could not be conclusively determined without further testing. Selective adrenal vein sampling performed under continuous ACTH stimulation revealed lateralization of aldosterone secretion to the right adrenal gland (see Table 1). The patient was referred for surgical removal of the right adrenal gland with the presumptive diagnosis of unilateral hyperplasia. This was performed laprascopically without complications, and the patient tolerated the procedure well. Pathologic examination revealed a single yellow nodule measuring $1.2 \times 1.1 \times 0.8$ cm. The remaining tissue was normal.

One month following surgery, the patient returned to clinic, and was noted to have a blood pressure of 130/80 mmHg while still requiring labetalol 300 mg daily, and 25 mg HCTZ daily. Spironolactone and losartan had been discontinued. He reported, however, new symptoms of lightheadedness upon standing, several times each day. Laboratory results revealed a sodium level of 131 mmol/L, as well as hyporeninemic hypoaldosteronism with aldosterone and renin levels of 5.9 ng/dL (normal = 3–25 ng/dL) and 1.1 ng/mL/h (normal = 0.4–8.8 ng/mL/h), respectively. Over the course of the following 6 mo, his symptoms improved, and his aldosterone, renin, and sodium levels normalized. He is currently 1 yr postsurgery, and continues on labetalol and HCTZ treatment. His blood pressure is 120/80 mmHg, and he no longer notes headaches.

Discussion

This case exemplifies some important considerations in the evaluation of the hypertensive patient. Essential hypertension is very prevalent with more than 25 million people currently diagnosed as having elevated arterial blood pressure in the United States. More attention, however, is being focused on possible secondary causes of hypertension. For example, recent data have suggested that primary aldosteronism is underdiagnosed, with up to 8% of all hypertensive patients possibly suffering from a hyperaldosterone state, even if normokalemic *(1,2)*. Other secondary causes of hypertension include renovascular hypertension, cortisol excess, and pheochromocytoma.

This patient was first noted by a physician to be hypertensive at age 14. The young age of onset of hypertension is unusual, and prompted an evaluation for secondary causes of hypertension. However, at that time, his physician only evaluated him for pheochromocytoma, and later for renal vascular disease with an IVP and nephrogram. Recent studies have shown that an IVP with nephrogram is suboptimal as a screening test, and consideration should be given to performing a captopril renogram, magnetic resonance angiogram, or an arteriogram when renal vascular disease is being investigated.

Ultimately, when this patient became hypokalemic, primary aldosteronism was diagnosed based on plasma renin and aldosterone values. The plasma aldosterone to plasma renin ratio is an effective screening test for this disorder *(3)*. In most series, a ratio of plasma aldosterone to renin of greater than 30:1 should raise suspicion of the disorder. Weinberger et al. *(4)*, have found that an aldosterone to renin ratio of >30 when found with a plasma aldosterone concentration of >20 ng/dL, is 90% sensitive and 91% specific for the diagnosis of primary aldosteronism. Confirmatory testing involves the demonstration of autonomous aldosterone production following volume expansion. Such testing includes oral salt loading, saline infusion, or Florinef administration while on a high salt diet, followed by a urine or blood aldosterone measurement. Failure to suppress aldosterone levels in these settings confirms autonomous hypersecretion. This patient subsequently underwent a saline suppression test, and had nonsuppressible aldosterone levels, confirming the diagnosis of hyperaldosteronism.

The five subtypes of primary hyperaldosteronism include: aldosterone-producing adenoma (APA), bilateral adrenal hyperplasia (BAH), adrenal carcinoma, glucocorticoid-remediable aldosteronism (GRA), and unilateral adrenal hyperplasia (UAH). All of these hyperaldosterone states are notable for the finding of an inappropriately high aldosterone level in the setting of a suppressed renin level. It can be very difficult, however, to diagnose the etiology of hyperaldosteronism in individual patients. Making the correct diagnosis, however, is of utmost importance given the differing treatments that are offered for each disorder. For APA and UAH, surgery is the treatment of choice, whereas for GRA and BAH, medical therapy is optimal. For most patients with primary aldosteronism, the difficulty is distinguishing between APA and BAH. In this setting, Blumenfeld et al. *(5)* have found that certain clinical findings correlate with APA. Specifically, these include: more severe hypertension (SBP >161 mmHg, DBP >105 mmHg); more profound hypokalemia; higher plasma (>27 ng/dL) and urinary aldosterone levels, and higher serum 18-hydroxycortisol levels (>70 ng/dL). Although patients with these findings are considered to have a high probability of APA, there is significant overlap with BAH, and correlation with radiographic findings is needed. This patient subsequently underwent CT scanning of the abdomen and adrenal glands. No adrenal nodule was noted. Note that the first scan in this patient used 5-mm slices; most experts would recommend a specific "adrenal" protocol with 1–2-mm slices, to ensure that small nodules are visualized (50% of APA are <1 cm in size) *(6)*. The second scan in this patient using such a protocol revealed bilateral micronodular adrenal glands.

Given the strong family history of juvenile onset hypertension, the possibility of GRA was appropriately considered. GRA is an autosomal dominant disorder characterized by a chimeric duplication whereby the 5'-regulatory region of the 11 β-hydroxylase gene (regulated by ACTH) is fused to the coding sequences of the aldosterone synthase gene *(7,8)*. Aldosterone synthesis is therefore abnormally and solely regulated by ACTH. Although this patient's family history was consistent with a diagnosis of GRA, direct genetic blood testing for the chimeric gene was negative. In general, this disorder should be considered in patients with early-onset hypertension, especially if there is suppressed PRA and an abnormal PA/PRA ratio. A strong family history of early cerebral hemorrhage (<35 yr) should also raise suspicion for GRA.

When faced with hyperaldosteronism in a patient without a unilateral adrenal mass, deciding on further testing can be difficult. As a result, adrenal vein sampling is used as the "gold standard" to diagnose unilateral vs bilateral aldosterone hypersecretion. It should be noted, however, that adrenal vein sampling is not needed for all patients. Data suggest that patients with a high probability of APA by clinical criteria, and a >1-cm unilateral adrenal nodule should be considered for unilateral adrenalectomy *(6)*. Other experts recommend adrenalectomy without further testing in patients with confirmed primary hyperaldosteronism, age less than 40 yr, and a unilateral, hypodense adrenal nodule on CT scanning in the setting of an anatomically normal contralateral adrenal gland. Even in this cohort, however, surgery nevertheless will reveal a small percentage of patients with BAH. As a result, patients with equivocal radiographic features should be considered for adrenal vein sampling. In this patient, the finding of primary hyperaldosteronism without evidence of a unilateral adrenal mass prompted adrenal venous sampling.

The protocol used for adrenal vein sampling, as well as the diagnostic cutoff points to confirm APA vs BAH, vary between authors. Young et al. have found the greatest predictive value associated with venous sampling during continuous ACTH infusion *(9)*. Simultaneous right and left adrenal vein samples, as well as a sample from the inferior vena cava (IVC) are collected for aldosterone and cortisol levels, and a ratio is subsequently calculated. This is termed the "cortisol-corrected" aldosterone ratio. The corresponding right and left "cortisol-corrected" aldosterone ratios are then compared. A high-side to low-side ratio of >4.0 strongly favors the diagnosis of APA, whereas a value of <3.0 suggests BAH. Using these criteria, a positive and negative predictive value of over 90% is obtained *(9)*.

This patient had significant lateralization to the right side, with a right-to-left cortisol-corrected ratio of greater than 30. This strongly suggested a right-sided APA that was not detected radiographically, or unilateral adrenal hyperplasia. He underwent removal of the right adrenal gland, with improvement in his blood pressure and correction of his potassium wasting. Pathology revealed the presence of an aldosterone-producing adenoma previously not detected by CT scanning, hidden in one limb of the right adrenal gland.

In this patient, blood pressure did not completely normalize postoperatively, and he continued to require antihypertensive medication. Presumably, this was a result of possible underlying, coexistent essential hypertension, or the effects of long-term hypertension and/or aldosterone excess on blood vessels and cardiac tissue. Interestingly, this patient experienced salt wasting, hyporeninemic hypoaldosteronism, and orthostatic symptoms for months following removal of his tumor. This was likely caused by long-standing hyperaldosteronism that led to atrophy of the juxtaglomerular apparatus in the kidneys, resulting in atrophy of the zona glomerulosa in the unaffected, contralateral adrenal gland. This situation is best managed conservatively with orthostatic precautions, and liberalizing sodium intake. With time, the renin-aldosterone axis recovered in the contralateral adrenal gland.

REFERENCES

1. Gordon RD, Stowasser M, Tunny TJ, et al. High incidence of primary aldosteronism in 199 patients referred with hypertension. Clin Exp Pharm Phys 1994;21:315–318.
2. Lim PO, Rodgers P, Cardale K, et al. Potentially high prevalence of primary aldosteronism in a primary-care population. Lancet 1999;353:40.
3. Mckenna TJ, Sequeira SJ, Heffernan A, et al. Diagnosis under random conditions of all disorders of renin-angiotensin-aldosterone axis, including primary hyperaldosteronism. J Clin Endocrinol Metab 1991;73: 952–957.
4. Weinberger MH, Fineberg NS. The diagnosis of primary aldosteronism and separation of the two major subtypes. Arch Intern Med 1993;153:2125–2129.
5. Blumenthal JD, Sealey JE, et al. Diagnosis and treatment of primary hyperaldosteronism. Ann Intern Med 1994;121:877–885.
6. Dunnick NR, Leight GS Jr, Roubidoux MA, et al. CT in the diagnosis of primary aldosteronism: sensitivity in 29 patients. Am J Roentgenol 1993;160:321–324.
7. Lifton RP, Dluhy RG, Powers M, et al. A chimaeric 11-beta-hydroxylase/aldosterone synthase gene causes glucocorticoid-remediable aldosteronism and human hypertension. Nature 1992;355:262–265.
8. Lifton RP, Dluhy RG, Powers M, et al. Hereditary hypertension caused by a chimeric gene duplication and ectopic expression of aldosterone synthase. Nat Genet 1993;2:66–74.
9. Young WF Jr, Stanson AW, Grant CS, et al. Primary aldosteronism: adrenal venous sampling. Surgery 1996;120:913–919.

CASE #3: ACUTE HYPERKALEMIA

Case Description

A 74-yr-old female with a history of type 2 diabetes and chronic obstructive pulmonary disease (COPD) was admitted to the hospital with unstable angina. During her second hospital day, the potassium level was noted to be 7.0 mmol/L (normal = 3.5–5.0 mmol/L). An urgent consult was requested to assist with the diagnosis and management of her hyperkalemia.

The patient was diagnosed with diabetes mellitus 17 yr ago, and she was initially managed with dietary therapy. Eight years ago, she was started on an oral sulfonylurea medication with good control of her glucose levels. At the present time, she is taking long-acting glipizide, 10 mg daily. A recent hemoglobin A1c was measured at 7.1% (normal 4.2–5.6%). She has no evidence of retinopathy, but a recent 24-h urine sample for microalbumin revealed a mild elevation (65 mg/24 h; normal <30.0 mg/24 h), suggesting early diabetic renal disease.

Her past medical history is notable for obesity, recurrent urinary tract infections, and COPD. There was no history of hypertension. Her current medications include albuterol (inhaled), long-acting glipizide, ibuprofen as needed, and trimethaprim/sulfamethoxazole as prophylaxis for recurrent urinary tract infections. She has no known allergies to any medication. There is a prior history of tobacco use, last noted 20 yr ago. Her family history is notable for diabetes mellitus and hypothyroidism.

On physical exam, her blood pressure was 132/84 mmHg, heart rate was 70 bpm, and she was afebrile. She weighed 60 kg, with a BMI of 28 kg/m^2. Notable findings included scant axillary and pubic hair, and a II of VI holosystolic heart murmur appreciated best at the cardiac apex. There was no abdominal guarding or flank tenderness. Her skin was normal and she was not hyperpigmented. Pertinent laboratory results showed: sodium 137 mmol/L, potassium 7.0 mmol/L, arterial pH 7.36, creatinine 1.2 mg/dL, HCO3 24 mg/dL, and glucose 140 mg/dL. Laboratory values 1 mo prior to admission revealed a potassium level of 5.0 mmol/L. Previous laboratory values over the last two years revealed potassium levels of 4.9–5.5 mmol/L.

Upon admission, the patient was initially managed with metoprolol, aspirin, intravenous heparin, simvastatin, and nitroglycerine overnight. She had received no potassium supplements. Trimethoprim/sulfamethoxazole was continued. Her chest pain resolved, and a cardiac catheterization was not performed. When the potassium level of 7.0 mmol/L was first noted, the housestaff administered insulin and glucose, and then instituted oral kayexalate. Repeat potassium level was 6.3 mmol/L later that day; the trimethoprim/sulfamethoxazole was discontinued.

The possibility of adrenal insufficiency was raised and the patient was given 2 mg of dexamethasone intravenously (iv) and underwent a rapid cosyntropin stimulation test (250 mcg iv as a bolus). The cortisol values were 5.6 mcg/dL, 16.5 mcg/dL, and 21.3 mcg/dL at 0, 30, and 60 min, respectively. The dexamethasone was stopped. It was subsequently recommended that plasma renin activity (PRA), and aldosterone levels should be checked 2 h after assuming an upright posture. The upright PRA was 0.5 ng/mL/h (normal 0.4–8.8 ng/mL/h, normal salt diet) with a simultaneous aldosterone level of 2.4 ng/dL (normal 3–35 ng/dL, normal salt diet), and potassium level of 6.7 mmol/L.

Heparin therapy was subsequently stopped, and the potassium level normalized over the subsequent 3 d as she recovered from her acute coronary event. She was discharged home on aspirin, metoprolol, simvastatin, nitroglycerine, long-acting glipizide, and albuterol (inhaled). She had multiple potassium levels checked over the following 6 mo, with values ranging between 4.9–5.4 mmol/L.

Discussion

This case provides an informative example of the causes of hyperkalemia, as well as adrenocortical dysfunction. This patient exhibited multiple factors that may have contributed to her hyperkalemia. The initial approach to hyperkalemia begins with consideration of three possible mechanisms of potassium excess: increased potassium intake, insufficient renal potassium excretion, or a disruption of normal serum/intracellular potassium equilibrium. In this case, there was a history of chronic, mild hyperkalemia (levels 5.0–5.5 mmol/L) over the past several years, with an acute increase in potassium levels upon admission. Such a history points toward an underlying abnormality that is acutely worsened by a secondary factor. There was no history of excess potassium intake and, in fact, hyperkalemia does not occur in such a setting unless there is significant reduction in creatinine clearance (<30 mL/min). There was also no evidence for acidosis to suggest an internal metabolic cause. It seems most likely, therefore, that this patient's hyperkalemia was caused by impairment of potassium excretion.

Close attention to this patient's history reveals mild hyperkalemia for several years (values of 5.0–5.5 mmol/L). The most likely cause of the prior persistent, mild hyperkalemia in this patient with long-standing diabetes mellitus is hyporeninemic hypoaldosteronism. Hyporeninemic hypoaldosteronism occurs commonly in the seventh decade of life, and is often found in the setting of mild to moderate renal insufficiency. Long-standing diabetes mellitus is the most common disease associated with hyporeninemic hypoaldosteronism, but other concurrent illnesses such as multiple myeloma, systemic lupus, amyloidosis, and sickle cell disease have also also been reported *(1)*. This patient had a history of diabetes for 20 yr, as well as evidence of a mild reduction in renal function. She also had evidence of a mild, nonanion gap, metabolic acidosis suggesting a possible type IV renal tubular acidosis, as is often seen in such patients. Although never documented, it is likely that she had a hyporeninemic hypoaldosterone state prior to her hospitalization. For such patients, the hyperkalemia is often mild, and can usually be managed with dietary potassium restriction.

The diagnosis of hyporeninemic hypoaldosteronism can be established by demonstrating subnormal stimulation of renin and aldosterone levels following provocation with upright posture and a low sodium diet, or with acute volume depletion using a diuretic such as furosemide. In most patients with long-standing diabetes, a presumptive diagnosis of hyporeninemic hypoaldosteronism can be made and laboratory confirmation is not commonly performed.

The next issue is to consider what secondary, acute process may have caused or contributed to her acute, severe hyperkalemia. When this patient was found to have acute hyperkalemia on her second day of admission, the medical team appropriately considered the possibility of primary adrenal insufficiency, and treated her with steroids while awaiting definitive testing following the cosyntropin stimulation test. The differential diagnosis of adrenal failure should include both *chronic* (autoimmune destruction, granulomatous disease), and *acute*, primary adrenal failure. This patient had no signs of hyperpigmentation, or a history of fatigue, orthostatis, or hypotension, which would have suggested chronic adrenal hypofunction. However, acute adrenal insufficiency can occur in patients who are anticoagulated in the setting of bilateral adrenal hemorrhage *(2)*. Secondary adrenal failure should not be considered as a cause of hyperkalemia as aldosterone secretion is preserved by the renin-angiotensin system. In this patient, acute and chronic primary adrenal failure was ruled out by normal cosyntropin testing (cortisol levels exceeding 18.0 mcg/dL at 60 min).

The use of trimethoprim/sulfmethoxazole (bactrim) by this patient is also important to note, as it is a possible contributory factor to her hyperkalemia. Trimethoprim (an organic cation) acts similar to amiloride and inhibits the apical membrane epithelial sodium channel in the distal nephron. As a consequence, the transepithelial voltage is reduced and potassium secretion is inhibited *(3)*. In addition, the use of ibuprofen could have contributed to a hypoaldosterone state by reducing prostaglandin levels, further reducing plasma renin levels. However, this patient had been on both trimethoprim/sulfamethoxazole and ibuprofen for several years without complications, and it therefore seems very unlikely that either medication is contributing to the acute process at the present time.

Therefore, given the normal cosyntropin stimulation test, as well as the absence of acute renal failure, attention should focus on acquired forms of selective hypoaldosteronism as the central factor causing the abrupt increase in potassium levels. The etiologies of aldosterone deficiency are numerous (*see* Table 2). The initial approach toward diagnosis should be based on the renin status of the patient; aldosterone deficiency can therefore be classified as hyporeninemic (secondary), or hyperreninemic (primary). Thus, a renin and aldosterone level in the setting of hyperkalemia can be useful diagnostically. In this patient, the PRA and aldosterone were clearly subnormal, and confirmed a hyporeninemic hypoaldosterone state. Oppositely, in patients with primary autoimmune adrenal insufficiency or adrenal hemorrhage, the renin level would be elevated. As aforemen-

Table 2
Etiologies of Aldosterone Deficiency/Resistance States

Secretagogue deficiency
  Hyporeninemia
    Diabetes mellitus
    Drugs [β-blockers, protaglandin synthase inhibitors (NSAIDS)]
  Angiotension II deficiency (ACE inhibitors) or blockade (AT1 receptor antagonist)
  Hypokalemia
Adrenocortical dysfunction
  Autoimmune destruction (idiopathic Addison's disease)
  Adrenal hemorrhage
  Infectious/infiltrative diseases (e.g., cytomegalovirus in AIDS patients; tuberculosis)
  Steroidogenic defects (aldosterone synthase deficiency[a]; 21-hydroxylase deficiency[b])
  Drugs (heparin)
Intrinsic renal abnormalities
  Mineralocorticoid receptor antagonism (spironolactone, eplerenone)
  Epithelial sodium channel (ENaC) dysfunction
    Mutation (pseudohypoaldosteronism type 1)
    Drugs (amiloride, trimethoprim, triamterene)

---

[a] Selective aldosterone deficiency.
[b] Cortisol and aldosterone deficiencies.
(Adapted from Litchfield WR, Dluhy RD. Mineralocorticoid deficiency syndromes. Contemporary Endocrinology: Hormone Replacement Therapy 1999;14:231–240; with permission.)

tioned, there are numerous medications that can further reduce the activity of the renin-angiotensin system, and can exacerbate the hypoaldosterone state. For example, prostaglandin synthase inhibitors, β-blockers, and ACE inhibitors interrupt the renin-angiotensin system at various loci, and worsen the hyporeninemic hypoaldosterone state in patients who have this disorder at baseline.

However, the most likely explanation of this patient's abrupt increase in potassium levels was heparin treatment, which is known to cause acute hypoaldosteronism (4,5). Heparin decreases angiotensin II-mediated aldosterone production by decreasing receptor numbers, as well as the binding affinity of angiotensin II receptors on adrenal glomerulosa cells. Higher doses of heparin can also impair ACTH and potassium-stimulated aldosterone production. Although aldosterone levels are probably reduced in all patients on heparin therapy, most subjects do not exhibit overt hypoaldosteronism because they are able to compensate by increasing renin release from the kidney. Individuals with long-standing diabetes mellitus, renal insufficiency or critical illness exhibit impaired compensation and are therefore at higher risk of developing heparin-induced hypoaldosteronism.

This patient did well, and had resolution of her hyperkalemia with appropriate initial therapy which included insulin and glucose, and an oral cation-exchange resin (such as Kayexalate®) administration. When the heparin was stopped, the potassium levels returned to the normal range. She was continued on metoprolol, given the important cardiac benefit of beta-blockers, although it was recognized by the clinician that these agents can further reduce renin secretion. Caution should be considered in the future when any medications that may effect aldosterone secretion or action are administered (e.g., spironolactone).

REFERENCES

1. Zipser RD, Davenport MW, Martin KL, et al. Hyperreninemic hypoaldosteronism in the critically ill: a new entity. J Clin Endocrinol Metab 1981;53:867–873.
2. Dahlberg PJ, Goellner MH, Pehling GB. Adrenal insufficiency secondary to adrenal hemorrhage. Two case reports and a review of cases confirmed by computed tomography. Arch Intern Med 1990;150: 905–909.
3. Velazauez H, Perazella MA, Wright FS, Ellison DH. Renal mechanism of trimethoprim-induced hyperkalemia. Ann Intern Med 1993;119:296–301.
4. Aull L, Chao H, Coy K. Heparin-induced hyperkalemia. DICP 1990;24:244–246.
5. Oster JR, Singer I, Fishman LM. Heparin-induced hypoaldosteronism and hyperkalemia. Am J Med 1995;98:575–586.

CASE #4: HIV AND ADRENAL DYSFUNCTION

Case Description

A 36-yr-old hispanic male with a known history of human immunodeficiency virus (HIV) infection was admitted to the hospital with recurrent fever and chills. He was diagnosed with HIV 10 yr ago, and has been treated with various drug regimens, currently consisting of zidovudine (AZT), didanosine (DDI), and nelfinivir. He had been hospitalized for *pneumocystis* pneumonia (PCP) 7 yr ago. His most recent CD4 count was 75 per cubic mm (normal >500 per cubic mm), and his viral load was measured at 24,000 copies (normal = undetectable). The patient was a known intravenous drug user, and his medical history was notable for a prior episode of *S. Aureus* endocarditis 17 yr ago, for which he underwent three months of antibiotic therapy.

The patient noted chills 2 mo ago, accompanied by fatigue and a mild cough. However, he was able to continue his present level of activity, and did not seek medical attention. His fatigue worsened and he noted frequent rigors. He then complained of progressive dyspnea on exertion, and symptoms consistent with orthopnea. He finally sought medical care where he was noted to have a temperature of 102.1°F. He was admitted to a hospital where he was found to have a blood pressure of 110/60 mmHg (lying), which fell to 90/65 mmHg standing. His pulse increased from 70 bpm lying to 90 bpm standing. His respiratory rate was 32 breaths per min (normal 12–16 breaths per min), and his temperature was 102.3°F. He was noted to have a new, III of VI holosystolic murmur heard best at the apex. His lung examination revealed rales halfway up both lung fields. His skin was slightly tanned, but felt to be "consistent" with his Hispanic heritage. There was an isolated 1.3×2.1 cm red, raised papule on his right forearm. His abdomen was soft and without tenderness; no masses could be palpated.

Blood cultures were drawn, and the patient was started on vancomycin and gentamicin for a presumed diagnosis of endocarditis. An echocardiogram confirmed the presence of valvular vegetations on both the mitral and aortic valves; significant mitral regurgitation, and aortic insufficiency were also noted. The ejection fraction was 25%. Subsequently, serologic studies confirmed prior cytomegalovirus (CMV) infection.

After 24 h, the patient's blood cultures revealed growth of *S. aureus*, sensitive to nafcillin. Upon recommendations from the Infectious Disease team, the patient's antibiotics were changed to nafcillin and gentamicin, and rifampin was added. The patient's fever improved, and rigors disappeared.

The following day, the patient was found confused and disoriented. His supine blood pressure was 68/40 mmHg, with a pulse of 100 bpm. The remainder of his physical exam was unchanged. He was transferred to the intensive care unit, and subsequently intubated. Intravenous fluids were given, but the patient required dopamine and neosynephrine to maintain a stable blood pressure. It was initially felt the patient was in septic shock, confounded by severe valvular dysfunction and congestive heart failure. His laboratory results revealed a potassium of 6.1 mmol/L, sodium of 137 mmol/L, creatinine 0.9 mg/dL, and the arterial blood gas revealed a pH of 7.39. The endocrine service was consulted regarding the possible diagnosis of adrenal insufficiency. He immediately was started on 2 mg of dexamethasone intravenously, and adrenal testing was performed. Approximately 4 h after receiving the dexamethasone, his blood pressure had risen to 120/74 mmHg, and the patient was able to be withdrawn from pressors over the next 12 h.

A rapid cosyntropin stimulation test was performed (250 mcg given IV as a bolus). The cortisol levels at 0, 30, and 60 min were 3.1 mcg/dL, 3.7 mcg/dL, and 2.9 mcg/dL, respectively. His ACTH level prior to dexamethasone administration was 80 ng/mL (normal 5–50 ng/mL). He was diagnosed with primary adrenal insufficiency, and prednisone 10 mg daily, was initiated. A CT scan of his abdomen and pelvis performed during his hospitalization revealed normal adrenal glands bilaterally without evidence of hemorrhage, calcification, or masses.

Further questioning revealed that he had no history of tuberculosis or other granulomatous diseases. There was no history of personal or family autoimmune disorders. His family had noted the patient's desire to apply salt liberally to his food for several months.

The patient recovered after a long hospital course, and surgical replacement of his aortic valve. Following discharge from the hospital in stable condition, he completed a 3-mo course of nafcillin. A follow-up cosyntropin stimulation test was performed, which revealed cortisol levels of 6.3 mcg/dL, 5.8 mcg/dL, and 5.9 mcg/dL, at 0, 30, and 60 min, respectively. Plasma aldosterone levels were 3.1 ng/dL and 3.8 ng/dL, at 0 and 60 min. He was instructed to continue taking prednisone replacement every morning, and was told to increase his dose during stressful situations, such as infections. A medialert bracelet was also provided to the patient. He is presently continuing his rehabilitation.

Discussion

The first description of the acquired immunodeficiency syndrome (AIDS) occurred in 1981 and was followed by the identification of the presumed etiologic agent, HIV. Since then, a number of alterations in endocrine function have been observed to occur in the HIV-infected person (1,2). This case provides an example of adrenal insufficiency in HIV disease, as well as the effects of various medications on cortisol metabolism.

The above patient first presented with fever and chills, and signs of infection. The risk of opportunistic infection was high given this patient's low CD4 count, and history of previous PCP pneumonia, as well as the lack of any prophylactic antibiotics such as trimethoprim. The medical team was appropriately concerned of the possibility of endocarditis given the signs of bacteremia and the findings of new cardiac murmurs. Blood cultures and an echocardiogram confirmed the diagnosis. However, in HIV-infected individuals, the possibility of adrenal insufficiency should always be considered especially in the setting of hypotension and fever, as was seen in this patient during his hospitalization.

This patient had no known history of any endocrinologic or autoimmune disorder, but when he was first examined, it was noted that he had orthostatic blood pressure readings. Although this symptom is nonspecific, it should raise suspicion for adrenal insufficiency. The appearance of hyperkalemia also supports this diagnosis.

Based on autopsy studies, the adrenal gland is the most commonly affected endocrine organ during the course of long-standing HIV infection *(3–5)*. Pathologic reports have found involvement of infectious agents (viral and fungal), malignancy, and hemorrhage *(4)*. Cytomegalovirus (CMV) is the most common infectious pathogen in the adrenal glands, having been found in 38–88% of HIV patients examined postmortem. Mycobacterium avium intracellulare has been demonstrated in the adrenal glands of 1–12% of cases. In addition, adrenal involvement with Kaposi's sarcoma and toxoplasmosis have been reported *(5)*. This patient had previous CMV pneumonitis, raising the suspicion of CMV adrenalitis.

However, although infectious involvement of the adrenal glands is very common in HIV-infected individuals, biochemical evidence of clinical adrenal insufficiency is rare. This is likely because of the fact that at least 90% of adrenal tissue must be destroyed before frank adrenal insufficiency occurs *(4)*. In several large series, normal, or more commonly, elevated basal cortisol levels have been noted in almost all HIV patients studied. Such individuals are presumed to be reacting with a chronic "stress response," and mild hypercortisolism ensues. Although CMV infection is the most common opportunistic infection found in these patients, necrotizing CMV adrenalitis rarely results in more than 50% destruction of the adrenal cortex. However, many patients with CMV adrenalitis probably have decreased adrenal reserve compared to normal subjects.

Note that this patient presented with a 2-mo history of severe infectious symptoms with high fevers. Yet, despite this, he showed no signs of hemodynamic collapse or adrenal crisis. Thus, it is likely that prior to hospitalization, he had sufficient adrenal reserve to avoid adrenal crisis.

Therefore, it is important to note the abrupt change in clinical status that ensued during his hospital stay, and to focus on potential causes. When the diagnosis of endocarditis was made, the antibiotics were changed to nafcillin, gentamicin, and rifampin. The patient subsequently became hypotensive and unresponsive. The possible causes of hypotension and shock in the patient are numerous, and the initial concern was for septic shock. However, other findings such as hyperkalemia suggested the possibility of hypoadrenalism. Subsequently, the cosyntropin stimulation test was abnormal, and secured the diagnosis of adrenal insufficiency. The elevated ACTH level also supported the diagnosis of primary adrenal insufficiency.

The key question is why acute adrenal insufficiency was precipitated in this patient. A number of medications that affect steroidogenesis are used in the treatment of disorders in patients with HIV and AIDS. Drugs such as ketoconazole inhibit steroidogenesis, whereas rifampin, and phenytoin accelerate steroid metabolism *(6,7)*. Patients with decreased adrenal reserve at the onset would be expected to be at risk for precipitating acute adrenal insufficiency when such medications are administered. In this case, the patient was started on rifampin prior to the appearance of adrenal crisis. Rifampin, which is increasingly used for treatment of mycobacterium tuberculosis, as well as severe cases of endocarditis, is a potent inducer of the hepatic mixed oxygenase enzymes. Studies have demonstrated that patients receiving rifampin have an increase in cytochrome *P450* activity and intense proliferation of smooth endoplasmic reticulum *(6)*, with a resultant increase in hormonal clearances which may have serious and profound effects. Numerous endocrinologic abnormalities such as hypothyroidism, decreased 25-hydroxyvitamin D levels, and severe adrenal insufficiency have been noted in patients treated with rifampin.

For example, Kyriazopoulou et al. also noted that mean plasma cortisol concentrations decreased 17% in cortisol-taking individuals on rifampin *(7)*. In addition, cortisol half-life decreased by 35%, and the systemic clearance of cortisol was increased by 35% *(7)*. Thus, it is postulated that the above patient had decreased adrenal reserve at baseline, but adrenal *crisis* was precipitated by rifampin. This is supported by the two cosyntropin stimulation tests in which higher cortisol levels were demonstrated during the second test after rifampin was discontinued.

This patient had a gratifying clinical improvement when glucocorticoids were administered, and he was quickly withdrawn from pressor medications. A CT scan of the adrenal glands showed no abnormalities, such as calcification, hemorrhage or masses that could represent fungal involvement. Thus, it is likely that this patient had underlying necrotizing CMV adrenalitis of the adrenal cortex with decreased adrenal reserve.

In long-term treatment of such patients, chronic glucocorticoid therapy would be recommended, even with the absence of medications that change steroid metabolism. This is based on the presumption that disease progression may ensue, and life-threatening adrenal crisis could occur unpredictably.

REFERENCES

1. Grinspoon SK, Bilezikian JP. HIV disease and the endocrine system. N Engl J Med 1992;327:1360–1365.
2. Sellmeyer DE, Gunfeld C. Endocrine and metabolic disturbances in human immunodeficiency virus infection and the acquired immune deficiency syndrome. Endocr Rev 1996;17:518–532.
3. Donovan DS, Dluhy RG. AIDS and its effect on the adrenal gland. Endocrinologist 1991;1:227–232.
4. Rotterdam H, Dembitzer F. The adrenal gland in AIDS. Endocr Pathol 1993;4:4–14.
5. Freda PU, Wardlaw SL, Brudney K, et al. Primary adrenal insufficiency in patients with the acquired immunodeficiency syndrome: a report of five cases. J Clin Endocrinol Metab 1994;79:1540–1545.
6. Mignet JP, Mavier P, Soussey CJ, Phumeaux D. Induction of hepatic enzymes after administration of rifampicin in man. Gastroenterology 1977;72:924.
7. Kyriazopoulou V, Parparousi O, Vagenakis AG. Rifampicin-induced adrenal crisis in addisonian patients receiving corticosteroid replacement therapy. J Clin Endocrinol Metab 1984;59:1204–1206.

9

Pheochromocytoma

Mary P. Gillam, MD and Lewis Landsberg, MD

CONTENTS

CASE #1: PHEOCHROMOCYTOMA CRISIS

Case Description

A 51-yr-old woman with neurofibromatosis was seen in the emergency room for symptoms of sinus congestion, productive cough, nausea with emesis, and malaise. She appeared flushed and was found to be profoundly orthostatic by both pulse and blood pressure. Her symptoms, physical exam, and sinus computed tomography (CT) films were all consistent with a diagnosis of sinusitis, and she was therefore admitted for intravenous hydration and antibiotics.

The patient had a medical history significant for hypertension, which had been diagnosed 1 yr earlier, and was treated with metoprolol 50 mg daily. In the month prior to her admission to the hospital, she underwent two surgical procedures for the excision of neurofibromas and a malignant schwannoma. Although her intra- and postoperative courses were uneventful, it was noted that she had become hypertensive and tachycardic with a maximum blood pressure and heart rate postoperatively of 210/92 mmHg and 118 beats per minute (bpm), respectively. Following her second surgery, the patient developed sinus congestion and thereafter she began using pseudoephedrine/chlorpheneramine on a daily basis for sinus relief.

Aggressive hydration, which began in the emergency room, continued on the medical floor. She was given a neosynephrine nasal spray, in addition to the pseudoephedrine she was taking prior to admission, to help control the copious nasal secretions that were nauseating and "gagging" her. Although she was not hypoxemic initially, she became progressively more dyspneic, tachypneic, and hypoxemic within the first 24 h. The morning after admission, an electrocardiogram (ECG) indicated ST segment elevations in the precordial leads and cardiac enzymes later confirmed that she had, in fact, suffered an anterior wall myocardial infarction (MI). She was transferred to the cardiac intensive care unit,

From: *Contemporary Endocrinology: Challenging Cases in Endocrinology*
Edited by: M. E. Molitch © Humana Press Inc., Totowa, NJ

and soon thereafter, developed atrial fibrillation with hemodynamic instability, requiring cardioversion. Obtundation and respiratory failure followed, leading to intubation and mechanical ventilation. Heparin, furosemide, lopressor, nitropaste, and aspirin were administered. Her chest X-ray, which was unremarkable on admission, now showed bilateral upper lobe pulmonary congestion and consolidation. Initially, her pulmonary edema was attributed to cardiogenic shock; however, pulmonary artery catheter monitoring revealed normal wedge and elevated pulmonary artery pressures. Later, an echocardiogram revealed an akinetic septum, but hyperdynamic wall motion throughout the remainder of the myocardium with mild left ventricular hypertrophy. As a result, her respiratory decompensation could not be solely attributed to cardiogenic edema resulting from the acute MI.

Meanwhile, over the next several days, she remained persistently tachycardic with heart rates climbing into the 150s on an esmolol infusion. Overall, her blood pressure tended to remain in the low-normal range, but occasionally, episodic hypertensive surges were noted. Her hemodynamic profile (tachycardia, relative hypotension, elevated cardiac index, and low systemic vascular resistance) was felt to reflect a state of impending sepsis. Simultaneously with these events, she developed spiking fevers, which continued despite broadening the antibiotic spectrum. Other perplexing findings surfaced, including rising liver transaminases and hyperamylasemia. A variety of explanations were proposed, such as rhabdomyolysis, pancreatitis, and "shock" liver. Finally, after cultures of blood, urine, sputum, and stool failed to identify the source of her fevers, an abdominal CT was obtained, searching for an occult abscess. A 7.2-cm mass was seen above the left kidney, and the diagnosis of pheochromocytoma was entertained (see Fig. 1).

The next day, while collecting urine for catecholamines, metanephrines, and vanillylmandelic acid, the patient developed a sudden pressor crisis during which her blood pressure rose to 210/130 mmHg. A test dose of 0.5 mg intravenous (iv) phentolamine dropped her systolic blood pressure into the 70s, lending further support for the diagnosis of a pheochromocytoma.

Upon the recommendation of the endocrinology service, α-blockade was initiated with phenoxybenzamine at a dose of 5 mg every 12 h. The next day, 30 min after 10 mg propranolol was given to help control tachycardia, the patient became diaphoretic, agitated, and flushed, and her blood pressure rose to 200/100 mmHg. Thereafter, β-blockade was withheld until it was certain that more complete α-blockade was established. Pressor crises, in the meantime, were treated with 1.0 mg boluses of iv phentolamine.

Very elevated catecholamine levels were found on plasma and 24 h urine testing, confirming the diagnosis (see Table 1). As titration of phenoxybenzamine proceeded, the patient remained tachycardic, but the lability in her blood pressure diminished. Her overall condition improved with resolution of her fevers and noncardiogenic pulmonary edema. Oxygen requirements diminished, and she was extubated on the 14th hospital day. After several days of α-blockade alone, a second attempt at β-blockade was made, this time successfully, starting with small doses of propranolol (5 mg every 8 h). Ultimately, her blood pressure and heart rate were controlled on 30 mg phenoxybenzamine qd and 20 mg propanolol qid.

As the patient's medical status stabilized, debate ensued over the optimal timing of surgery to remove the pheochromocytoma. The surgical service, concerned about her risk for perioperative mortality with her recent MI, initially advised medical management for 6 mo followed by surgical resection. On the other hand, the medical services felt that even with a recent MI, postponing surgery would pose greater risk, given the size of

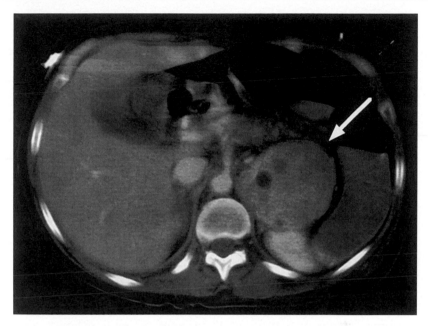

Fig. 1. CT scan of 7.2 cm heterogeneous left adrenal mass.

Table 1
Laboratory Evaluation

	Day #5	Day #6	Normal range
Plasma			
Norepinephrine (pg/mL)	45,175	76,000	70–750 supine
Epinephrine (pg/mL)	26,860	47,474	undetectable-110
Dopamine (pg/mL)	2116	2406	<30
24 hour Urine			
Vanillylmandelic acid (mg)	111.5		2–10
Norepinephrine (µg)		1744	0–100
Epinephrine (µg)		1659	0–25
Total catecholamines (µg)		3403	20–120
Dopamine (µg)		364	80–440
Metanephrines (µg)		44,168	44–300
Normetanephrines (µg)		25,401	110–620
Total metanephrines (µg)		69,569	140–820
Creatinine (g)		0.736	0.8–1.6

her tumor, elevated catecholamine levels, and the possibility of tumor necrosis, which might result in recurrent hypertensive crises, and ultimately death. To assess her cardiovascular surgical risk, she underwent a DP thallium stress test to evaluate myocardial viability and ischemia. No perfusion defects were found. Therefore, in view of her negative DP thallium study and normal overall left ventricular function, postponement of surgery seemed unwarranted. All involved agreed to have her proceed to surgery after restoring blood and plasma volume, and completing 2 wk of preoperative α-blockade.

Table 2
Neuropeptides in the Adrenal Medulla

Adrenomedullin
Calcitonin gene-related peptide
Chromogranins
Endorphins/enkephalins
Erythropoetin
Natriuretic peptides
Neuropeptide Y
Parathyroid hormone-related protein
Histamine
ACTH
Corticotropin-releasing hormone (CRH)
Somatostatin
Substance P
Vasoactive intestinal peptide (VIP)

The pheochromocytoma was successfully resected without difficulty. She remained hemodynamically stable throughout, guided by pulmonary artery catheter monitoring. Postoperatively, she became normotensive off adrenergic blockade, and transient tachycardia resolved with intravascular volume repletion. She was discharged home off antihypertensive medications 5 d after surgery.

Discussion

Experience with cases such as the one described here has led endocrinologists to allege that pheochromocytomas create some of the most dramatic and life-threatening crises in all of endocrinology (1). The danger of pheochromocytomas lies only rarely in their malignant oncologic potential. Rather, it is their ability to synthesize, store, and secrete large amounts of catecholamines, which in turn produce multiple physiologic effects, and leads to serious and often fatal outcomes. This feature was astutely recognized by Esperson and Dahl-Iversen more than 50 yr ago in their description of pheochromocytomas as being "morphologically benign, yet physiologically malignant" (2).

One of the most fascinating aspects of pheochromocytomas is the extreme variety of clinical manifestations associated with these tumors (3). In the literature, more than 80 different presentations have been described (4). Pheochromocytomas may present with symptoms that are directly attributable to excess catecholamines, or they may present with manifestations attributable to complications of the tumor that then dominate the clinical picture. To add to the confusion, the presentation of a pheochromocytoma may be modified by the effects of various biologically active hormones or neuropeptides that are ectopically produced and secreted by these tumors (see Table 2) (5). Although the heterogeneous manifestations of pheochromocytomas give rise to interesting anecdotes, such diversity can occasionally be bewildering to the clinician (6). In this case, the diagnosis of pheochromocytoma was not entertained until a clue was discovered on an abdominal CT performed as part of an evaluation for fevers of unknown origin. Yet once the diagnosis was suggested, it became clear that a pheochromocytoma was the likely unifying diagnosis to explain the patient's clinical course. The difficulty and delay in making the diagnosis illustrate well the concept that the most critical and challenging element in the management of a pheochromocytoma is the initial consideration of the disease in the differential diagnosis *(7)*.

The rapid clinical deterioration of the patient in this case typifies the sudden hemodynamic decompensation that may develop in a patient with a previously unsuspected pheochromocytoma. Occasionally, a patient who is minimally symptomatic for years will suddenly present with a major cardiovascular or cerebrovascular complication, such as hypertensive crisis, acute MI, hemorrhagic stroke, arrythmia, or circulatory shock *(5)*. This explosive potential is emphasized throughout the literature. Aranow, for example, characterized the pheochromocytoma as a "veritable pharmacologic bomb" *(8)*. Likewise, Robinson compared the tumor to a "metabolic volcano" that suddenly erupts after a quiescent state *(9)*.

Although uncommon, the development of multiorgan system failure and noncardiogenic pulmonary edema are well-recognized consequences of pheochromocytoma *(10)*. In rare circumstances, these complications may present as the initial manifestations of the tumor *(11–16)*. Noncardiogenic pulmonary edema is believed to result from transient increases in pulmonary capillary pressure because of pulmonary venoconstriction and to altered pulmonary capillary permeability *(11,17,18)*. In addition to multiorgan failure with noncardiogenic pulmonary edema, a subset of patients will also develop fever, obtundation, and extremely labile blood pressure. The highly lethal tetrad of multiorgan decompensation, pyrexia, blood pressure lability, and obtundation has been referred to as the pheochromocytoma multisystem crisis *(19)*. When noncardiogenic pulmonary edema coexists with fever as part of pheochromocytoma multisystem crisis, the clinical picture and hemodynamic profile resemble, and therefore masquerade as septic shock *(20–24)*. If unrecognized, this syndrome frequently results in a prolonged search for an infectious source, only to delay the diagnosis and retard the institution of appropriate therapy.

The mechanisms underlying an acute pheochromocytoma crisis are not known for certain. Pheochromocytomas, unlike the normal adrenal medulla, are not innervated, and catecholamine release is not initiated from neural impulses. Some stimuli that may stimulate catecholamine release, and thereby trigger paroxsyms include changes in tumor blood flow, hemorrhagic necrosis, release of vasoactive substances, or use of certain drugs. A knowledge of these stimuli may be useful in suspecting pheochromocytoma when they are discovered in a patient's history (see Table 3). Proprietary cold medicines and decongestants which contain sympathomimetic amines can increase blood pressure by releasing catecholamines from augmented stores in nerve endings. They are common precipitators, and may have contributed to the development of the crisis in this case *(5)*.

Both nonspecific diagnostic clues and explanations for previously inexplicable findings are often identifiable in a retrospective analysis of perplexing cases of pheochromocytoma. This case is no exception. Hyperamylasemia, which falsely suggested acute pancreatitis, was likely secondary to damaged pulmonary endothelium associated with noncardiogenic pulmonary edema, as has been demonstrated in similar cases *(12,25)*. The patient's profound orthostasis on presentation was not an unrelated sign. In fact, orthostatic hypotension, which is found in up to 70% of patients with pheochromocytoma, can be a valuable diagnostic clue *(26)*. The mechanism for postural changes in blood pressure is not certain, but is thought to be secondary to both a dimunition in plasma volume, as well as a depression of sympathetic vasomotor reflexes that usually maintain

Table 3
Triggers of Paroxysms
in Patients with Pheochromocytomas

Medications
  Opiates
  Histamine
  Corticotropin
  Saralasin
  Glucagon
  Metaclopramide
  Tricyclic antidepressants
  Phenothiazines
  Monoamine oxidase inhibitors
  Guanethedine
  Methyldopa
  Sympathomimetic amines
  Anesthetic agents
Radiographic contrast media
Diagnostic procedures
  Arteriogram
  Lumbar puncture
  Presacral aerogram
  Percutaneous biopsy
Endotracheal intubation/anesthesia induction
Mechanical compression of tumor
  Pregnancy
  Uterine contraction
  Abdominal palpation
Food or alcoholic beverages containing tyramine
Cigarette smoking

upright blood pressure *(27)*. An explanation for the patient's prolonged non-infectious diarrhea became evident when an elevated serum VIP level confirmed the ectopic secretion of this hormone originating from the pheochromocytoma *(28,29)*.

Not to be ignored is the well-known association between neurofibromatosis and pheochromocytoma. Neurofibromatosis type 1 is one of the most common autosomal dominant disorders in which affected individuals develop both benign and malignant tumors at an increased frequency. The underlying molecular basis for the disease involves inactivating mutations in the *NF1* gene, a putative tumor suppressor gene that encodes the gene product, neurofibromin *(30)*. This tumor suppresor appears to be involved in the regulation of *ras* protooncogenes *(31)*. Interestingly, mutations in the *NF1* gene may contribute to the development of pheochromocytomas in patients without neurofibromatosis, as demonstrated by the loss of *NF1* expression in sporadic tumors *(32,33)*.

Whereas neurofibromatosis occurs in approximately 5% of patients with pheochromocytoma, these tumors are present in roughly 1% of patients with type 1 neurofibromatosis *(34)*. However, among hypertensive patients with neurofibromatosis, the prevalence may be as high as 50% *(35)*. Therefore, the presence of neurofibromatosis in a patient with hyper-tension or classic symptoms should heighten the index of suspicion for pheochromocytoma.

Surgical intervention merits comment in this case. Although recent MI is a condition in which postponement of surgery is often prudent, two strong arguments favored expeditious surgery in this case. First, there was no evidence that the patient's MI resulted in permanent myocardial injury, and it was likely that in the absence of coronary artery disease, coronary vasospasm could have provoked the event *(36)*. Second, the presence of recent myocardial injury should not serve as an absolute contraindication to prompt surgical resection of a pheochromocytoma, because removal of the source of excess catecholamines is likely to improve the cardiac condition *(19)*.

REFERENCES

1. Keiser HR. Pheochromocytoma and related tumors. In: De Groot L, ed. Endocrinology. W.B. Saunders, New York, 1995, pp. 1853–1877.
2. Espersen T, Dahl-Iversen E. The clinical picture and treatment of tumors of the suprarenal. Acta Chir Scand 1946;94:271–290.
3. Gifford R, Kvale W, Maher F. Clinical features, diagnosis, and treatment of pheochromocytoma: a review of 76 cases. Mayo Clinic Proc 1964;39:281–302.
4. De Courcy JL, De Courcy CB. Pheochromocytomas and the General Practitioner. Barclay Newman, Cincinatti, OH, 1952, p. 163.
5. Landsberg L, Young J. Catecholamines and the adrenal medulla. In: Foster D, Wilson J, eds. Williams Textbook of Endocrinology, WB Saunders, Philadelphia, PA, 1998, pp. 665–728.
6. Manger WM, Gifford RW. Clinical and Experimental Pheochromocytoma. Blackwell Science, New York, 1996, p. 570.
7. Landsberg L. The sympathoadrenal system. In: Bagdade JD, ed. The Yearbook of Endocrinology. Mosby Year Book, St. Louis, MO, 1996, pp. 178, 179.
8. Aranow H Jr. Pheochromocytoma. In: Bean WB, ed. Monographs in Medicine. Series 1. Williams and Wilkins, Baltimore, MD, 1952, pp. 179–224.
9. Robinson R. Tumours that Secrete Catecholamines: Their Detection and Clinical Chemistry. John Wiley, Chichester, 1980, p. 65.
10. Landsberg L, Young JB. Pheochromocytoma. In: Braunwald E, ed. Principles of Internal Medicine. McGraw-Hill, New York, 2001, pp. 2105–2109.
11. de Leeuw PW, Waltman FL, Birkenhager WH. Noncardiogenic pulmonary edema as the sole manifestation of pheochromocytoma. Hypertension 1986;8:810–812.
12. Gan TJ, Miller RF, Webb AR, Russell RC. Phaeochromocytoma presenting as acute hyperamylasaemia and multiple organ failure. Can J Anaesth 1994;41:244–247.
13. Joshi R, Manni A. Pheochromocytoma manifested as noncardiogenic pulmonary edema. South Med J 1993;86:826–828.
14. Okada Y, Suchi M, Takeyama H, Hodgson ME, Kato T, Manabe T. Noncardiogenic pulmonary edema as the chief manifestation of a pheochromocytoma: a case report of MEN 2A with pedigree analysis of the RET proto-oncogene. Tohoku J Exp Med 1999;188:177–187.
15. Lorz W, Cottier C, Imhof E, Gyr N. Multiple organ failure and coma as initial presentation of pheochromocytoma in a patient with multiple endocrine neoplasia (MEN) type II A. Intensive Care Med 1993;19:235–238.
16. van der Kleij FG. Adult respiratory distress syndrome due to pheochromocytoma as the initial presentation of multiple endocrine neoplasia type IIA syndrome [letter]. Am J Med 1999;107:401.
17. Case records of the Massachusetts General Hospital. Weekly clinicopathological exercises. Case 15-1988. A 26-year-old woman with cardiomyopathy, multiple strokes, and an adrenal mass. N Engl J Med 1988;318:970–981.
18. Berk JL, Hagen JF, Koo R, et al. Pulmonary insufficiency caused by epinephrine. Ann Surg 1973;178:423–435.
19. Newell KA, Prinz RA, Pickleman J, et al. Pheochromocytoma multisystem crisis. A surgical emergency. Arch Surg 1988;123:956–959.
20. Mok CC, Ip TP, So CC. Phaeochromocytoma with adult respiratory distress syndrome mimicking septicaemic shock. Med J Aust 1997;166:634–635.

21. Page LB, Raker JW, Berberick FR. Pheochromocytoma with predominant epinephrine secretion. Am J Med 1969;47:648–652.
22. Fred HL, Allred DP, Garber HE, et al. Pheochromocytoma masquerading as overwhelming infection. Am Heart J 1967;73:149–154.
23. Ford J, Rosenberg F, Chan N. Pheochromocytoma manifesting with shock presents a clinical paradox: a case report. CMAJ 1997;157:923–925.
24. Gordon DL, Atamian SD, Brooks MH, et al. Fever in pheochromocytoma. Arch Intern Med 1992;152: 1269–1272.
25. Perrier NA, van Heerden JA, Wilson DJ, Warner MA. Malignant pheochromocytoma masquerading as acute pancreatitis—a rare but potentially lethal occurrence. Mayo Clin Proc 1994;69:366–370.
26. Ross EJ, Griffith DN. The clinical presentation of phaeochromocytoma. Q J Med 1989;71:485–496.
27. Engelman K, Zelis R, Waldmann T, Mason DT, Sjoerdsma AM. Mechanisms of orthostatic hypotension in pheochromocytoma. Circulation 1968;38(Suppl 6):1–72.
28. Fisher BM, MacPhee GJ, Davies DL, McPherson SG, Brown IL, Goldberg A. A case of watery diarrhoea syndrome due to an adrenal phaeochromocytoma secreting vasoactive intestinal polypeptide with coincidental autoimmune thyroid disease. Acta Endocrinol (Copenh) 1987;114:340–344.
29. Sackel SG, Manson JE, Harawi SJ, Burakoff R. Watery diarrhea syndrome due to an adrenal pheochromocytoma secreting vasoactive intestinal polypeptide. Dig Dis Sci 1985;30:1201–1207.
30. Wallace MR, Marchuk DA, Andersen LB, et al. Type 1 neurofibromatosis gene: identification of a large transcript disrupted in three NF1 patients. Science 1990;249:181–186.
31. Li Y, O'Connell P, Breidenbach HH, et al. Genomic organization of the neurofibromatosis 1 gene (NF1). Genomics 1995;25:9–18.
32. Gutmann DH, Geist RT, Rose K, Wallin G, Moley JF. Loss of neurofibromatosis type I (NF1) gene expression in pheochromocytomas from patients without NF1. Genes Chromosomes Cancer 1995;13: 104–109.
33. Xu W, Mulligan LM, Ponder MA, et al. Loss of NF1 alleles in phaeochromocytomas from patients with type I neurofibromatosis. Genes Chromosomes Cancer 1992;4:337–342.
34. Colman SD, Wallace MR. Neurofibromatosis type 1. Eur J Cancer 1994;13:1974–1981.
35. Kalff V, Shapiro B, Lloyd R, et al. The spectrum of pheochromocytoma in hypertensive patients with neurofibromatosis. Arch Intern Med 1982;142:2092–2098.
36. Gupta KK. Letter: Phaeochromocytoma and myocardial infarction. Lancet 1975;1:281–282.

CASE #2: PHEOCHROMOCYTOMA OR METASTASIS?

Case Description

A 45-yr-old woman with a history of mild hypertension underwent a lumpectomy and 1 mo later, a left radical mastectomy for breast cancer. Histopathology revealed an infiltrating ductal carcinoma with local lymphatic spread. During these surgeries, the patient was noted to be mildly hypertensive, with systolic blood pressures varying from 140–160 mmHg and diastolic blood pressures ranging from 80–100 mmHg. After surgery, her blood pressure was controlled by doubling her dose of enalapril (the only medication she was taking) from 5 to 10 mg/day.

Following these surgeries, as a part of the staging evaluation of her cancer, she had a CT scan of her abdomen and pelvis, which revealed a 4.8 × 3.7 cm nonhomogeneous right suprarenal mass, suspicious for a metastatic lesion (see Fig. 2). Because of the concern for metastatic disease, an ultrasound-guided fine needle aspiration biopsy (FNAB) of the suprarenal mass was performed. After the first pass of the needle, the patient developed severe pounding occipital headaches and palpitations. Her blood pressure rapidly increased from 120/80 mmHg to 185/90 mmHg and her heart rate rose from 72 to 90 beats/min. She vomited twice. Her blood pressure responded to intravenous (iv) sedation with Fentanyl, and it eventually fell to 120/80 mmHg after several hours of observation. Further attempts

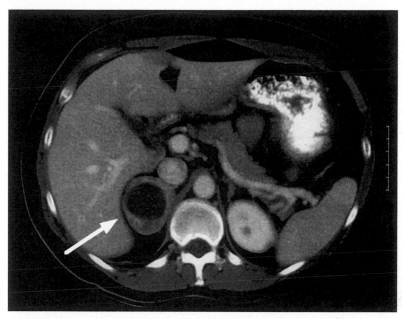

Fig. 2. CT scan of 4 × 4 cm right suprarenal mass with large cystic central component, initially reported as suspicious for metastatic disease.

at biopsy were not made and the suspicion for a pheochromocytoma was raised. Plasma catecholamines collected at the time of this event revealed a norepinephrine level of 699 pg/mL (normal 70–750), an epinephrine level of 490 pg/mL (normal <110), and a dopamine level of 12 pg/mL (normal < 30). Unfortunately, FNAB results were nondiagnostic.

The patient had been diagnosed with hypertension at age 30 based upon routine blood pressure measurements done at office visits to her internist. Her blood pressure was well controlled with 5 mg enalapril qd. Her family history was notable for her mother, who was diagnosed with hypertension in her 40s, and her maternal grandmother who died of a cerebrovascular accident at age 54. There was no other family history of endocrinopathies. Her review of systems was notable only for mild intermittent headaches. She denied palpitations, heat intolerance, and diaphoresis.

A 24 h collection for urinary catecholamines, vanillylmandelic acid, and metanephrines revealed an epinephrine level of 115.8 µg (normal <20), norepinephrine level of 180.6 µg (normal <80), dopamine level of 187.6 µg (normal 88–420), vanillylmandelic acid level of 15.0 mg (normal 2–10), and metanephrine level of 1.6 µg (normal 44–300). MRI showed a right adrenal mass with a characteristic high signal intensity on T2 weighted images (see Fig. 3). Meta-iodobenzylguanidine (MIBG) scintigraphy localized uptake in the right adrenal gland. These findings were all compatible with a diagnosis of pheochromocytoma.

Two weeks prior to her scheduled surgery, the patient was initiated on α-blockade with phenoxybenzamine, which was gradually titrated to a dose of 20 mg q am, and 30 mg q pm at the same time monitoring for symptoms of orthostasis; 10 mg propranolol tid was added to control mild tachycardia during the second week. On this regimen, her systolic blood pressure ranged from 110–132 mmHg, and diastolic blood pressure ranged from 80–86 mmHg. Surgical excision of the tumor was uneventful. Intraoperatively, the

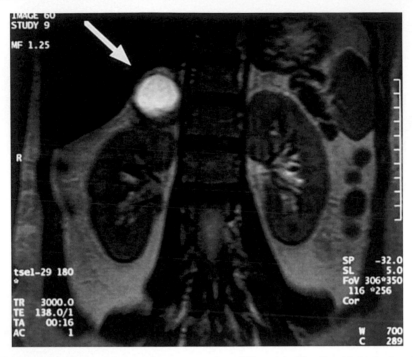

Fig. 3. MR image of suprarenal mass demonstrated on CT scan in Fig. 2, with high signal intensity displayed on the T_2-weighted image.

patient received 5 L of lactated ringer's intravenous fluid. Total blood loss was estimated at 150 mls. She developed an episode of transient mild hypotension after the last adrenal vein was ligated. Blood pressure quickly recovered with a bolus of intravenous fluid, and remained stable throughout the remainder of her 4 h surgery.

The patient's postoperative course was uncomplicated as well. She was observed overnight in the surgical intensive care unit for hemodynamic monitoring. Mild incisional abdominal pain was controlled with an epidural infusion of Fentanyl. She remained normotensive and was discharged from the hospital off antihypertensives. Two-week and 1-yr follow-up 24 h collections for urinary catecholamines, metanephrines, and vanillylmandelic acid have been normal.

Discussion

The diagnosis of pheochromocytoma is easily suspected in a hypertensive individual exhibiting paroxysmal symptoms of headache, excessive perspiration, and diaphoresis. Although only half of all patients with pheochromocytomas will experience paroxysms, most patients harboring the tumor will report some chronic or intermittent symptoms that are associated with the tumor (see Table 4). Indeed, in one series of greater than 21,000 hypertensive patients, Plouin et al. found that the absence of headache, diaphoresis, and palpitations virtually excluded the diagnosis of pheochromocytoma. Nevertheless, as emphasized by this case, at times, symptoms of the disease can be subtle, and it is often only in retrospect that their significance and relationship to the diagnosis are recognized. Such subtlety of symptoms may lead to the incidental discovery of pheochromocytomas

Table 4
Frequency of Symptoms in 100 Patients with Pheochromocytoma

Symptom	%	Symptom	%
Headache	80	Anxiety	22
Diaphoresis	71	Epigastric abdominal pain	22
Palpitations	64	Chest pain	19
Pallor	42	Dyspnea	19
Nausea	42	Flushing	18
Tremor	31	Parethesias or numbness	11
Generalized weakness	28	Blurring of vision	11

Adapted from (5).

at unrelated surgery, during abdominal imaging, or at autopsy. The paucity of associated signs and symptoms may also lead to missed diagnoses with tragic consequences.

The case under discussion exemplifies the presentation of an incidentally discovered, clinically unsuspected pheochromocytoma. Here the patient had controllable hypertension and mild headaches—common problems that ordinarily would not warrant evaluation for a pheochromocytoma. Had it not been for the staging evaluation for her breast cancer, it is likely that her pheochromocytoma would have remained undiagnosed, at least until catecholamine production and secretion increased to the point that paroxysms developed or blood pressure worsened. Several studies of routine autopsies have emphasized that a large number of "silent" pheochromocytomas escape detection and are first discovered postmortem (3–10). A Mayo Clinic study of 54 proven cases of pheochromocytoma revealed that 41 (76%) of these tumors were clinically unsuspected during life (11). Interestingly, over 90% of these same patients were retrospectively noted to have reported symptoms during life that are characteristic of pheochromocytoma. Such observations indicate that a large number of patients with pheochromocytomas may present with minor signs and symptoms, the significance of which are not readily apparent. Furthermore, the rare incidence and protean manifestations associated with pheochromocytoma contribute to the elusive nature of its diagnosis.

In hindsight, there were two clues in this patient's history that were suggestive of a diagnosis of pheochromocytoma. The first hint dated back 15 yr prior at age 30, when she was first discovered to have hypertension. Because pheochromocytoma is a rare cause of hypertension, the relatively young age of onset in this patient might have suggested a secondary cause, albeit in the absence of any other features, a pheochromocytoma would not have been suspected at this point. Hypertension, which is found in 90% of patients with pheochromocytomas, is sustained in one-half of patients, paroxysmal in one-third, and absent in one-tenth (12). The second clue in her history was the unusual elevation in blood pressure that occurred during the mastectomy. A paradoxical blood pressure response to anesthesia and surgery is a well-documented observation in an unrecognized pheochromocytoma, one which should prompt consideration of its possibility, even in asymptomatic individuals (13).

This patient was fortunate to have had such a smooth operative course at the time of her mastectomy, for when the diagnosis of pheochromocytoma escapes detection, potentially disastrous consequences may result. In the Mayo Clinic autopsy series, 11/41 (27%)

of the patients with an unsuspected pheochromocytoma died during or immediately after surgery for unrelated conditions *(14)*. These findings underscore the danger of surgery in undiagnosed patients who are not prepared with adrenergic blockade.

Although the incidental discovery of pheochromocytoma is an atypical presentation of the disease, it is one that is not rare. It is estimated that approximately 5% of all pheochromocytomas present as adrenal incidentalomas *(15,16)*. Furthermore, in some series, pheochromocytomas account for up to 13% of all serendipitously discovered adrenal masses *(17–19)*.

The method of laboratory diagnosis in this case deserves comment. Once suspected, pheochromocytoma can usually be confirmed without difficulty by careful analysis of a properly collected 24 h sample of urinary catecholamines, metanephrines, and/or vanillylmandelic acid (VMA). As was done here, commencing the collection after the onset of a paroxysmal attack can increase the diagnostic yield *(20)*. With the availability of highly sensitive measurements of catecholamines and their metabolites, provocative testing has been rendered virtually obsolete. Measurements of plasma catecholamine levels are generally not useful in screening for sporadic pheochromocytomas because of the inherent difficulty in their proper collection. Plasma catecholamines also lack the advantage of an integrated assessment of catecholmine levels over a 24-h time span. In the patient under discussion, plasma catecholamines were collected at the time the paroxysm was triggered by biopsy. Here, only the epinephrine level was elevated, and then only to a modest degree. Even if frankly elevated catecholamine levels were detected, one would have to interpret them cautiously, given the stressful conditions under which they were collected. It was for this reason that a second 24-h urine sample was critical, to verify that the first results were accurate and diagnostic.

This case is instructive because it is relevant to issues regarding the evaluation and management of incidentally discovered adrenal masses. As radiologic technology has improved and advanced abdominal imaging has increased in frequency, greater numbers of both benign and malignant adrenal lesions are being discovered, leading to the common clinical problem of the adrenal incidentaloma. The challenge centers on distinguishing the small fraction of malignant and/or hypersecretory masses from those that are nonfunctioning, benign, and require no intervention.

In the case under discussion, the adrenal mass was serendipitously discovered as part of a staging evaluation for cancer. CTs and MRIs are widely used for this purpose, and adrenal masses are often found. In a patient with a history of cancer, metastases are the most common cause of an incidental adrenal mass, regardless of size *(21)*. Indeed, because carcinomas of the breast are one of the most common sources for adrenal gland metastases, this patient's adrenal mass was highly suspicious for a metastasis. Nevertheless, it is a mistake to assume that such masses are always metastases, because a considerable proportion are benign *(22)*. In the setting of a known extraadrenal primary cancer, malignancy rates of incidental adrenal masses discovered by CT range from 32 to 73%, whereas rates of benign lesions range from 27 to 68% of cases *(18)*. Although there is a tremendous overlap in these rates, it is nonetheless clear that either is possible. When an adrenal mass is the only finding suspicious for metastatic disease in a patient with a known extraadrenal cancer, the distinction between a metastasis and other causes of adrenal masses may be critical in determining whether curative therapy of the primary neoplasm is feasible. Such was the scenario for this patient. In her case, there were no other systemic metastases evident, and therefore, confirmation of the nature of this adrenal lesion was imperative in determining appropriate chemotherapy. Often, in the urgency of establishing a pathologic diagnosis, assessment of functional status is forgotten.

Recent attention has focused on identifying certain adrenal imaging features to characterize incidental adrenal masses in an attempt to differentiate among adenomas, carcinomas, pheochromocytomas, and cancer metastases. Neither CT nor MRI, however, can reliably distinguish a metastasis from either a benign adenoma or from a primary adrenal malignancy based solely upon the radiologic appearance (23). Once biochemical data has established the diagnosis of pheochromcytoma, MRI is particularly useful in confirmation and localization of the tumor, because they exhibit a pathognomonic high signal intensity on enhanced T-2 weighted images (24). However, MRI is not always helpful in distinguishing malignancy from pheochromocytoma, because 65% of pheochromocytomas have an overlap with adrenal metastases in relative signal intensity on T-2 weighted images (25,26).

Scintigraphic localization with radiolabeled ^{131}I MIBG was reassuring in this case because it verified the functional nature of the mass, and together with the biochemical data, established the diagnosis with finality. [131]I MIBG is an analogue of norepinephrine that is taken up by chromaffin cells. In general, ^{131}I MIBG scanning is useful when biochemical evidence is positive and results of abdominal imaging are negative (27). However, it is not the suggested imaging procedure for initial localization because of its inferior sensitivity, as compared with CT and MRI (28).

Finally, this case underscores the importance of carefully evaluating every incidental adrenal mass for hormonal hypersecretion, even in patients with known primary extra-adrenal malignancies who do not have clinical features of hormonal excess. Neither lack of hypertension nor lack of typical symptoms precludes the diagnosis of a pheochromocytoma. Percutaneous adrenal biopsy of a pheochromocytoma may precipitate a hypertensive crisis, retroperitoneal hemorrhage, and even death (16,29–32). Therefore, all patients with adrenal incidentalomas should undergo biochemical testing for pheochromocytoma before proceeding to FNAB of the adrenals.

REFERENCES

1. Plouin PF, Chatellier G, Delahousse M, et al. [Detection, diagnosis and localization of pheochromocytoma. 77 cases in a population of 21,420 hypertensive patients]. Presse Med 1987;16:2211–2215.
2. Miyajima A, Nakashima J, Baba S, Tachibana M, Nakamura K, Murai M. Clinical experience with incidentally discovered pheochromocytoma. J Urol 1997;157:1566–1568.
3. Gifford R, Kvale W, Maher F. Clinical features, diagnosis, and treatment of pheochromocytoma: a review of 76 cases. Mayo Clinic Proceedings 1964;39:281–302.
4. Hartley L, Perry-Keene D. Phaeochromocytoma in Queensland—1970–83. Aust N Z J Surg 1985;55: 471–475.
5. Kasperlik-Zeluska AA, Roslonowska E, Slowinska-Srzednicka J, et al. Incidentally discovered adrenal mass (incidentaloma): investigation and management of 208 patients. Clin Endocrinol (Oxford) 1997; 46:29–37.
6. Minno A, Bennett W, Kvale W. Pheochromocytoma. A study of 15 cases diagnosed at autopsy. N Engl J Med 1954;251:959–965.
7. Modlin IM, Farndon JR, Shepherd A, et al. Phaeochromocytomas in 72 patients: clinical and diagnostic features, treatment and long term results. Br J Surg 1979;66:456–465.
8. Stenstrom G, Svardsudd K. Pheochromocytoma in Sweden 1958–1981. An analysis of the National Cancer Registry Data. Acta Med Scand 1986;220:225–232.
9. Goldstein RE, O'Neill JA Jr, Holcomb GW III, et al. Clinical experience over 48 years with pheochromocytoma. Ann Surg 1999;229:755–764; discussion 764–766.

10. Krane NK. Clinically unsuspected pheochromocytomas. Experience at Henry Ford Hospital and a review of the literature. Arch Intern Med 1986;146:54–57.

11. Sutton DM, Hauser R, Kulapongs P, Bachmann F. Intravascular coagulation in abruptio placentae. Am J Obstet Gynecol 1971;109:604–614.

12. Landsberg L, Young J. Catecholamines and the adrenal medulla. In: Foster D, Wilson J, eds. Williams Textbook of Endocrinology, WB Saunders, Philadelphia, PA, 1998, pp. 665–728.

13. Cross DA, Meyer JS. Postoperative deaths due to unsuspected pheochromocytoma. South Med J 1977;70:1320–1321.

14. Sutton MG, Sheps SG, Lie JT. Prevalence of clinically unsuspected pheochromocytoma. Review of a 50-year autopsy series. Mayo Clin Proc 1981;56:354–360.

15. Barzon L, Scaroni C, Sonino N, et al. Incidentally discovered adrenal tumors: endocrine and scintigraphic correlates. J Clin Endocrinol Metab 1998;83:55–62.

16. Young WF, Jr. Management approaches to adrenal incidentalomas. A view from Rochester, Minnesota. Endocrinol Metab Clin North Am 2000;29:159–185.

17. Angeli A, Osella G, Ali A, Terzolo M. Adrenal incidentaloma: an overview of clinical and epidemiological data from the National Italian Study Group. Horm Res 1997;47:279–283.

18. Kloos RT, Gross MD, Francis IR, Korobkin M, Shapiro B. Incidentally discovered adrenal masses. Endocr Rev 1995;16:460–484.

19. Ross NS, Aron DC. Hormonal evaluation of the patient with an incidentally discovered adrenal mass. N Engl J Med 1990;323:1401–1405.

20. Daly PA, Landsberg L. Phaeochromocytoma: diagnosis and management. Baillieres Clin Endocrinol Metab 1992;6:143–166.

21. Belldegrun A, Hussain S, Seltzer SE, Loughlin KR, Gittes RF, Richie JP. Incidentally discovered mass of the adrenal gland. Surg Gynecol Obstet 1986;163:203–208.

22. Hussain S, Belldegrun A, Seltzer SE, Richie JP, Abrams HL. CT diagnosis of adrenal abnormalities in patients with primary non-adrenal malignancies. Eur J Radiol 1986;6:127–131.

23. Doppman JL, Reinig JW, Dwyer AJ, et al. Differentiation of adrenal masses by magnetic resonance imaging. Surgery 1987;102:1018–1026.

24. Boland GW, Lee MJ. Magnetic resonance imaging of the adrenal gland. Crit Rev Diagn Imaging 1995; 36:115–174.

25. Reinig JW, Doppman JL, Dwyer AJ, Frank J. MRI of indeterminate adrenal masses. AJR Am J Roentgenol 1986;147:493–496.

26. van Gils A, Falke T, van Erkel A, van de Velde C, Pauwels E. Non-invasive imaging of functioning paragangliomas (including phaeochromocytomas). Frontiers in European Radiology 1990;7:1–38.

27. Maurea S, Cuocolo A, Reynolds JC, et al. Iodine-131-metaiodobenzylguanidine scintigraphy in preoperative and postoperative evaluation of paragangliomas: comparison with CT and MRI. J Nucl Med 1993;34:173–179.

28. van Gils AP, Falke TH, van Erkel AR, et al. MR imaging and MIBG scintigraphy of pheochromocytomas and extraadrenal functioning paragangliomas. Radiographics 1991;11:37–57.

29. Candel AG, Gattuso P, Reyes CV, Prinz RA, Castelli MJ. Fine-needle aspiration biopsy of adrenal masses in patients with extraadrenal malignancy. Surgery 1993;114:1132–1136; discussion 1136–1137.

30. Casola G, Nicolet V, vanSonnenberg E, et al. Unsuspected pheochromocytoma: risk of blood-pressure alterations during percutaneous adrenal biopsy. Radiology 1986;159:733–735.

31. Lambert MA, Hirschowitz L, Russell RC. Fine needle aspiration biopsy: a cautionary tale. Br J Surg 1985;72:364.

32. McCorkell SJ, Niles NL. Fine-needle aspiration of catecholamine-producing adrenal masses: a possibly fatal mistake. AJR Am J Roentgenol 1985;145:113–134.

CASE #3: PHEOCHROMOCYTOMA IN PREGNANCY

Case Description

A 28-yr-old Hispanic G_3P_2 female with a previous history of gestational diabetes presented to the gestational diabetes clinic with a blood pressure of 140/98 mmHg at 13 wk gestation. During prior pregnancies and prenatal visits she had been normotensive. She

Table 5
Laboratory Evaluation

24 h urine	Specimen 1	Specimen 2	Normal range
Vanillylmandelic acid (mg)	17.6		2–10
Norepinephrine (µg)	1453.1	728.1	15–80
Epinephrine (µg)	7.2	7.0	0–20
Dopamine (µg)	519.7	326.7	88–420
Metanephrines (µg)		2.2	44–300
Creatinine (mg)	1208	1271	800–1800

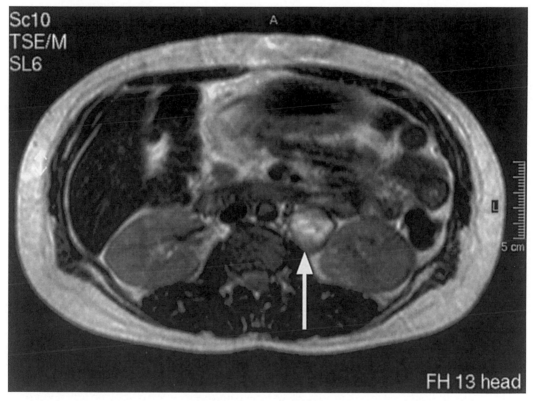

Fig. 4. Transverse section of adrenal MR image demonstrating a 2 × 3 cm right suprarenal mass, with high signal intensity displayed on the T_2-weighted image.

had no symptoms of headache, palpitations, or diaphoresis. With the exception of the management of her gestational diabetes, the pregnancy had proceeded unremarkably to that point. Given her first trimester presentation and the absence of edema or proteinuria, secondary causes for hypertension were appropriately considered. Further evaluation with a 24-h collection of urine revealed elevated levels of norepinephrine, and an MRI of the abdomen demonstrated a 2 × 3 cm mass near the hilum of the left kidney consistent with an extraadrenal pheochromocytoma (see Table 5 and Fig. 4).

By the time testing was complete and the diagnosis was established, the patient was in her 23rd wk of pregnancy, and it was at this time that she was admitted for initiation of adrenergic blockade and blood glucose monitoring. Although asymptomatic, she was found to be markedly orthostatic by both pulse and blood pressure. With a rise from the supine to standing position, her systolic and diastolic blood pressures of 190 and 100 mmHg each fell 30 mmHg, and her pulse increased 45 bpm. Phenoxybenzamine was introduced at a dose of 10 mg bid and gradually titrated to a dose of 20 mg bid. As alpha adrenergic blockade proceeded, intravenous fluids expanded her plasma volume and her insulin requirements diminished such that by the ninth day of adrenergic blockade, insulin doses had been reduced by two thirds.

Not surprisingly, issues over the timing of delivery and the timing of surgical intervention surfaced and were deliberated at length. Because several important factors needed to be considered in the management of her case, a multidisciplinary team of high risk obstetricians, endocrinologists, endocrine surgeons, and neonatologists met to discuss the most appropriate management plan. Postponement of surgery was associated with the maternal risk of hypertensive crises and with fetal risks of hypoxia and intrauterine fetal growth retardation from prolonged vasoconstriction. Immediate tumor resection, however, was attended with surgical technical difficulty. Owing to the location of her particular tumor, a transabdominal surgical approach was necessary, but one which would be technically difficult to perform in the third trimester with a gravid uterus obstructing the operative field. A cesarean section followed by tumor resection seemed the most prudent strategy, but this would still have to be postponed until fetal lung maturity had been reached, during which time potentially inadequate blockade could lead to the above mentioned complications. Ultimately, three options were proposed:

1. terminate the pregnancy and resect the tumor immediately;
2. resect the tumor immediately and manage the remainder of pregnancy expectantly;
3. medically manage the patient then perform a combined cesarean section/ tumor resection when maternal and fetal indicators suggested delivery was appropriate and fetal lung maturity had been reached.

The consensus of the multidisciplinary group was to recommend the third option; the patient was in agreement.

In the meantime, alpha blockade had proceeded well, and propranolol was added to control mild supine tachycardia. On the 10th hospital day, she was discharged with strict instructions to liberalize salt intake, monitor blood sugars, and maintain bed rest.

At home, daily orthostatic blood pressure measurements were performed by a visiting nurse and the patient was seen at weekly intervals in the maternal/fetal medicine clinic. Although her blood pressure was reasonably well controlled on 20 mg bid phenoxybenzamine and 10 mg tid propranolol, over the next few weeks, she developed symptomatic orthostasis, necessitating a reduction in the dose of phenoxybenzamine to 10 mg bid. At 30 wk gestation, when an ultrasound revealed that fetal growth rate was only 10% of normal, she was readmitted for fetal monitoring, administration of intravenous fluids, and maximization of adrenergic blockade.

Once admitted, phenoxybenzamine was pushed to a total dose of 30 mg qd as intravenous fluids were administered. The fetus was monitored daily with nonstress tests and amniotic fluid indices.

Early in the morning on the third day of admission, the patient began experiencing uterine contractions. She was rushed to labor and delivery, but as operative preparations were being made, the fetal heart rate declined from 100 to 80 bpm. Ten minutes later, heart tones were absent, and an ultrasound confirmed intrauterine fetal demise owing to placental abruption. Initially, the obstetrics team had planned to postpone delivery of the fetus until after tumor resection, but 2 h later, coagulation studies indicated that she had entered a state of disseminated intravascular coagulation. Prompt delivery of the fetus was therefore urgent. After 2 h of labor during which hypertensive surges were treated with nitroprusside and esmolol infusions, the patient delivered a nonviable fetus with a placenta that exhibited multiple areas of infarction and adherent blood clots.

Thereafter, the patient's condition rapidly deteriorated. Despite meticulous attention to blood pressure, hemodynamics, and blood losses during delivery, she nonetheless developed oliguric renal failure. Resection of the pheochromocytoma again had to wait until her coagulopathy resolved, renal function improved, and adequate adrenergic blockade was established. Therefore, nitroprusside was tapered and the esmolol infusion was predominantly used to control blood pressure at the same time reinstating escalating phenoxybenzamine doses.

Over the next few days, the patient's serum creatinine continued to rise. On the second day postpartum, she became acutely agitated and restless, then confused and verbally unresponsive. An extensive evaluation to explain her clinical status was unenlightening—metabolic, infectious, and hemorrhagic etiologies were all systematically investigated and excluded on the basis of appropriate testing. In the meantime, her blood pressure, which was stable on phenoxybenzamine, soon became labile when she became unable to take oral medications. Intravenous labetolol was temporarily substituted.

Serious consideration was given to dialysis when her creatinine rose to 3.7 mg/dL. Many involved in her care suspected that, in the absence of any other explanation, her neurologic status was a result of thiocyanate toxicity. However, dialysis (in the face of adrenergic blockade) was fraught with the potential for severe hypotension that might further endanger recovery of her renal function. As her urine output improved in the diuretic phase of acute tubular necrosis, the decision was made to observe her. Soon a thiocyanate level returned—a normal level was found.

Then, just as DIC seemed to be resolving and renal function started to improve, the patient developed seizure activity. High doses of labetolol used for blood pressure control and adrenergic blockade were implicated as the etiologic agent, and therefore, this was tapered. Phenoxybenzamine was administered through a nasogastric tube. Propranolol and prazosin were needed in addition to 40 mg bid phenoxybenzamine to optimally control her blood pressure.

After several days of intensive care monitoring and general supportive measures, her coagulopathy resolved, renal function normalized, and neurologic status returned to baseline. She was taken to surgery where a $3.5 \times 4.0 \times 1.8$ cm pheochromocytoma at the left renal hilum was resected without complications. Postoperatively, her course was uneventful. She was discharged home without pharmacologic agents in good condition, and has remained normotensive with normal catecholamine excretion ever since.

Discussion

Pheochromocytoma complicating pregnancy is a rare event. Yet, as demonstrated by Case 3, its presence has grave implications, both for management of the pregnancy and for the prognosis of the mother and offspring. Undiagnosed, the mortality for both approaches 50% (1). Antepartum diagnosis substantially reduces maternal mortality to 11%, and in recent years, treatment with alpha adrenergic blockade has reduced maternal mortality even further, to 3% *(2)*. However, despite treatment, fetal morbidity and mortality remain high, at approximately 15% *(3,4)*. The devastating consequences of pheochromocytomas discovered during pregnancy are clearly demonstrated in this case. Furthermore, this case shows that even with antepartum diagnosis, intensive monitoring, and careful pharmacological treatment, untoward fetal and maternal outcomes are still very possible.

The symptoms and signs of a previously quiescent pheochromocytoma may first manifest during pregnancy. The presenting features of pheochromocytoma in pregnancy are pleomorphic—just as they are in the nonpregnant state. During pregnancy, some patients present with classic hypertensive paroxysms associated with typical symptoms of headaches, palpitations, and diaphoresis. Others may present with postural hypotension, arrythmias, or sudden cardiovascular collapse that is either spontaneous, or induced by anesthesia or delivery *(1)*. In asymptomatic cases, pheochromocytoma may come to attention during pregnancy because of prenatal blood pressure monitoring. In the present case, the diagnosis was suspected because of the first trimester onset of hypertension and the coexistence of gestational diabetes mellitus.

Approximately 60% of patients with pheochromocytomas develop hyperglycemia or impaired glucose intolerance *(5)*. The mechanisms underlying hyperglycemia are multifactorial, and related to the various metabolic effects of catecholamines. For example, catecholamines directly inhibit pancreatic insulin secretion through an alpha$_2$ adrenergic receptor mediated inhibition *(6,7)*. They also stimulate glycogenolysis and impair peripheral insulin sensitivity by elevating free fatty acids *(8,9)*. The diabetic state associated with pheochromocytomas is reversible, as supported by the improvement in glucose tolerance with administration of alpha blockade, and as demonstrated by the resolution of hyperglycemia following surgical resection of these tumors *(10,11)*.

One of the major obstacles in making an early diagnosis of pheochromocytoma in pregnancy is the difficulty in differentiating it from pregnancy-induced hypertension and preeclampsia *(12,13)*. This distinction is crucial, because the treatment of preeclampsia, i.e., delivery of the fetus, may have catastrophic consequences in undiagnosed pheochromocytoma *(14)*. In this case, the absence of edema and proteinuria were extremely helpful clues. Later in pregnancy, the differentiation of a pheochromocytoma from toxemia of pregnancy is challenging, because both are associated with a wide variety of clinical manifestations *(15,16)*. When pheochromocytoma is suspected during pregnancy, appropriate analysis of a 24-h urine sample for catecholamines and catecholamine metabolites will usually confirm the diagnosis as it did here. Urinary catecholamine levels are unaffected by normal pregnancy except in unusually stressful situations, or in the period between the onset of labor and the second postpartum day *(17,18)*. Noteworthy in this particular case is the markedly elevated norepinephrine level accompanied by the quite normal epinephrine level—a typical biochemical finding in extra-adrenal pheochromocytomas *(19)*. This predominance of norepinephrine secretion in extra-adrenal tumors is suspected to result from the absence of high glucocorticoid levels necessary to induce full expression and activity of phenyl-ethanolamine-N-methyltransferase, which methylates norepinephrine to epinephrine *(20,21)*.

Localization of pheochromocytoma is especially important for operative planning in pregnancy. MRI is the preferred imaging modality for several reasons. As in the nonpregnant patient, it is highly sensitive, it is capable of detecting extraadrenal pheochromocytomas, and it has the superior ability to distinguish pheochromocytoma from other adrenal lesions by virtue of its hyperintense signal emitted on T_2-weighted images (22,23). In pregnancy, it has the further advantage over CT of avoiding exposure to ionizing radiation and contrast material. Nuclear medicine scintigraphy with ^{131}I MIBG is generally contraindicated in pregnancy.

Interestingly, fetal morbidity associated with maternal pheochromocytoma is not likely to be the direct consequence of elevated maternal catecholamines acting in the fetus. The placenta, which has high levels of catechol-O-methyl transferase and monoamine oxidase, metabolizes catecholamines, and therefore protects the fetus (24). This placental clearance of catecholamines implies that the essential element involved in adverse *in utero* effects is catecholamine-induced placental vasoconstriction, leading to ischemia with attendant effects on fetal oxygenation and nutrition. These effects in turn may result in hypoxia and intrauterine growth retardation (25,26). The therapeutic implication of this observation is the recognition that maintaining good control of maternal blood pressure is crucial to maximize the chances for fetal survival.

Issues regarding the timing of surgery for pheochromocytomas diagnosed during pregnancy have generated considerable controversy. There are no prospective controlled data to judge the optimal timing of surgery. Most authorities advocate surgical excision of the tumor in early pregnancy following preparation with alpha adrenergic antagonists (27,28). In the third trimester, medical treatment with adrenergic blocking agents continues and surgery is delayed until the fetus is of sufficient size and maturity that Cesarean section may be followed by extirpation of the tumor. The rationale for this approach is that before 28 wk gestation, surgery can be performed safely, and resection of the pheochromocytoma removes the fetus from exposure to the deleterious effects of catecholamines. In later pregnancy, uterine enlargement impairs localization of the pheochromocytoma and impedes its removal (29,30).

The basis for the above recommendations is derived from retrospective analyses of case reports that overall indicate improved maternal and fetal outcomes when the tumor is resected early in pregnancy, and poor surgical outcomes when tumor resection is attempted in late pregnancy (3,12,31). The gestational age at which the diagnosis of pheochromocytoma was firmly established proved to be particularly problematic in the patient presented here, for it was made within a time window wherein surgical resection would have been technically difficult, and would put the fetus at high risk for abortion. Yet, she was also at a gestational age at which medical management to bring the fetus to viability could potentially be lengthy. Although experience with long term treatment with alpha antagonists is limited, medical management of pheochromocytoma with delayed tumor removal has been successful. Successful outcomes with alpha adrenergic blockade administered for as long as 25 wk have been reported repeatedly in the literature (2,32–39).

Severe placental abruption occurred in this case, despite inpatient blood pressure monitoring, close fetal surveillance, and vigilant efforts to maximize adrenergic blockade. Two other cases of placental abruption developing in pregnancies complicated by pheochromocytomas have been reported in the literature (40,41). Although it is impossible to prove a causal relationship between catecholamine excess and the placental abruption in this case, it is plausible that placental vasoconstriction associated with hypertension may have contributed to the event, given that maternal hypertension is the most consistently identified factor predisposing to placental abruption (42–45).

If one assumes that placental vasoconstriction associated with the pheochromocytoma did contribute to the development of the abruption, this would imply that the degree of adrenergic blockade was suboptimal, despite what appeared to be reasonable blood pressure control. One could speculate that transient paroxysmal rises in blood pressure associated with catecholamine surges were not detected with periodic blood pressure measurements. All of this underscores the hazards of harboring a pheochromocytoma in pregnancy, even while under the protection of alpha blockade, and emphasizes that postponement of surgery is not without risk. Moreover, pressure from the uterus, hemorrhage into the tumor, uterine contractions, and even vigorous fetal movements can provoke catecholamine surges, leading to hypertensive crises, fetal hypoxia, and the potential deaths of the mother and fetus *(3)*.

Disseminated intravascular coagulation (DIC) complicates greater than 50% of cases of abruptio placentae, and the degree of placental abruption correlates with the severity of the coagulopathy *(46)*. Given the severity of this abruption, the development of DIC was not surprising. Nevertheless, the onset of DIC significantly complicated an already tenuous situation, and it led to a second major dilemma: weighing the risks of surgery in the face of a profound bleeding diathesis versus the risks of provoking hypertensive crises associated with vaginal delivery. Even in the presence of adequate adrenergic blockade, vaginal delivery can be dangerous because the physiologic stresses of labor may provoke massive catecholamine release leading to severe or fatal paroxysms *(12)*.

Finally, whereas the final outcome was not ideal for the fetus in this case, it is nevertheless clear that a multifaceted team approach to management of pheochromocytoma in pregnancy is critical in determining a plan that will optimize fetal and maternal outcomes.

REFERENCES

1. Schenker JG, Chowers I. Pheochromocytoma and pregnancy. Review of 89 cases. Obstet Gynecol Surv 1971;26:739–747.
2. Stenstrom G, Swolin K. Pheochromocytoma in pregnancy. Experience of treatment with phenoxybenzamine in three patients. Acta Obstet Gynecol Scand 1985;64:357–361.
3. Harper MA, Murnaghan GA, Kennedy L, Hadden DR, Atkinson AB. Phaeochromocytoma in pregnancy. Five cases and a review of the literature. Br J Obstet Gynaecol 1989;96:594–606.
4. Keely E. Endocrine causes of hypertension in pregnancy—when to start looking for zebras. Semin Perinatol 1998;22:471–484.
5. Manger WM, Gifford RW. Clinical and Experimental Pheochromocytoma. Blackwell Science, New York, 1996, p. 570.
6. Wilber JF, Turtle JR, Crane NA. Inhibition of insulin secretion by a phaeochromocytoma. Lancet 1966; 2:733.
7. Isles CG, Johnson JK. Phaeochromocytoma and diabetes mellitus: further evidence that alpha 2 receptors inhibit insulin release in man. Clin Endocrinol (Oxford) 1983;18:37–41.
8. Rosen SG, Clutter WE, Shah SD, Miller JP, Bier DM, Cryer PE. Direct alpha-adrenergic stimulation of hepatic glucose production in human subjects. Am J Physiol 1983;245:E616–E626.
9. Spergel G, Bleicher SJ, Ertel NH. Carbohydrate and fat metabolism in patients with pheochromocytoma. N Engl J Med 1968;278:803–809.
10. Stenstrom G, Sjostrom L, Smith U. Diabetes mellitus in phaeochromocytoma. Fasting blood glucose levels before and after surgery in 60 patients with phaeochromocytoma. Acta Endocrinol (Copenh) 1984;106:511–515.
11. Balestrieri PG, Spandrio S, Romanelli G, Giustina G. Diabetes mellitus as presenting feature in extra-adrenal pheochromocytoma: report of a case. Acta Diabetol Lat 1990;27:261–265.
12. Schenker JG, Granat M. Phaeochromocytoma and pregnancy—an updated appraisal. Aust N Z J Obstet Gynaecol 1982;22:1–10.
13. Zuspan FP. Catecholamines. Their role in pregnancy and the development of pregnancy-induced hypertension. J Reprod Med 1979;23:143–150.
14. Easterling TR, Carlson K, Benedetti TJ, Mancuso JJ. Hemodynamics associated with the diagnosis and treatment of pheochromocytoma in pregnancy. Am J Perinatol 1992;9:464–466.

15. el-Minawi MF, Paulino E, Cuesta M, Ceballos J. Pheochromocytoma masquerading as pre-eclamptic toxemia. Current concepts of diagnosis and treatment. Am J Obstet Gynecol 1971;109:389–395.
16. Hendee AE, Martin RD, Waters WC. Hypertension in pregnancy: toxemia or pheochromocytoma? Am J Obstet Gynecol 1969;105:64–72.
17. Zuspan FP. Urinary excretion of epinephrine and norepinephrine during pregnancy. J Clin Endocrinol Metab 1970;30:357–360.
18. Goodall M, Diddle AW. Epinephrine and norepinephrine in pregnancy. A comparative study of the adrenal gland and catechol output in different species of animals and man. Am J Obstet Gynecol 1971; 111:896–904.
19. Kimura N, Miura Y, Nagatsu I, Nagura H. Catecholamine synthesizing enzymes in 70 cases of functioning and non-functioning phaeochromocytoma and extra-adrenal paraganglioma. Virchows Arch A Pathol Anat Histopathol 1992;421:25–32.
20. Evinger MJ, Towle AC, Park DH, Lee P, Joh TH. Glucocorticoids stimulate transcription of the rat phenylethanolamine N-methyltransferase (PNMT) gene in vivo and in vitro. Cell Mol Neurobiol 1992; 12:193–215.
21. Funahashi H, Imai T, Tanaka Y, et al. Discrepancy between PNMT presence and relative lack of adrenaline production in extra-adrenal pheochromocytoma. J Surg Oncol 1994;57:196–200.
22. Greenberg M, Moawad AH, Wieties BM, et al. Extraadrenal pheochromocytoma: detection during pregnancy using MR imaging. Radiology 1986;161:475–476.
23. Udelsman R, Fishman EK. Radiology of the adrenal. Endocrinol Metab Clin North Am 2000;29: 27–42.
24. Breuer H. The metabolism of the natural estrogens. Vitamins and Hormones 1962;20:285.
25. Dahia PL, Hayashida CY, Strunz C, Abelin N, Toledo SP. Low cord blood levels of catecholamine from a newborn of a pheochromocytoma patient. Eur J Endocrinol 1994;130:217–219.
26. Landsberg L. Pheochromocytoma complicating pregnancy [comment]. Eur J Endocrinol 1994;130:215–216.
27. Landsberg L, Young J. Catecholamines and the Adrenal Medulla. In: Foster D, Wilson J, eds. Williams Textbook of Endocrinology, WB Saunders, Philadelphia, PA, 1998, pp. 665–728.
28. Bravo EL. Evolving concepts in the pathophysiology, diagnosis, and treatment of pheochromocytoma. Endocr Rev 1994;15:356–368.
29. Freier DT, Thompson NW. Pheochromocytoma and pregnancy: the epitome of high risk. Surgery 1993; 114:1148–1152.
30. Fudge TL, McKinnon WM, Geary WL. Current surgical management of pheochromocytoma during pregnancy. Arch Surg 1980;115:1224–1225.
31. Burgess GE. Alpha blockade and surgical intervention of pheochromocytoma in pregnancy. Obstet Gynecol 1979;53:266–270.
32. Griffith MI, Felts JH, James FM, Meyers RT, Shealy GM, Woodruff LF Jr. Successful control of pheochromocytoma in pregnancy. JAMA 1974;229:437–439.
33. Lyons CW, Colmorgen GH. Medical management of pheochromocytoma in pregnancy. Obstet Gynecol 1988;72:450–451.
34. Simanis J, Amerson JR, Hendee AE, Anton AH. Unresectable pheochromocytoma in pregnancy. Pharmacology and biochemistry. Am J Med 1972;53:381–385.
35. Venuto R, Burstein P, Schneider R. Pheochromocytoma: antepartum diagnosis and management with tumor resection in the puerperium. Am J Obstet Gynecol 1984;150:431–432.
36. Sukenik S, Biale Y, Ben-Aderet N, Khodadadi J, Levi D, Stern J. Successful control of pheochromocytoma in pregnancy. Case report. Eur J Obstet Gynecol Reprod Biol 1979;9:249–251.
37. Oliver MD, Brownjohn AM, Vinall PS. Medical management of phaeochromocytoma in pregnancy. Aust N Z J Obstet Gynaecol 1990;30:268–271.
38. Mastboom JL. [Treatment of pheochromocytoma during pregnancy]. Geburtshilfe Frauenheilkd 1966; 26:568–571.
39. Chukwuemeka AC, Paton AM, Gebbie DA, Ayim EN, Dhall DP. Phaeochromocytoma in pregnancy. East Afr Med J 1974;51:496–499.
40. Batts JA Jr, Tchilinguirian NG, Passmore J. Pheochromocytoma in pregnancy: a case report and review of the pathophysiology. Am J Obstet Gynecol 1974;118:576–577.
41. Pestelek B, Kapor M. Pheochromocytoma and abruptio placentae. Am J Obstet Gynecol 1963;85:538–540.
42. Pritchard JA, Mason R, Corley M, Pritchard S. Genesis of severe placental abruption. Am J Obstet Gynecol 1970;108:22–27.

43. Naeye RL, Harkness WL, Utts J. Abruptio placentae and perinatal death: a prospective study. Am J Obstet Gynecol 1977;128:740–746.
44. Kramer MS, Usher RH, Pollack R, Boyd M, Usher S. Etiologic determinants of abruptio placentae. Obstet Gynecol 1997;89:221–226.
45. Ananth CV, Smulian JC, Vintzileos AM. Incidence of placental abruption in relation to cigarette smoking and hypertensive disorders during pregnancy: a meta-analysis of observational studies. Obstet Gynecol 1999;93:622–628.
46. Sutton DM, Hauser R, Kulapongs P, Bachmann F. Intravascular coagulation in abruptio placentae. Am J Obstet Gynecol 1971;109:604–614.

CASE #4: IT'S ALL IN THE GENES

Case Description

A 56-yr-old Russian woman with a history of hypertension went to an emergency room (ER) with a severe headache that was unrelieved by over-the-counter analgesics. Ten years prior to this, while living in the Ukraine, she began experiencing intense throbbing bifrontal headaches that occurred two to three times a week. The headaches were accompanied by visual changes, pallor, and generalized weakness. Over the next 5 yr, the headaches became more severe and were accompanied by symptoms of sweating and palpitations. A few months prior to the ER visit, she sought medical attention when the headaches began to disturb her on a daily basis. Her blood pressure was noted to be elevated, and she started treatment with hydrochlorthiazide and methyldopa. Although her blood pressure apparently normalized with this therapy, she continued to experience heat intolerance. One week prior to her ER visit, she was given pseudoephedrine for a "sinus" headache.

In the ER, the patient's blood pressure was found to be 210/100mmHg. She was treated with meperidine and phenergan. After instruction to take her antihypertensives the next morning, she was discharged. Three hours later, she returned when her headache worsened. Her blood pressure had risen to 240/140 mmHg and an electrocardiogram revealed ST segment depressions in the inferior leads. After she showed no response to morphine, nitropaste, and furosemide, she was admitted to the medical intensive care unit with an hypertensive emergency.

Shortly after admission, the patient's blood pressure was noted to be labile and pheochromocytoma was considered in the differential diagnosis. Elevated catecholamine levels and an abdominal CT scan showing bilateral adrenal masses confirmed this diagnosis (see Table 6). She began alpha adrenergic blockade with phenoxybenzamine, followed by beta blockade with propranolol, and was discharged home to complete a two-week preoperative course.

As she was awaiting surgery, information regarding the patient's family history was obtained. Upon further questioning, the patient related that both her mother and 25-yr-old son had described similar "spells" of headaches, palpitations, and diaphoresis, raising the suspicion for a hereditary form of pheochromocytoma. When a serum basal calcitonin level of 13,299 ng/L returned, the syndrome of multiple endocrine neoplasia was confirmed.

The patient was taken to surgery where she underwent a bilateral total adrenalectomy. The right adrenal contained a pheochromocytoma with a diameter of 3 cm and the left adrenal contained a pheochromocytoma with a 6.5 cm diameter. She recovered well postoperatively and was discharged home, relieved of the adrenergic symptoms, with a normal blood pressure. Six weeks later, she underwent total thyroidectomy. At surgery, hard nodules were found in both lobes of the thyroid gland. Two superior parathyroid glands

Table 6
Laboratory Evaluation

24 h urine		Normal range
VMA (mg)	24.4	(1–8)
Catecholamines (μg)	3620	(0–100)
Metanephrines (mg)	8.3	(0.3–0.9)
Plasma		
Norepinephrine (ng/L)	3955	(65–400)
Epinephrine (ng/L)	15.92	(0–70)

were identified, but not removed. Histopathologic analysis established the diagnosis of medullary carcinoma of the thyroid.

Over the next several years, the patient suffered multiple episodes of nephrolithiasis and her serum calcium level was noted to rise. Eighteen years after the initial surgeries, her calcium level has risen to 12 mg/dL, phosphorus level has declined to 2.8 mg/dL, and the intact parathyroid hormone level is 146 pg/mL. She has not yet undergone a parathyroidectomy.

The index patient's only child, a 25-yr-old son, was evaluated for MEN 2, and was found to have medullary carcinoma of the thyroid and bilateral pheochromocytomas. He has undergone bilateral adrenalectomy, total thyroidectomy, and a left modified neck dissection. Recently, calcitonin levels of up to 2000 ng/L have been found in a follow up visit. In order to search for metastases, a CT, an MRI, and an octreotide nuclear medicine scan were performed. The only identifiable site of possible medullary carcinoma was found in the right superior mediastinum, an area with a known mass of 2 cm that has been stable in size for several years. After much discussion, the patient proceeded to a diagnostic laparoscopy to exclude hepatic metastases, mediastinal resection of the mass, and to a right modified radical neck dissection. Histopathology confirmed metastatic medullary carcinoma of the thyroid in the mediastinal mass; 2/14 lymph nodes were positive for metastatic disease. His recovery has been uncomplicated. Postoperative pentagastrin stimulated calcitonin levels are unavailable.

Discussion

The syndrome of multiple endocrine neoplasia type 2 (MEN 2) was first described 40 yr ago by J. Sipple in his article that described several cases of thyroid cancer associated with pheochromocytomas (1). During the last half century, progress in the understanding of the MEN 2 syndromes has led to the evolution of a fascinating chronicle that began with the identification of the clinical features of MEN 2. This was followed by the characterization of the biochemical abnormalities and culminated with the elucidation of its molecular basis. MEN 2 is an inherited cancer syndrome defined by the concurrence of hyperplasia or tumor in the adrenal glands, thyroid, and/or parathyroids. It is characterized by autosomal dominant inheritance with nearly complete penetrance and variable expressivity of each component (2). The subclassification of MEN into its three distinct syndromes is shown in Table 7.

Pheochromocytomas are found in approximately 50% of patients with MEN 2A and MEN 2B, although this frequency varies widely among different kindreds and is greater when surveillance of individuals is extended over long durations (3,4). As seen in the

Table 7
Clinical Varieties of MEN 2

Men 2A	Men 2B
MTC 100%	MTC 100%
Pheochromocytoma 50%	Pheochromocytoma 50%
Hyperparathyroidism 20%	Enteric ganglia hyperplasia 100%
	Marfanoid habitus !00%
	Intestinal ganglioneuromatosis/
	Mucosal neuromas 100%
MEN 2A variants	
FMTC	
MEN 2A with cutaneous lichen amyloidosis	
MEN 2A with Hirschsprung disease	

Legend: MTC, medullary thyroid carcinoma; FMTC, familial medullary thyroid carcinoma.

present case, pheochromocytomas associated with MEN are typically located within the adrenal gland bed, are frequently bilateral, and are rarely malignant (5–8). Prior to the recognition of the syndrome in the early 1960s, at least half of all deaths in MEN 2A were attributed to cardiovascular disease—many of which were likely related to pheochromocytomas (2). Furthermore, before prospective screening, patients often presented with large pheochromocytomas accompanied by hypertension, headaches, and cardiac arrythmias. Now that many MEN patients are screened regularly for the development of pheochromocytoma, the presentation of pheochromocytoma has changed, such that most MEN patients are asymptomatic or oligosymptomatic (9). Nevertheless, pheochromocytomas in MEN may cause palpitations, headaches, or anxiety attacks early in the course of the development of these tumors, prior to the detection of significant hypertension (3). Such may have been the scenario for the son, who although normotensive, described a history of "spells" and was also found to have pheochromocytomas.

In screened individuals from kindreds with known MEN 2, medullary thyroid carcinoma usually precedes the development of pheochromocytoma. However, pheochromocytoma is still frequently the first manifestation of MEN 2 in a newly discovered index case, as illustrated by this patient. For example, pheochromocytoma was the first manifestation of the MEN 2 syndrome in the index case in 35 (64%) families studied by Calmettes et al. who followed a series of 55 kindreds (10).

Although the presentation of pheochromocytoma and MEN 2 in these individuals preceded the era of genetic testing, this patient, nevertheless, serves as a basis for a discussion of the prospects for the clinical application of knowledge regarding the molecular basis of the MEN 2 syndromes. MEN 2 is caused by activating germline mutations in the RET protooncogene, which encodes a tyrosine kinase receptor expressed in tissues and tumors of neural crest origin. This receptor appears to transduce signals for diverse processes, including cell growth, differentiation, survival, and death. Mutations in the RET protooncogene result in constiutitive activation of the tyrosine kinase receptor, rendering cells susceptible to neoplastic transformation (11). In MEN 2A and familial medullary thyroid carcinoma, mutations most commonly affect cysteine residues of the extracellular domain of the receptor, whereas in MEN 2B, mutations affect one of three codons in the intracellular domain (see Fig. 5) (12).

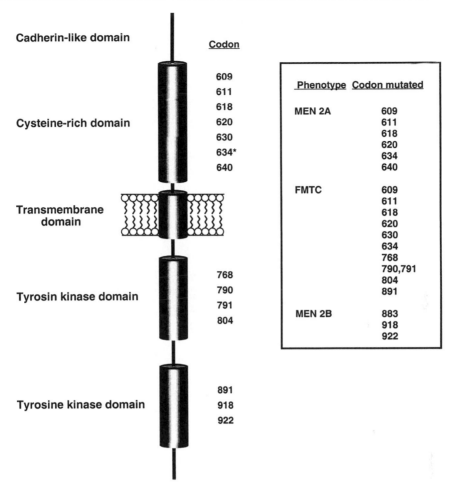

Fig. 5. Schematic representation of the product of the *RET* protooncogene product, a tyrosine kinase receptor that is rendered constitutively active by mutations at codons indicated above. A continuously updated listing of nucleotide substitutions in the *RET* protooncogene is available on the Human Gene Mutation Database at www.uwcm.ac.uk/uwcm/mg/ns/1/120346.html

The identification of germline mutations in the *RET* protooncogene in MEN 2 has profoundly changed the approach to the diagnosis and management of MEN 2 syndromes. Mutational analysis of the *RET* protooncogene to identify carrier status for the mutation is now the clinical standard of care, and permits definitive identification of individuals at risk in afflicted families *(13)*. The major impact of genetic testing in identifying affected individuals involves offering early prophylactic thyroidectomy to prevent the development of medullary thyroid carcinoma, because it affects virtually all those with MEN 2 and is potentially lethal *(13,14)*. In the management of adrenal medullary disease, genetic testing is useful because it enables identification of gene carriers, who are at risk for the development of pheochromocytomas, and who therefore require biochemical screening.

Interestingly, genotype-phenotype correlation studies have suggested that mutations of specific residues of the *RET* protooncogene may be highly predictive of developing pheochromocytoma. For example, any substitution at codon 634 has been associated with an increased frequency of pheochromocytoma, especially the C634R mutation. MEN 2A families that rarely develop pheochromocytoma are more likely to have mutations in codons 609, 611, 618, or 620 *(15–19)*. These studies suggest that the variability in the penetrance of pheochromocytomas among different kindreds with MEN 2 might be explained by differences in the biochemical consequences of the particular mutation involved. The precise mechanism of genotype/phenotype effects is not known for certain, but theoretically, different *RET* mutations could cause *RET* to signal at different intensities, or different mutations could result in altered signaling of *RET* down distinct pathways *(20)*. Some experts speculate that targeted screening based upon specific codon mutations may be possible in the future to determine the vigilance with which one should screen for pheochromocytoma within a certain kindred *(18)*. In the authors' opinion, results of genotype–phenotype correlations should be interpreted cautiously, since ascertainment biases can affect results. Targeted screening is only appropriate if a perfect genotype–phenotype correlation is found.

Because at least 50% of patients with MEN 2 are likely to develop adrenal medullary abnormalities, annual screening for pheochromocytoma in patients with known *RET* protooncogene mutations and in patients with previously diagnosed MEN is recommended beginning between the ages of 5–10 yr *(2)*. The goal of screening for pheochromocytoma in individuals with MEN 2 is to detect the tumor before it causes significant or life-threatening consequences of catecholamine excess.

Pheochromocytomas associated with MEN 2 cause distinctive biochemical features that have important implications in performing and interpreting screening tests. Familial pheochromocytomas are more likely to secrete large amounts of epinephrine *(21)*. For this reason, an increase in urinary epinephrine or an increased ratio of epinephrine to norepinephrine in a 24-h urine sample may be the only abnormalities detectable early in the course of the disease *(18,22)*. Urinary vanillylmandelic acid excretion is usually normal in the early stages of the disease and is therefore less valuable for early detection. Measurement of plasma metanephrines and normetanephrines for the early detection of pheochromocytomas in MEN 2 is an investigational approach that has been studied in small numbers of individuals *(23)*. At the present time, assays for plasma metanephrine and normetanephrines are not widely available, and further data will be needed to establish their validity as screening tools.

Two interesting questions arise from the discovery of *RET* protooncogene mutations in MEN 2 syndromes:

1. Do mutations in *RET* play a role in the development of sporadic pheochromocytomas?
2. Should individuals who develop sporadic pheochromocytomas undergo mutational analysis of the *RET* gene to detect *de novo* or previously unidentified heritable MEN 2?

Somatic mutations of *RET* have been discovered in the tumor tissue of some sporadic pheochromocytomas, a finding which is conceptually interesting because it confirms that *RET* mutations are involved in tumorigenesis *(24.25)*. However, germline mutations of *RET* have not been identified in patients with apparently sporadic cases of pheochromocytomas. Specifically, combined data from five studies analyzing 156 patients have not identified a single germline *RET* mutation among patients with sporadic pheochromocytomas *(26–30)*. These data indicate that mutational analysis of *RET* in an individual with an apparently sporadic pheochromocytoma is not likely to be useful in detecting a previously unsuspected MEN 2 syndrome. However, patients with bilateral or family history of pheochromocytomas, should be evaluated for MEN 2, and genetic testing for *RET* may be indicated.

In general, the treatment of pheochromocytoma in MEN 2 does not differ from the treatment of sporadic pheochromocytoma. However, because of the proclivity for bilateral pheochromocytomas to develop in the MEN 2 syndromes, controversy has arisen over how extensive the initial adrenal resection should be. Bilateral adrenalectomy is clearly indicated in individuals with bilateral tumors. Controversy ensues, however, when a unilateral tumor is found, because available data demonstrate a 30–50% probability that a pheochromocytoma will develop in the unaffected adrenal within 10 yr. Advocates of unilateral adrenalectomy reason that unilateral surgery forestalls the need for exogenous replacement glucocorticoids, and cite data indicating that no deaths have occurred as a result of catecholamine crises in patients who underwent unilateral surgery and later developed bilateral disease *(3,31–34)*. The pivotal issue in the controversy involves weighing the risk of the Addisonian state following bilateral adrenalectomy against the risk of complications which might occur as a result of a second pheochromocytoma developing in the contralateral gland. Given the rarity of malignant pheochromocytomas in the MEN 2 syndromes and the potential risks attendant to dependence upon exogenous glucocorticoid replacement, the majority of experts favor unilateral adrenalectomy with careful surveillance of the contralateral gland for tumor development *(31,35)*.

Although the clinical presentation of pheochromocytoma has changed, pheochromocytomas continue to contribute to the morbidity and mortality associated with MEN 2. This is illustrated by reports of hypertensive crises leading to cerebrovascular hemorrahage, hypertensive encephalopathy, and deaths in individuals known to be at risk for developing pheochromocytomas *(33,36)*. In a survey of 100 cases of MEN 2A, pheochromocytoma was the cause of death in 11 of 17 patients who ultimately died. Ten of these 11 died suddenly, emphasizing the necessity of systematic biochemical screening in at-risk individuals, even in the absence of clinical symptoms *(37)*.

One can foresee that in the future, because most individuals with MEN will have undergone prophylactic thyroidectomy at an early age and thus have prevented its development, screening for the other manifestations of MEN 2A will become the most challenging aspect of care of these patients.

Aside from special issues associated with MEN 2A, there are two notable aspects of this case which deserve comment. Perhaps most remarkable is the prolonged duration over which the index patient was symptomatic prior to seeking medical attention. Such a delay has been observed often, because of the insidious onset of symptoms which seem relatively unalarming to patients. Engelman fittingly referred to this delay as the "diagnosis gap" *(38)*. Second, this case serves as yet another reminder of the adverse effects certain medications can have on patients who harbor a pheochromocytoma. Here, the sympathomimetic amine, pseudoephedrine, probably triggered a catecholamine-induced hypertensive crisis which worsened further after the administration of meperidine. Catecholamine crises triggered by opiates in patients with pheochromocytomas are frequently observed, but their untoward effects have received insufficient emphasis in the literature *(39)*.

REFERENCES

1. Sipple J. The association of pheochromocytoma with carcinoma of the thyroid gland. Am J Med 1961; 31:163–166.

2. Gagel R. Multiple Endocrine Neoplasia. In: Foster D, Wilson J, eds. Williams Textbook of Endocrinology. WB Saunders, Philadelphia, PA, 1998, pp. 1627–1649.

3. Gagel RF, Tashjian AH Jr, Cummings T, et al. The clinical outcome of prospective screening for multiple endocrine neoplasia type 2a. An 18-year experience. N Engl J Med 1988;318:478–484.

4. Vasen HF, Nieuwenhuijzen Kruseman AC, Berkel H, et al. Multiple endocrine neoplasia syndrome type 2: the value of screening and central registration. A study of 15 kindreds in The Netherlands. Am J Med 1987;83:847–852.

5. Howe JR, Norton JA, Wells SA Jr. Prevalence of pheochromocytoma and hyperparathyroidism in multiple endocrine neoplasia type 2A: results of long-term follow-up. Surgery 1993;114:1070–1077.

6. Carney JA, Sizemore GW, Sheps SG. Adrenal medullary disease in multiple endocrine neoplasia, type 2: pheochromocytoma and its precursors. Am J Clin Pathol 1976;66:279–290.

7. Keiser HR, Beaven MA, Doppman J, Wells S Jr, Buja LM. Sipple's syndrome: medullary thyroid carcinoma, pheochromocytoma, and parathyroid disease. Studies in a large family. NIH conference. Ann Intern Med 1973;78:561–579.

8. Modigliani E, Vasen HM, Raue K, et al. Pheochromocytoma in multiple endocrine neoplasia type 2: European study. The Euromen Study Group. J Int Med 1995;238:363–367.

9. Pomares FJ, Canas R, Rodriguez JM, Hernandez AM, Parrilla P, Tebar FJ. Differences between sporadic and multiple endocrine neoplasia type 2A phaeochromocytoma. Clin Endocrinol (Oxf) 1998;48:195–200.

10. Calmettes C, Rosenberg-Gourgin M, Caron J, Feingold N. Pheochromocytoma: a frequent indicator for MEN 2. Henry Ford Hosp Med J 1992;40:276–277.

11. Santoro M, Melillo RM, Carlomagno F, et al. Molecular biology of the MEN2 gene. J Intern Med 1998; 243:505–508.

12. Eng C. RET proto-oncogene in the development of human cancer. J Clin Oncol 1999;17:380–393.

13. Gagel RF, Cote GJ, Martins Bugalho MJ, et al. Clinical use of molecular information in the management of multiple endocrine neoplasia type 2A. J Intern Med 1995;238:333–341.

14. Lips CJ, Landsvater RM, Hoppener JW, et al. Clinical screening as compared with DNA analysis in families with multiple endocrine neoplasia type 2A [see comments]. N Engl J Med 1994;331:828–835.

15. Mulligan LM, Eng C, Healey CS, et al. Specific mutations of the RET proto-oncogene are related to disease phenotype in MEN 2A and FMTC. Nat Genet 1994;6:70–74.

16. Eng C, Clayton D, Schuffenecker I, et al. The relationship between specific RET proto-oncogene mutations and disease phenotype in multiple endocrine neoplasia type 2. International RET mutation consortium analysis. JAMA1996;276:1575–1579.

17. Frank-Raue K, Hoppner W, Frilling A, et al. Mutations of the ret protooncogene in German multiple endocrine neoplasia families: relation between genotype and phenotype. German Medullary Thyroid Carcinoma Study Group. J Clin Endocrinol Metab 1996;81:1780–1783.

18. Frank-Raue K, Kratt T, Hoppner W, Buhr H, Ziegler R, Raue F. Diagnosis and management of pheochromocytomas in patients with multiple endocrine neoplasia type 2-relevance of specific mutations in the RET proto-oncogene. Eur J Endocrinol 1996;135:222–225.

19. Schuffenecker I, Billaud M, Calender A, et al. RET proto-oncogene mutations in French MEN 2A and FMTC families. Hum Mol Genet 1994;3:1939–1943.

20. Ponder BA. The phenotypes associated with ret mutations in the multiple endocrine neoplasia type 2 syndrome. Cancer Res 1999;59:1736s–1741s; discussion 1742s.

21. Vistelle R, Grulet H, Gibold C, et al. High permanent plasma adrenaline levels: a marker of adrenal medullary disease in medullary thyroid carcinoma. Clin Endocrinol (Oxf) 1991;34:133–138.

22. Hamilton BP, Landsberg L, Levine RJ. Measurement of urinary epinephrine in screening for pheochromocytoma in multiple endocrine neoplasia type II. Am J Med 1978;65:1027–1032.

23. Eisenhofer G, Lenders JW, Linehan WM, Walther MM, Goldstein DS, Keiser HR. Plasma normetanephrine and metanephrine for detecting pheochromocytoma in von Hippel-Lindau disease and multiple endocrine neoplasia type 2. N Engl J Med 1999;340:1872–1879.

24. Beldjord C, Desclaux-Arramond F, Raffin-Sanson M, et al. The RET protooncogene in sporadic pheochromocytomas: frequent MEN 2-like mutations and new molecular defects [see comments]. J Clin Endocrinol Metab 1995;80:2063–2068.

25. Zedenius J, Wallin G, Hamberger B, Nordenskjold M, Weber G, Larsson C. Somatic and MEN 2A de novo mutations identified in the RET proto-oncogene by screening of sporadic MTC:s. Hum Mol Genet 1994;3:1259–1262.

26. Brauch H, Hoeppner W, Jahnig H, et al. Sporadic pheochromocytomas are rarely associated with germ-line mutations in the vhl tumor suppressor gene or the ret protooncogene. J Clin Endocrinol Metab 1997; 82:4101–4104.

27. Bar M, Friedman E, Jakobovitz O, et al. Sporadic phaeochromocytomas are rarely associated with germ-line mutations in the von Hippel-Lindau and RET genes. Clin Endocrinol (Oxf) 1997;47:707–712.

28. Eng C, Crossey PA, Mulligan LM, et al. Mutations in the RET proto-oncogene and the von Hippel-Lindau disease tumour suppressor gene in sporadic and syndromic phaeochromocytomas. J Med Genet 1995;32:934–937.

29. Lindor NM, Honchel R, Khosla S, Thibodeau SN. Mutations in the RET protooncogene in sporadic pheochromocytomas. J Clin Endocrinol Metab 1995;80:627–629.

30. Hofstra RM, Stelwagen T, Stulp RP, et al. Extensive mutation scanning of RET in sporadic medullary thyroid carcinoma and of RET and VHL in sporadic pheochromocytoma reveals involvement of these genes in only a minority of cases. J Clin Endocrinol Metab 1996;81:2881–2884.

31. Lairmore TC, Ball DW, Baylin SB, Wells SA Jr. Management of pheochromocytomas in patients with multiple endocrine neoplasia type 2 syndromes. Ann Surg 1993;217:595–601; discussion 601–603.

32. Jansson S, Tisell LE, Fjalling M, Lindberg S, Jacobsson L, Zachrisson BF. Early diagnosis of and surgical strategy for adrenal medullary disease in MEN II gene carriers. Surgery 1988;103:11–18.

33. Lips KJ, Van der Sluys Veer J, Struyvenberg A, et al. Bilateral occurrence of pheochromocytoma in patients with the multiple endocrine neoplasia syndrome type 2A (Sipple's syndrome). Am J Med 1981; 70:1051–1060.

34. Tibblin S, Dymling JF, Ingemansson S, Telenius-Berg M. Unilateral versus bilateral adrenalectomy in multiple endocrine neoplasia IIA. World J Surg 1983;7:201–208.

35. de Graaf JS, Dullaart RP, Zwierstra RP. Complications after bilateral adrenalectomy for phaeochromocytoma in multiple endocrine neoplasia type 2—a plea to conserve adrenal function. Eur J Surg 1999; 165:843–846.

36. Jadoul M, Leo JR, Berends MJ, et al. Pheochromocytoma-induced hypertensive encephalopathy revealing MEN-IIa syndrome in a 13-year old boy. Implications for screening procedures and surgery. Horm Metab Res Suppl 1989;21:46–49.

37. Casanova S, Rosenberg-Bourgin M, Farkas D, et al. Phaeochromocytoma in multiple endocrine neoplasia type 2 A: survey of 100 cases. Clin Endocrinol (Oxf) 1993;38:531–537.

38. Engelman K. Principles in the diagnosis of pheochromocytoma. Bull N Y Acad Med 1969;45:851–858.

39. Landsberg L, Young J. Catecholamines and the adrenal medulla. In: Foster D, Wilson J, eds. Williams Textbook of Endocrinology, WB Saunders, Philadelphia, PA, 1998, pp. 665–728.

ACKNOWLEDGMENT

The authors wish to acknowledge the contributions of Johanna Palotta, MD for providing clinical information for the final case of this chapter, and of Peter Kopp, MD for his assistance with the figures and critical review of this manuscript.

10

Hypercalcemia and Hyperparathyroidism

Bart L. Clarke, MD and Sundeep Khosla, MD

CONTENTS

CASE #1: PRIMARY HYPERPARATHYROIDISM

Case Description

A 62-yr-old woman presented in the outpatient clinic with a serum calcium of 10.6 mg/dL (normal, 8.9–10.1 mg/dL) and phosphate of 2.8 mg/dL (normal, 2.5–4.5 mg/dL). Her serum total alkaline phosphatase was 160 U/L (normal, 108–282 U/L), and serum creatinine 0.8 mg/dL (normal, 0.6–0.9 mg/dL). Her whole-molecule parathyroid hormone (PTH) by immunochemiluminometric assay (ICMA) was increased at 5.5 pmol/L (normal 1.0–5.2 pmol/L). Her 24-h urine calcium was 260 mg (normal, 20–275 mg), with 24-h urine creatinine 1100 mg. The calculated calcium to creatinine clearance ratio (24-h urine calcium × serum creatinine/24-h urine creatinine × serum total calcium) was 0.018, consistent with a diagnosis of primary hyperparathyroidism.

Further evaluation showed that she had forearm osteopenia with a one-third distal radius bone mineral density (BMD) of 0.873 gm/cm^2 (T-score: −1.8, Z-score: −2.0), vertebral osteoporosis with an L2–L4 lumbar spine BMD of 0.650 gm/cm^2 (T-score: −2.5, Z-score: −2.0), and left femoral neck osteopenia with BMD of 0.755 gm/cm^2 (T-score: −1.9, Z-score: −1.5). An X-ray of the kidneys, ureters, and bladder with tomograms showed no calcium-containing kidney stones. She denied any complaint of abdominal pain, esophageal reflux, heartburn, or history of peptic ulcer disease. She complained of mild fatigue and difficulty maintaining concentration, and wondered whether her mild hypercalcemia was contributing to her lack of energy or declining mental acuity.

From: *Contemporary Endocrinology: Challenging Cases in Endocrinology*
Edited by: M. E. Molitch © Humana Press Inc., Totowa, NJ

Past medical history was significant for mild essential hypertension for 5 yr, easily controlled with hydrochlorothiazide 25 mg/d, hypercholesterolemia diagnosed 2 yr earlier and treated to goal range with atorvastatin 10 mg/d without hepatitis or myositis, and deep venous thrombosis (DVT) with pulmonary embolus (PE) 10 yr ago associated with bed rest recommended for a traumatic vertebral compression fracture. She underwent spontaneous menopause at age 52 yr, but was never prescribed hormone replacement therapy (HRT) or raloxifene because of her history of DVT and PE. Her uterus was intact and she had no history of calcium-containing kidney stones.

Current medications included hydrochlorothiazide 25 mg/d, atorvastatin 10 mg/d, aspirin 81 mg/d, calcium carbonate 500 mg elemental calcium/d, and multivitamin containing vitamin D 400 IU/d. She had never taken alendronate, risedronate, etidronate, salmon calcitonin nasal spray, or fluoride. She denied known drug allergies.

Family history was unremarkable for known hypercalcemia, hypercalciuria, calcium-containing kidney stones, osteoporosis, or other metabolic bone disease. She stopped smoking cigarettes 20 yr ago after 12 pack-years, and denied any history of alcohol use or excessive caffeine intake.

Her vital signs included height 188 cm, weight 72.0 kg, right arm blood pressure (sitting) 158/88 mmHg, and regular pulse (sitting) of 76/min. Physical examination was within normal limits except for mild arcus senilis bilaterally, mild upper thoracic kyphosis, and mild superficial lower extremity varicose veins. She had no bone pain with palpation or percussion, and no costovertebral angle tenderness to percussion.

She was given a tentative diagnosis of mild primary hyperparathyroidism, complicated by mild lumbar spine osteoporosis, and advised to discontinue her hydrochlorothiazide for 1 mo in order to determine her serum total calcium and whole-molecule PTH off thiazide. When she returned 1 mo later, her repeat serum total calcium was 10.4 mg/dL and PTH 6.2 pmol/L, confirming the diagnosis of mild primary hyperparathyroidism. Treatment options were reviewed with the patient, including conservative management, traditional elective parathyroidectomy, and minimally invasive parathyroidectomy. She preferred minimally invasive parathyroidectomy because of unwillingness to live with the knowledge that she had a benign tumor in her neck, and concern about her osteoporosis and inability to take HRT. Parathyroid sestamibi scan showed uptake in the region of the right inferior parathyroid gland, and she underwent unilateral neck exploration with removal of a right inferior parathyroid adenoma of wet weight 200 mg. Her preoperative whole-molecule PTH level was 8 pmol/L, and her PTH level immediately after adenoma removal was 0.4 pmol/L, confirming removal of the source of her excess parathyroid hormone. Her postoperative serum calcium 6 h after surgery was 8.5 mg/dL, with repeat serum calcium of 9.2 mg/dL 24 h after surgery. She was dismissed from hospital on a total daily elemental calcium intake of 1500 mg and instructed to continue her vitamin D supplement of 400 IU/d.

Discussion

Primary hyperparathyroidism is estimated to occur in 1:1000 in men and in 2–3:1000 women, making it the most common cause of outpatient hypercalcemia (1,2). Primary hyperparathyroidism occurs at all ages, but most commonly is reported in 50–60-yr-old postmenopausal women. Wermers et al. reported that the incidence of primary hyperparathyroidism was declining in Olmsted County, MN, but it has not yet been confirmed that this is a national trend (3). Modern health care management practices have restricted routine measurement of serum calcium in asymptomatic patients, which will likely reduce the incidence of recognized primary hyperparathyroidism further.

Primary hyperparathyroidism is caused by oversecretion, or inappropriate secretion, of PTH for a given level of serum ionized calcium. Solitary parathyroid adenomas are the cause of PTH oversecretion in 80–85% of cases, whereas four-gland hyperplasia is found in 15–20% of cases, and parathyroid cancer in less than 0.5% of cases. As with other endocrine tumors, the pathologic diagnosis of parathyroid carcinoma is difficult, and is usually based on evidence of local tissue or vascular invasion or metastatic disease *(4)*. The majority of single parathyroid adenomas represent sporadic disease, whereas four-gland hyperplasia most often implies a familial disorder, which may be due to multiple endocrine neoplasia (MEN) types I or IIA. Excess PTH secretion by an adenoma is a result of loss of feedback control of PTH secretion by extracellular calcium at the cellular level (resulting from an increased setpoint), whereas excess PTH secretion by hyperplastic cells appears due simply to an increased number of cells with normal calcium setpoint.

The molecular etiology of sporadic primary hyperparathyroidism is not well understood. Previous exposure to neck irradiation contributes to a minority of cases, typically 20–30 yr after exposure. Most commonly, adenomas are thought to represent clonal expansion of a single or several abnormal cells, because of a genetic abnormality resulting either in stimulation of cell proliferation or loss of inhibition of cell proliferation *(5)*. A small number of adenomas have been reported to have a *PRAD1* (cyclin D1) proto-oncogene rearrangement, in which the *PRAD1* gene is inserted close to enhancer elements of the PTH gene, resulting in stimulation of parathyroid cell division whenever PTH secretion is stimulated by low ionized calcium. *PRAD1* protein expression has been found to be increased in about 20% of parathyroid adenomas. About 17% of parathyroid adenomas have been reported to contain a mutation in the *MEN*-I (menin) gene, which functions as a tumor suppressor gene. Parathyroid adenomas evaluated by loss of heterozygosity analysis have been found to have a number of other potential sites for parathyroid oncogenes on chromosomes 16*p* and 19, and loss of tumor suppressor genes on chromosomes 1*p*, 1*q*, 6*q*, 13*q*, and other sites. No study of parathyroid adenomas to date has shown detectable abnormalities in the calcium-sensing receptor (CaSR).

Most patients currently diagnosed with primary hyperparathyroidism have asymptomatic mild hypercalcemia, typically with serum calcium levels less than 1.0 mg/dL above the upper end of the normal range. More severe cases occasionally are diagnosed with more classical bone features, including osteitis fibrosa cystica. Bone changes associated with osteitis fibrosa cystica include distal phalangeal subperiosteal resorption, distal clavicular resorption, "salt and pepper" skull, bone cysts, and long bone brown tumors. Occasional patients will meet criteria for osteoporosis, predominantly at cortical sites such as the distal one-third radius, but also at more cancellous sites such as the lumbar spine. Fractures at a number of skeletal sites were reported to be increased in one epidemiological study *(6)*. Bone disease is currently recognized clinically in less than 5% of patients. Calcium-containing kidney stones may be found in up to 20% of patients, but nephrocalcinosis or renal insufficiency may also be present, and hypercalciuria is reported in up to 30% of patients. Psychological symptoms are often reported, typically as mild fatigue or weakness or subtle cognitive impairment *(7)*. Peptic ulcer disease or pancreatitis may not be causally related to primary hyperparathyroidism, unless associated with MEN syndromes. Mild hypertension, coronary artery calcifications, cardiac valvular calcification, and septal and left ventricular hypertrophy may be seen in more symptomatic hyperparathyroidism, but it is also not yet clear that these are causally related. Other classical abnormalities of primary hyperparathyroidism, such as gout, pseudogout, anemia, band keratopathy, or loose teeth because of lamina densa resorption, are virtually never seen today. Occasional patients still present with severe hypercalcemia, as a form of acute primary hyperparathyroidism or parathyroid crisis.

Patients with newly diagnosed primary hyperparathyroidism typically have mildly increased serum total calcium and ionized calcium, with minimal variation around an average value over time. Serum phosphate is usually low normal or mildly decreased, with normal or mildly increased serum total or bone alkaline phosphatase, and normal serum creatinine. Intact PTH, measured by two-site immunoradiometric (IRMA) or ICMA assays, is mildly increased or inappropriately high normal for the level of serum calcium. There is no crossreactivity between PTH and PTHrp in current assays. Patients treated with thiazides or lithium may have increased PTH levels secondary to drug effect, without coexisting primary hyperparathyroidism. To ensure that hypercalcemic patients treated with thiazides or lithium do not also have primary hyperparathyroidism, it is necessary to document persistent hypercalcemia and increased whole-molecule PTH levels after discontinuing thiazides or lithium for 1–2 mo. Markers of bone turnover may be increased without obvious bone disease, possibly driven by increased interleukin 6 (IL-6) or tumor necrosis factor-α (TNF-α). PTH renal tubular effects may lead to mildly increased serum chloride and decreased bicarbonate. 1,25-dihydroxyvitamin D levels are typically upper normal or mildly increased, and 25-hydroxyvitamin D levels are usually low normal. Twenty-four-hour urinary calcium is increased in 25–30% of patients.

Surgical intervention is usually necessary for symptomatic primary hyperparathyroidism. The more difficult situation is often whether to recommend surgery to patients with asymptomatic or mildly symptomatic primary hyperparathyroidism. The 1991 NIH Consensus Development Conference recommended surgery for patients with serum calcium >1.0 mg/dL above the upper limit of normal, recognized complications such as nephrolithiasis or overt bone disease, acute primary hyperparathyroidism with life-threatening hypercalcemia, 24-h urine calcium in excess of 400 mg/d, one-third distal radial bone density Z-score of less than –2.0, or age younger than 50 yr (8). About half of all patients currently diagnosed with asymptomatic primary hyperparathyroidism meet at least one of these criteria. Some of these asymptomatic patients have increased urine calcium or low bone mass. Patients with asymptomatic primary hyperparathyroidism who elect to defer surgery generally have stable mild hypercalcemia without progression, at least over ten years of follow-up (9).

When elective parathyroidectomy is necessary, it is best performed by an experienced surgeon because of the notorious variability in parathyroid gland location. Preoperative location of parathyroid adenomas before initial neck exploration may be unnecessary in major referral centers because of extremely high cure rates (95–98%) with standard neck exploration, but many physicians practicing outside major centers perform at least one imaging study prior to surgical referral because of preference by less experienced surgeons. Patient or physician interest in minimally invasive parathyroid surgery of necessity leads to parathyroid imaging studies including neck ultrasound, technetium[99]-thallium or technetium[99]-sestamibi subtraction scanning, or CT or MRI of the neck prior to first neck exploration. False-negative and false-positive results are relatively common, however, making this approach difficult to recommend routinely. Patients identified to have single adenomas typically undergo adenoma resection and identification of the remaining normal glands, whereas patients with parathyroid hyperplasia either have removal of three and one-half glands, or removal of all four glands followed by autotransplantation of part of a gland in the forearm or neck. Patients cured of their primary hyperparathyroidism normalize their serum calcium within a short time, often after a brief period of asymptomatic relative hypocalcemia. "Hungry bones" syndrome may develop in patients with severe or extensive bone disease with rapid skeletal mineral uptake after surgery, and usually requires both intravenous and oral calcium and vitamin D supplementation for days to weeks to prevent symptomatic hypocalcemia. Complications of parathyroid surgery include postoperative hypocalcemia because of chronic surgical hypoparathyroidism, or recurrent laryngeal nerve damage. Bone mass improves rapidly in most patients after surgery, predominantly at the lumbar spine but less impressively at the radius *(10)*.

A major reason to choose an experienced parathyroid surgeon for primary neck exploration is that reoperation for persistent or recurrent primary hyperparathyroidism is technically challenging. Most surgeons mandate preoperative imaging to localize abnormal parathyroid tissue before attempting a second exploration. Invasive arteriography and selective venous sampling may be helpful if available, although this is expensive and time consuming. Reconfirmation of the diagnosis of primary hyperparathyroidism is necessary before a second surgery, to make sure that patients do not have unsuspected familial benign hypercalcemia. Intraoperative technetium[99]-sestamibi scanning with a hand-held gamma counter, coupled with rapid intraoperative PTH assay, may help in difficult cases. Other surgical techniques, including endoscopic parathyroidectomy, are being investigated.

Medical options for patients with symptomatic hypercalcemia not able to tolerate surgery are limited *(11)*. Patients should generally maintain hydration and remain physically active. Thiazides or lithium should be avoided. Dietary calcium intake of 800–1000 mg/d is advised to minimize bone loss and not worsen hypercalcemia or hypercalciuria, because dietary calcium intake of <600 mg/d will paradoxically stimulate physiologic hyperparathyroidism and worsen hypercalcemia and hypercalciuria. Oral or intravenous phosphate should be avoided because of risk of precipitation of ectopic calcification. Estrogen replacement therapy (ERT) may improve hypercalcemia and prevent bone loss in postmenopausal women, probably by direct effects on bone, because PTH and phosphate levels have not been found to improve. Oral bisphosphonates may be beneficial in lowering hypercalcemia or preventing bone loss, but etidronate and clodronate have not shown long-term benefit. Alendronate, risedronate, raloxifene, and salmon calcitonin by nasal spray or injection have not been rigorously investigated for treatment of primary hyperparathyroidism. CaSR agonists (calcimimetics) show promise and are under active investigation for treatment of primary and secondary hyperparathyroidism *(12)*. Occasional patients with adenomas localized by ultrasound may benefit from alcohol ablation of their tumor under ultrasound guidance, particularly in situations where surgical intervention is contraindicated or refused by the patient.

REFERENCES

1. Al Zahrani A, Levine MA. Primary hyperparathyroidism. Lancet 1997;349:1233–1238.
2. Bilezikian JP. Primary hyperparathyroidism. In: Favus MJ, ed. Primer on the Metabolic Bone Diseases and Disorders of Mineral Metabolism. 4th ed. Lippincott Williams and Wilkins, Philadelphia, PA, 1999, pp. 187–192.

3. Wermers RA, Khosla S, Atkinson EJ, et al. The rise and fall of primary hyperparathyroidism: a population-based study in Rochester, Minnesota 1965–1992. Ann Int Med 1997;126:433–440.

4. Wynne AG, Van Heerden J, Carney JA, Fitzpatrick LA. Parathyroid carcinoma: clinical and pathological features in 43 patients. Medicine 1992;71:197–205.

5. Tominaga Y, Takagi H. Molecular genetics of hyperparathyroid disease. Curr Opin Nephrol Hyperten 1996;5:336–341.

6. Khosla S, Melton LJ III, Wermers RA, et al. Primary hyperparathyroidism and the risk of fracture: a population-based study. J Bone Miner Res 1999;14:1700–1707.

7. Okomoto T, Gerstein HC, Obara T. Psychiatric symptoms, bone density and non-specific symptoms in patients with mild hypercalcemia due to primary hyperparathyroidism: a systematic overview of the literature. Endocrine J 1997;44:367–374.

8. Consensus Development Conference Panel. Diagnosis and management of asymptomatic primary hyperparathyroidism: Consensus Development Conference Statement. Ann Intern Med 1991;114:593–597.

9. Silverberg SJ, Shane E, Jacobs TP, Siris E, Bilezikian JP. A 10-year prospective study of primary hyperparathyroidism with or without parathyroid surgery. N Engl J Med 1999;341:1249–1255.

10. Silverberg SJ, Gartenberg F, Jacobs TP, et al. Increased bone density after parathyroidectomy in primary hyperparathyroidism. J Clin Endocrinol Metab 1995;80:729–734.

11. Silverberg SJ, Bilezikian JP, Bone HG III, et al. Therapeutic controversies in primary hyperparathyroidism. J Clin Endocrinol Metab 1999;84:2275–2285.

12. Silverberg SJ, Bone HG III, Marriott TB, et al. Short-term inhibition of parathyroid hormone secretion by a calcium-receptor agonist in patients with primary hyperparathyroidism. N Engl J Med 1997;337: 1506–1510.

CASE #2: HYPERCALCEMIA

Case Description

A 60-yr-old man presented to the emergency room with dehydration, fatigue, malaise, and mild confusion and disorientation. His serum total calcium was 14.0 mg/dL (normal, 8.9–10.1 mg/dL), serum phosphate 4.5 mg/dL (normal, 2.5–4.5 mg/dL), serum total alkaline phosphatase 250 U/L (normal, 98–251 U/L), and serum creatinine 1.0 mg/dL (normal, 0.8–1.2 mg/dL). The patient and his family denied that he had any previous history of hypercalcemia or similar symptoms.

Past medical history was significant for three primary malignancies. He had been diagnosed with prostate cancer 10 yr ago and treated with radical retropubic prostatectomy, bilateral orchiectomy, and local radiation therapy, with apparent cure. His most recent prostate specific antigen was undetectable 2 mo ago. He had undergone partial left colectomy for an early colon cancer diagnosed on flexible sigmoidoscopy 5 yr ago, without need for chemotherapy or other intervention, and on subsequent yearly colonoscopies had no evidence of recurrence. Two years ago, he had been diagnosed with an early squamous cell lung cancer without lymph node involvement, and had undergone left upper lobectomy without complication. Subsequent yearly CT scans of his chest had been without evidence of recurrence. He had been relatively healthy his entire life, otherwise, and without history of osteoporosis, other metabolic bone disease, bone pain, or calcium-containing kidney stones.

Current medications included verapamil SR 240 mg/d, pravastatin 10 mg/d at bedtime, vitamin E 400 IU/d, vitamin C 500 mg/d, and aspirin 325 mg/d. He specifically denied any supplemental vitamin D, vitamin A, or calcium. He was allergic to sulfa antibiotics, which caused hives.

Family history was unremarkable for hypercalcemia, hypercalciuria, osteoporosis, other metabolic bone disease, or malignancy in general. There was no history of tuberculosis or other fungal disease in the family. The patient was employed as an insurance agent, and had no recent travel or known infectious disease exposures. He had smoked cigarettes one pack per day for 10 yr before quitting 30 yr ago and he denied alcohol use.

Systems review was otherwise remarkable for intermittent drenching night sweats over the last several months, with undocumented low-grade nocturnal fevers without chills or rigors. He noted that his fatigue had been of gradual onset beginning 3 mo earlier, but that his appetite was good and that his weight had been stable. He denied problems with headache, visual changes, neck or back pain, chest pain or shortness of breath, abdominal pain, change in bowel habit, skin rash, or arthralgias or myalgias.

Vital signs at admission included a height of 190 cm, weight of 76.0 kg, supine blood pressure in the left arm of 120/70 mmHg, and regular pulse of 96/min. On sitting his blood pressure in the left arm decreased to 90/50 mmHg and his pulse increased to 120/min, and he developed lightheadedness and dizziness. Physical exam revealed only dry mucous membranes and decreased skin turgor, mild tachycardia, and toenail onychomycosis.

Laboratory studies at admission, prior to rehydration, showed mild anemia consistent with chronic disease, with hemoglobin 11.5 gm/dL (normal, 13.5–17.5 gm/dL) and MCV 87.5 fL (normal, 81.2–95.1 fL), normal serum electrolytes, and normal serum protein electrophoresis. Whole-molecule PTH drawn at admission was later reported to be undetectable. Chest X-ray showed old calcified granulomas and mild diffuse fibrosis, without evidence of active tuberculosis, fungal, or other granulomatous disease.

He was admitted to the hospital for treatment of symptomatic hypercalcemia, and given intravenous rehydration in the form of 2 L of normal saline over the next 4 h, with frequent cardiac and respiratory evaluation. This was followed by furosemide 40 mg intravenously, and intravenous (iv) normal saline was continued at 200 mL/h, with furosemide repeated at the same dose 6 h later. Repeat serum total calcium after 8 h of saline diuresis was 12.5 mg/dL, and he remained mildly confused and disoriented. Hydration was subsequently maintained with half-normal saline at a rate of 150 mL/h, and he was given pamidronate 60 mg intravenously over 4 h without difficulty. Over the next 3 d, his serum total calcium gradually decreased to 9.8 mg/dL with marked improvement in his mental status and fatigue.

Evaluation during his hospitalization revealed suppressed serum PTH-related peptide (PTHrp), and normal or unremarkable sensitive TSH, random cortisol, 25-hydroxy-vitamin D, free retinol (vitamin A), angiotensin converting enzyme, antineutrophilic cytoplasmic antibody (c- and p-ANCA), fungal serologies, and PPD skin test with appropriate controls. His serum 1,25-dihydroxyvitamin D level was increased at 85 pg/mL (normal, 15–60 pg/mL), suggesting extrarenal 1α-hydroxylase activity. In view of the fact that he had no serologic or imaging evidence of active granulomatous disease, he was suspected to have lymphoma, and was referred for bone marrow aspirate and biopsy. His aspirate and biopsy confirmed non-Hodgkin's B-cell lymphoma, and he was referred for chemotherapy including prednisone, which subsequently controlled his hypercalcemia without further iv pamidronate or saline diuresis.

Discussion

Hypercalcemia is estimated to occur in 1–3.9% of the general adult population, and 0.2–2.9% of hospitalized populations, with a variable clinical presentation depending on severity *(1)*. Most commonly it is asymptomatic, but it may become life threatening. The range of normal serum calcium ranges between 8.5–10.5 mg/dL in most assays, with different laboratories reporting slightly different normal ranges based on assay method.

Circulating serum calcium is bound to protein, primarily albumin (50%), and anions such as citrate or sulfate (5%), but also is found as free ionized calcium (45%). Only the free ionized fraction of calcium is physiologically active.

Several factors affect measured serum total and ionized calcium. Alterations in serum albumin increase or decrease serum total calcium without affecting free ionized calcium. Decreases in serum albumin below 4.0 mg/dL decrease total calcium by 0.8 mg/dL for each 1.0 mg/dL decrease in serum albumin. Dehydration may increase serum total calcium by causing hemoconcentration. Acidemia increases free ionized calcium, and alkalemia decreases free ionized calcium, without affecting serum total calcium. Free ionized calcium should generally be measured in patients with complicated medical illness associated with changes in albumin concentration (owing to stress or poor nutrition) or blood pH (owing to acid-base disturbances), but under less complicated circumstances serum total calcium measurement is adequate (2).

Serum calcium reflects the balance between calcium influx into extracellular fluid and calcium efflux from extracellular fluid. Sources of calcium influx into extracellular fluid include intestinal absorption, skeletal resorption, and renal resorption. Sources of calcium efflux from extracellular fluid include intestinal secretion, skeletal uptake, and renal excretion. Hypercalcemia usually results from increased skeletal resorption or intestinal absorption with normal or decreased renal excretion, but may also result from normal influx with decreased renal excretion or skeletal mineralization. Increased skeletal resorption typically is due to accelerated osteoclast recruitment and activation, most often under the influence of PTH, PTHrp, or 1,25-dihydroxyvitamin D (3). Other cytokines that may stimulate osteoclast recruitment or function include interleukin (IL)-1α, IL-1β, IL-6, tumor necrosis factor-α (TNF-α), lymphotoxin, or transforming growth factor-β (TGF-β). Increased intestinal absorption of calcium is less common, although this may occur with increased 1,25-dihydroxyvitamin D production or absorptive hypercalciuria. Regardless of the cause of increased calcium influx into extracellular fluid, serum calcium levels do not usually increase unless the kidneys simultaneously fail to excrete calcium in a compensatory fashion for some reason.

Other factors may indirectly affect serum calcium. Increased PTH and PTHrp directly stimulate renal tubular resorption of filtered calcium, limiting the ability of the kidneys to excrete calcium. Hypercalcemia interferes with antidiuretic hormone (ADH)-stimulated free water reabsorption in the distal renal tubule, resulting in mild nephrogenic diabetes insipidus. Nausea and vomiting resulting from increased serum calcium may cause further hemoconcentration, and prerenal volume depletion may interfere with renal calcium clearance. Immobilization or lack of physical activity, especially when Paget's disease of bone is present, or astronauts in space, may directly increase bone resorption.

The G-protein-coupled extracellular CaSR plays a major role in regulation of extracellular calcium (4). This receptor is found on parathyroid cells, renal tubular cells, osteoblasts, and intestinal mucosal cells, as well as other cells in many tissues. The CaSR specifically regulates PTH secretion by parathyroid cells and renal tubular calcium resorption, and probably regulates bone turnover and intestinal calcium absorption as well. The CaSR is a member of the 7-transmembrane segment receptor family, with a large extracellular portion that binds ionized calcium, and a shorter intracellular portion that interacts with a variety of G-proteins and signal-transduction pathways. It may be part of a larger family of yet to be discovered calcium- or cation-binding receptors.

Table 1
Parathyroid Hormone-Mediated Hypercalcemia

Primary Hyperparathyroidism
   Parathyroid adenoma
   Parathyroid lipoadenoma
   Parathyroid hyperplasia
   Parathyroid carcinoma
   Mediastinal parathyroid cyst
Secondary Hyperparathyroidism
Tertiary Hyperparathyroidism
Ectopic PTH Production (small cell lung cancer,
   small cell ovarian carcinoma, squamous cell
   lung carcinoma, ovarian adenocarcinoma,
   thymoma, papillary thyroid carcinoma,
   hepatocellular carcinoma, undifferentiated
   neuroendocrine tumor)

Clinical manifestations of hypercalcemia are widely variable, and include a spectrum of neurologic dysfunction, ranging from mild cognitive impairment and drowsiness to apparent depression, confusion, delirium, or obtundation (5). Muscle weakness may be prominent with severe hypercalcemia. Constipation is typical, and anorexia, nausea, or vomiting are frequent complaints. Pancreatitis or peptic ulcer disease are relatively uncommon but may occur in association with primary hyperparathyroidism, although the causality of these disorders is still controversial. Frequent urination and thirst are not uncommon, and kidney stones and nephrocalcinosis may occur if the hypercalcemia is chronic. Cardiac manifestations include rapid repolarization associated with shortened QT interval, bradycardia, first-degree AV block, and other dysrhythmias. Chronic hypercalcemia may be associated with osteopenia or osteoporosis with fractures. Most patients with hypercalcemia are asymptomatic unless the serum calcium is $\geq$12 mg/dL or rapidly increasing, and virtually all patients are symptomatic with serum calcium >14 mg/dL.

There are many disorders in the differential diagnosis of hypercalcemia, but the condition can be divided into PTH-mediated (see Table 1) and non-PTH-mediated (see Table 2) hypercalcemia. The most common cause of PTH-mediated hypercalcemia is primary hyperparathyroidism, and the most common cause of non-PTH-mediated hypercalcemia is malignancy. The most common cause of malignancy-associated hypercalcemia is humoral hypercalcemia of malignancy (HHM) because of PTHrp oversecretion. Benign tumors also appear able to occasionally oversecrete PTHrp (6). A number of endocrine disorders are associated with hypercalcemia. Thyrotoxicosis may cause hypercalcemia due to thyroid hormone-mediated increased bone resorption. Pheochromocytoma may cause hypercalcemia owing to associated primary hyperparathyroidism in MEN-IIA, or directly due to PTHrp oversecretion or catecholamine excess. Adrenal insufficiency or crisis causes hypercalcemia by causing hemoconcentration because of diarrhea or nausea and vomiting. VIPomas may cause hypercalcemia by causing dehydration and metabolic acidosis. Granulomatous disorders cause hypercalcemia by extrarenal granuloma macrophage 1α-hydroxylase activity, which directly increases 1,25-dihydroxyvitamin D levels. Vitamin D excess may stimulate increased calcium absorption, whereas thiazide diuretics

Table 2
Nonparathyroid Hormone-Mediated Hypercalcemia

Malignant Tumors
   PTHrp (lung, esophagus, head and neck, renal cell, ovary, bladder, pancreas, uterine fibroid,
      thymic carcinoma, islet cell carcinoma, carcinoid, sclerosing hepatic carcinoma)
   Ectopic 1,25-dihydroxyvitamin D (B-cell lymphoma, Hodgkin's disease, lymphomatoid
      granulomatosis)
   Lytic bone metastases (Multiple myeloma, lymphomas, breast cancer, invasive sarcoma)
Tumor production of other cytokines (T-cell lymphoma/leukemia, non-Hodgkin's lymphoma,
      other hematologic malignancies)
   Benign Tumors: PTHrp (ovarian dermoid cyst)
   Endocrine Diseases
   Thyrotoxicosis
   Pheochromocytoma
   Addison's disease
   Islet cell pancreatic tumors
   VIPoma
Granulomatous Disorders
   Sarcoidosis
   Wegener's granulomatosis
   Berylliosis
   Silicone- and paraffin-induced granulomatosis
   Eosinophilic granuloma
   TB (focal, disseminated, MAC in AIDS)
   Histoplasmosis
   Coccidioidomycosis
   Nocardia asteroides
   Candidiasis
   Leprosy
   Cat-scratch disease
Drugs
   Vitamin D excess (oral or topical)
   Vitamin A excess
   Thiazide diuretics
   Lithium
   Estrogens and antiestrogens
   Androgens
   Aminophylline, theophylline
   Gancyclovir
   Recombinant growth hormone treatment of AIDS patients
   Foscarnet
   8-chloro-cyclic AMP
Miscellaneous
   Immobilization with or without Paget's disease of bone
   End-stage liver failure
   Total parenteral nutrition
   Milk-alkali syndrome
   Hypophosphatasia
   Systemic lupus erythematosus
   Juvenile rheumatoid arthritis
   Recent hepatitis B vaccination
   Gaucher's disease with acute pneumonia
   Aluminum intoxication (chronic hemodialysis)
   Manganese intoxication
   Primary oxalosis

stimulate increased renal tubular calcium reabsorption and thereby block renal excretion. Lithium interferes with the ability of calcium to interact with parathyroid and renal calcium sensing receptors, resulting in increased PTH secretion. Vitamin A excess is thought to directly stimulate bone resorption by actions on osteoclasts. Estrogens, antiestrogens, androgens, aminophylline, or theophylline affect other physiologic mechanisms causing hypercalcemia. A variety of other miscellaneous drugs and disorders may also be associated with hypercalcemia.

Hypercalcemia should be treated initially with rehydration with normal saline, followed by furosemide- or other loop diuretic-induced diuresis. Thiazide diuretics should be discontinued during treatment if previously used by the patient, and specifically avoided during aggressive saline diuresis. If rehydration and diuresis are insufficient to normalize serum calcium, as in the case presented, or to maintain normalization of serum calcium, intravenous pamidronate (Aredia®) 30–90 mg infused over 4 h or etidronate (Didronel®) 5 mg/kg infused over 24 h should be used. Other options used in the past include intravenous plicamycin (mithramycin) at 15–25 µg/kg over 4–6 h, intramuscular or subcutaneous calcitonin 4–8 U/kg every 6–8 h, or intravenous gallium nitrate at 200 mg/m^2/d over 5 d. Occasional patients may require combination therapy with these older agents, or require them because of resistance to the intravenous bisphosphonates. Glucocorticoids, given as hydrocortisone or equivalent 200–300 mg/d for 3–5 d, may also be used to decrease hypercalcemia, as in the case presented, especially if it is because of lymphoma, multiple myeloma, granulomatous disease, or vitamin D toxicity. Intravenous phosphate should never be used to lower serum calcium because of potential for severe organ dysfunction and death. Hemodialysis with low or zero calcium dialysate should be reserved for extreme hypercalcemia not responding to other measures.

Humoral hypercalcemia of malignancy (HHM) is caused by excess tumoral production of a circulating factor that causes hypercalcemia (7). In the usual situation, HHM implies tumoral production of PTHrp, but technically HHM includes production of other recognized factors such as 1,25-dihydroxyvitamin D and other as yet unidentified factors that cause hypercalcemia. Tumors causing hypercalcemia by overproduction of PTHrp typically have limited or no known skeletal involvement. The syndrome was first described in 1941 in a patient with renal cell carcinoma with a solitary skeletal metastasis. Subsequent investigation showed that HHM resolves after tumor resection, and factors originally proposed to explain the syndrome included prostaglandin E_2, a variety of vitamin D-like compounds, and PTH. PTHrp was finally identified in 1987 as the cause of about 70% of cases of HHM.

Patients with HHM associated with overproduction of PTHrp are typically in the later stages of clinically evident malignancy, and often within weeks to months of death. However, some patients with PTHrp produced by well-differentiated pheochromocytomas or islet cell tumors do well and have long-term survival. Tumors associated with HHM include squamous cell carcinomas of the lung, esophagus, cervix, vulva, skin, or head and neck, as well as renal cell, bladder, ovarian, or breast carcinomas and human T-cell leukemia virus I (HTLV I)-associated lymphomas.

Patients with PTHrp-mediated HHM typically manifest hypercalcemia, hypophosphatemia, hypercalciuria, hyperphosphaturia, low or suppressed PTH levels, increased urinary cAMP production, and increased osteoclastic bone resorption as measured by bone histomorphometry. In contrast to patients with primary hyperparathyroidism, however, these patients have more marked hypercalciuria, reduced 1,25-dihydroxyvitamin

D levels, reduced intestinal calcium absorption, and decreased osteoblastic activity. Differences between HHM and primary hyperparathyroidism are not completely understood because PTH and PTHrp both interact with the same PTH/PTHrp receptor, with similar in vitro and in vivo animal effects. PTHrp may be useful as a tumor marker for following responses to therapy. Treatment of HHM involves reducing tumor burden, blocking increased osteoclastic activity with bisphosphonates, calcitonin, or mithramycin, and stimulating renal calcium clearance with saline hydration and diuretics.

About 30% of patients with HHM do not have increased levels of PTHrp. Rare renal cell carcinomas causing HHM secrete prostaglandin E_2, but other potential factors are not currently well characterized. It is important to exclude other coexisting causes of hypercalcemia, such as sarcoid, TB, or fungal disease, in these patients.

REFERENCES

1. Frolich A. Prevalence of hypercalcemia in normal and hospitalized populations. Danish Med Bull 1998; 45:436–439.
2. Shane E. Hypercalcemia. In: Favus MJ, ed. Primer on the Metabolic Bone Diseases and Disorders of Mineral Metabolism. 4th ed. Lippincott Williams and Wilkins, Philadelphia, PA, 1999, pp. 183–187.
3. Mundy GR, Guise TA. Hormonal control of calcium homeostasis. Clin Chem 1999;45;1347–1352.
4. Brown EM, Vassilev PM, Quinn S, Hebert SC. G-protein-coupled, extracellular Ca^{2+}-sensing receptor: a versatile regulator of diverse cellular functions. Vitamin Horm 1999;55:1–71.
5. Bushinsky DA, Monk RD. Calcium. Lancet 1998;352:306–311.
6. Knecht TP, Behling CA, Burton DW, et al. The humoral hypercalcemia of benignancy. A newly appreciated syndrome. Am J Clin Pathol 1996;105:487–492.
7. Rankin W, Grill V, Martin TJ. Parathyroid hormone-related protein and hypercalcemia. Eur J Cancer 1998;34;222–229.

CASE #3: FAMILIAL HYPOCALCIURIC HYPERCALCEMIA WITH RECURRENT PANCREATITIS

Case Description

A 19-yr-old woman with a known family history of familial hypocalciuric hypercalcemia (FHH) presented in the outpatient endocrine clinic for further evaluation and management of recurrent hypercalcemia associated with pancreatitis.

Two years earlier, she had presented to the local emergency trauma unit with an episode of acute periumbilical pain radiating through to her back, subsequently diagnosed as acute pancreatitis, documented by moderately increased serum lipase and amylase. She denied previous episodes of similar acute pain, although she admitted having some occasional intermittent periumbilical pain of minor consequence over several months prior to presentation. She denied recent abdominal trauma, alcohol use or overuse, history of gallstones, excessive dietary fat intake, recent viral syndromes, or any other factor that might explain her pancreatitis.

At hospital admission her initial serum total calcium was found to be 12.5 mg/dL (normal, 8.9–10.1 mg/dL), and serum phosphate 3.5 mg/dL (normal, 2.5–4.5 mg/dL). She had not previously had a serum calcium measurement, and had refused screening when her paternal aunt and father had initially been diagnosed with FHH several years earlier. Her whole-molecule PTH level was mildly increased at 6.5 pmol/L (normal, 1.0–5.2 pmol/L). Serum triglycerides were mildly increased at 250 mg/dL (goal, less than 150 mg/dL).

Because her father and paternal aunt had previously been diagnosed with FHH, with well-documented serum total calcium levels measured in the 10.0–10.5 mg/dL range over time, it was felt that the patient's degree of hypercalcemia was in excess of that expected for her kindred, and the possibility that she might have primary hyperparathyroidism was considered. Her calcium to creatinine clearance ratio (24-h urine calcium × serum creatinine/24-h urine creatinine × serum total calcium) was calculated to be 0.009, supportive of a diagnosis of FHH, because patients with this disorder typically have values below 0.01, whereas patients with primary hyperparathyroidism typically have values above 0.01.

Conservative management of her pancreatitis, including withholding oral intake and providing intravenous rehydration, resulted in gradual improvement in her abdominal pain and a decrease in her serum total calcium to 10.5 mg/dL. Ultrasound of her abdomen showed no evidence of gallstones or gall bladder sludge, or common bile duct or pancreatic duct abnormalities. Computed tomography (CT) scan of her abdomen showed no evidence of abscess or pseudocyst formation, and no other pancreatic abnormalities, so she was dismissed from hospital with advice to avoid alcohol and fat-rich meals in the future.

Over the next 18 mo, she returned to the local emergency trauma unit twice for recurrent episodes of pancreatitis, each time presenting similarly to her initial episode. At each presentation, her serum total calcium initially was in the 12.5–13.5 mg/dL range, with subsequent improvement with rehydration and conservative management. Between hospitalizations, her serum total calcium typically ranged from 11.0–12.0 mg/dL during pain-free intervals. At each hospitalization, no precipitating cause for pancreatitis was discovered, and she continued to deny abdominal trauma, alcohol use or overuse, excess dietary fat intake, or recent viral syndromes. Outpatient ERCP was eventually undertaken without diagnosis of any pancreatic duct abnormalities or precipitation of pancreatitis.

At the time of her initial outpatient endocrine clinic visit, she had recently been dismissed from the hospital after her third episode of pancreatitis. She complained of gradually increasing periumbilical pain, more or less persistent most of the time, over the preceding 6 mo prior to her clinic evaluation. Her primary care physicians could find no obvious cause for her abdominal pain, including pancreatitis, during her outpatient evaluations and had referred her for chronic pain management. Her serum total calcium in the clinic was 11.5 mg/dL (normal, 8.9–10.1 mg/dL), with serum phosphate 2.8 mg/dL (normal, 2.5–4.5 mg/dL), and normal serum total alkaline phosphatase and serum creatinine. Her whole-molecule PTH level was mildly increased at 8.2 pmol/L (normal, 1.0–5.2 pmol/L). Her repeat calculated outpatient calcium to creatinine clearance ratio was 0.011, just above the threshold of 0.01 for distinguishing primary hyperparathyroidism from FHH. Because of her recurrent pancreatitis, developing chronic abdominal pain syndrome, and unexpectedly high serum total calcium for her kindred and other typical cases of FHH, nuclear isotopic imaging of her neck was undertaken. Her parathyroid sestamibi scan showed uptake in both inferior parathyroid glands, suggestive of adenomas. Neck ultrasound confirmed the presence of nodular lesions in the inferior thyroid lobe regions, distinct from the thyroid, and consistent with parathyroid adenomas.

Traditional elective parathyroidectomy by a very experienced parathyroid surgeon revealed four slightly enlarged parathyroid glands. Two-and-one-half glands were resected, and the other gland biopsied. The pathology report indicated only normal-appearing parathyroid tissue, without evidence of parathyroid adenoma or hyperplasia. Her initial postoperative serum total calcium 6 h after surgery was 10.0 mg/dL, but this gradually drifted up to 11.0 mg/dL within 3 mo after her neck exploration. Over two subsequent years of follow-up, she has had no further episodes of pancreatitis, although she still has occasional periumbilical pain. She no longer requires narcotics for pain control, and overall feels well. She has been advised that complete parathyroidectomy may eventually be required if she develops further episodes of recurrent pancreatitis.

Discussion

FHH, also known as familial benign hypercalcemia (FBH), is an autosomal dominant, highly penetrant disorder characterized by mild to moderate hypercalcemia and relative hypocalciuria from birth onward (1). Unless part of a known kindred, most patients are detected in young adulthood. Most kindreds are asymptomatic, but individuals within kindreds may develop mild fatigue, neuropsychiatric imbalances, or polydipsia. Occasional patients develop severe pancreatitis or relapsing pancreatitis, as demonstrated by this case, and there may be an increased risk of gallstones, diabetes mellitus, or early myocardial infarction (2). No study to date has demonstrated an increased risk of nephrolithiasis, nephrocalcinosis, peptic ulcer disease, low bone mass, or fractures.

FHH families usually have mildly increased serum total and ionized calcium, mildly decreased serum phosphate, high normal or mildly increased serum magnesium, normal serum creatinine and creatinine clearance, mildly increased renal calcium and magnesium reabsorption causing relative hypocalciuria and hypomagnesiuria, renal calcium to creatinine clearance ratio <0.01, high normal to mildly increased PTH and 1,25-dihydroxyvitamin D, and mild parathyroid gland hyperplasia (3). It should be noted that patients with primary hyperparathyroidism may occasionally have a calcium to creatinine clearance ratio <0.01, and that patients with FHH may occasionally have a ratio >0.01, as was apparent in this case. In addition, the calcium to creatinine clearance ratio may vary somewhat over time, also demonstrated by this case. At least one patient has been reported to have coexisting FHH and idiopathic hypercalciuria, and rare patients have been reported with surgically proven coexisting primary hyperparathyroidism and FHH. Patients typically have normal imaging studies, although mild chondrocalcinosis and early vascular calcification may be seen. Markers of bone turnover may be mildly increased, but bone density is usually normal and fracture risk is not increased.

Subtotal parathyroidectomy in FHH results in transient lowering of hypercalcemia, as demonstrated in this case, with recurrence of hypercalcemia usually within a week. Total parathyroidectomy causes the expected chronic hypoparathyroidism with hypocalcemia and low 1,25-dihydroxyvitamin D levels. For these reasons, it is usually unnecessary and inadvisable to recommend parathyroidectomy for patients with FHH. However, patients with FHH and severe hypercalcemia (>14 mg/dL), recurrent pancreatitis, or neonatal severe hyperparathyroidism are generally advised to undergo total parathyroidectomy without autotransplantation. Several FHH patients undergoing total parathyroidectomy with autotransplantation have developed recurrent hypercalcemia after autotransplantation. Diuretics, estrogen, and phosphate therapy appear to have no significant effect on serum total calcium in patients with FHH. There is no current evidence to suggest that FHH shortens life expectancy, and patients have been reported with this disorder who lived into their ninth decade.

Pregnancy in an FHH carrier or the spouse of an FHH carrier may result in a variety of outcomes. The FHH infant of an FHH mother should have asymptomatic hypercalcemia at birth, whereas the normal infant of an FHH mother may have symptomatic hypocalcemia after birth because of transient suppression of fetal PTH secretion by maternal-fetal hypercalcemia during pregnancy. The FHH infant of a normal mother may have significant neonatal hypercalcemia at birth because of fetal secondary hyperparathyroidism during pregnancy, but this should resolve over time to asymptomatic hypercalcemia without neonatal parathyroidectomy.

The prevalence of FHH is unknown, but thought to be similar to MEN-I, probably accounting for about 2% of cases of asymptomatic hypercalcemia. FHH heterozygotes have virtually 100% penetrance for hypercalcemia at birth, with the degree of hypercalcemia usually constant within kindreds, although the patient presented demonstrated that this is not always the case. Most kindreds have mild hypercalcemia in all affected members, but several kindreds with moderate (12.5–14 mg/dL) hypercalcemia have been reported. Genetic analysis has linked the FHH gene to chromosome $3q13.3–q21$ in eight families, chromosome $19q$ in one family, and chromosome $19q$ in another family, implying heterogeneity in the genetic basis of the disorder. Most cases linked to chromosome $3q$ are thought due to single allelic inactivating mutations of the CaSR, whereas cases linked to chromosome $19p$ or $19q$ are due to other mutations in genes not yet described. Patients with double allelic inactivating mutations of the CaSR develop neonatal severe primary hyperparathyroidism, with severe hypercalcemia and massive parathyroid gland hyperplasia.

REFERENCES

1. Brown EM. Mutations in the calcium-sensing receptor and their clinical implications. Horm Res 1997; 48:199–208.
2. Law WM Jr, Heath H III. Familial benign hypercalcemia (hypocalciuric hypercalcemia): clinical and pathogenetic studies in 21 families. Ann Intern Med 1985;102:511–519.
3. Marx SJ, Attie MF, Levine MA, et al. The hypocalciuric or benign variant of familial hypercalcemia: clinical and biochemical features in fifteen kindreds. Medicine 1981;60:397–412.

11

Hypoparathyroidism and Hypocalcemia

Elena I. Barengolts, MD
and Subhash C. Kukreja, MD

Contents

CASE #1: PARATHYROID AUTOTRANSPLANTATION IN POSTSURGICAL HYPOPARATHYROIDISM

Case Description

This 33-yr-old man presented with recurrent kidney stones and hypercalcemia, and was diagnosed as having primary hyperparathyroidism (serum Ca 10–12 mg/dL, serum PTH 95 pg/mL). Further work-up demonstrated a growth hormone and prolactin secreting pituitary tumor, a spinal cord ependymoma, and an insulinoma; therefore, a diagnosis of MEN 1 Syndrome was made. During the parathyroidectomy in May 1999, parathyroid hyperplasia was discovered and total parathyroidectomy with autotransplantation to the left forearm was performed.

Postoperatively, the patient complained of numbness and tingling involving the circumoral region, fingertips, and toes and muscle cramps. Physical examination revealed a blood pressure of 135/80 mm Hg, a pulse 88, and positive Chvostek's and Trousseau's signs. Treatment was initiated with 2 ampules of 10 mL calcium gluconate diluted in 100 mL of 5% dextrose (180 mg elemental calcium) and 2 g MgSO$_4$ intramuscularly while awaiting laboratory results. The laboratory results showed a serum calcium of 6.1 mg/dL, an ionized calcium of 3.5 mg/dL, a magnesium of 1.5 mg/dL, a phosphorus of 1.2 mg/dL, a potassium of 3.3 mg/dL, an albumin of 3.2 g/dL and a bicarbonate of 22 mEq/L. The serum calcium initially increased to 8.2 mg/dL (ionized 4.3 mg/dL), but later decreased to 6.4 mg/dL (ionized 3.8 mg/dL) with recurrence of symptoms. A calcium drip was initiated with 10 ampules of calcium gluconate in 500 mL of 5% dextrose infused at a rate

From: *Contemporary Endocrinology: Challenging Cases in Endocrinology*
Edited by: M. E. Molitch © Humana Press Inc., Totowa, NJ

100 mL/h (180 mg of elemental calcium/h). Oral therapy was started with calcium carbonate (500 mg of elemental calcium every 6 h) and calcitriol 0.25 μg a day. The patient's symptoms resolved and he was discharged with a serum calcium of 8.2 mg/dL (ionized 4.2 mg/dL).

The serum calcium was monitored twice a week and the dose of oral calcium carbonate was increased from 2 g to 5 g elemental calcium a day with calcitriol continued at 0.25 μg/d. Over the next several weeks, the serum calcium ranged between 8.3 and 8.8 mg/dL. An attempt to decrease the calcium dose to 2 g of elemental calcium a day resulted in a decline of the serum calcium to 7.2 mg/dL. The patient complained of occasional twitches in his leg muscles, a bitter taste, and abdominal discomfort. Calcium citrate was tried for better palatability, but after the symptoms resolved, it was changed back to calcium carbonate providing 4 g of elemental calcium a day. Calcitriol was increased to 0.5 μg/d. A repeat serum calcium was 8.8 mg/dL and the serum magnesium was 1.6 mg/dL. The patient was then supplemented with oral magnesium oxide, 200 mg daily.

The patient required two operations for his MEN 1 syndrome, transsphenoidal adenomectomy and distal pancreatectomy. His preoperative evaluation showed high prolactin (PRL) (214 ng/mL), insulin-like growth factor (IGF-1) (809 ng/mL), growth hormone (GH) (3.2 ng/mL), and proinsulin (51.8 pmol/L); low testosterone (141 ng/dL), follicle-stimulating hormone (FSH) (3.9 mIU/mL), and luteinizing hormone (LH) (1.3 mIU/mL); and normal cortisol (19.6 μg/dL), and gastrin (46 pg/mL). At the time of transsphenoidal surgery in October 1999 the patient's ionized calcium dropped to 3.7 ng/mL and he was supplemented with intravenous calcium gluconate. A calcium infusion was required again for symptomatic hypocalcemia at the time of the distal pancreatectomy when the calcium fluctuated between to 6.1 and 7.7 mg/dL. The postoperative hormonal evaluation showed a prolactin of 96.1 ng/mL, a growth hormone of <0.1 ng/mL, an IGF-1 of 157 ng/mL, and a proinsulin 28.3pmol/L. Treatment with cabergoline 2.5 mg twice a week was initiated.

In January 2000, an attempt to decrease the oral calcium supplement to 2 g daily was associated with the development of circumoral and fingertip tingling and a drop in the serum calcium level to 6.1 mg/dL. Hydrochlorthiazide, 25 mg/day was added, but the patient still required 4–8 g of elemental calcium per day to maintain his serum calcium in the low normal range. A serum PTH level was low at 3 pg/mL (normal range 10–65 pg/mL). It was decided that the previous parathyroid implantation had failed. In March 2000, approximately 0.5 g of the patient's cryopreserved parathyroid tissue was transplanted to the left forearm. Two months after transplantation on 4 g of elemental calcium (calcium carbonate), 0.5 μg of calcitriol, and 25 mg hydrochlorthiazide daily, the patient had serum calcium in the normal range (9.3 mg/dL). A tapering of these medications has been initiated.

Discussion

Acute transient hypocalcemia has been reported in 20–85% of patients after total parathyroidectomy including neck exploration for MEN 1 syndrome *(1–2)*. Neck surgery is the most common cause of prolonged hypocalcemia and permanent hypoparathyroidism, occurring in 1% to 30% of cases *(1–5)*. Parathyroid hormone (PTH) is the principal regulator of calcium homeostasis via enhancing bone resorption, calcium re-absorption in the distal tubule of the kidney, and synthesis of 1,25-dihydroxyvitamin D, which directly increases calcium absorption in the duodenum and jejunum *(6)*. Although it is clear that this patient had hypocalcemia due to surgically-induced hypoparathyroidism, other contributing causes of hypocalcemia should be considered, including vitamin D-related problems, hypomagnesemia, and renal failure *(7)*. Indeed, this patient had hypomagnesemia that may have contributed to hypocalcemia via decreased PTH secretion and resistance to PTH action in skeletal and renal tissue *(6)*. Because magnesium is an intracellular cation, a serum concentration below the normal value of 1.8 mg/dL suggests significant depletion and warrants treatment.

Postoperative monitoring of serum calcium levels simplifies the diagnosis but treatment should be started before laboratory values are available if the patient develops symptoms and signs of hypocalcemia. Muscular irritability characteristic of hypocalcemia may progress from paresthesias and muscle cramps to laryngospasm, bronchospasm, tetany, and seizures, especially in children. Mental status changes, prolongation of the QT interval on the electrocardiogram, and congestive heart failure may complicate hypocalcemia, particularly when there is a precipitous fall of calcium and with the concurrent presence of alkalosis that decreases the availability of ionized calcium.

Treatment of acute, symptomatic hypocalcemia starts with intravenous administration of calcium. Calcium gluconate, calcium chloride, and calcium gluceptate contain 90, 272, and 180 mg of elemental calcium per 10 mL solution, respectively. Calcium gluconate causes less tissue irritation and is preferred. For symptomatic hypocalcemia 1 to 2 ampules of calcium gluconate diluted in 50–100 mL of 5% dextrose can be infused over 5–10 min. This can be repeated and followed by a calcium drip, 10–15 mg/kg body weight. Five ampules of calcium gluconate in 500 mL of 5% dextrose infused at a rate 100 mL/h will deliver 90 mg of elemental calcium per hour. Approximately 1000 mg of elemental calcium infused over 5–10 h will increase the serum calcium by 2–3 mg/dL.

Multiple calcium preparations are available for oral use. Elemental calcium content in the commonly used preparations is as follows: 40% in calcium carbonate, 21% in calcium citrate, 9% in calcium gluconate, and 39% in tricalcium phosphate. Calcium carbonate is used most widely, providing the least expensive form of calcium supplement. Though calcium citrate and tricalcium phosphate may have slightly better taste, studies do not support their better absorption *(8)*. Approximately 30–40% of ingested calcium is absorbed. Dividing doses and taking calcium with meals improves absorption, particularly in achlorhydric subjects. Constipation is the most common side effect of calcium. Magnesium oxide can relieve constipation and improve magnesium deficiency.

Vitamin D supplementation is often necessary in hypoparathyroidism. Calcitriol (1,25 dihydroxyvitamin D), 0.25 to 1.0 µg/d, is the drug of choice because renal 1-α-hydroxylation of 25 hydroxyvitamin D is impaired in hypoparathyroidism. Vitamin D enhances intestinal calcium absorption and may result in hypercalciuria, as there is a loss of calcium-re-absorbing effect of PTH on the distal renal tubule *(9)*. In cases of hypercalciuria associated with hypocalcemia, addition of a thiazide diuretic will enhance calcium reabsorption and increase serum calcium levels. Thiazide diuretics alone may also correct hypocalcemia in mild cases.

Maintaining calcium in the low normal range and avoiding hypercalciuria are the goals of therapy in chronic hypoparathyroidism. Our patient required calcium and magnesium supplements, 1,25 dihydroxyvitamin D, and a thiazide diuretic to maintain his calcium level in the low normal range. He developed symptomatic hypocalcemia when he missed his medications during surgery and during attempts to taper calcium supplements. It became obvious that parathyroid implantation at the time of total parathyroidectomy failed and implantation of cryopreserved parathyroid tissue was performed.

Total parathyroidectomy has become treatment of choice for patients with MEN 1 syndrome because long-term studies have shown recurrence rate of 30–66% after partial parathyroidectomy *(1–3)*. Cure of hyperparathyroidism, however, is achieved at the price of a higher incidence of surgically induced hypoparathyroidism. Permanent hypoparathyroidism has been reported in 8%–36% of patients with MEN 1 *(1–3)* comparing unfavorably with 0%–20% reported after surgery for sporadic hyperplasia *(4)*. Autotransplantation of parathyroid tissue introduced by Lahey and advanced by Wells *(11,12)*, has become an established strategy for preventing permanent hypoparathyroidism after total parathyroidectomy *(11–16)*. This strategy allows easy access in case of recurrent hyperparathyroidism and delayed transplantation in case of persistent hypoparathyroidism.

Autotransplantation of fresh parathyroid tissue resulted in full recovery (no calcium supplementation) in more than 80% of patients *(11–16)*. Review of studies reporting separate results for MEN 1 shows full recovery in only 10%–20% of patients *(13,14)*. Difficulties in achieving better results in MEN 1 are probably explained by the multiplicity of genomic defects of the calcium-sensing receptor, resulting in highly variable PTH release in MEN 1-related parathyroid hyperplasia *(17)*.

Patients with permanent hypoparathyroidism may have a second chance of recovery with transplantation of cryopreserved tissue. Cure rates of hypoparathyroidism of 50%–70% were reported initially, but later series showed only 8%–20% success rates *(12–15)*; these studies did not provide separate data for patients with MEN 1. Investigation of the pathophysiology of the higher failure rates of cryopreserved parathyroid autografts suggests that total number of live parathyroid cells may be reduced owing to the freezing and thawing process and by dispersion of cryopreserved cells, but is unrelated to the duration of storage *(14,18)*. In cases of improved parathyroid function, vitamin D supplements can be discontinued first followed by calcium tapering a few months after surgery. Our patient had his best serum calcium level two months after transplantation of cryopreserved parathyroid tissue, suggesting that at least partial restoration of parathyroid function should be expected.

REFERENCES

1. Kraimps JL, Duh QY, Demeure M, et al. Hyperparathyroidism in multiple endocrine neoplasia syndrome. Surgery 1992;112:1080–1088.
2. O'Riordan DS, O'Brien T, Grant CS, et al. Surgical management of primary hyperparathyroidism in multiple endocrine neoplasia types 1 and 2. Surgery 1993;114:1031–1039.
3. Hellman P, Skogseid B, Oberg K, et al. Primary and reoperative parathyroid operations in hyperparathyroidism of multiple endocrine neoplasia type 1. Surgery 1998;124:993–999.
4. Proye C, Carnaille B, Quievreux JL, et al. Late outcome of 304 consecutive patients with multiple gland enlargement in primary hyperparathyroidism treated by conservative surgery. World J Surg 1998;22: 526–530.
5. Olson JA, DeBenedetti MK, Bauman DS et al. Parathyroid autotransplantation during thyroidectomy. Results of long-term follow-up. Ann Surg 1996;223:472–480.
6. Broadus AE. Mineral balance and homeostasis. In: Favus MJ, ed. Primer on the metabolic bone disease, 4th ed. Lippincott, Philadelphia, PA, 1999, pp. 74–80.
7. Guise TA, Mundy GR. Evaluation of hypocalcemia in children and adults. J Clin Endocrinol Metab 1995;80:1473–1478.
8. Heaney RP. Absorption of calcium as the carbonate and citrate salts, with some observation on method. Osteoporosis Int 1999;9:19–23.
9. Vieth R. Vitamin D supplementation, 25-hydroxyvitamin D concentrations, and safety. Am J Clin Nutr 1999;69:842–856.
10. Veldhuis JD, Norton JA, Wells SA Jr, et al. Theraputic controversy. Surgical versus medical management of multiple endocrine neoplasia (MEN) type I. J Clin Endocrinol Metab 1997;82:357–364.

11. Wells SA Jr, Ellis GJ, Gunnells JC, et al. Parathyroid autotransplantation in primary parathyroid hyperplasia. N Engl J Med 1976;195:57–62.

12. Wells SA Jr, Gunnels JC, Gutman RA, et al. The successful transplantation of frozen parathyroid tissue in man. Surgery 1977;81:86–90.

13. Saxe AW, Brennan MF. Reoperative parathyroid surgery for primary hyperparathyroidism caused by multiple-gland disease: total parathyroidectomy and autotransplantation with cryopreserved tissue. Surgery 1982;91:616–621.

14. Herrera M, Grant C, vanHeerden JA, et al. Parathyroid autotransplantation. Arch Surg 1992;127:825–830.

15. Caccitolo J, Farley DR, vanHeerden JA, et al. The current role of parathyroid cryopreservation and autotransplantation in parathyroid surgery: an institutional experience. Surgery 1997;122:1062–1067.

16. Mallette LE, Blevins T, Jordan P, et al. Autogenous parathyroid grafts for generalized primary parathyroid hyperplasia: contrasting outcome in sporadic hyperplasia versus multiple endocrine neoplasia type I. Surgery 1987;101:738–745.

17. Carling T, Rastad J, Ridefelt P, et al. Hyperparathyroidism of multiple endocrine neoplasia type 1: candidate gene and parathyroid calcium sensing protein expression. Surgery 1995;118:924–931.

18. McHenry CR, Stenger DB, Calandro NK. The effect of cryopreservation on parathyroid cell viability and function. Am J Surg 1997;174:481–484.

CASE #2: HYPOPARATHYROIDISM DURING PREGNANCY

Case Description

A 22-yr-old female was brought to the emergency room (ER) by her mother because of seizures. Laboratory evaluation showed hypocalcemia and hypomagnesemia and she was admitted for evaluation and treatment. By history, she had been diagnosed with mental retardation in early childhood, with epilepsy at age 16, and with idiopathic hypoparathyroidism at age 19. She had never taken prescribed medications regularly.

Review of her records revealed that she had recently been seen at 6-mo gestation when her obstetrician noticed hypocalcemia during a prenatal visit. At that time she denied paresthesias but had muscle cramps in her lower back, legs, and feet. Her examination showed a positive Chvostek's sign and a negative Trousseau's sign. Laboratory data were as follows: serum calcium 5.1 mg/dL, ionized calcium 2.4 mg/dL, magnesium 1.2 mg/dL, phosphorus 5.1 mg/dL, potassium 4.8 mEq/L, albumin 3.3 g/dL and bicarbonate 27 mEq/L. She was started on oral calcium carbonate to provide 1.2 g of elemental calcium/d and magnesium oxide 1 g/d.

At 7 months gestation she remained asymptomatic except for occasional muscle cramps. Her serum calcium was 5.3, phosphorus 4.9 mg/dL, magnesium 1.5 mg/dL, and albumin 3.4 g/dL. She was instructed to increase her calcium intake to 1.5 g of elemental calcium/d and calcitriol 0.25 µg/d was added.

In her eighth month of pregnancy she complained of weakness and generalized tingling. She stated she could not take medications because of nausea, abdominal discomfort, and intermittent diarrhea. The serum calcium was 4.9 mg/dL, magnesium 1.6 mg/dL, phosphorus 4.9 mg/dL, and previously sent intact PTH 5.1 pg/mL (normal range 10–65 pg/mL). Hospital admission was recommended but declined by the patient. Her oral dose of calcium was increased to 2 g/d, calcitriol to 0.5 µg/d, and magnesium oxide continued at 1 g/d.

When first seen in the emergency department for seizures, she complained of weakness and muscle cramps. Her mother reported that the patient had a seizure 4 d earlier and twice on the day of presentation. Seizures involved shaking of the head and arms with urinary incontinence and postictal stupor. She had intermittent diarrhea, but no fever, chills, respiratory infection, vomiting, abdominal pain, visual problems, or tinnitus. Two weeks previously the patient gave birth to a normal boy after labor induction for fetal bradycardia. She was not breast feeding her child. Her medications included phenytoin 300 mg/d, ferrous sulfate 325 mg/d, and calcium carbonate 1 g/d.

Physical examination on admission revealed mental retardation, short stature (1.45 m), dry skin, coarse hair, prominent nose, gingival hyperplasia, prognathism with normal teeth, a positive Chvostek's sign, a negative Trousseau's sign, normal thyroid size, normal fingernails, and no evidence of metacarpal or metatarsal shortening. Her blood pressure was 110/70 mmHg, pulse 76 bpm, and temperature 97.6°F.

At the time of admission, the serum calcium was 4.7 mg/dL, ionized calcium 2.0 mg/dL, magnesium 1.1 mg/dL, phosphorus 5.5 mg/dL, potassium 4.7 mg/dL, albumin 3.3 g/dL, CO_2 27, and phenytoin 3.3 µg/mL (normal range 10–20 µg/mL). Her serum PTH was 3 pg/mL and 1,25 dihydroxyvitamin D was 30 pg/mL (normal range 15–60 pg/mL). To increase her serum calcium and magnesium acutely, she was given intravenous calcium gluconate and magnesium sulfate. She was also treated with intravenous phenytoin. The patient had no further seizures. Oral calcitriol 0.25 µg every 6 h was given for four doses and then 0.25 µg daily and her serum calcium increased to 8.1 mg/dL over 3 d. The patient was discharged on calcium carbonate 1 g/d, calcitriol 0.25 µg/d, and phenytoin 300 mg/d.

Discussion

Idiopathic hypoparathyroidism and phenytoin use are the probable underlying causes for chronic hypocalcemia in this patient. Seizures are a rare manifestation of hypocalcemia and are predominantly seen in children. Hypocalcemic seizures may be focal, petit mal, or grand mal. Our patient had history of epilepsy and underlying hypocalcemia which probably lowered the seizure threshold. A more characteristic clinical manifestation of hypocalemia is tetany. It includes sensory and muscular components. The sensory component involves a tingling sensation in the fingers and around the mouth that may spread to the body. The muscular component is a spontaneous tonic muscular contraction (1). Muscular spasm initiated with adduction of the thumb progresses to the characteristic "d'accoucheur" pose; uncommonly it involves the feet in combined carpopedal spasm, and rarely it advances to life-threatening laryngeal spasm. Tonic seizures of generalized tetany are characterized encephalographically by bursts of high voltage slow waves (2–5 Hz) with the frequency correlated with the serum calcium level (1).

Pregnancy increases calcium demands, but does not produce hypocalcemia in healthy women. The growing fetal skeleton accumulates 20–35 g of calcium, most of it in the third trimester. The main adjustment during pregnancy is a doubling of 1,25 dihydroxyvitamin D levels, resulting in a doubling of maternal calcium absorption and absorptive hypercalciuria (2). The level of PTH is decreased while that of parathyroid hormone-related protein (PTHrP) is increased, the latter being produced by several maternal and fetal tissues including the placenta, amnion, decidua, umbilical cord, fetal parathyroids, and breast. Increased PTHrP contributes to higher 1,25 dihydroxyvitamin D levels and regulates placental calcium transport (3). Although the total serum calcium is decreased owing to decreased albumin, ionized calcium and phosphorus remain normal during pregnancy. In women with hypoparathyroidism, vitamin D requirements are increased during pregnancy, particularly after the 20th wk and in the third trimester (4–6). A recent report showed that calcium and calcitriol doses had to be increased from 1 g/d to 4 g/d and from 0.25–0.5 µg/d to 0.75–3.25 µg/d, respectively, in hypoparathyroid pregnant women in order to maintain serum calcium levels in the low normal range (4). These data suggest that increased PTHrP is unable to compensate for the lack of PTH during pregnancy in hypoparathyroid women.

Increased bone turnover during lactation protects women from hypocalcemia and also provides 300–1000 mg of calcium daily in breast milk (2). The major hormonal change is an increased level of PTHrP produced in the breast. The level of PTHrP in breast milk is 10,000 times higher than the serum concentrations of normal people or even patients with hypercalcemia of malignancy (7). In women with hypoparathyroidism, PTHrP stimulates 1,25 dihydroxyvitamin D synthesis independent of PTH (8), explaining low calcitriol requirements during the early postpartum period, especially if the woman breastfeeds. Spontaneous remission of hypoparathyroidism (9) and hypercalcemia in a calcitriol-treated hypoparathyroid (6) woman was reported during lactation, emphasizing the important physiological role of PTHrP.

Despite poor compliance with medications, this patient had a successful pregnancy. Previous reports have shown serious adverse events in nearly half of hypoparathyroid pregnancies (10). Maternal hypocalcemia can lead to uterine irritability, preterm labor or abortion (11). In the fetus it can cause reactive hyperparathyroidism, intrauterine fractures and intracranial bleeding (11,12). Use of calcitriol has dramatically improved pregnancy outcome in hypoparathyroid women. In a recent series of 12 women (4), 10 of them carried pregnancy to the term and delivered healthy babies. The adverse events in the other two women included premature closure of the frontal fontanels, and stillbirth in the 20th wk because compex fetal malformation. High doses of vitamin D have been shown to be teratogenic in experimental animals (13) and caution is recommended for its use in pregnancy. Short duration of action providing reversal of possible toxicity just a few days after discontinuation of calcitriol improves safety and makes calcitriol the vitamin D preparation of choice for hypoparathyroid women during pregnancy and lactation. The goal is to keep the serum calcium in the low normal range. Monitoring treatment with urinary calcium excretion is not helpful because hypercalciuria is expected even in healthy pregnant women.

This patient was taking phenytoin for epilepsy. Anticonvulsants are well known to cause hypocalcemia and osteomalacia. Reports indicate that 10–40% of patients receiving long-term anticonvulsant therapy have reduced levels of serum 25 hydroxyvitamin D and serum and urinary calcium (14–16). The main mechanism is induction of liver microsomal mixed oxidase activity with increased metabolism and clearance of vitamin D (17). In vitro, phenytoin inhibits intestinal calcium absorption (18) and PTH-mediated bone resorption (19), but the contribution of these effects to calcium metabolism in vivo needs further clarification.

The association of idiopathic hypoparathyroidism with a short stature, some peculiarity of the face, mental retardation and epilepsy suggests the chromosomal defect of DiGeorge syndrome in this patient. Hypoparathyroidism was a major manifestation in two patients with velocardiofacial syndrome (VCFS), one of the conditions associated with DiGeorge syndrome (20). These two patients with mental retardation, minimal facial abnormalities and normal sexual development presented in their late teens with epilepsy and hypoparathyroidism but without congenital cardiac defects or T-cell deficiency. A microdeletion of chromosome region 22q11 was demonstrated in both patients confirming the diagnosis of VCFS. Although our patient did not have a chromosomal evaluation, her clinical presentation closely resembles the described cases and makes diagnosis of VCFS an interesting possibility.

REFERENCES

1. Strewler GJ, Rosenblatt M. Mineral metabolism. In: Felig P, Baxter JD, Frohman LA, eds. Endocrinology and Metabolism, 3rd ed, McGraw-Hill, New York, 1995, pp. 1407–1516.
2. Kovacs CS, Kronenberg HM. Maternal-fetal calcium and bone metabolism during pregnancy, puerperium and lactation. Endocr Rev 1997;18:832–872.
3. Cornish J, Callon KE, Nicholson GC, Reid IR. Parathyroid hormone-related protein-(107-139) inhibits bone resorption in vivo. Endocrinology 1997;138:1299–1304.
4. Callies F, Arlt W, Scholz HJ, et al. Management of hypoparathyroidism during pregnancy—report of twelve cases. Eur J Endocrinol 1998;139:284–289.
5. Salle BL, Berthezene F, Glorieux FH, et al. Hypoparathyroidism during pregnancy: treatment with calcitriol. J Clin Endocrinol Metab 1981;52:810–813.
6. Caplan RH, Beguin EA. Hypercalcemia in a calcitriol-treated hypoparathyroid woman during lactation. Obstet Gynecol 1990;76:485–489.
7. Dobnig H, Kainer F, Stepan V, et al. Elevated parathyroid hormone-related peptide levels after human gestation: relationship to changes in bone and mineral metabolism. J Clin Endocrinol Metab 1995;80: 3699–3707.
8. Mather KJ, Chik CL, Corenblum B. Maintenance of serum calcium by parathyroid hormone-related peptide during lactation in a hypoparathyroid patient. J Clin Endocrinol Metab 1999;84:424–427.
9. Cundy T, Haining SA, Guilland-Cumming DF, et al. Remission of hypoparathyroidism during lactation: evidence for a physiological role for prolactin in the regulation of vitamin D metabolism. Clin Endocrinol 1987; 26:667–674.
10. Hoper K, Pavel M, Dorr G, et al. Calcitriol-Gabe in der Scwangerschaft bei partieller Di-Geroge-Anomalie. Deutsche Medizinische Wochenschrift 1994;119:176–178.
11. Eastell R, Edmonds CJ, deDhayal RCS, McFadyen IR. Prolonged hypoparathyroidism presenting as second trimester abortion. Br Med J 1985;291:955–956.
12. Loughead JL, Mughal Z, Mimouni F, et al. Spectrum and natural history of congenital hyperparathyroidism secondary to maternal hypocalcemia. Am J Perinatol 1990;7:350–355.
13. Friedman WF, Mills LF. The relationship between vitamin D and craniofacial and dental anomalies of the supravalvular aortic stenosis syndrome. Pediatrics 1969;43:12–18.
14. Pylypchuk G, Oreopoulos, Wilson DR, et al. Calcium metabolism in adult outpatients with epilepsy receiving long-term anticonvulsant therapy. Can Med Assoc J 1978;118:635–638.
15. Weinstein RS, Bryce GF, Sappington LJ, et al. Decreased serum ionized calcium and normal vitamin D metabolite levels with anticonvulsant drug treatment. J Clin Endocrinol Metab 1984;58:1003–1009.
16. Hahn TJ, Hendin BA, Scharp CR, Haddad JGJ. Effect of chronic anticonvulsant therapy on serum 25-hydroxycalciferol levels in adults. N Engl J Med 1972;287:900–904.
17. Matheson RT, Herbst JJ, Jubiz W, et al. Absorption and biotransformation of cholecalciferol in drug-induced osteomalacia. J Clin Pharmacol 1976; 16:426–432.
18. Corradino RA. Diphenylhydantoin: direct inhibition of the vitamin D_3-mediated calcium absorptive mechanism in organ-cultured duodenum. Biochem Pharmacol 1976;25:863–864.
19. Hahn TJ, Scharp CR, Richardson CA, et al. Interaction of diphenylhydantoin (phenytoin) and phenobarbital with hormonal mediation of fetal rat bone resorption in vitro. J Clin Invest 1978;62:406–414.
20. Scire G, Dallapiccola B, Iannetti P, et al. Hypoparathyroidism as the major manifestation in two patients with 22q11 deletion. Am J Med Genet 1994;52:478–482.

CASE #3: OSTEOBLASTIC METASTASES IN PROSTATE CANCER

Case Description

An 88-yr-old African-American male diagnosed as having carcinoma of the prostate in 1978 was admitted in July 1980. He had a previous history of type 2 diabetes mellitus, inactive Paget's disease of the bone, status post-right nephrectomy, and chronic renal failure since 1973. His physical examination was remarkable for a generalized decrease in muscle strength and an enlarged prostate. Chvostek's and Trousseau's signs were negative. His admission laboratory data revealed a hemoglobin of 7.6 g/dL, WBC 7900/mm^3, and normal differential. Other laboratory values were as follows: serum Na 142 mEq/L, K 6.9 mEq/L, glucose 320 mg/dL, Cl 116 mEq/L, bicarbonate 17 mEq/L, creatinine 2.3 mg/dL, total calcium (Ca) 4.7 mg/dL (normal 8.6–10.2), phosphorus 3.9 mg/dL (normal 2.5–4.1), magnesium (Mg) 0.9 mEq/L (normal 1.5–2.4), and alkaline phosphatase 1641 mU/mL (normal = 77–260). His plasma ionized Ca was 2.16 mg/dL (normal 3.78–4.66), serum 25(OH) vitamin D_3 ($25OHD_3$) 10 ng/mL (normal 10–55) and serum 1,25 dihydroxyvitamin D_3 26.1 pg/mL (normal 21–44). His serum parathyroid hormone (PTH) level was at the upper limit or normal. Twenty-four hour urine calcium excretion was 12 mg (normal <200 mg). Selected laboratory data from his previous admission in 1978 were as follows: serum Ca 8.4 mg/dL, phosphorus 3.9 mg/dL, and creatinine 2.5 mg/dL.

X-rays of the skeleton revealed widespread osteoblastic lesions. A bone scan revealed markedly increased generalized skeletal uptake and absent renal uptake. However, a bone scan performed earlier in October 1978 was essentially normal (see Fig. 1). Bone marrow biopsy revealed extensive infiltration by adenocarcinoma cells.

His hypocalcemia failed to respond to treatment with intravenous and oral magnesium replacement despite normalization of the serum magnesium level. The patient received intravenous calcium (15 mg/kg elemental calcium in normal saline over 6 h with minimal change in serum calcium levels (normal expected response is 2.0–3.0 mg/dL increase). The patient was started on oral calcium carbonate (1 g elemental Ca q6hr) and 1,25 dihydroxyvitamin D_3 0.5 µg b.i.d. and stilbesterol 1 mg daily. In October 1980, his serum Ca was 5.1 mg/dL and serum Mg was 1.65 meq/L and the patient remained asymptomatic. He was subsequently lost to follow up.

Discussion

The association of hypercalcemia with cancer is well known. On the other hand, the presence of hypocalcemia in association with malignancy is less well recognized. In several studies of unselected cancer patients hypocalcemia has been observed more frequently than hypercalcemia. Raskin et al. *(1)* observed that hypocalcemia occurred in 16% of patients with cancer with bone metastases, as compared to the occurrence of hypercalcemia in 9% of patients. In other studies, the prevalence of hypocalcemia ranged from 5–13% in patients with bone metastases, depending on the correction formula used to adjust serum calcium values for protein concentrations *(2)*. However, true hypocalcemia based on ionized calcium measurements is less common *(3)*.

Decreased serum albumin levels are frequently observed in cancer patients. Approximately 45% of serum calcium is bound to proteins, predominantly albumin. Therefore, serum total calcium values may be decreased, whereas serum ionized calcium values are normal in these patients. Various correction formulas have been devised to calculate corrected serum total calcium levels. Most commonly applied formulas make adjustment for serum albumin concentrations. For each 1 g/dL change in serum albumin (from the normal mean value), 0.8 mg/dL is added or subtracted from the observed serum calcium value. While these formulas may accurately reflect the ionized calcium status in certain disease states such as cirrhosis of the liver, they do not perform as well in cancer patients *(3–6)*. Therefore, ionized calcium measurements are frequently necessary to determine whether the patient has true hypocalcemia.

Our patient had hypomagnesemia and renal insufficiency, both of which could lead to hypocalcemia. In magnesium deficiency, there is a defect in parathyroid hormone secretion, which is corrected within minutes of magnesium infusion *(7)*. In addition, there is evidence that skeletal effects of parathyroid hormone are impaired in the presence of

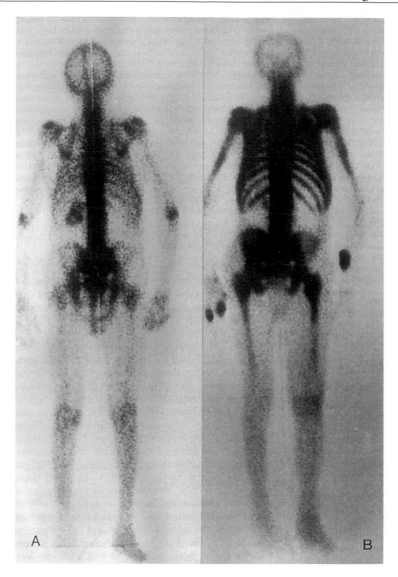

Fig. 1. Posterior views of the bone scan were done in October 1978 (**A**) revealing a normal skeletal study (right kidney is absent due to previous nephrectomy) and in July 1980, (**B**) revealing extensive generalized skeletal uptake. (Reprinted with permission from ref. *3*.)

magnesium deficiency *(7)*. Hypomagnesemic patients may continue to have tetany, even if serum calcium values are corrected by calcium infusions. Magnesium deficiency is best corrected by parenteral administration of magnesium sulfate (2g $MgSO_4$ as 50% solution Q8h via IM injection or iv infusion 48 meq over 24 h) or oral supplementation with magnesium oxide (300–600 mg/d elemental Mg in divided doses). Our patient received supplementation with both intravenous and oral magnesium with normalization of serum magnesium levels. However, the hypocalcemia persisted. Parenteral, magnesium should be administered very cautiously to patients with impaired renal function to avoid hypermagnesemia.

The hypocalcemia associated with renal insufficiency is multifactoral (8). Patients with renal insufficiency may have a metabolic acidosis, which increases the ionized fraction and therefore, the decrease in serum total calcium may be out of proportion to the decrease in ionized calcium. Hyperphosphatemia resulting from inability to excrete phosphorus leads to a decrease in serum calcium levels. Impaired synthesis of 1,25 dihydroxy-vitamin D by the kidney results in poor calcium absorption from the gut. In addition, there is resistance to the actions of parathyroid hormone. The hypocalcemia seen in renal insufficiency responds to treatment with phosphate binders and 1,25 dihydroxyvitamin D. Our patient had low normal serum 1,25-dihydroxyvitamin D levels, however, the hypocalcemia did not respond to a relatively high dose of $1,25(OH)_2$ vitamin D_3 (0.5 µg BID).

Despite a marked decrease in serum ionized calcium levels, our patient was asymptomatic, and Chvostek's and Trousseau's signs were negative. Acute manifestations of hypocalcemia are related to increased neuromuscular irritability and include paresthesias, muscle cramps, carpopedal spasms, tetany, and seizures. In addition to hypocalcemia, the neuromuscular threshold is decreased by alkalosis and hypomagnesemia and if these are present, the clinical manifestations of tetany may occur at minimally decreased or even normal serum ionized calcium levels. The severity of symptoms is related to whether hypocalcemia is acute or chronic. In some patients with chronic hypocalcemia, there may be a striking paucity of symptoms. In adults, cardiac decompensation with congestive heart failure or cardiogenic shock may develop; these manifestations resolve after successful treatment of hypocalcemia (9).

There are several possible explanations for true hypocalcemia in patients with malignancy. Patients who are critically ill because of sepsis or other conditions, may develop hypocalcemia. The mechanisms that are responsible for this hypocalcemia are poorly understood, although cytokines such as interleukin-1 (IL-1) released by macrophages may be responsible. The frequency of hypocalcemia in critically ill patients varies from 12 to 23% (10). Serum parathyroid hormone levels in these patients may be inappropriately low for the degree of hypocalcemia. There is no clear evidence that demonstrates that correction of hypocalcemia in critically ill patients results in better clinical outcomes. However, it is generally agreed that when hypocalcemia is severe, and especially if heart failure is present, parenteral calcium should be given (11). The presence of large concentrations of citrate in preserved blood may contribute to some decrease in ionized calcium, although in clinical practice, this is not a significant problem.

Patients with malignancy often receive chemotherapeutic agents that might cause hypocalcemia. Common among these is cisplatinum, which directly inhibits bone resorption. In addition, its administration results in renal magnesium losses, resulting in hypomagnesemia and thus inducing hypocalcemia (12). Parenteral bisphosphonates are used for treatment of hypercalcemia, as well as for prevention of bone disease in normocalcemic patients with multiple myeloma. In general, clinically significant hypocalcemia is uncommon. However, there are a few case reports of patients with underlying hypoparathyroidism who developed hypocalcemia following bisphosphonate therapy. In these patients, the normal compensatory mechanisms, i.e., an increase in parathyroid hormone did not occur, thus resulting in hypocalcemia (13).

In patients with acute leukemia and Burkitt's lymphoma, tumors that are relatively sensitive to chemotherapy, rapid tumor lysis results in sudden release of uric acid, phosphate, and potassium into the circulation. As a consequence of the hyperphosphatemia, there is a precipitation of calcium and phosphate salts as the blood concentration exceeds the calcium phosphate stability product *(14)*. Hypocalcemia during treatment of acute leukemia is especially common in children. The hyperphosphatemia should be managed by adequate fluid administration; in severe cases, dialysis may be indicated for the hyperphosphatemia.

There are several case reports of true hypocalcemia occurring in patients with extensive osteoblastic bone metastases. The tumors that have been associated with this phenomenon are lung, breast, and prostate cancer *(15–19)*. Of these, prostate cancer is the most common. The association of hypocalcemia in patients with acute monocytic leukemia with osteoblastic bone formation and hypocalcemia has also been reported *(20)*. Calcium balance studies have shown that hypocalcemia in patients with osteoblastic metastases results from excessive accretion of calcium into bone. Increased uptake of radioactive calcium in strontium has been demonstrated in these patients. Bone scanning with Technetium-99m labeled bisphosphonates reveals extensive skeletal uptake and appearance of "super-scan," as seen in our patient *(21)*. Patients with this syndrome frequently have hypomagnesemia and hypophosphatemia, presumably because of accretion of these ions into the skeleton as well. Urinary calcium excretion is decreased, as was the case in our patient. Serum parathyroid hormone levels may be inappropriately normal for the degree of hypocalcemia, possibly owing to low serum magnesium levels. When serum magnesium is corrected, serum parathyroid hormone levels may increase appropriately.

In prostate cancer, extensive osteoblastic and metabolic consequences appear related to the production of osteoblast stimulating factors by tumor cells. Extracts of hyperplastic and neoplastic prostate tissue stimulate thymidine uptake and collagen synthesis by fibroblasts and osteoblasts *(22,23)*. Some studies suggest that the factors may be similar to urokinase *(24,25)*. In a more recent study, culture media from various stages of prostate cancer tissue were shown to stimulate proliferation and activity of osteoblasts in culture. This stimulation was greater with tissues from advanced stages and was not blocked by urokinase inhibitors *(26)*. The exact nature of these factors remains unknown. There are no cases reported where the response of the hypocalcemia to antiandrogen therapy in these patients with prostate cancer has been evaluated.

REFERENCES

1. Raskin P, McClain CJ, Medsger TA. Hypocalcemia associated with metastatic bone disease. A retrospective study. Arch Intern Med 1973;132:539–543.
2. Riancho JA, Arjona R, Valle R, Sanz J, Gonzalez-Macias J. The clinical spectrum of hypocalcemia associated with bone metastases. J Intern Med 1989;226:449–452.
3. Kukreja SC, Shanmugam A, Lad TE. Hypocalcemia in patients with prostate Cancer. Calcif Tissue Int 1988;43:340–345.
4. Ladenson JH, Lewis JW, Boyd JC. Failure of total calcium corrected for protein, albumin, and pH to correctly assess free calcium status. J Clin Endocrinol Metab 1978;46:986–993.
5. Shemerdiak WP, Kukreja SC, Lad TE, York PA, Henderson WJ. Evaluation of routine ionized calcium determination in cancer patients. Clin Chem 1981;27:1621–1622.
6. Thode J, Juul-Jorgensen B, Bhatia HM, Kjaerulf-Nielsen M, Bartels PD, Fogh-Andersen N, Siggaard-Andersen O. Comparison of serum total calcium, albumin-corrected total calcium, and ionized calcium in 1213 patients with suspected calcium disorders. Scand J Clin Lab Invest 1989;49:217–223.
7. Chase LR, Slatopolsky E. Secretion and metabolic efficacy of parathyroid hormone in patients with severe hypomagnesemia. J Clin Endocrinol Metab 1974;38:363–371.
8. Hanley DA, Sherwood LM. Secondary hyperparathyroidism in chronic renal failure: pathophysiology and treatment. Med Clin North Am 1978;62:1319–1339.
9. Suzuki T, Ikeda U, Fujikawa H, Saito K, Shimada K. Hypocalcemic heart failure: a reversible form of heart muscle disease. Clin Cardiol 1998; 21:227–228.

10. Zaloga GP. Hypocalcemia in critically ill patients. Crit Care Med 1992;20:251–262.
11. Jankowski S, Vincent JL. Calcium administration for cardiovascular support in critically ill patients: when is it indicated? J Intensive Care Med 1995;10:91–100.
12. Kukla LJ, Abramson EC, McGuire WP, Shevrin DH, Lad T, Kukreja SC. Cis-platinum treatment for malignancy-associated humoral hypercalcemia in an athymic mouse model. Calcif Tissue Int 1984; 36:559–562.
13. Comlekci A, Biberoglu S, Hekimsoy Z, Okan I, Piskin O, Sekeroglu B, Alakavuklar M. Symptomatic hypocalcemia in a patient with latent hypoparathyroidism and breast carcinoma with bone metastasis following administration of pamidronate. Intern Med 1998;37:396–397.
14. Cadman EC, Lunberg WB, Bertino JR. hyperphosphatemia and hypocalcemia accompanying rapid cell lysis in a patient with Burkitt's lymphoma and Burkitt cell leukemia. Am J Med 1977;62:283–290.
15. Sackner MA, Apivack AP, Balian LJ. Hypocalcemia in the presence of osteoblastic metastases. N Engl J Med 1960;262:173–176.
16. Randall RE Jr, Lirenman DS. Hypocalcemia and hypophosphatemia accompanying osteoblastic metastases. J Clin Endocrinol Metab 24:1331–1334.
17. Hall TC, Griffiths CT, Petranek JR. Hypocalcemia—an unusual metabolic complication of breast cancer. N Engl J Med 1966;275:1474–1477.
18. Tommaso CL, Tucci JR. Metabolic studies in a case of hypocalcemia and osteoblastic metastases. Arch Intern Med 1979;139:238–241.
19. Smallridge RC, Wray HL, Schaaf M. Hypocalcemia with osteoblastic metastases in patient with prostate carcinoma. A cause of secondary hyperparathyroidism. Am J Med 1981;71:184–188.
20. Schenkein DP, O'Neill WC, Shapiro J, Miller KB. Accelerated bone formation causing profound hypocalcemia in acute leukemia. Ann Intern Med 1986;105:375–378.
21. Sy WM, Patel D, Faunce H. Significance of absent or faint kidney sign on bone scan. J Nucl Med 1975; 16:454–456.
22. Jacobs SC, Pikna D, Lawson RK. Prostatic osteoblastic factor. Invest Urol 1979;17:195–198.
23. Simpson E, Harrod J, Eilon G, Jacobs JW, Mundy GR. Identification of a messenger ribonucleic acid fraction in human prostatic cancer cells coding for a novel osteoblast-stimulating factor. Endocrinology 1985;117:1615–1620.
24. Rabbani SA, Xing RH. Role of urokinase (uPA) and its receptor (uPAR) in invasion and metastasis of hormone-dependent malignancies. Int J Oncol 1998;12:911–920.
25. Achbarou A, Kaiser S, Tremblay G, Ste-Marie LG, Brodt P, Goltzman D, Rabbani SA. Urokinase overproduction results in increased skeletal metastasis by prostate cancer cells in vivo. Cancer Res 1994;54: 2372–2377.
26. Festuccia C, Teti A, Bianco P, Guerra F, Vicentini C, Tennina R, Villanova I, Sciortino G, Bologna M. Human prostatic tumor cells in culture produce growth and differentiation factors active on osteoblasts: a new biological and clinical parameter for prostatic carcinoma. Oncol Res 1997;9:419–431.

12

Metabolic Bone Disease

Michael Kleerekoper, MD, FACE,
Hisham Alrefai, MD, Louis Afonso, MD,
and Bharat Raman, MD

CONTENTS

CASE #1: PAGET'S DISEASE OF BONE

Case Description

The patient is an 80-yr-old woman who was referred because of findings on a head CT "suggestive of Paget's disease." She gave a history of generalized vague headache for 6–8 mo as well as decreased hearing in both ears for the last year. There were no complaints of dizziness or visual changes. She also had a history of bilateral leg pains over the same time period. The pain was described as constant, deep, and dull in nature, not related to exercise or position. It was poorly localized but mainly in the distal portion of the legs. She obtained partial relief with nonsteroidal antiinflammatory drugs (NSAIDs). She had a chronic 4 yr history of bilateral hip pains, which she and her physician attributed to "arthritis," but she denied any back pain or sensory symptoms, and she had no sphincter disturbances. Lately, the patient has been having difficulty chewing because of a poorly fitting lower denture. Review of symptoms was otherwise negative.

The patient lives alone caring for herself but leads a sedentary life. Her brother had been diagnosed with Paget's disease (PD) and there was a family history of hypertension. Medications were amlodipine, acetaminophen, ibuprofen. She was ambulant with the aid of a cane.

On examination, she looked generally healthy. Blood pressure: 145/89 mmHg; pulse: 65 bpm; weight 157 lb; height 5'1" (unchanged from 2 yr ago), afebrile. She was edentulous but the remainder of her head and neck exam was normal. Bedside audiometric

From: *Contemporary Endocrinology: Challenging Cases in Endocrinology*
Edited by: M. E. Molitch © Humana Press Inc., Totowa, NJ

testing was consistent with sensorineural impairment in both ears. The examination of the extremities revealed no edema or clubbing. There was a marked increase in the temperature over the anterior aspect of the right thigh, and also increased warmth over the forehead. The musculoskeletal exam showed mild kyphosis with normal range of motion of the spine. There were no gross extremity deformities and there was no leg-length discrepancy. There was a slight decrease in range of motion along with tenderness in the hip joints. Neurological examination did not reveal abnormalities.

A complete blood count was normal. The total alkaline phosphatase was 580 U/L (50–180 U/L), but her AST, ALT, total bilirubin, and prothombin time were normal.

Scintigraphy was consistent with PD, demonstrating intense increased uptake involving the skull, right scapula, sacrum, cervicothoracic junction spine, right proximal femur, and hip (see Fig. 1). Radiographs of the femurs showed a flame-shaped lytic lesion in the right femur characteristic of PD (see Fig. 2). The skull X-ray was suggestive of osteitis frontalis interna (see Fig. 3). Computed tomography (CT) scan of the head (the reason for the referral) showed thickened and edematous small rounded sclerotic areas consistent with PD of the occipital region. Audiometry confirmed the sensorineural hearing loss.

Therapy was initiated with risedronate 30 mg orally daily and 2 mo later she felt better and the alkaline phosphatase was 271 U/L.

Discussion

The diagnosis of PD of bone was easy to confirm, once it had been suggested by the initial radiographic study (head CT) *(1)*. The vast majority of patients are diagnosed incidentally by X-rays or elevated alkaline phosphatase levels. Most patients are asymptomatic with this presentation. The important clinical teaching point of this case is the delay between initial symptomatic presentation (4 yr of arthritis *(2)*, 1 yr of progressive deafness *(3)*, and 6–8 mo of worsening headache) and ultimate diagnosis. In retrospect this constellation of symptoms is very typical of symptomatic PD *(4,5)* and perhaps the diagnosis should not have been delayed. However, at age 76, degenerative arthritis is far more common than PD, and at age 79–80 deafness and headache are common complaints. The rapidly progressive nature of these symptoms alerted the clinician that this was out of the ordinary, hence the initial CT.

Once a diagnosis has been established clinically, biochemically, and radiographically, a radionuclide bone scan should be performed in all patients *(6)*. The features on the scan are usually diagnostic, as in our patient, but there is a more important reason to obtain the scan even after the diagnosis has been well established. There are few documented reports of patients with PD developing a lesion in a new bone once the diagnosis has been established *(7)*. Thus, should a new suspicious lesion appear on X-ray or scan while the patient is under observation, it is more likely to represent a different disease (such as a sclerotic metastasis of prostate cancer). If the diagnosis of PD is initially suspected because of the incidental finding of an elevated alkaline phosphatase, it is better to obtain a bone scan before plane radiographs. The scan will detect those areas of the skeleton most likely to be involved in PD. Subsequently radiographs of the "hot spots" should be obtained *(8,9)*.

The goal in treating PD is to control the symptoms and prevent the complications. Although many therapies have been tried in the past, often with significant benefit as is seen with calcitonin or mithramycin therapy, the current treatment of choice is one of the available bisphosphonate class of drugs [alendronate *(10)*, etidronate *(11)*, pamidronate *(12)*, risedronate *(13)*, or tiludronate *(14)*]. Very few head-to-head comparisons of these

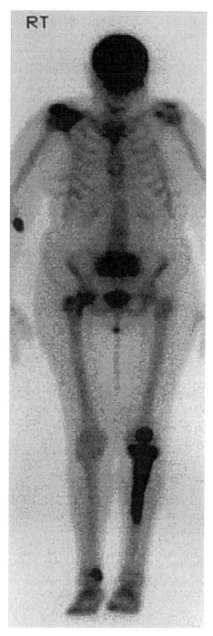

Fig. 1. Bone scan in **Case 1**, patient with Paget's disease. Note the intense isotope uptake in the skull, the right shoulder, sacrum, right femoral head, and left tibia. A typical bone scan for polyostotic Paget's disease of bone.

different bisphosphonates have been studied in formal clinical trials, and the cost of a course of treatment is comparable for all of them. Pamidronate in the United States is only available as an intravenous infusion and several protocols for its safe and effective use in PD have been reported. Of the oral bisphosphonates the shortest course of therapy required to achieve sustained remission (6 mo or longer) is with risedronate (30 mg daily for 2 mo) or alendronate (40 mg daily for 3 mo). Symptomatic relief can be seen as early as 1 wk

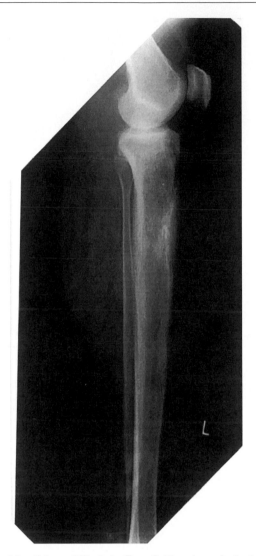

Fig. 2. Plane radiograph of the tibia and fibula in **Case 1**. Note how the lesion compares to the lesion in the left tibia in the bone scan in Fig. 1. The "flame-shaped" or "blade of grass" appearance to the advancing edge of bone lysis corresponding to the blade appearance on the scan is well demonstrated.

after initiating therapy with a decrease in local warmth and a decrease in bone pain. Nerve compression syndromes may also respond to therapy although hearing loss is likely to be permanent. Rarely a patient with vertebral body involvement will develop an acute paraplegia as the growing vertebra impinges on the spinal cord. This is clearly a medical emergency and may require urgent surgical decompression. However, it is appropriate to delay surgery for several days and begin therapy with intravenous pamidronate. Some, perhaps most, patients will have rapid and sustained relief of the paraplegia with this medical therapy alone. Additionally, as already noted, the skeleton lesions of PD are very vascular and this medical therapy decreases this vascularity quickly. Bone deformity does not change after effective medical treatment of PD and surgical correction may be needed. The patient may require joint replacement because of arthritis secondary to the skeletal

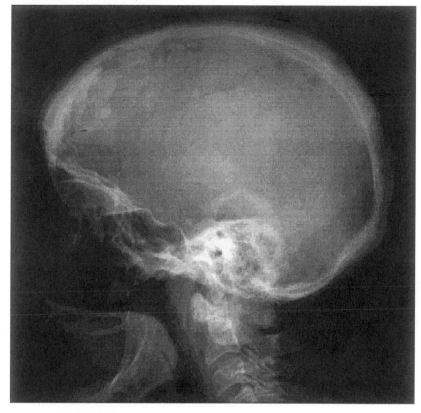

Fig. 3. Plain radiograph of the skull in **Case 1**. Note the changes of osteitis frontalis on the X-ray and the corresponding intense isotope uptake on the scan (Fig. 1).

deformity of PD. Surgical repair of a fracture through a segment of bone affected by PD may be needed but here too surgery should be delayed if possible until medical therapy has reduced the vascularity.

REFERENCES

1. Tehranzadeh J, Fung Y, Donohue M, Anavim A, Pribram HW. Computed tomography of Paget disease of the skull versus fibrous dysplasia. Skeletal Radiol 1998;27:664–672.
2. Helliwell PS, Porter G. Controlled study of the prevalence of radiological osteoarthritis in clinically unrecognised juxta-articular Paget's disease. Ann Rheum Dis 1999;58:762–765.
3. Monsell EM, Cody DD, Bone HG, Divine GW. Hearing loss as a complication of Paget's disease of bone. J Bone Miner Res 1999;14(Suppl 2):92–95.
4. Ankrom MA, Shapiro JR. Paget's disease of bone (osteitis deformans). J Am Geriatr Soc 1998;46:1025–1033.
5. Gold DT, Burchett BM, Shipp KM, Pieper CF, Lyles KW. Factors associated with self-rated health in patients with Paget's disease of bone. J Bone Miner Res 1999;14(Suppl 2):99–102.
6. Pons F, Alvarez L, Peris P, Guanabens N, Vidal-Sicart S, Monegal A, Pavia J, Ballesta AM, Munos-Gomez J, Herranz R. Quantitative evaluation of bone scintigraphy in the assessment of Paget's disease activity. Nucl Med Commun 1999;20:525–528.
7. Renier JC, Audran M. Polyostotic Paget's disease. A search for lesions of different durations and for new lesions. Rev Rhum Engl Ed 1997;64:233–242.
8. Mirra JM, Brien EW, Tehranzadeh J. Paget's disease of bone: review with emphasis on radiologic features, Part I. Skeletal Radiol 1995;24:163–171.

9. Mirra JM, Brien EW, Tehranzadeh J. Paget's disease of bone: review with emphasis on radiologic features, Part II. Skeletal Radiol 1995;24:173–184.

10. Lombardi A. Treatment of Paget's disease of bone with alendronate. Bone 1999;24:59S–61S.

11. Miller PD, Brown JP, Siris ES, Hoseyni MS, Axelrod DW, Bekker PJ. A randomised, double-blind comparison of risedronate and etidronate in the treatment of Paget's disease of bone. Paget's Risedronate/ Etidronate Study Group. Am J Med 1999;106:513–520.

12. Gutteridge DH, Retallack RW, Ward LC, Stuckey BG, Stewart GO, Prince RL, Kent GN, Bhagat CI, Price RI, Thompson RI, Nicholson GC. Clinical, biochemical, hematologic, and radiographic responses in Paget's disease following intravenous pamidronate disodium: a 2-year study. Bone 1996;19:387–394.

13. Brown JP, Chines AA, Myers WR, Eusebio RA, Ritter-Hrncirik C, Hayes CW. Improvement of pagetic bone lesions with risedronate treatment: a radiologic study. Bone 2000;26:263–267.

14. Fraser WD, Stamp TC, Creek RA, Sawyer JP, Picot C. A double-blind, multicentre, placebo-controlled study of tiludronate in Paget's disease of bone. Postgrad Med J 1997;73:496–502.

CASE #2: SYSTEMIC MASTOCYTOSIS

Case Description

A 34-yr-old male felt a sudden "pop" in his back as he was lifting a bundle of wires in his usual occupation as an electrician. He had experienced similar episodes on two previous occasions but neither was as severe. He gave a history of chronic back pain for 5 yr, but this only minimally interfered with his employment. Six years prior to this presentation he was involved in a motor vehicle accident in which he sustained fractures of the pelvis, ribs, and second cervical vertebra. He had attributed his chronic back pain to that accident. He was certain that no other vertebral fractures had been sustained during that accident. Initial history was essentially unrevealing for possible causes of osteoporotic fracture. There was no family history of osteoporosis or fragility fractures, and he had normal thyroid and gonadal function by history. He had a 15+-yr smoking history at one pack per day, drank only moderately, and did not use other recreational drugs. He was on no chronic medication.

Physical examination revealed a maculopapular rash over the trunk and upper extremities. On the possibility that this was a manifestation of systemic mastocytosis, dermatographia was elicited and further history obtained. He stated that the rash had been present for about 4 yr and was intensely pruritic at night or after a warm shower. He also complained of epigastric burning and dyspeptic symptoms that were aggravated in the supine position, but denied vomiting, abdominal cramps, or diarrhea. He denied any weight loss although he had lost approximately 2 in in height. He had experienced two episodes of unexplained (and unevaluated) syncope in the past. He denied any known drug allergies. He had used no medication for his rash.

The remainder of the physical examination included height 70.3 in, weight 91.3 kg, and blood pressure 140/90 mmHg (no postural changes). There was a normal thoracic kyphosis but a slight decrease in the lumbar lordotic curve. There was no spinal or paraspinal tenderness and reasonable preservation of range of motion of the spine. There was normal abdominal examination without hepatosplenomegaly. Cardiac, lung, and neurologic exams were normal.

He was evaluated by a dermatologist who agreed with the clinical diagnosis of urticaria pigmentosa that was confirmed on skin biopsy. Urine excretion of histamine was elevated at 577 nmol/g (reference interval, 0–321). This same 24-h urine collection contained 419 mg calcium, 85.1 pmol pyridinoline/μmol creatinine (reference value <61), and 23.8 pmol deoxypyridinoline/μmol creatinine (reference value <19). Serum bone specific alkaline phosphatase was 31 μ/mL (reference interval 3–12) and serum osteocalcin 2.6 ng/mL (reference 3–13). Serum calcium, 8.8 mg/dL; inorganic phosphate, 4.3 mg/dL; and intact PTH, 16 pg/mL were normal as were the liver enzymes. Hemoglobin 14.4 g/dL; WBC 6.800; platelets, 208,000; neutrophils 69%; lymphocytes 23%; monocytes 6%; eosinophils 1%; basophils, 1%.

Spine radiographs revealed compression fractures of T12, L1, and L2 with diffuse osteopenia. No sclerotic lesions were seen. Bone mineral density was measured by dual energy X-ray absorptiometry (DEXA). Only L3 and L4 could be evaluated in the lumbar spine because of the fractures and the value of 0.66 g/cm^2 was 4.2 standard deviations (SD) below the mean for young adult males. In the radial midshaft (a measure of predominantly cortical bone), the value of 0.81 g/cm^2 was 0.2 SD below the mean for this age group. In the femoral neck, the value of 0.7 g/cm^2 was 1.9 SD below the mean for this age group.

Upper gastrointestinal endoscopy revealed esophagitis and duodenitis without ulceration. No biopsy was performed. Therapy was begun with astemizole and omeprazole with prompt relief of skin and gastrointestinal symptoms.

The patient was unable to resume his former work because of the back pain and he was denied a disability claim because of "the preexisting condition of osteoporosis." He has relied on supplies of medication from clinic resources and has been only intermittently on therapy. Every lapse in therapy is associated with return of symptoms that are again relieved when he resumes therapy.

Discussion

Osteoporosis occurring in men or in premenopausal women should always prompt a search for potentially treatable secondary causes of accelerated bone loss. This is also the case when the severity of the disease is greater than can be accounted for by the patient's age, sex, and menopausal status. Indexes of disease severity include bone mineral density (BMD) below the reference interval adjusted for age, sex, ethnicity (Z score), or fragility fractures occurring at unusual sites. Often the cause is readily apparent, as in patients receiving chronic corticosteroid therapy, but in many cases the cause is far less obvious, requiring extensive laboratory investigation. This is the case of a 34-yr-old man referred for evaluation of osteoporosis after he had sustained three vertebral compression fractures following trivial trauma.

This case illustrates quite dramatically the importance of obtaining a complete history and performing a comprehensive examination. The story of episodic profuse itching was not elicited initially but the diagnosis became very apparent when the patient disrobed and the typical rash of urticaria pigmentosa was observed. The dermatographia, skin biopsy, and elevated urine histamine quickly confirmed the diagnosis.

Systemic mastocytosis is a very uncommon secondary cause of osteoporosis in a young man in whom the diagnosis would not have been considered in the absence of the skin rash. A simple clinical maneuver is to check for dermatographia in any patient examined for osteoporosis although this finding has limited specificity. It would appear from the literature that the absence of skin manifestations is more common than the presence. Chines et al. *(1)* reported none of the four males in their series of 10 osteoporotic patients with systemic mastocytosis had skin lesions and only two had any systemic manifestations. A recent abstract report of a specific evaluation for systemic mastocytosis in 1110 bone biopsies obtained from osteoporotic subjects revealed 12 cases previously unrecognized *(2)*. Of the six males, only one had urticaria pigmentosa. Accordingly, it is imperative to inquire about all of the possible symptoms of mast cell excess. Even in the absence of these symptoms it would seem prudent to collect a 24-h urine specimen for determination of histamine.

Therapy is directed at alleviating symptoms, preventing complications and just as importantly, reassuring patients about the usually benign nature of the disease. An important aspect of treatment is the avoidance of factors that may potentially trigger mediator release such as temperature changes, friction, physical exertion and ethanol ingestion. Pharmacologic treatment is generally directed at stabilizing mast cells or blocking mediator effects on target organs. Itching and flushing are primarily H1 receptor mediated and can be effectively alleviated by standard antihistamines such as hydroxyzine or chlorpheniramine *(3)*. Gastrointestinal manifestations of hyperchlohydria generally improve with H2 receptor blockade *(4)* using cimetidine, ranitidine, or proton pump inhibitors such as omeprazole. Salicylates have proved helpful in patients with flushing or episodic vascular collapse *(5)*. Prompt intervention with epinephrine and volume repletion is critical in the management of mastocytosis associated vascular collapse *(6)*. Orally administered cromolyn sodium is useful in the management of patients with Gl symptoms, especially those with diarrhea and abdominal pain *(7)*. Psoralens and ultraviolet A photochemotherapy provides temporary benefit in cases of urticaria pigmentosa, but, relapses after cessation of therapy are common and the associated risk of skin cancer limit its therapeutic value *(8)*. Recently, three cases of SM have been reported in whom intravenous pamidronate therapy has both increased spine BMD and reduced bone pain Similar responses have been reported in three patients treated with interferon α 2-B—associated with a significant decrease in bone marrow mast cells. A fourth patient similarly treated has been reported—with the additional observation that trabecular BMD was also increased.

REFERENCES

1. Chines A, Pacifici R. Avioli LV, Teitelbaum SL, Lorenblat PK. Systemic mastocytosis presenting as osteoporosis: a clinical and histomorphometric study. J Clin Endocrinol Metab 1991;72:1404.
2. Lazarescu AD, Hass K, Delling G. Minne HW. Systemic mastocytosis—a hidden cause of severe osteoporosis. Clinic Dr Fuerstenhof Bad Pymont, German, Dept. Osteopathol, Univ Hamburg, Germany. 1997;20(4S):1–122S.
3. Metcalfe DD. Mastocytosis syndromes. In: Middleton E, Reed CE, Ellis EF, Adkinson NF, Yunginger JW, Buse WW, eds. Allergy: Principles and Practice, 4 ed. Mosby, St. Louis, MO, 1993, pp. 1537–1551.
4. Metcalfe DD. The treatment of mastocytosis: an overview. J Invest Dermatol 1991;96(Suppl):55S–59S.
5. Roberts LJ II, Sweetman BJ, Lewis RA, Austen KF, Oates JA. Increased production of prostaglandin D2 in patients with systemic mastocytosis. N Engl J Med 1980;303:1400–1404.
6. Turk J, Oates JA, Roberts LJ II. Intervention with epinephrine in hpotension associated with mastocytosis. J Aller Clin Immunol 1983;71:189–192.
7. Horan RF, Sheffer AL, Austen KF. Cromolyn sodium in the management of systemic mastocytosis. J Aller Clin Immunol 1990;85:852–855.
8. Christophers E, Honigsman H. Wolff K, et al. PUVA-treatment of urticaria pigmentosa. Br J Dermatol 1978;98:701–702.

CASE #3: TERTIARY HYPERPARATHYROIDISM

Case Description

A 42-yr-old woman was referred to the endocrine clinic for evaluation of hyperparathyroidism. Her chief complaint had been generalized arthralgias and progressive weakness over the last 3 yr. She was unable to climb stairs without a tremendous effort and walking on level ground had also become difficult and painful to the point that she now used a cane and walked with a significant limp. Combing her hair was difficult because of weakness and pain. There never was a history of joint swelling or fractures. She had been on various analgesics over the years with only minimal improvement in her symptoms. A diagnosis of lupus had been entertained but she did not respond to symptomatic therapy. She had undergone a Roux en Y gastrojejunostomy 10 yr earlier (jejunum transected 6" distal to the ligament of Trietz with a jejunojejunostomy 18" distal to the G–J junction) for treatment of morbid obesity. Her preoperative weight was 266 lbs. She lost more than 100 lb. as a result of the surgery and was initially very satisfied with the result. She had been diagnosed as having vitamin B_{12} deficiency 2 yr before the current presentation.

She had a history of deep venous thrombosis 4 yr prior to the gastric surgery. She had undergone multiple D&Cs for dysfunctional uterine bleeding and ultimately underwent a hysterectomy with left and partial right oophorectomy 3 yr prior to this presentation. The family history included breast cancer in her mother, but there was no family history of any endocrinopathy.

On physical examination her height was 5'2" and her weight 151 lbs. There was no goiter or neck masses, no joint swelling, synovitis, or restriction of movement. She had a pronounced proximal myopathy and was unable to get of a chair without using her arms. She had bilateral groin, shin, and rib tenderness. There was no skin rash.

Laboratory data which accompanied the patient included: sedimentation rate 19 mm/h (0–18 mm/h Westergren); rheumatoid factor none detected; ANA < 1:40 (normal <1:40); hemoglobin 12.3 g/dL; hematocrit 37.5%; MCV 100.9 fl (80–100); WBC 5100, and platelets 295,000; alkaline phosphatase 1379 µU/L (25–130); ALT 9 µU/L (0–53); 24-h urine hydroxyproline 208 mg (7–49), creatinine 0.7 g (0.63–2.5), calcium 69 mg (50–250) total volume 500 mL; intact PTH 1595 pg/mL (10–65); serum calcium 11.1 mg/ dL (8.6–10.2); phosphorous 1.9 mg/dL (2.4–4.9); magnesium 1.3 mg/dL (1.6–2.5); electrolytes normal; creatinine 0.5 mg/dL (0.5–1.5); albumin 4.1 g/dL (3.5–5.2). Thyroid function tests were normal. Plasma 25 hydroxyvitamin D was low at 6 ng/mL (14–42).

A bone scan obtained before she was referred had documented increased uptake in the ribs, wrists, and SI joints bilaterally had been erroneously reported as showing Paget's disease of bone. Plane radiographs of the skull revealed typical salt and pepper changes of hyperparathyroidism and subperiosteal resorption of the phalanges was noted.

A diagnosis of vitamin D deficiency secondary to her gastric surgery and tertiary hyperparathyroidism was made and the patient was started on calcediol 20 mcg daily without supplemental calcium, whereas her serum and urine chemistries were closely monitored for hypercalciuria, hypercalcemia, and renal insufficiency. Prior to therapy the 24 h urine calcium was 119 mg. A dramatic improvement was noted by the patient in her arthralgias and myopathy within a few days of initiation of therapy. Over the next several months the dose of calcediol was frequently reduced to maintain the serum calcium below 12.0 mg/ dL (after albumin correction). After 6 mo of this therapy the patient was symptom free and her serum calcium was 10.3 mg/dL, albumin 4.1 g/dL, intact PTH 553 pg/mL, and alkaline phosphatase 294 IU/mL.

Four months later, the patient was admitted to a local hospital with acute abdominal pain felt to result from intestinal obstruction secondary to adhesions. On admission she was markedly hypercalcemic with serum calcium of 14.8 mg/dL and the phosphorous of 2.0 mg/dL. At that hospital, without further consultation, a parathyroidectomy was performed with removal of the right inferior and left superior glands in addition to the left thyroid lobe. The remaining parathyroid glands were felt to be normal at the time of surgery as was the remainder of the thyroid. The right inferior parathyroid weighed 3300 mg with hypercellular parathyroid tissue, and the left superior parathyroid weighed 33mg with hypercellular tissue. The left thyroid lobe contained a colloid nodule. Within 24 h of surgery she developed profound symptomatic hypocalcemia for which she required prolonged intravenous (iv) calcium, often receiving as much as 30 mg/kg/h to remain normocalcemic and symptom free. The intact PTH decreased to 11 pg/mL with calcium of 5.9 mg/dL, phosphorous 4.1 mg/dL, and albumin of 3.1 gm/dL, and alkaline phosphatase of 310 U/L on the ninth postoperative day. She was discharged from the hospital 4 wk postoperatively on calcium carbonate 7.0 gm/d and calcitriol 2 mg/d and the following chemistries: intact PTH 36 pg/mL, calcium 7.1 mg/dL, phosphorous 5.6 mg/dL, alkaline phosphatase 211 U/L and albumin of 4.4 g/dL.

Discussion

Tertiary hyperparathyroidism (HPT) was a term originally coined to describe the hypercalcemic HPT that persisted after successful renal transplantation. Patients with long-standing end-stage renal disease (ESRD) developed severe secondary HPT from both phosphate retention and the absence of calcitriol production by nonfunctioning kidneys. Transplantation corrected the phosphate retention and the graft kidney synthesized calcitriol but the parathyroid glands had become so hyperplastic that the serum parathyroid hormone remained elevated even after the cause of the hyperplasia had been corrected. Occasionally parathyroid hyperplasia is so pronounced in patients with secondary HPT that hypercalcemia is manifest even before the cause of the secondary HPT has been corrected. This was seen infrequently in patients with ESRD and also in patients with hypophosphatemic rickets or osteomalacia treated with adequate phosphate and inadequate vitamin D. Here we report a case of a patient with severe secondary HPT resulting from malabsorption that progressed to tertiary HPT in the absence of therapy.

This patient had been referred initially because of the "unusual combination of Paget's disease and primary hyperparathyroidism," an error perpetuated by the erroneous bone scan report. Had the bone scan been followed by plain radiographs, the diagnosis would have been more readily apparent. Of interest, when plain radiographs were obtained, the radiologic diagnosis was renal osteodystrophy because of the very dramatic changes of hyperparathyroidism. The normal serum creatinine quickly eliminated that diagnosis.

The patient did not initially report her history of previous bariatric surgery (1–5). However, when she was asked to move from the consultation office to the examination room her profound proximal myopathy was very apparent and further history was obtained prior to the physical examination. Proximal myopathy is seen in a number of endocrinopathies (6,7) but is probably most pronounced with vitamin D deficiency (8–11). Of interest, the "waddling gait" of vitamin D deficiency rickets is not seen in some other forms of rickets such as X-linked hypophosphatemic rickets where vitamin D stores are normal and there is no myopathy.

Initial treatment decisions in our patient, once the correct diagnosis was established, were quite difficult. Adequate vitamin D replacement quickly corrected the proximal myopathy and began to relieve the diffuse bone pain and tenderness but this occurred at the expense of aggravating the hypercalcemia. It was our goal to delay definitive parathyroidectomy for as long as possible to forestall a "hungry bone" syndrome in the immediate postoperative period, given the clinical extent of her bone involvement with HPT.

When parathyroidectomy was performed, the operative and pathologic findings of one very large "hyperplastic" gland, with one smaller "hyperplastic" gland and two "normal appearing" glands left intact was unexpected *(12–14)*, and strongly suggests that the large gland had undergone clonal transformation. It is unlikely that vitamin D replacement, as we had planned, would have ultimately corrected this "tertiary" HPT.

REFERENCES

1. Parfitt AM, Miller MJ, Frame B, Villanueva AR, Rao DS, Oliver I, Thomson DL. Metabolic bone disease after intestinal bypass for treatment of obesity. Ann Int Med 1978;89:193–199.
2. Taylor HC, Teitelbaum SL, Lambert PW. Symptomatic osteomalacia after jejunoileal bypass surgery in a patient with primary hyperparathyroidism. Gastroenterology 1983;85:735–742.
3. Shaker JL, Norton AJ, Woods MF, Fallon MD, Findling JW. Secondary hyperparathyroidism and osteopenia in women following gastric exclusion surgery for obesity. Osteoporosis Int 1991;1:177–181.
4. Kikuchi H, Ujiie S, Kanamaru R. Osteomalacia that became symptomatic 13 years after a total gastrectomy. Intern Med 2000;39:394–396.
5. Seshadri MS, Qurttom MA, Sivanandan R, Shihab-al-Mohannadi, S. Tertiary hyperparathyroidism in nutritional osteomalacia. Postgrad Med J 1994;70:595–596.
6. Schneider C, Grimm T, Kress W, Sommer C, Muller CR. Hyperparathyroidism in a patient with proximal myotonic myopathy. (PROMM). Neuromusc Disord 2000;10:481–483.
7. Sansone V, Griggs RC, Moxley RT III. Hypothyroidism unmasking proximal myotonic myopathy. Neuromusc Disord 2000;10:165–172.
8. Russell JA. Osteomalacic myopathy. Muscle Nerve 1994;17:578–580. Comment in: Muscle Nerve 1995;18:360–361.
9. Ziambaras K, Dagogo-Jack S. Reversible muscle weakness in patients with vitamin D deficiency. West J Med 1997;167;435–439.
10. Reginato AJ, Falasca GF, Pappu R, McKnight B, Agha A. Musculoskeletal manifestations of osteomalacia: report of 26 cases and literature review. Semin Arth Rheum 1999;28:287–304.
11. Prabhala A, Garg R, Dandona P. Severe myopathy associated with vitamin D deficiency in Western New York. Arch Intern Med 2000;160:1199–1203.
12. Krause MW, Hedinger CE. Pathologic study of pararthyroid glands in tertiary hyperparathyroidism. Hum Pathol 1985;16:772–784.
13. Kilgo MS, Pirsch JD, Warner TF, Starling JR. Tertiary hyperparathyroidism after renal transplantation: surgical strategy. Surgery 1998;124:677–683; discussion 683–684.
14. Pasieka JL, Parsons LL. A prospective surgical outcome study assessing the impact of parathyroidectomy on symptoms in patients with secondary and tertiary hyperparathyroidism. Surgery 2000;128:531–539.

CASE #4: HETEROTOPIC OSSIFICATION

Case Description

The patient is a 55-yr-old man who has been partially paraplegic since the age of 17, secondary to a fall-related T12 vertebral fracture. He was doing reasonably well until late 1998, when he began experiencing progressive weakness and decreased sensation in the right upper extremity. The neurological evaluation confirmed a diagnosis of cervicothoracic syringomyelia, and in early 1999 he underwent cervical subarachnoid shunt, which left him with moderate weakness and decreased sensation. His neurologic condition was stable postoperatively; however, a few months later, he started complaining of right shoulder pain and stiffness with decreased range of motion. On further questioning, he said that his pain was aggravated by motion and partially relieved with ibuprofen. He has noted some swelling of the proximal part of the right upper extremity. He denied any trauma or recent fall, no fever or chills, no headache or neck pains, and had no other new complaints.

He is a single, unemployed, wheel-chair dependent person, living on his own. He has no sexual partner, and no tobacco, alcohol, or drug use. Medications were verapamil for long-standing well-controlled hypertension, and ibuprofen. He had no known drug allergy. The family history included type 2 diabetes and hypertension.

On physical examination, he was a pleasant, healthy appearing man driving the wheel-chair mainly by using his left arm. Blood pressure 128/80 mmHg; pulse 80 bpm, body mass index (BMI) 32, temperature 97°F. There was no thyromegaly or neck adenopathy. Heart, lung, and abdominal examinations were normal. Peripheral pulses were normal. There was no clubbing or cyanosis, and there was scant pitting edema in lower extremities and right upper extremity. Musculoskeletal examination revealed limited range of motion in the right shoulder (flexion to 90°, extension to 30°, and abduction to 60°) with moderate tenderness. There was a slight increase in temperature of the skin over the right shoulder and deltoid region. Neurologic examination revealed that the cranial nerves were intact. There was decreased sensation of all modalities below T10 level along with power (3–4/5) in the lower extremities. There was normal sensation and power in left arm, but decreased sensation and power (2/5) in the right arm.

A complete blood count with differential was normal, as was the biochemical profile. Right shoulder radiographs showed marked destruction of the right numeral head (consistent with either a septic process or a Charcot's joint). Irregular heterotopic ossification (HO) was noticed around the proximal humeral shaft (see Fig. 4). The patient underwent Tc-99 MDP bone scan that revealed an intense tracer uptake in the region where the HO was described radiographically (see Fig. 5). To rule out any possibility of an infectious process, a CT-guided arthrocentesis was performed. A few milliliters of bloody fluid was obtained and this was negative for infection. The CT scan confirmed the HO findings. The total alkaline phosphatase was within normal limits. In order to complete the workup, bone-specific alkaline phosphatase was ordered and was 20.4 U/mL (reference interval 4.3–19.0 U/mL).

Discussion

This case illustrates the clinical setting of HO and the difficulty in establishing the correct diagnosis from plain radiographs early in the course of the disease. The case also highlights the limited value of routine laboratory studies or even more esoteric tests of skeletal metabolism. Finally the limitations of medical therapy for HO must be emphasized.

HO cannot be distinguished histologically from callus in the healing bone. However, HO osteoblast cells exhibit elevated levels of activities traditionally ascribed to osteoblasts, such as collagen synthesis and alkaline phosphatase activity *(1)*. Most series report an incidence of 20 to 30% in spinal cord injury patients and the incidence is greater in patients after total hip arthroplasty. Severe functional limitations develop in 8 to 10% of all patients who develop HO. There is a good correlation between the severity of the initial injury and the size and the incidence of HO *(2)* The most commonly involved joints are hip and knee in the lower extremities, and shoulder and elbow in the upper extremities. Other medical conditions should be considered such as venous thrombosis, septic arthritis, and cellulitis. In paraplegic patients, HO can be an incidental finding during a routine radiological study.

The laboratory evaluation includes elevated alkaline phosphatase; particularly bone-specific alkaline phosphatase in most cases, and this can be used as a marker of the activity of the disease. Osteocalcin is not a valuable adjunct in confirming or assessing

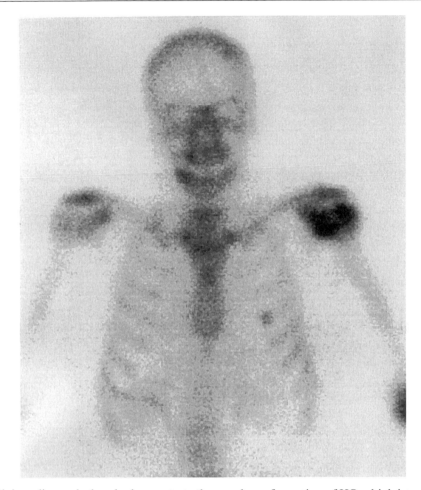

Fig. 4. Plain radiographs barely demonstrate the new bone formation of HO which is much more clearly seen in a CT image.

the maturity of HO *(3)*. C-reactive protein and the sedimentation rate are also usually elevated. Whereas plain X-rays can detect late HO, it is important to note that one should not wait to initiate therapy until the X-ray is positive. Therapy should be started once symptoms occur and the bone scan is positive. Triple-phase bone scan using Tc-99 MDP is very helpful in making the diagnosis as well as monitoring the activity or maturity *(4)* of the disease and in planning for surgical resection. Having inactive disease (HO on plain X-ray, negative bone scan) is essential in reducing the risk of recurrence postsurgically. Ultrasound *(5)*, CT scan, and MRI can be helpful as well.

Perioperative irradiation or NSAIDs have been used as prophylactic measures in high-risk patients. In one retrospective study HO, incidence was reduced in patients receiving indomethacin preoperatively for 5 to 11 d *(6)*. In a direct comparison study, radiation prophylaxis was slightly more successful than NSAIDs *(7)*, however both of them were effective in reducing the incidence of HO. Both modalities have been used together in other studies. Fractionated irradiation was preferred to a dose-equivalent single-dose radiation in a rat study *(8)*. Once HO has developed, the earlier treatment is started the

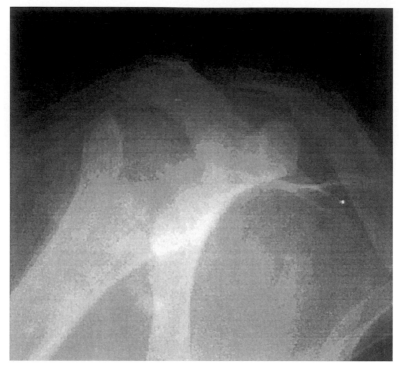

Fig. 5. The bone scan in this patient with heterotopic ossification (**Case 4**) is similar to the appearance of the shoulder in the patient with Paget's disease of bone.

better the results. Etidronate has been used with good results, especially in patients with symptoms and a positive bone scan but with negative X-rays *(9)*. Other modalities include NSAIDS, surgical resection, and irradiation *(10)*. Osteonecrosis of the femoral head has been reported after combined treatment with surgery, irradiation, and NSAIDs in the hip joint *(11)*. It is advisable to not prescribe forcible mobilization until the acute inflammatory phase has subsided. In one study, it was concluded that passive stretching of the periarticular structures during the acute phase of HO is detrimental to the final outcome *(12)*.

REFERENCES

1. Kaysinger KK, Ramp WK, Gruber HE. Comparison of human osteoblasts and osteogenic cells from heteropic bones. Clin Orthop 1997:342:181–191.
2. Tally AB. Heterotopic Ossification in non-traumatic myelopathies. Spinal Cord 1999;37:47–49.
3. Mysiw WJ, Tan J, Jackson RD. Heterotopic ossification. The utility of osteocalcin in diagnosis and management.
4. Freed JH, Hahn H, Menter R, Dillon T. The use of three-phase bone scan in the early diagnosis of HO and in the evaluation of Didronel therapy. Paraplegia 1982;20:208–216.
5. Thomas EA, Cassar-Pullicino VN, McCall IW. The role of ultrasound in the early diagnosis and management of heterotopic bone formation. Clinical Radiology 1991;43:190–196.
6. Vastel L, Kerboull L, Dejean O, Courpied JP, Kerboul M. Prevention of HO in hip arthroplasty. Int Orthop 1999;23:107–110.
7. Kolbl O. Preoperative irradiation versus the use of NSAIDS for prevention of HO following total hip replacement. Int J Radiat Oncol Biol Phys 1998 42:397–401.

8. Esenwein SA. Effects of single-dose versus fractionated irradiation on the suppression of heterotopic bone formation-an animal model-based follow-up study in rats. Arch Orthop Trauma Surg 2000;120: 575–581.
9. Banovac K, Gonzalez F. Evaluation and management of HO in patients with spinal cord injury. Spinal Cord 1997;35:158–162.
10. Sautter-Bihl ML, Liebermeister E, Nanassy A. Radiotherapy as a local option for HO in patients with spinal cord injury. Spinal Cord 2000;38:33–37.
11. Van Kuijk AA. Osteonecrosis after treatment for HO in spinal cord injury with the combination of surgery, irradiation, and NSAIDS. Spinal Cord 2000;38:319–324.
12. Crawford CM, Varghese G, Mani MM, Neff JR. HO. are range of motion exercise contraindicated. J Burn Care Rehabil 1986;7:323–327.

13

Male Reproductive Endocrinology

Shalender Bhasin, MD, Atam B. Singh, MD, and Robert Christiansen, MD

Contents

CASE #1: 23-YR-OLD MAN WITH ADRENAL INSUFFICIENCY AND HYPOGONADOTROPIC HYPOGONADISM

Case Description

This 23-yr-old man was referred to our Endocrinology Clinic for the management of adrenal insufficiency. The patient was born of a full-term uncomplicated delivery, and grew up normally in early childhood. At 6 yr of age, he became ill, stopped growing, and developed increased pigmentation of the skin. He was evaluated at a local hospital in Mexico and diagnosed as having adrenal insufficiency. After initiation of glucocorticoid replacement therapy with 5 mg prednisone daily, his condition improved and growth resumed, but the increased skin pigmentation persisted.

At age 17, he was evaluated at a Los Angeles Hospital for failure to develop secondary sex characteristics, and started on testosterone injections, which he takes infrequently. At the time of his clinic visit at age 23, he had not been sexually active, reported very little sexual desire, and did not shave or masturbate.

He had had mild bronchial asthma for 3 yr; his asthma was controlled with intermittent use of a metered-dose inhaler. His medications included prednisone 5 mg twice daily, 9-α fludrocortisone 0.2 mg daily, albuterol inhaler as required for bronchial asthma, sustained release theophylline 300 mg daily, and testosterone enanthate 200 mg intramuscularly every 2 wk. At the time of his clinic visit, he had not received his testosterone injections for several months.

From: *Contemporary Endocrinology: Challenging Cases in Endocrinology*
Edited by: M. E. Molitch © Humana Press Inc., Totowa, NJ

FAMILY TREE

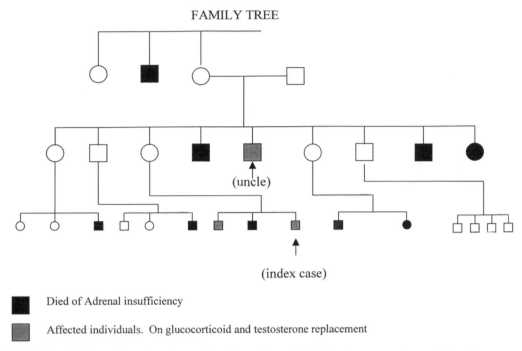

Fig. 1. Family Tree. Note that almost all of the affected individuals were males, and that they were sons of clinically unaffected mothers, who were presumably carriers.

One maternal uncle had a similar medical condition, and was being treated in our clinic with prednisone and testosterone injections (Fig. 1). His uncle's testosterone level was 145 ng/dL in 1985, and 40 ng/dL at a recent clinic visit in 1999, and his testicular volume had decreased from 12 mL to about 4 mL over the same period. One brother and a first cousin (son of maternal aunt) have similar problems. The other affected members of the family (Fig. 1) were being followed at different hospitals in Mexico and Los Angeles, CA. The patient's mother reported that two of her brothers, one sister, one maternal uncle, and a niece had died during early childhood. The exact cause of their death was not ascertained.

The patient was 161 cm tall, and weighed 167 pounds (76 kg). His blood pressure was 112 / 70 mmHg, with no orthostatic changes, and pulse rate was 90 beats per minute. He had dark brown pigmentation on the skin, which was especially increased around the elbows, knees, and knuckles. He also had patchy pigmentation on the tongue and buccal mucosa inside the lips. He had sparse, fine hair in the sideburn area, but no axillary hair. He had a female pattern escutcheon with sparse pubic hairs shaped in the form of an inverted triangle. He had bilateral breast enlargement (see Fig. 2). His penis was 6 cm in length, with a terminally located meatus. Both testicles were 5 mL in volume, and firm in consistency. His sense of smell was normal. The rest of his physical examination revealed no abnormalities.

His hemoglobin was 12.9 g/L with mean corpuscular volume of 84 u^3. His serum total testosterone concentration was 73 ng/dL, luteinizing hormone (LH) 1.7 IU/L, and follicle-stimulating hormone (FSH) 1.3 IU/L. His total serum thyroxine concentration was

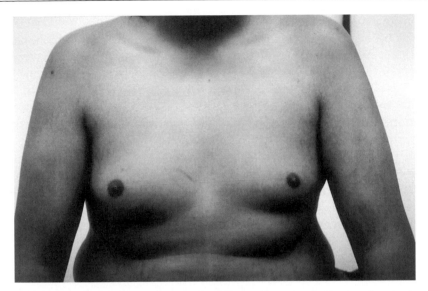

Fig. 2. A photograph of the patient demonstrating bilateral breast enlargement, hyperpigmentation of the skin, and lack of chest and abdominal hair.

8.3 µg/dL, free thyroxine index 9.2 µg/dL, and thyroid-stimulating hormone (TSH) 4.8 U/L. During an adrenocorticotropic hormone (ACTH) stimulation test, his plasma cortisol concentration was 1.2 µg/dL at baseline, and 1.3 µg/dL 60 min after the intravenous (iv) injection of 250-µg cosyntropin. His plasma ACTH concentration at baseline was 3355 pg/mL.

A magnetic resonance imaging (MRI) scan of the hypothalamic-pituitary region did not reveal any space-occupying lesion. A dual energy X-ray absorptiometry (DEXA) scan of the body reported vertebral bone density to be –2 standard deviations below the mean for healthy young men (T score = –2).

Discussion

This 23-yr-old man has adrenal insufficiency, as indicated by the low baseline cortisol, and failure of serum cortisol levels to increase appropriately in response to ACTH stimulation. The presence of hyperpigmentation and markedly increased ACTH concentrations are consistent with the diagnosis of primary adrenal insufficiency. He has been on replacement therapy with prednisone, although the 10-mg daily dose of prednisone being used by this patient is higher than the typical replacement dose used in the treatment of adrenal insufficiency. There is increasing recognition that cortisol production rates in healthy men and women are lower than previously estimated *(1)* and that the 30-mg dose of hydrocortisone typically used for replacement is supraphysiological *(1,2)*. There is concern that these supraphysiological doses of glucocorticoids might be associated with decreased bone mineral density and predispose these patients to an increased risk of bone fractures *(2–4)*.

It is apparent that this patient has marked delay in his pubertal development. Even at 23-yr of age, he has very sparse facial and axillary hair and a female escutcheon, consistent with androgen deficiency. A very low serum testosterone level confirmed the presence of androgen deficiency. Low LH and FSH levels in the presence of low testosterone levels indicate that he has hypogonadotropic hypogonadism and that the pathophysiologic defect resides at the hypothalamic-pituitary site. Further workup with MRI scan and measurement of a prolactin level did not reveal any space-occupying lesion of the hypothalamic-pituitary site. The process of exclusion leaves us with the diagnosis of idiopathic hypogonadotropic hypogonadism. His sense of smell was intact, and he did not have any of the dysmorphic features of other hypothalamic syndromes associated with hypogonatropic hypogonadism, such as Prader Willi syndrome.

How can we explain the cooccurrence of primary adrenal insufficiency with hypogonadotropic hypogonadism in this individual? Patients with multiple autoimmune endocrinopathies can have deficiencies of multiple endocrine end organs. Based on the constellation of endocrinopathies, these patients can be classified into one of two main categories. Polyglandular autoimmune endocrinopathy syndrome, type 1, is characterized by mucocutaneous candidiasis, autoimmune hypoparathyroidism and adrenal insufficiency, and ectodermal dystrophy *(5)*. There is increasing evidence linking this syndrome to mutations in the APECED (autoimmune polyendocrinopathy-candidiasis-ectodermal-dystrophy) or AIRE (autoimmune regulator) gene *(5)*. This candidate gene codes for a putative transcription factor that has two zinc-finger motifs. Typically, onset of type 1 autoimmune polyglandular failure syndrome occurs in childhood and failures of multiple endocrine organs evolve throughout the lifetime. Type 2 autoimmune polyglandular failure syndrome is characterized by adult-onset adrenal failure associated with type 1 diabetes mellitus and autoimmune thyroid disease. Type 2 polyglandular endocrinopathy is believed to be polygenic, and is characterized by dominant inheritance and association with HLA DR3 *(5)*. Patients with both type 1 and 2 multiple autoimmune endocrinopathy syndromes can present with adrenal insufficiency in association with Leydig cell failure *(5)*. However, androgen deficiency in these patients is a result of primary testicular dysfunction, and therefore associated with increased LH and FSH concentrations. Hypogonadotropic hypogonadism in conjunction with primary adrenal insufficiency has not been reported in multiple autoimmune endocrinopathy.

A number of homeodomain transcription factors are involved in the development and differentiation of the different hormone-producing cells within the pituitary gland *(6–15)*. Abnormalities of multiple endocrine systems caused by deficiencies of pituitary tropic hormones are well known in patients with mutations of homeo-domain-containing transcription factors, such as *Pit-1, Prop-1, Lhx 3*, and *Gsx-1* (see Table 1). Thus, patients with *Prop-1* mutations have deficiencies of multiple anterior pituitary hormones, including LH and FSH, GH, prolactin, and TSH. ACTH secretion is normal at birth, but corticotropes may degenerate secondarily. Mutations in the *Pit-1* homeodomain transcription factor have been associated with deficiencies of GH, prolactin and TSH *(6–8)*, but not ACTH. Mutations of *Pit-1, Gsx-1*, and *Lhx3* are typically not associated with ACTH deficiency, whereas those of *Ptx2a* and *Ptx2b*, and *Hesx1* present with specific craniofacial, dental, and eye anomalies or septooptic dysplasia, which this patient did not have. Also, the elevated ACTH concentrations and normal TSH in this patient are incompatible with *Prop-1* mutation. In fact, his clinical phenotype is inconsistent with mutations of any of the known pituitary homeodomain transcription factors.

To date, mutations in at least four genes have been implicated in the pathophysiology of idiopathic hypogonadotropic hypogonadism in the human: *KALIG-1* (the gene for X-linked Kallmann syndrome), *DAX1* (the gene for X-linked adrenal hypoplasia congenita),

Table 1
Mutations of Homeodomain Transcription Factors
are Associated with Heritable Disorders of Pituitary Development

Gene Mutation	PIT1	PROP1	HESX1
GH	Absent	Low	Low
PRL	Absent	Low	?
TSH	Low	Low	?
LH, FSH	Normal	Absent	?
ACTH	Normal	Low in 1/3	?
ADH	Normal	Normal	Normal/Low
Pituitary Size	Small/Medium	S/M/L/XL/XXL	Small
Complex Phenotype	No	No	Septooptic dysplasia

Reproduced with permission from ref. *(10)*.

GnRH receptor, and the gene for prohormone convertase 1 that causes a syndrome of hypogonadotropic hypogonadism and defects in prohormone processing (see *(16)* for review). Of these, mutations of *DAX-1* are known to be associated with primary adrenal insufficiency and hypogonadotropic hypogonadism, and best explain the phenotype of this patient *(17–23)*.

X-linked congenital adrenal hypoplasia presents classically with adrenal insufficiency within the first 6 mo of life, as the fetal adrenal cortex progressively involutes *(17–19)*. However, some patients may have delayed presentation of adrenal insufficiency in late childhood, as was the case in our patient, or even in adulthood *(20)*. Hypogonadotropic hypogonadism in these patients is usually recognized when these children fail to experience normal progression of pubertal development *(20)*.

A quick look at this patient's family tree (see Fig. 1) reveals that almost all of the affected individuals were males, and that they were sons of clinically unaffected, mothers who were presumably carriers. This is typical of X-linked mode of inheritance. The *DAX-1* gene has been mapped to the human X-chromosome, and the pattern of inheritance displayed by this patient's family is consistent with mutations of this X-linked gene.

The DAX-1 protein, a member of the nuclear hormone receptor family, inhibits transcriptional activators by direct protein–protein interactions and indirectly by binding DNA hairpin structures *(21–23)*. *DAX-1*, steroidogenic factor (*SF-1*), and *Sry* are involved in determination of sexual differentiation. At least in the mouse, the products of the *DAX-1* and *Sry* genes appear to act antagonistically; increased expression of *DAX-1* leads to female development and increased activity of *Sry* to male development *(21)*. The mouse and human proteins appear to behave differently. Absence of *DAX-1* in humans is associated with adrenal insufficiency and hypogonadotropic hypogonadism; however, *DAX-1*-deficient, XY mice have normal levels of corticotropins and adrenal hormones, but are sterile *(21)*.

Although patients with *DAX-1* mutations (see Fig. 3) have hypogonadotropic hypogonadism, some affected men also have impaired testicular responses to LH *(17–19)*. These observations suggest that androgen deficiency in men with *DAX-1* mutations is because

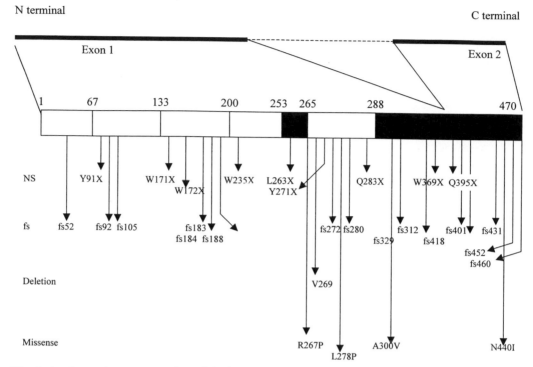

Fig. 3. A schematic representation of the human *DAX-1* gene showing the relative positions of the introns and exons, and several reported mutations. Human *DAX1* gene consists of 2 exons that code for a 470 amino acid protein. Exon 1 is 1168 bp in length and encodes the DNA binding domain and 63% of the ligand-binding domain. Exon 2 is 245 bp in size and encodes the 80 aminoacids of the C-terminal portion of the ligand-binding domain. The locations of some of the reported mutations are shown. The amino acids are shown by single letter code: Alanine (A); Isoleucine (I); Leucine (L); Asparagine (N); Proline (P); Glutamine (Q); Arginine (R); Valine (V); Tryptophan (W); Tyrosine (Y), and stop codon X. Adapted with permission from *(20–23)*.

of a combined hypothalamic-pituitary-gonadal defect and that the *DAX-1* gene product may play a critical role in regulating both pituitary and testicular function.

SF-1, another member of the nuclear receptor family, was initially cloned as a transcriptional regulator of several steroidogenic enzyme genes in the adrenal and the gonad. However, gene-targeting experiments in mice have revealed that *SF-1* is an essential factor in adrenal and gonadal development. SF-1 protein is also required for the proper functioning of the hypothalamic-pituitary-gonadal axis and the formation of the ventromedial nucleus of the hypothalamus. Although mutations of the *SF-1* gene could theoretically result in adrenal insufficiency and hypogonadism, such mutations have not yet been discovered in humans.

In summary, the co-occurrence of primary adrenal insufficiency and hypogonadotropic hypogonadism in this patient in conjunction with a family tree that is consistent with an X-linked mode of inheritance, support the diagnosis of *DAX-1* mutation. Final confirmation of the diagnosis would require the testing of the patient's genomic DNA for *DAX-1* mutation.

REFERENCES

1. Brandon DD, Isabelle LM, Samuels MH, Kendall JW, Loriaux DL. Cortisol production rate measurement by stable isotope dilution using gas chromatography-negative ion chemical ionization mass spectrometry. Steroids 1999;64:372–378.
2. Jeffcoate W. Assessment of corticosteroid replacement therapy in adults with adrenal insufficiency. Ann Clin Biochem 1999;36:151–157.
3. Peacey SR, Guo CY, Robinson AM, Price A, Giles MA, Eastell R, Weetman AP. Glucocorticoid replacement therapy: are patients over treated and does it matter? Clin Endocrinol (Oxf) 1997;46:255–261.
4. Valero MA, Leon M, Ruiz Valdepenas MP, Larrodera L, Lopez MB, Papapietro K, Jara A, Hawkins F. Bone density and turnover in Addison's disease: effect of glucocorticoid treatment. Bone Miner 1994; 26:9–17.
5. Obermayer-Straub P, Manns MP. Autoimmune polyglandular syndromes. Baillieres Clin Gastroenterol 1998;12:293–315.
6. Pfaffle RW, Blankenstein O, Wuller S, Kentrup H. Combined pituitary hormone deficiency: role of Pit-1 and Prop-1. Acta Paediatr Suppl 1999;88:33–41.
7. Castrillo JL, Theill LE, Karin M. Function of the homeodomain protein GHF1 in pituitary cell proliferation. Science 1991;253:197–199.
8. Dattani MT, Martinez-Barbera JP, Thomas PQ, Brickman JM, Gupta R, Martensson IL, et al. Mutations in the homeobox gene HESX1/Hesx1 associated with septo-optic dysplasia in human and mouse. Nat Genet 1998;19:125–133.
9. Parks JS, Brown MR. Transcription factors regulating pituitary development. Growth Horm IGF Res 1999;9(Suppl B):2–8.
10. Parks JS, Brown MR, Hurley DL, Phelps CJ, Wajnrajch MP. Heritable disorders of pituitary development. J Clin Endocrinol Metab 1999;84:4362–4370.
11. Pfaffle RW, DiMattia GE, Parks JS, Brown MR, Wit JM, Jansen M, et al. Mutation of the POU-specific domain of Pit-1 and hypopituitarism without pituitary hypoplasia. Science 1992;257:1118–1121.
12. Radovick S, Nations M, Du Y, Berg LA, Weintraub BD, Wondisford FE. A mutation in the POU-homeo-domain of Pit-1 responsible for combined pituitary hormone deficiency. Science 1992;257:1115–1118.
13. Semina EV, Reiter R, Leysens NJ, Alward WL, Small KW, Datson NA, et al. Cloning and characterization of a novel bicoid-related homeobox transcription factor gene, RIEG, involved in Rieger syndrome. Nat Genet 1996;14:392–399.
14. Wu W, Cogan JD, Pfaffle RW, Dasen JS, Frisch H, O'Connell SM, et al. Mutations in PROP1 cause familial combined pituitary hormone deficiency. Nat Genet 1998;18:147–149.
15. Sadeghi-Nejad A, Senior B. Autosomal dominant transmission of isolated growth hormone deficiency in iris-dental dysplasia (Rieger's syndrome). J Pediatr 1974;85:644–648.
16. Seminara SB, Hayes FJ, Crowley WF Jr. Gonadotropin-releasing hormone deficiency in the human (idiopathic hypogonadotropic hypogonadism and Kallmann's syndrome): pathophysiological and genetic considerations. Endocr Rev 1998;19:521–539.
17. Reutens AT, Achermann JC, Ito M, Ito M, Gu WX, Habiby RL, et al. Clinical and functional effects of mutations in the DAX-1 gene in patients with adrenal hypoplasia congenita. J Clin Endocrinol Metab 1999;84:504–511.
18. Kaiserman KB, Nakamoto JM, Geffner ME, McCabe ER. Minipuberty of infancy and adolescent pubertal function in adrenal hypoplasia congenita. J Pediatr 1998;133:300–302.
19. Binder G, Wollmann H, Schwarze CP, Strom TM, Peter M, Ranke MB. X-linked congenital adrenal hypoplasia: new mutations and long-term follow-up in three patients. Clin Endocrinol (Oxf) 2000;53: 249–255.
20. Tabarin A, Achermann JC, Recan D, Bex V, Bertagna X, Christin-Maitre S, et al. A novel mutation in DAX1 causes delayed-onset adrenal insufficiency and incomplete hypogonadotropic hypogonadism. J Clin Invest 2000;105:321–328.
21. Goodfellow PN, Camerino G. DAX-1, an 'antitestis' gene. Cell Mol Life Sci 1999;55:857–863.
22. Burris TP, Guo W, McCabe ER. The gene responsible for adrenal hypoplasia congenita, DAX-1, encodes a nuclear hormone receptor that defines a new class within the superfamily. Recent Prog Horm Res 1996;51:241-259; discussion 259–260.
23. Zanaria E, Muscatelli F, Bardoni B, Strom TM, Guioli S, Guo W, Lalli E, Moser C, Walker AP, McCabe ER, et al. An unusual member of the nuclear hormone receptor superfamily responsible for X-linked adrenal hypoplasia congenita. Nature 1994;372:635–641.

CASE #2: TOPICAL STEROID USE
ASSOCIATED WITH SECONDARY ADRENAL
INSUFFICIENCY, ANDROGEN DEFICIENCY, AND OSTEOPOROSIS

Case Description

This 38-yr-old man presented to the emergency room (ER) with nausea, vomiting, and fever of 2 d duration. He had suffered from psoriasis since age 7. The initial diagnosis of psoriasis was made in Mexico, where he was prescribed topical betamethasone cream. Extensive areas of the skin (approximately 80%) were involved with psoriasis, and only the face and the neck were spared. For 17 yr, he has lived in the USA and used the betamethasone topical preparation on a daily basis.

On examination in the ER, he was noted to have ecchymoses, thin fragile skin over all extremities, psoriatic skin lesions on the trunk, arm, and legs, telangiectasia, and a Cushingoid appearance (see Fig. 4). His heart rate was 120/min, and blood pressure 90/60 mmHg.

His random cortisol was 0.6 µg/dL (normal 2–25 µg/dL). A diagnosis of adrenal insufficiency was made, and oral prednisone was started at a dose of 5 mg in the morning and 2.5 mg in the evening. The patient was referred to Dermatology Clinic for management of psoriasis where betamethasone was replaced with triamcinolone acetonide 0.1% cream and cyclosporine 75 mg daily orally was commenced. Prednisone was gradually tapered off over a 12-mo period.

A short ACTH stimulation test (Cosyntropin-250 µg) was performed 1 mo after discontinuation of prednisone (cortisol levels 0'–4.5 µg/dL, 30'–8.7 µg/dL, 60'–12.0 µg/dL). The results were consistent with partial adrenal insufficiency.

A DEXA scan to assess bone mineral density showed severe osteoporosis with a bone mineral density (BMD) at the spine (L1–L5) of 0.774 gm/cm^2, T score (in relation to peak BMD) of −2.89 and Z score (age matched normal) = −2.83 and BMD at the hip of 0.713 gm/cm^2, T score of −2.59 and Z score of −2.30. His total testosterone was 363 ng/dL (normal range 300–1200 ng/dL) and free testosterone 30 pg/mL (normal 50–240 pg/mL).

The patient was started on alendronate, 10 mg daily, calcium carbonate 500-mg thrice daily, and testosterone enanthate 200 mg intramuscularly every 2 wk. The patient was advised not to take prednisone on a regular basis, but was instructed to commence hydrocortisone treatment in case of illness of any form. A relative was taught how to inject hydrocortisone injection in the event of vomiting or loss of consciousness. When seen in the clinic 1 mo later, the patient complained of aches and pains in the bones. An ACTH stimulation test was repeated at this time and again showed inadequate adrenal response (0'–1.5 µg/dL, 30'–6.7 µg/dL, 60'–8.2 µg/dL). He was started on hydrocortisone. His psoriasis improved with topical emollient and cyclosporine.

Discussion

Systemic corticosteroid use over prolonged periods of time is associated with a number of side effects. Although osteoporosis and suppression of the hypothalamo-pituitary-adrenal (HPA) axis are widely recognized as common complications of prolonged oral steroid therapy, these complications are rare with topical steroid use (1–8). This case illustrates that topical corticosteroids, such as betamethasone, that are effective in the treatment of corticosteroid-responsive dermatoses primarily because of their antiinflammatory and antipruritic actions, can cause androgen deficiency, osteoporosis, and long-term suppression of the HPA axis in men.

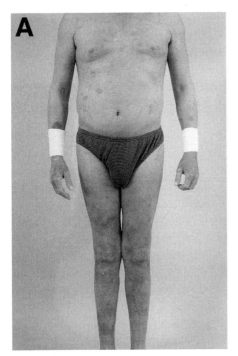
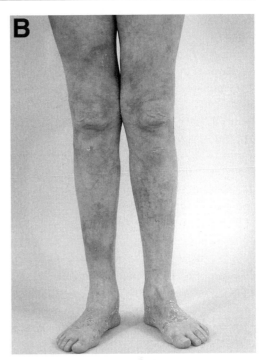

Fig. 4. (A) and **(B)** Photographs of the patient's trunk and lower extremities demonstrating ecchymoses, psoriatic skin lesions, thinning of the skin resulting in prominence of veins, telangiectasia, and wasting of muscles around the shoulder girdle.

This patient had used betamethasone topical cream on a large area of his skin for many years; he developed not only suppression of his HPA axis, but also osteoporosis and androgen deficiency. He presented to the ER with manifestations of adrenal insufficiency, and ACTH stimulation testing confirmed the presence of partial adrenal insufficiency, presumably resulting from the suppression of his HPA axis by the topical betamethasone. The extent of systemic absorption of topically applied steroids is determined by a number of factors, including the vehicle, integrity of the epidermal barrier, and the use of occlusive dressings. Topical steroids are absorbed into the systemic circulation only to a small extent through the normal skin, but the presence of inflammation can significantly increase percutaneous absorption. Once absorbed through the skin, topical steroids enter pharmacokinetic pathways similar to systemically administered corticosteroids. Conditions that augment systemic absorption include application of more potent corticosteroids, application over a large surface area, occlusive dressings, and prolonged use *(1–7)*.

Systemic effects of topical corticoids include suppression of the HPA axis, manifestations of Cushing's syndrome, hyperglycemia, and increased susceptibility to infections *(2–7)*. Chronic glucocorticoid therapy also lowers serum testosterone levels by its effects at all levels of the hypothalamic-pituitary-gonadal asix *(10,11)*. Glucocorticoids suppress GnRH secretion from the hypothalamus, attenuate the LH response to GnRH, and also directly suppress Leydig cell steroidogenesis. Several reports have shown that patients with Cushing's syndrome often have low testosterone levels *(10,11)*.

HPA suppression with exogenous oral corticosteroids and Cushing's features are well described but such features are rare with the use of topical, inhaled, and nasal steroids

(6–8). Acute adrenal crisis has been reported after inadvertent cessation of high doses of potent, topically applied steroids *(9)*. Although the risk of the suppression of hypothalamic-pituitary axis cannot be entirely eliminated, the regimens that employ intermittent administration of topical steroids are believed to cause lesser degree of adrenal suppression *(9)*.

Osteoporosis is a frequent complication of oral steroid administration, but has not been commonly described in association with topical or inhaled steroid therapy *(12)*. Glucocorticoid therapy is an important cause of osteoporosis, and substantially increases the risk of bone fractures *(12)*. After institution of glucocorticoid therapy, patients may lose as much as 10–40% of their bone mass within months *(12)*. About 30% of patients receiving long-term glucocorticoid therapy will develop bone fractures *(12)*; the fracture risk depends on the patient's age, initial bone density, the dose and duration of steroid use, and past history of fracture.

Our patient had significant degree of osteoporosis as indicated by markedly decreased bone mineral density in both the lumbar spine and the femoral neck. There are several possible factors that could have contributed to the pathophysiology of osteoporosis in this patient. In addition to the well-known deleterious effects of glucocorticoid therapy on bone mineral density, he also had partial androgen deficiency, as indicated by low free testosterone levels. In addition, he was receiving cyclosporine, which can cause high turnover bone loss, with bone resorption exceeding bone formation. Thus, all three factors—corticosteroids, low testosterone levels, and cyclosporine—working in concert, could have contributed to osteoporosis in our patient.

Glucocorticoids cause osteoporosis by affecting calcium and bone mineral metabolism at many levels *(12–16)*. These drugs inhibit gastrointestinal calcium absorption, and reduce calcium reabsorption in the renal tubule. Glucocorticoids also stimulate bone resorption and decrease bone formation *(12–16)*. Although glucocorticoids stimulate osteoblastic differentiation, they have important inhibitory actions on bone formation. Glucocorticoids affect the expression of many osteoblast genes, including the downregulation of type I collagen and osteocalcin, and upregulation of interstitial collagenase *(12)*. The synthesis and activity of osteoblast growth factors can be modulated by glucocorticoids as well. For example, the expression of insulin-like growth factor 1 (IGF-1), an important stimulator of osteoblast function, is decreased by glucocorticoids. The synthesis of IGF binding proteins (IGFBPs) is also regulated by glucocorticoids within bone cells. Glucocorticoids increase the apoptotic rates of osteoblasts and osteocytes *(16)*. The net result is a decrease in number of bone cells and that translates into lower rates of bone formation and decreased trabecular width. Recent studies have shown that osteoprotegrin ligand and soluble neutralizing receptor, osteoprotegerin, play an important role in osteoclastogenesis. Hofbauer et al. *(14)* have reported that dexamethsone stimulates osteoprotegerin ligand and inhibits osteoprotegerin production in human osteoblastic cells in culture. These findings provide a potential paracrine mechanism by which glucocorticoids induce osteoporosis *(12–16)*.

The risk of glucocorticoid-induced osteoporosis can be reduced by administration of bisphophonates, testosterone, or vitamin D metabolites *(17–19)*. In a 48-wk, randomized, placebo-controlled study of men and women who were receiving glucocorticoid therapy *(17,18)*, alendronate therapy was associated with a greater increase in bone mineral density than that associated with placebo-treatment alone. There were fewer new vertebral fractures in the alendronate group than in the placebo group. Several studies *(17,18)* are in agreement that alendronate is an effective and safe treatment for the prevention and treatment of glucocorticoid-induced osteoporosis. All patients receiving long-term gluco-corticoid therapy should receive calcium and vitamin supplementation. The efficacy of calcitriol, calcitonin, and flouride in prevention or treatment of glucocorticoid-induced osteoporosis has not been convincingly demonstrated in randomized trials.

Testosterone supplementation in men receiving glucocorticoids is also associated with greater increments in bone mineral density than those associated with placebo-administration alone (19). Testosterone administration may have the additional benefit of increasing muscle mass and strength and thereby reducing fall propensity. Large-scale clinical trials to determine the effects of testosterone supplementation on fracture risk in glucocorti-coid-treated men and women have not been performed.

In our patient, calcium supplementation, alendronate, and testosterone administration were effective in increasing the bone mineral density in this patient. The repeated DEXA scan demonstrated a significant improvement in bone mineral density.

Because of the substantial morbidity associated with glucocorticoid-induced osteo-porosis, a baseline bone mineral density should be measured prior to initiation of gluco-corticoid therapy (see Fig. 5). These patients should receive calcium, vitamin D, and a bisphosphonate. In men receiving glucocorticoid therapy, serum testosterone levels should be measured and if testosterone levels are low, consideration should also be given to androgen supplementation.

REFERENCES

1. Lipworth BJ. Systemic adverse effects of inhaled corticosteroids therapy: a systemic review and meta-analyses. Arch Int Med 1999;159:941–955.
2. Walsh P, Aeling JL, Huff L, and Weston WL. Hypothalamus-pituitary-adrenal axis suppression by superpotent topical steroids. J Am Acad Dermatol 1993;29:501–503.
3. Homer JJ, Gazis TG. Cushing's syndrome induced by betamethasone nose drops: in rhinological disease betamethasone should be regarded as systemic corticosteroid. Br Med J 1999;318:1355–1357.
4. Vargas R, Dockhorn RJ, Findlay SR, Korenblat PE, Field EA, Kral KM. Effect of fluticasone propionate aqueous nasal spray versus oral prednisone on the e hypothalamic-pituitary-adrenal axis. J Aller Clin Immunol 1998;102:191–197.
5. Taylor AV, Laoprasert N, Zimmerman D, and Sachs MI. Adrenal suppression secondary to inhaled fluticasone propionate. Ann Aller Asthma Immunol 1999;83:68–70.
6. Krasner AS. Glucocorticoid-induced adrenal insufficiency. JAMA 1999;282:671–676.
7. Laroche M, Porteau L, et al. Osteoporotic vertebral fractures in a man under high-dose inhaled gluco-corticoid therapy. A case-report with review of literature. Rev Rhum Engl Ed 1997;64:267–270.
8. Young CA, Williams IR, and McFarlane IA. Unrecogonized Cushing's syndrome and adrenal suppres-sion due to topical clobetasol propionate. Br J Clin Pract 1991;45:61–62.
9. Gilbertson EO, Spellman MC, Piacquadio DJ, Mulford MI. Superpotent topical corticosteroid use with adrenal suppression: clinical considerations. J Am Acad Derm 1998;38:318–321.
10. MacAdams MR, White RH, and Bradley CE. Reduction in serum testosterone levels during chronic glucocorticoid therapy. Ann Int Med 1986;104:648–646.
11. McKenna TJ, Lorber D, Lacroix A, Rabin D. Testicular activity in Cushing's disease. Acta Endocrinol (Copenh) 1979;91:501–510.
12. Reid IR. Glucocorticoid osteoporosis—mechanisms and management. Eur J Endocrinol 1997;137:209–217.
13. Hofbauer LC, Gori F, Riggs BL, Lacey DL, Dunstan CR, Spelsberg TC, Khosla S. Stimulation of osteoprotegerin ligand and inhibition of osteoprotegerin production by glucocorticoids in human osteo-blastic lineage cells: potential paracrine mechanisms of glucocorticoid-induced osteoporosis. Endocri-nology 1999;140:4382–4389.
14. Kim CH, Cheng SL, Kim GS. Effects of dexamethasone on proliferation, activity, and cytokine secre-tion of normal human bone marrow stromal cells: possible mechanisms of glucocorticoid-induced bone loss. J Endocrinol 1999;162:371–379.

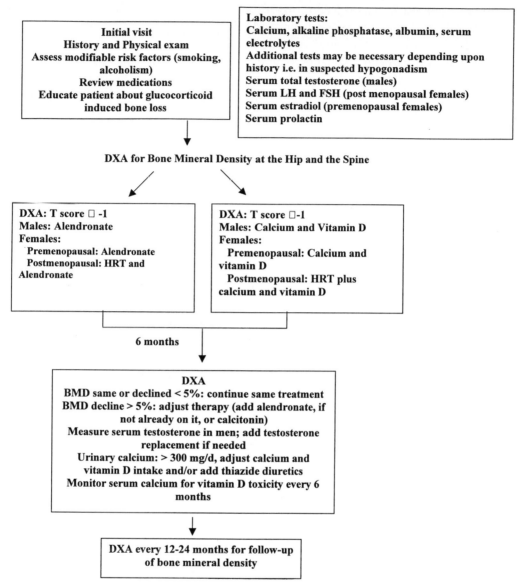

Fig. 5. Recommendation for osteoporosis prevention in patients who are being considered for long-term glucocorticoid therapy (modified from American College of Rheumatology, *20*).

15. Weinstein RS, Jilka RL, Parfitt AM, Manolagas SC. Inhibition of osteoblastogenesis and promotion of apoptosis of osteoblasts and osteocytes by glucocorticoids. Potential mechanisms of their deleterious effects on bone. J Clin Invest 1998;102:274–282.

16. Adachi JD, Saag KG, Delmas PD, Liberman UA, Emkey RD, Seeman E, et al. Two-year effects of alendronate on bone mineral density and vertebral fracture in patients receiving glucocorticoids: a randomized, double-blind, placebo-controlled extension trial. Arthritis Rheum 2001;44:202–211.

17. Saag KG, Emkey R, Schnitzer TJ, Brown JP, Hawkins F, Goemaere S, et al. Alendronate for the prevention and treatment of glucocorticoid-induced osteoporosis. Glucocorticoid-Induced Osteoporosis Intervention Study Group. N Engl J Med 1998;339:292–299.

18. Boutsen Y, Jamart J, Esselinckx W, Devogelaer JP. Primary prevention of glucocorticoid-induced osteoporosis with intravenous pamidronate and calcium: a prospective controlled 1-year study comparing a single infusion, an infusion given once every 3 months, and calcium alone. J Bone Miner Res 2001; 16:104–112.
19. Reid IR, Wattie DJ, Evans MC, Stapleton JP. Testosterone therapy in glucocorticoid-treated men. Arch Intern Med 1996;156:1173–1177.
20. Recommendations for the prevention and treatment of glucocorticoid-induced osteoporosis. American College of Rheumatology task force on osteoporosis guidelines. Arthritis Rheumat 1996;39:1791–1801.

CASE #3: GONADOTROPIN-INDEPENDENT PRECOCIOUS PUBERTY

Case Description

This 7-yr-old boy was evaluated in the Endocrinology Clinic because of precocious sexual development and, as his legal guardian described, "behavioral problems at school." The patient, an orphan living in a foster home, was brought to the clinic by his foster mother who was concerned about his precocious sexual development and behavior. The patient had been born of a full-term delivery in a Los Angeles hospital, and was healthy at birth. Shortly after birth, he was placed in a foster home because of the incarceration of his mother. The whereabouts of his father are not known. Until 1 yr prior to his clinic visit, his growth had been normal in comparison to other children at the foster home. In the year preceding the visit, he started to develop facial hair, phallic growth, and acne on his face. Also, he started to masturbate and his foster parent was concerned about his excessive attention to girls in his classroom. His grades at school deteriorated over the previous year. He did not have any other medical problems, and denied taking any medications. There was no history of head trauma or meningitis. The only family history that was available indicated that his mother was a single woman who used multiple drugs and was incarcerated because of some drug charges.

He was 123 cm tall (50th percentile), and weighed 25 kg (75th percentile) (see Fig. 6). He had dark hair on the upper lip, chin, and side burns, axillae, and pubic region. The pubic hair extended up to the top of his pubic bone in an inverted triangle. He had acne on his face. The penile length was 7.5 cm. His scrotum was rugated and darkly pigmented. The testicular volume was 12 cm^3, and testicular palpation did not reveal the presence of a mass. The skin did not have any hyperpigmented spots. There was no palpable breast tissue. The rest of his physical examination was normal. In particular, there was no neurological deficit or papilledema.

Laboratory evaluation revealed a serum testosterone of 350 ng/dL, an LH < 0.1 IU/L, an FSH < 0.5 IU/L, an estradiol of 20 pg/mL, and a DHEA of 100 ng/dL. hCG β-subunit was undetectable. Upon intravenous administration of 100 µg GnRH, his LH increased from <0.1 IU/L to 0.3 IU/L, and FSH from <0.5 IU/L to 1.0 IU/L. His bone age was 9 yr, and bone X-rays did not show polyostotic fibrous dysplasia. A computerized tomography (CT) scan of the head was normal and did not reveal any evidence of either hydrocephalus or space occupying lesion. Ultrasound of the testes did not show any mass lesion.

Discussion

This 7-yr-old boy has precocious sexual development. Based on pubic hair, phallic size, scrotal development, and testicular size, he is at Tanner stage IV to V in his sexual

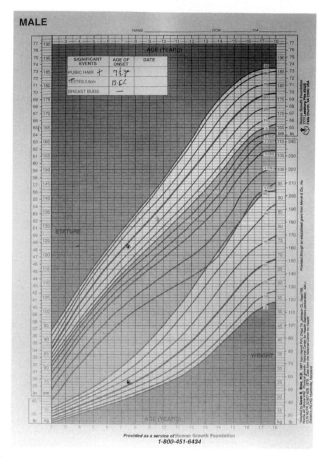

Fig. 6. A growth chart showing the patient's height and weight in relation to the normative range.

maturation. His bone age is more advanced than his chronological age, but his sexual development has advanced far more than his chronological and bone age. His testosterone levels are in the adult range. The DHEAS concentration is appropriate for his age and not increased, suggesting that the source of increased androgen production in this patient is his testis.

Serum LH and FSH levels are below the limit of assay detection, and demonstrated subnormal increases in response to GnRH. In addition, the circulating concentrations of hCG is not increased. Thus, we are unable to explain the premature stimulation of testosterone secretion on the basis of ectopic hCG production. Taken together, these data indicate that our patient has premature stimulation of testosterone production by the testis without the activation of gonadotropin secretion by the pituitary. These are hallmarks of the syndrome of gonadotropin-independent precocious puberty. This syndrome is predominantly seen in boys, and is often familial. A family history of sexual precocity can be elicited in half of these patients.

The distinction between gonadotropin-dependent and gonadotropin-independent precocious puberty is not always straightforward. Many commercial assays for the measurement of LH and FSH have suboptimal sensitivity for the measurement of the low circulating concentrations that are prevalent in prepubertal children. However, the use of highly sensitive, fluorometric and chemiluminescent assays for LH and FSH, and the assessment of responses to GnRH or GnRH agonist can help distinguish these two conditions *(1–3)*.

The work-up of children with precocious puberty, whose LH and FSH levels are very low or below the limit of assay detection, should include diagnostic tests to exclude the presence of autonomous, androgen secreting tumors in the adrenal glands or the testes, and ectopic hCG secreting neoplasms. The diagnosis of idiopathic, gonadotropin-independent, precocious puberty is made by the exclusion of adrenal or testicular neoplasms and by demonstration of premature activation of testicular steroidogenesis in the face of very low or undetectable LH concentrations. In this patient, this diagnosis seems likely because appropriate diagnostic work-up failed to reveal the presence of an adrenal or testicular neoplasm or evidence of ectopic hCG secretion.

Recent studies have provided important insights into the molecular and genetic basis of premature activation of testicular testosterone secretion in patients with idiopathic, gonadotropin-independent precocious puberty *(4–13)*. At least two mutations have been described in patients presenting with this syndrome. McCune Albright Syndrome is a clinical disorder characterized by gonadotropin-independent precocious puberty in association with hormone-secreting ovarian cysts, hyperpigmented, café-au-lait skin lesions, and polyostotic fibrous dysplasia *(4–8)*. The pathophysiology of unregulated hormone production in a significant proportion of patients with McCune Albright syndrome is best explained by somatic, activating mutations of the α-subunit of the stimulatory guanine nucleotide binding protein (G protein) *(6–9)*. Guanyl nucleotide proteins function as transducers of biologic signal between hormone receptors and the effector systems within the cell (see Fig. 7). For instance, after binding of LH or FSH to their respective receptors on the surface of the steroidogenic cell, the receptor undergoes a transformational change that results in dissociation of the Gs α-subunit. The Gs α-subunit in the presence of GTP activates adenylyl cyclase, resulting in the production of cyclic AMP, and stimulation of hormone production. Some mutations of the Gs subunit result in constitutive activation of adenylyl cyclase with increased intracellular cyclic AMP production. The net result is ligand-independent unregulated, autonomous hormone production by the steroidogenic cells that is clinically manifested as premature sexual development in the absence of an appropriate regulatory signal from the hypothalamus and the pituitary. McCune-Albright syndrome is predominantly a disorder seen in girls, and in the absence of café-au-lait spots and polyostotic fibrous dysplasia in this male patient, the diagnosis of McCune-Albright Syndrome does not appear likely.

Activating mutations of the luteinizing hormone receptor (see Fig. 8, Table 2) have been associated with male-limited gonadotropin-independent precocious puberty *(10–14)*. Almost all of the known, activating mutations of the LH receptor have been missense mutations caused by single base substitution (see Table 2) *(10–14)*. The most frequent mutation found in association with gonadotropin-independent precocious puberty is the replacement of Asp-578 by *Gly* due to A to G substitution at position 1733 *(9–14)*. Most of these activating mutations have been located in exon 11 of the LH receptor, which encodes the sequence for the transmembrane domain of the LH receptor. The activating mutations of the LH receptor produce a clinical phenotype only in boys; they appear to produce no clinically detectable effects in affected females. Some patients with testicular neoplasms have also been found to have activating mutations of the LH receptor *(10,12)*.

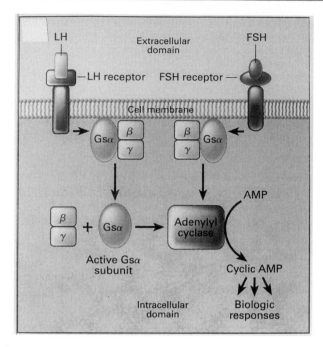

Fig. 7. A schematic representation of the Gs α-protein and its role in transducing intracellular signaling [Adapted with permission from Farfel et al. *(15)*]. The G nucleotide protein is a trimeric protein consisting of α, β, and γ subunits, and is associated with the receptor on the cell surface. The hormone binding to its receptor causes the G protein to dissociate from the receptor and release the α subunit. The active α subunit and GTP bind to the regulatory subunits of adenylyl cyclase, resulting in activation of its catalytic subunits. The catalytic subunits of adenylyl cyclase in turn catalyze the conversion of ATP to 3', 5', cyclic AMP, which serves as the second messenger within the cell to transduce the biological signal. Activating mutations of the α subunit have been associated with McCune Albright syndrome.

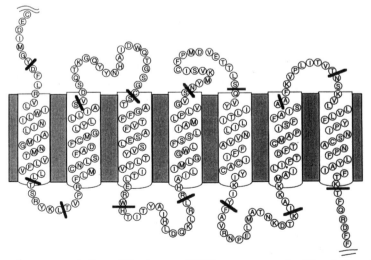

Fig. 8. A schematic representation of the human LH Receptor protein. The deduced amino acid sequence and topology of the hLHR. The receptor is a G protein coupled receptor that has an extracellular domain, seven transmembrane regions, and an intracellular carboxy-terminal tail. Bolded lines indicate the proposed transmembrane boundaries. The extracellular domain and the cytoplasmic tail have been truncated (Minegishi et al.) *(16)*.

Table 2
Some of the Previously Reported Inactivating and Activating Mutations of the hLH Receptor*

LH receptor gene		Males	Females
Inactivating	Cys 545 Stop	Leydig cell hypoplasia	
Mutations	Arg 554 Stop	Leydig cell hypoplasia	secondary amenorrhea
	Ala 593 Pro	Leydig cell hypoplasia	primary amenorrhea
	Ser 616 Tyr	micropenis	
Activating	Met 398 Thr	male precocious puberty	
Mutations	Ile 542 Leu	male precocious puberty	
	Asp 564 Gly	male precocious puberty	
	Ala 568 Val	male precocious puberty	
	Ala 572 Val	male precocious puberty	
	Met 575 Ile	male precocious puberty	
	Thr 577 Ile	male precocious puberty	
	Asp 578 Gly	male precocious puberty	
	Asp 578 Tyr	male precocious puberty	
	Cys 581 Arg	male precocious puberty	
	Asp 582 Gly	male precocious puberty	

*Reproduced with permission from ref. (17).

The clinical phenotype of this patient is most consistent with the diagnosis of an activating mutation of the human LH receptor. However, in the absence of the confirmatory mutation analysis, this diagnosis remains presumptive.

The treatment options for the treatment of gonadotropin-independent precocious puberty are limited. These patients do not respond to GnRH agonist administration because their testosterone secretion is not under the control of pituitary LH secretion. Only limited information is available about the effectiveness of androgen antagonists and inhibitors of androgen production. Thus, ketoconazole, an inhibitor of *Cyp450*-linked steroidogenic enzymes, has been used to suppress endogenous testosterone secretion. However, there is concern about adrenal suppression and liver toxicity at high doses of ketoconazole. Similarly, cyproterone acetate, an androgen antagonist, has not been shown to increase final height or improve clinical outcomes. Long-term clinical trials with more potent and selective androgen antagonists are needed to determine the impact of therapy on clinical outcomes and final height.

REFERENCES

1. Albano MC, Latronico AC, Arnhold IJ, Domenice S, Bloise W, Mendonca BB. Long-acting GnRH agonists in the differential diagnosis of male precocious puberty. J Pediatr Endocrinol Metab 1997;105: 499–503.
2. Apter D. Ultrasensitive new immunoassays for gonadotropins in the evaluation of puberty. Curr Opin Pediatr 1993;5:481–487.
3. Garibaldi LR, Aceto T Jr, Weber C, Pang S. The relationship between luteinizing hormone and estradiol secretion in female precocious puberty: evaluation by sensitive gonadotropin assays and the leuprolide stimulation test. J Clin Endocrinol Metab 1993;76:851–856.
4. Lauue L. Ligand-independent hormone secretion. Curr Opin Pediatr 1995;7:434–439.
5. DiMeglio LA, Pescovitz OH. Disorders of puberty: inactivating and activating molecular mutations. J Pediatr 1997;131(1 Pt 2):S8–S12.

6. Schwindinger WF, Francomano CA, Levine MA. Identification of a mutation in the gene encoding the alpha subunit of the stimulatory G protein of adenylyl cyclase in McCune-Albright syndrome. Proc Natl Acad Sci USA 1992;89:5152–5156.

7. Weinstein LS, Shenker A, Gejman PV, Merino MJ, Friedman E, Spiegel AM. Activating mutations of the stimulatory G protein in the McCune-Albright syndrome. N Engl J Med 1991;325:1688–1695.

8. Latronico AC, Lins TS, Brito VN, Arnhold IJ, Mendonca BB. The effect of distinct activating mutations of the luteinizing hormone receptor gene on pituitary-gonadal axis in both sexes. Clin Endocrinol (Oxf) 2000;53:609–613.

9. Kremer H, Martens JW, van Reen M, Verhoef-Post M, Wit JM, Otten BJ, et al. A limited repertoire of mutations of the LH receptor gene in familial and sporadic patients with male LH-independent precocious puberty. J Clin Endocrinol Metab 1999;84:1136–1140.

10. Wu SM, Leschek EW, Rennert OM, Chan WY. Luteinizing hormone receptor mutations in disorders of sexual development and cancer. Front Biosc 2000;5:D343–D352.

11. Bertelloni S, Baroncelli GI, Lala R, Cappa M, Matarazzo P, De Sanctis C, Saggese G. Long-term outcome of male-limited gonadotropic-independent precocious puberty. Horm Res 1997;48:235–239.

12. Martin MM, Wu SM, Martin AL, Rennert OM, Chan WY. Testicular seminoma in a patient with a constitutively activating mutation of the luteinizing hormone/chorionic gonadotropin receptor. Eur J Endocrinol 1998;139:101–106.

13. Laue L, Chan WY, Hsueh AJ, Kudo M, Hsu SY, Wu SM, Blomberg L, Cutler GB Jr. Genetic heterogeneity of constitutively activating mutations of the human luteinizing hormone receptor in familial male-limited precocious puberty. Proc Natl Acad Sci USA 1995;92:1906–1910.

14. Shenker A, Laue L, Kosugi S, Merendino JJ Jr, Minegishi T, Cutler GB Jr. A constitutively activating mutation of the luteinizing hormone receptor in familial male precocious puberty. Nature 1993;365:652–654.

15. Farfel Z, Bourne HR, Liri T. The expanding spectrum of G protein diseases. N Engl J Med 1999;340:1012–1020.

16. Minegishi T, Nakamura K, Takakura K, et al. Cloning and sequencing of human LH/hCG receptor cDNA. Biochem Biophys Res Commun 1990;172:1049–1054.

17. Conway GS. Clinical manifestations of genetic defects affecting gonadotropins and their receptors. Clin Endocrinol 1996;45:657–663.

CASE #4: DELAYED PUBERTAL DEVELOPMENT AND NONPALPABLE TESTES

Case Description

This 19-yr-old man was evaluated because of failure of normal sexual development. The patient was born at home in Mexico and, according to his mother, he was healthy and had normal male external genitalia. He grew up normally in comparison to his two brothers. He developed some axillary hair around age 10, but did not develop facial hair. He did not shave or masturbate, is not sexually active, and denies having any penile erections. His voice has continued to be high pitched. His two brothers, 24 and 20 yr of age, respectively, started shaving around the age of 15. The oldest brother is married. He has two older sisters, 26 and 23, who are married and have children.

His height was 170 cm, arm span 176 cm, and weight 68 kg. He had sparse brown hair on the face, dark axillary hair, and very sparse pubic hair below the symphysis pubis. His voice was high pitched. His penis was 7 cm in length. The scrotum was hypopigmented, and no testicular tissue was palpable in the scrotum or the inguinal canal. Breast tissue was palpable on both sides. His sense of smell was normal and the rest of his examination was normal.

Laboratory tests showed that his serum testosterone level was 20 ng/dL, LH 34 IU/L, FSH 36 IU/L, and estradiol 24 pg/mL. In response to 1500 U of human chorionic gonadotropin (hCG) administered by intramuscular injection, his serum testosterone levels did not increase (baseline 15 ng/dL, 24 h 18 ng/dL, 48 h 15 ng/dL). hCG administration at a dose of 1500 U three times weekly for 4 wk increased his serum testosterone levels from a baseline of 20 ng/dL to 24 ng/dL. Karyotype on peripheral blood was 46, XY. An ultrasound of the pelvis did not reveal any testicular tissue either in the pelvis or in the inguinal canal. No Mullerian structures were seen. A magnetic resonance imaging (MRI) scan of the abdomen did not show the presence of intraabdominal testicular tissue.

Discussion

This patient had normal male external genitalia, a well-developed scrotum and phallus, and a normally placed urethral meatus. These clinical findings indicate that the patient underwent normal sexual differentiation during fetal life. Therefore, one can assume normal function of *Sry*, *DAX-1*, and SF-1 proteins that play an important role in determining sexual differentiation. In addition, testosterone is required for the development of Wolffian structures along male lines. Dihydrotestosterone, derived from 5-α-reduction of testosterone, is required for the development of the genital tubercle into the glans penis. It is reasonable to assume that in this patient, the urogenital sinus and genital tubercle were exposed to normal testosterone and DHT concentrations during critical periods of sexual differentiation during fetal life. The absence of structures that normally develop from Mullerian ducts is also consistent with the proposal that, at least during prenatal life, the testes developed normally and were producing appropriate amounts of androgens and Mullerian inhibitory hormone. Presumably, both testes atrophied at some unknown time after completion of the process of sexual differentiation.

In an individual with male external genitalia, in whom the testes are not palpable in the scrotum, it is essential to determine whether the testes are present in the abdomen (see Fig. 9). Although there is no foolproof method, short of exploratory laparotomy, to exclude the presence of intraabdominal testes, several noninvasive tests can be helpful *(1–3)*. The serum testosterone response to human chorionic gonadotropin can help confirm the presence of testicular tissue. Although a normal testosterone response to hCG is indicative of the presence of testicular tissue, an absent or suboptimal response does not necessarily exclude the presence of intraabdominal testicular tissue *(1–3)*. Leydig cell function in cryptorchid testis is often attenuated and sometimes severely impaired. In this patient, baseline testosterone concentrations were very low and did not increase significantly in response to hCG. Thus, the absence of a testosterone response to hCG favors the diagnosis of anorchia, although it does not completely exclude the possibility of abdominal testes.

Measurement of serum Mullerian inhibiting hormone levels has been proposed as a diagnostic test for the evaluation of children with nonpalpable gonads *(4,5)*. In one study *(4)*, the sensitivity and specificity of serum Mullerian inhibiting hormone levels for detecting the absence of testicular tissue were 92% and 98%, respectively, as compared with 69% and 83% for testosterone levels. Thus, measurements of serum Mullerian inhibiting hormone can be useful in detecting the presence of testicular tissue and differentiating anorchia from undescended testes in phenotypic males with nonpalpable testes. However, Mullerian inhibiting hormone concentrations may be misleading in patients with dysgenetic testes in whom there can be a discrepancy between the degree of anatomical Mullerian duct regression and serum levels *(5)*. Mullerian inhibiting hormone concentrations may be normal in male pseudohermaphrodites with dysgenetic testes and persis-

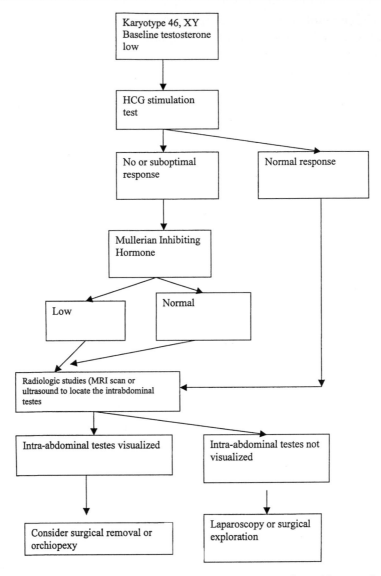

Fig. 9. An algorithm for the work-up of phenotypic males presenting with nonpalpable testes.

tence of Mullerian structures *(5)*. Also, Mullerian inhibiting hormone assays are not readily available from many commercial laboratories and the clinical experience with this diagnostic test remains limited.

An MRI scan and an ultrasound examination did not show the presence of testicular tissue within the abdomen of this patient. Both MRI and ultrasound can occasionally miss abdominal gonads, especially if the gonads are markedly atrophied. Therefore, a search for intraabdominal testicular tissue by laparoscopy or by surgical exploration is sometimes necessary.

Collectively, the very low baseline testosterone levels, the absence of a testosterone response to hCG, and the failure to detect any intraabdominal tissue by MRI and ultrasound favor the diagnosis of anorchia, although we cannot fully exclude bilateral cryptorchidism. The genetic basis of anorchia is not known. The presence of normal male external genitalia suggests that the genetic and hormonal elements necessary for sexual differentiation during fetal life are intact in these individuals *(6–14)*. The karyotype is typically normal in patients with anorchia, and previous studies have failed to find mutations of the coding region of the *Sry* gene in these patients *(8–14)*. Others have proposed the occurrence of *in utero* torsion of the testis as the pathophysiologic basis *(8)*. However, many patients with anorchia have normal testis at birth that gradually shrink and disappear over time, giving rise to the term "vanishing testis syndrome." The molecular basis of the process that results in insidious destruction of testicular tissue remains unclear. Several case reports of anorchia occurring in association with idiopathic hypogonadotropic hypogonadism have been reported. It is possible that at least some of these patients have *DAX-1* mutations *(11,15)*.

The treatment of patients with congenital bilateral anorchia includes life-long testosterone replacement. In addition, placement of testicular implants in the scrotum is esthetically appealing to many men. Once androgen replacement has been initiated, these patients need periodic evaluation to monitor the potential adverse effects of testosterone. Achievement of fertility is not possible at present, but adoption or insemination of the female partner by donor sperm are effective options that should be discussed with these patients.

REFERENCES

1. Hamidinia A, Nold S, Amankwah KS. Localization and treatment of nonpalpable testes. Surg Gynecol Obstet 1984;159:439–441.
2. Bartone FF, Huseman CA, Maizels M, Firlit CF. Pitfalls in using human chorionic gonadotropin stimulation test to diagnose anorchia. J Urol 1984;132:563–567.
3. Lee MM, Donahoe PK, Silverman BL, Hasegawa T, Hasegawa Y, Gustafson ML, Chang YC, MacLaughlin DT. Measurements of serum mullerian inhibiting substance in the evaluation of children with nonpalpable gonads. N Engl J Med 1997;336:1480–1486.
4. Forrest MG. Serum mullerian inhibiting substance assay—a new diagnostic test for disorders of gonadal development. N Engl J Med 1997;336:1519–1521.
5. Mendoza-Morfin F, Rodriguez-Lopez M, Oliveros-Rodriguez A, Altamirano-Bustamante P, Navarrete-Lopez R, Gutierrez-Perez H, Oseguera-Valladares R. Circulating gonadotropin pattern in anorchia syndrome. Response to treatment. Arch Invest Med 1980;11:239–247.
6. Bernasconi S, Ghizzoni L, Panza C, Volta C, Caselli G. Congenital anorchia: natural history and treatment. Horm Res 1992;37(Suppl 3):50–54.
7. Smith NM, Byard RW, Bourne AJ. Testicular regression syndrome—a pathological study of 77 cases. Histopathology 1991;19:269–272.
8. Kulin HE, Santner SJ. The assessment of diminished testicular function in boys of pubertal age. Clin Endocrinol (Oxf) 1986;25:283–292.
9. Parigi GB, Bardoni B, Avoltini V, Caputo MA, Bragheri R. Is bilateral congenital anorchia genetically determined? Eur J Pediatr Surg 1999;9:312–315.
10. Suzuki Y, Sasagawa I, Izumiya K, Nakada T, Sato J. A genotypic male with anorchia in conjunction with isolated idiopathic hypogonadotropic hypogonadism. Scand J Urol Nephrol 1999;33:347–349.
11. Flett ME, Jones PF, Youngson GG. Emerging trends in the management of the impalpable testis. Br J Surg 1999;86:1280–1283.
12. De Rosa M, Lupoli G, Mennitti M, Zarrilli S, Mirone V, Lombardi G. Congenital bilateral anorchia: clinical, hormonal and imaging study in 12 cases. Andrologia 1996;28:281–285.
13. Lobaccaro JM, Medlej R, Berta P, Belon C, Galifer RB, Guthmann JP, Chevalier C, Czernichow P, Dumas R, Sultan C. PCR analysis and sequencing of the SRY sex determining gene in four patients with bilateral congenital anorchia. Clin Endocrinol (Oxf) 1993;38:197–201.
14. Sasagawa I, Nakada T, Kubota Y, Kato T, Sawamura T. Anorchia associated with gonadotropin deficiency. Urol Int 1993;51:231–233.

14 Disorders of Female Reproduction

Jared C. Robins, MD and Robert Rebar, MD

CONTENTS

CASE #1: HIRSUTISM

Case Description

This 19-yr-old nulligravid woman presented with the chief complaint of facial hirsutism for 5 yr. Thelarche began at 8.5 yr of age and menarche occurred at 13 yr of age. Her menses were irregular, heavy, and associated with dysmenorrhea. To "regulate her cycles," her general medical doctor placed her on combination oral contraceptive pills (ethinyl estradiol 35 mcg and norethindrone 1 mg). Although effective in controlling her bleeding, the contraceptives did not affect her facial hair. She denied symptoms of an endocrinopathy, including excessive thirst or urination, temperature intolerance, and weight changes. She was not taking any medication. There was no significant past medical history, past surgical history, family history, or history of childhood illnesses. Her review of systems was negative.

On examination, this patient was 65 in (1.67 m) tall and weighed 125 lbs (56.7 kg) (body mass index = 21). She had 3+ out of 4+ facial hair noted on her chin, upper lip, and sideburn area. Hair growth was also noted on her midline chest and abdomen. There were no signs of thyroid disease or glucocorticoid excess. Breast development was Tanner stage 4 and there were no masses or galactorrhea. A pelvic exam revealed Tanner stage 5 pubic hair; external and internal genitalia were normal, and there was no clitoromegaly. There were no other pertinent findings.

In an effort to rule out an androgen-producing tumor and to help differentiate among familial idiopathic hirsutism, polycystic ovarian syndrome (PCOS), and nonclassic adrenal hyperplasia (NCAH), a blood sample was obtained for the measurement of testosterone, dehydroepiandrosterone sulfate (DHEA-S) and 17α hydroxyprogesterone (17-OHP) levels. Testosterone was 68 ng/dL (normal range 0–83), and DHEA-S was 326 ng/dL (normal 20–394), and 17-OHP was 1377 ng/dL (normal 20–500). To rule out congenital

From: *Contemporary Endocrinology: Challenging Cases in Endocrinology*
Edited by: M. E. Molitch © Humana Press Inc., Totowa, NJ

Table 1
ACTH Stimulation Test Results

Time	Cortisol µg/dL	17-OHP ng/dL
Baseline	1.3	80
30 min	9.2	6494
60 min	13.5	6635

adrenal hyperplasia, an adrenocorticotropic hormone (ACTH) stimulation test was performed with 250 µg of synthetic $ACTH_{1-24}$ after overnight adrenal suppression with 0.5 mg of dexamethasone. The results are summarized in Table 1. The low baseline cortisol is a result of dexamethasone suppression. The rise of cortisol >7 µg/dL above the baseline after ACTH stimulation demonstrates the adrenal's ability to produce adequate cortisol; however, the peak cortisol level of less than 20 µg/dL may suggest a mild defect in cortisol production. More impressive is her elevation of 17-OHP which, being >1500 ng/dL from baseline, is diagnostic for nonclassic adrenal hyperplasia (1).

After discussion of treatment options, the patient was started on a combination oral contraceptive (30 mcg ethinyl estradiol and 0.015 mg desogestrel) and 200 mg of spironolactone (100 mg bid) for three months. On her return, she stated that she noticed a small improvement in her hirsutism. Her potassium level was normal and her spironolactone dose was decreased to 100 mg daily. Her hirsutism continued to improve and, within 1 yr, she no longer required depilatory treatment. Hirsutism was noted to be effectively absent at the time of her next yearly visit.

Discussion

Hirsutism is defined as excessive facial and body hair caused by androgen stimulation. This definition can be misleading because hirsute women do not have an increase in the number of hair follicles. Rather, they have an increase in the proportion of terminal to vellus hair follicles. Vellus hair follicles are small follicles that produce fine, unpigmented hair. When vellus follicles are exposed to androgens, they are converted to terminal follicles that produce thick and pigmented hair. Hirsutism, therefore, is a manifestation of increased androgens in women.

The evaluation of the hirsute woman begins by eliminating the most serious conditions that may lead to increased androgen production. These conditions include neoplasms of the ovary and adrenal gland, Cushing's syndrome, and congenital adrenal hyperplasia (CAH). These diseases are generally apparent on visual inspection. Cushing's syndrome is a disease of excess cortisol production, most commonly from either an ACTH-secreting pituitary adenoma or a cortisol-producing adrenal adenoma or carcinoma. This endocrinopathy leads to distinctive physical findings including obesity, particularly of the face and cervicodorsal region, abdominal striae, thickened skin, easy bruisability, and purpura of the forearms and legs. Patients with Cushing's syndrome will often present with muscle weakness, hypertension, and diabetes. A concomitant increase in adrenal androgen production may result in mild hirsutism.

Virilization is also present in classic CAH; CAH is the result of an enzyme deficiency in the glucocorticoid synthesis pathway, most commonly (>90%) in 21-hydroxylase, resulting in hypocortisolemia and hypoaldosteronism. The lack of aldosterone production; if unrecognized in a newborn, will result in salt-wasting, fluid imbalance, and shock within 2 wk after birth. ACTH production is stimulated by the loss of negative feedback on the pituitary. This increase in ACTH drives the production of steroids, proximal to the enzyme deficiency, which may be converted into androgens. During *in utero*, this increase in androgens may cause severe virilization of female fetuses and result in ambiguous genitalia.

There is a wide range of clinical variation in patients with CAH. Classic CAH results from a virtually complete block in the synthetic pathway of glucocorticoids. So-called simple virilizing CAH is thought to be the result of point mutations in the cytochrome P450c21 that catalyzes 21-hydroxylase activity. The diminished enzyme activity decreases the production of cortisol with little effect on aldosterone. Therefore, although these newborns do not suffer from salt-wasting, females will be virilized and may have ambiguous genitalia.

In the absence of significant virilization, or in the absence of a rapid onset and progression of symptoms, the differential diagnosis of the hirsute woman includes idiopathic hirsutism, polycystic ovarian syndrome, and nonclassic adrenal hyperplasia (NCAH). All three of these diseases have very similar phenotypic presentations although their etiologies are very different. Idiopathic hirsutism is associated with an increase in 5α-reductase activity in the skin and hair follicles. This leads to a local increase in dihydrotestosterone, the active metabolite of testosterone *(2)*. Typically, there are no associated endocrinopathies with this syndrome. However, the increased enzyme activity results in an increase in 3α-androstanediol glucuronide that is measurable in peripheral blood samples.

Polycystic ovarian syndrome (PCOS), typified by hyperandrogenism and chronic anovulation, is one of most common causes of oligo- and amenorrhea. The exact pathophysiology is not clear, however, a neuroendocrine-metabolic dysfunction has been clearly associated with this disorder. Anovulation is likely secondary to low and unvarying levels of follicle-stimulating hormone (FSH) leading to follicular arrest *(3,4)*. Hyperandrogenism may results either from chronic stimulation of the ovarian theca cells by luteinizing hormone (LH) or by theca cell hypersensitivity to LH *(5)*. Recently, PCOS has been found to be associated with insulin resistance and hyperinsulinemia. This association is most dramatic in obese PCOS patients (representing about 50% of all PCOS patients). Interestingly, a positive correlation between hyperinsulinemia and hyperandrogenism has been noted and correction of the abnormality with insulin sensitizing drugs will significantly decrease serum testosterone *(6)*.

Nonclassic adrenal hyperplasia often presents identically to PCOS. However, as in classic CAH, the etiology of NCAH is an abnormality in the glucocorticoid synthesis pathway. In contrast to classic CAH, patients with NCAH have mild dysfunction resulting in minimal symptomatology. This disease is common among Ashkenazic Jews, Hispanics, and Italians. Genetic linkage studies have demonstrated that 75–85% of women with NCAH carry the human leukocyte antigen HLA-B14 *(7,8)*. The carrier frequency of this locus in women with NCAH is 250 times greater than in unaffected individuals *(9)*. Therefore, this disorder should be considered in any patient presenting with the symptoms and ethnicity of the patient illustrated.

The laboratory evaluation of women with hirsutism should be directed at confirming clinically established diagnoses. A random total testosterone and dehyroepiandrosterone sulfate (DHEA-S) should be obtained. Testosterone elevations greater than 200 ng/dL are suspicious for an androgen producing ovarian neoplasm and pelvic ultrasound should be performed. Values between 80 and 200 ng/dL, while usually benign, warrant close follow-up in 3–6 mo intervals. Likewise, DHEA-S levels more than two times normal are suggestive of adrenal neoplasm; computed tomography (CT) scanning or magnetic resonance imaging (MRI) are the best radiologic tests to evaluate for this tumor. Cortisol measurements are not useful unless Cushing's syndrome is suspected.

Stimulating the adrenal gland with ACTH and measuring the precursors of cortisol production makes the diagnostic distinction between PCOS and NCAH. Commonly, 250 µg of synthetic $ACTH_{1-24}$ is given by intravenous bolus. Cortisol and 17-hydroxyprogesterone (17-OHP) are measured at baseline and at 60 min. An elevation of 17-OHP $\geq$ 1500 ng/ dL is diagnostic for NCAH. Carriers tend to have elevations of approximately 1000 ng/dL.

The conventional treatment for NCAH is glucocorticoid therapy (10). This therapy is effective at suppressing androgen secretion, even when significant adrenal insufficiency is not diagnosed. Despite suppresion, little improvement in hirsutism is often noted. Consequently, some investigators have used antiandrogens to treat the associated hirsutism. Spritzer et al. demonstrated that cyproterone acetate will significantly decrease hirsutism when compared to conventional therapy (11). This drug is a potent antiandrogen that competes with testosterone for the androgen receptor and inhibits translocation of the hormone receptor complex into the cell nucleus (12). Cyproterone is potentially teratogenic to male fetuses. However, when combined with 35 mcg of ethinyl estradiol, it is effective in treating hirsutism and as an oral contraceptive (Diane-35) (13). Despite its effectiveness, cyproterone containing drugs are not approved by the United States Food and Drug Administration and are not available in the United States. Spironolactone also competes for the androgen receptor and is an effective treatment for hirsutism. When compared to Diane 35, in one study 50 mg of spironolactone was more effective at reducing hair growth (14). Generally, 200 mg daily is the starting dose and the dose is reduced to 100 mg after about 1 yr. The patient should be told that little effect will be seen until 6–12 mo of use. Like cyproterone, spironolactone can affect male fetal development and should be used with caution in women of reproductive age and never used during pregnancy.

Ovarian suppression alone has been shown to decrease hirsutism. Carmina and Lobo, noting the similarities between NCAH and PCOS, demonstrated that the use of a gonadotropin-releasing hormone (GnRH) agonist improves androgen levels and hirsutism (15). However, long-term clinical use of GnRH agonists is not practical. Oral contraceptives pills will suppress ovarian function and increase sex hormone binding globulin. Studies have shown that their use will improve hirsutism in more than 60% of cases (16).

Because our patient was leaving for college, we thought it would be both safer and more practical for her to avoid therapy with glucocorticoids. Side effects associated with the inappropriate use of glucocortocoids are not trivial and may include manifestation of Cushing's syndromes. Rather, we started her on spironolactone and oral contraception. She noted significant improvement at three months and did not require electrolysis by 1 yr of treatment.

REFERENCES

1. New MI, Lorenzen F, Lerner AJ, Kohn B, Oberfield SE, Pollack MS, Dupont B, Stoner E, Levy DJ, Pang S, Levine LS. Genotyping steroid 21-hydroxylase deficiency: hormone reference data. J Clin Endocrinol Metab 1983;57:320.
2. Horton R, Hawks D, Lobo R. 3a,17b-androstanediol glucuronide in plasma: a marker of androgen action in idiopathic hirsutism. J Clin Invest 1982;69:1203–1206.

3. Brown JB. Pituitary control of ovarian function-concepts derived from gonadotropin therapy. Aust N Z J Obstet Gynaecol 978;18:46.

4. Yen SSC. Polycystic ovary syndrome. In: Yen SSC, Jaffe RB, Barbieri RL, eds. Repoductive Endocrinology: Physiology, Pathophysiology and Clinical Management, 4th edition. WB Saunders, Philadelphia, PA, 1999, pp. 436–478.

5. Gilling-Smith C, Willis DS, Beard RW, Franks S. Hypersecretion of androstenedione by isolated thecal cells from polysystic ovaries. J Clin Endocrinol Metab 1994;79:1159–1165.

6. Dunaif A. Insulin resistance and the polycystic ovary syndrome: mechanism and implication for pathogenesis. Endocrin Rev 1997;81:942.

7. Kutten F, Coullin P, Girard F, Billand L, Vincencs M, Boucekkine C, Thalabard JC, Maudelonde T, Pritzer P, Mowszowicz I, et al. Late onset adrenal hyperplasia in hirsutism. N Engl J Med 1985;313:224–231.

8. Speiser PW, Dupont B, Rubinstein P, Piazza A, Kastelan A, New MI. High frequency of non-classical steroid 21-hydroxylase deficiency. Am J Hum Genet 1985;37:650–667.

9. Holler W, Scholz S, Knorr D, Bidlilgmaier F, Keller E, Albert ED. Genetic differences between the salt-wasting, simple virilizing and non-classical types of congenital adrenal hyperplasia. J Clin Endocrinol Metab 1985;60:757–763.

10. White PC, New MI, Dupont B. Congenital adrenal hyperplasia (I). N Engl J Med 1987;316:519–524.

11. Spritzer P, Billaud L, Thalabard JC, Birman P, Mowszowicz I, Raux-Demay MC, Clair F, Kuttenn F, Mauvais-Jarvis P. Cyproterone acetate versus hydrocortisone treatment in late-onset adrenal hyperplasia. J Clin Endocrinol Metab 1990;70(3):642–646.

12. Sciarra F, Toscano V, Concolino G, Di Silvierio F. Androgens: clinical apllicaitons. J Steroid Biochem Mol Biol 1990;37:349–362.

13. Vermeulen A, Rubens R. Effects of cyproterone acetate plus ethinylestradiol low dose on plasma androgens and lipids in mildly hirsute or acneic young women. Contraception 1988;38:419–428.

14. Lunde O, Djoseland O. A comparative study of Aldactone and Diane in the treatment of hirsutism. J Steroid Biochem 1987;28:161–165.

15. Carmina E, Lobo RA. Gonadotrophin-releasing hormone agonist therapy for hirsutism is as effective as high dose cyproterone acetate but results in a longer remission. Hum Reprod 1997;12:663–666.

16. Burkman RT. The role of oral contraceptives in the treatment of hyperandrogenic disorders. Am J Med 1995;98(1A):130S–138S.

CASE #2: AMENORRHEA AND PITUITARY NEOPLASM

Case Description

This 20-yr-old woman presented for the evaluation of primary amenorrhea. Pubarche and thelarche began at age 13 with little progression. Her growth and developmental milestones were normal. She denied excessive thirst or urination, temperature intolerance, anosmia, weight changes, or other symptoms suggestive of an endocrinopathy. She had never experienced cyclic abdominal pain or moliminal symptoms. She was not taking any medication. There was no significant past medical history, past surgical history, family history, or history of childhood illness. Her review of systems was negative except for a complaint of insertional dyspareunia.

On examination, she had normal vital signs. She was 62 in tall and weighed 104 lbs. There were no signs of thyroid disease, glucocorticoid imbalance, or androgen excess. Breast development was Tanner stage 3 and there were no masses or galactorrhea. A pelvic exam revealed Tanner stage 3 pubic hair development. Her vagina was hypoestrogenic; she had an unremarkable uterus and cervix. Neurologic exam was normal and there were no other pertinent findings.

A central abnormality was suspected because of interrupted pubertal development. LH, FSH, TSH, prolactin, cortisol, and thyroxine were all within normal limits for a woman in early puberty. Estradiol was low, but within normal limits for development.

A coned-down lateral X-ray of the sella turcica showed a 2 cm area of calcification in the hypothalamus. A follow-up contrast-enhanced MRI study showed a 2 cm solid and cystic mass below the floor of the third ventricle without involvement of the pituitary gland. The optic tracts were laterally displaced around this tumor. Visual field testing was normal. Dynamic pituitary testing with GnRH (100 mcg intravenous bolus), thyrotropin-stimulating hormone (500 mcg intravenous bolus), growth-hormone releasing hormone (1 mcg/kg), and corticotropin-releasing hormone (1 mcg/kg) resulted in normal FSH, LH, thyrotropin, prolactin, growth hormone, ACTH, and cortisol responses.

A consultation was obtained with a neurosurgeon; the size and the location of the tumor made a biopsy inadvisable. However, the cystic nature made craniopharyngioma the most likely diagnosis. Because the patient was not having any significant symptoms except for amenorrhea, expectant management was advised. This plan included yearly visual field testing, pituitary stimulation testing, and MRI.

The patient was started on 0.3 mg/d of conjugated equine estrogens (CEE) and 5 mg of medroxyprogesterone acetate days 1–12 of the calendar month. The CEE was increased to 0.6 mg/day and then 1.25 mg/d in 6 mo intervals. There was no progression of the tumor over 10 yr of observation. During that time period, the patient developed frontal headaches diagnosed as migraines. She was tried on variety of therapies without relief. These headaches increased in severity and became disabling. Despite stable radiologic findings, the neurologist, neurosurgeon, and a radiotherapist made the decision to treat her with 3-D conformational radiotherapy and she received 5040 cGy. No significant change in symptoms has yet been noted.

Discussion

Primary amenorrhea is defined as the absence of menarche by age 16 yr (1). The etiologies can be grouped into three categories based on the hypothalamic–pituitary–ovarian axis (HPO): hypergonadotropic, normogonadotropic and hypogonadotropic. Hypergonadotropic hypogonadism is seen with primary ovarian failure such as in Turner's syndrome. Normogonadotropic amenorrhea encompasses a variety of etiologies including anatomic abnormalities and chronic anovulation syndromes. Decreased gonadotropin secretion is noted in both functional and anatomic disorders of the hypothalamus and pituitary such as Kallmann's syndrome and isolated gonadotropin deficiency; it is also noted in association with anorexia, malnutrition, and exercise-associated amenorrhea.

In our patient, amenorrhea presented with arrested puberty. This is suggestive of a disorder within the HPO axis. Further testing is necessary to determine the etiology. A normal FSH level excludes ovarian failure. Patients with central causes for the amenorrhea typically have low to normal levels of gonadotropins (2). Relative gonadotropin deficiencies may be congenital or acquired. Acquired syndromes include histiocytosis X, inflammatory or vascular diseases, infections involving the central nervous system, trauma, and tumors. Therefore, it is obvious that a study for CNS lesions is an essential part of the evaluation of these patients. A thorough evaluation includes a neurologic exam, fundoscopic exam and imaging study. The introduction of CT scanning and MRI has minimized the value of plain skull films (3). Plain skull films may be helpful in identifying calcification, bony erosion, or hyperostosis (4). However, CT scans and MRI are required to exclude the presence of a mass lesion in the hypothalamic/pituitary area. Although less sensitive than MRI, the CT appearance of many tumors has been characterized and may, in many cases, be quite useful. MRI is highly sensitive and may detect small tumors that would be missed with CT scan. Further, its sensitivity for tumor enlargement and composition makes it an essential tool during conservative management of a brain tumor.

Craniopharyngiomas are benign tumors that occur in the suprasellar and hypothalamic-third ventricular region of the brain. They account for 1.2–4% of all intracranial tumors and 5–10% of all tumors in children (5). At the time of diagnosis, most patients present with endocrine dysfunction, visual disturbance or increased intracranial pressure. It is the most common neoplasm associated with HPO dysfunction and pubertal delay (2). Craniopharyngiomas affect reproductive function by compressing the hypothalamus, the portal system, and/or the pituitary gland. They are relatively slow-growing tumors. Therefore, endocrinologic manifestations of tumor growth may not be acute. Clearly then, it is essential to monitor tumor growth and pituitary function if no intervention is undertaken. The primary therapeutic management is surgical. These tumors, however, can be highly adherent to adjacent structures. Therefore, surgical procedures can be extremely challenging. Operative mortality can be as high as 10%. Surgical morbidity includes stroke, blindness, and permanent endocrine disorders. The majority of patients have permanent postoperative pituitary deficiencies (5). Radiotherapy is effective at shrinking tumor bulk and is often used in combination with surgical management (6). Typical dose requirements are approximately 5500 cGy and may result in significant morbidity. Reported side effects associated with radiation include learning disabilities, visual problems, hypopituitarism, and the development of secondary tumors (7). The patient presented did not have any life-threatening complications from her tumor. Therefore, conservative management was elected. Her headaches worsened and, although not clearly a result of the tumor, surgical management was contemplated. However, because the tumor was not enlarging on MRI and a surgical approach would require a major craniotomy, radiation therapy was performed.

A main management issue in this patient is hormone replacement. Because she is hypoestrogenic, she is at significant risk for osteoporosis and cardiac disease. Estrogen replacement should begin slowly and gradually increased to mimic normal pubertal development. If estrogen is increased too rapidly, normal breast development will not occur. In the patient presented, estrogen is currently being maintained with 1.25 mg of conjugated equine estrogens. It is important to note that young hypoestrogenic women may require doses of estrogen replacement therapy (ERT) twice those administered to postmenopausal women in order to maintain libido and sexual satisfaction. Progestin therapy is essential to prevent endometrial hyperplasia. Although progestin is recommended every month, some studies indicate that less frequent administration is acceptable (8). To assure protection, the progestin should be administered for a minimum of 12 d per administration cycle (9). This patient is receiving 10 mg of medroxyprogesterone acetate for fourteen days every other month.

REFERENCES

1. ACOG. Amenorrhea. In: Technical Bulletin. 1989; No. 128.
2. Grumbach MM, Styne DM. Puberty: ontogeny, neuroendocrinology, physiology, and disorders. In: Wislon JD, Foster DW, eds. Williams Textbook of Endocrinology. WB Saunders, Philadelphia, PA, 1992, pp. 1139–1221.
3. Brody AS. New perspectives in CT and MRI imaging. Nuerol Clin 1991;9:273–286.
4. Black P, Wen PY. Clinical, imaging and laboratory diagnosis of brain tumors. In: Kaye AH, Laws ER, eds. Brain Tumors. Churchill Livingstone, Edinburgh, UK, 1995, pp. 191–214.

5. Samii M, Tatagiba M. Craniopharyngiom. In: Kaye AH, Laws ER, eds. Brain Tumors. Churchill Livingstone, Edinburgh, UK, 1995, pp. 783–894.
6. Wara WM, Sneed PK, Larson DA. The role of radiation therapy in the treatment of craniopharyngioms. Pediatr Neurosurg 1994;21(Suppl 1):98–100.
7. Al-Mefty O, Kersh JE, Routh A, Smith RR. The long-term side effects of radiation therapy for benign brain tumors in adults. J Neurosurg 1990;73:502–512.
8. Ettinger B, Selby J, Citron JT, Vangessel A, Ettinger VM, Hendrickson MR. Cyclic hormone replacement therapy using quarterly progestin. Obstet Gynecol 1994;83:693–700.
9. Whitehead MI. Prevention of endometrial abnormalities. Acta Obstet Gynecol Scand Suppl 1986;134: 81–91.

CASE #3: PREMATURE OVARIAN FAILURE

Case Description

This patient was born at 35 wk's gestation to a diabetic mother. At birth, she was noted to have a slightly enlarged liver; however, this was thought to be an incidental finding attributed to maternal diabetes. At 6 mo, she presented to the emergency room (ER) with a protuberant abdomen and shortness of breath. She was noted to have a large abdominal mass that was diagnosed as a neuroblastoma by biopsy. The mass was surgically excised. Subsequently, she was administered 1800 rads of whole abdominal radiation therapy and did well during her childhood.

Her adolescence was complicated by short stature. An endocrinologic and metabolic source for her slowed growth was investigated and no abnormalities were found. Interval growth remained adequate. In addition, during her adolescence, she underwent two corrective surgeries for strabismus and had multiple episodes of otitis media.

At the age of 11, she presented for the evaluation of the lack of sexual development. An examination at that time revealed Tanner stage 1 breast and pubic hair development. The patient and her mother were reassured that this was not abnormal for her age. However, FSH was measured. She was noted to be hypergonadotropic, consistent with ovarian failure. At the age of 13.5 yr, she was started on 0.3 mg of conjugated equine estrogens. At 14.5 yr, this dose was increased to 0.625 mg and a progestin was added for 12 d each month. Approximately 6 mo later, she was placed on an oral contraceptive pill containing 20 mcg of ethinyl estradiol.

At age 18, she presented to the office with a positive home pregnancy test. A transvaginal ultrasound revealed a 6 wk gestation with cardiac activity. At 16 wk, she began to experience pelvic pressure and spontaneously aborted. A dilation and curettage was performed to deliver the placenta and suggested an intrauterine abnormality. Pathological examination of the fetus revealed an age-appropriate male without obvious anomalies.

In 1993, several months after her spontaneous abortion, she underwent a hysterosalpingogram to evaluate the etiology of her second trimester pregnancy loss. A slight fundal defect was noted consistent with a partial septum vs bicornuate uterus. Because this was a mild defect, no intervention was planned. She was maintained on her hormone replacement regimen.

A second pregnancy was diagnosed in 1996. A cerclage was placed during the beginning of the second trimester. Despite this, she had spontaneous rupture of membranes at 22 wk's gestation. The cerclage was removed and she delivered her fetus without complication. Again, no significant pathology was noted.

Subsequently, she was taken to the operating room to further evaluate her uterine abnormality. Laparoscopy and hysteroscopy confirmed a partial septum that was hysteroscopically resected. In 1999, a third pregnancy was conceived and a cerclage was placed. Each of these pregnancies was conceived as she was taking oral contraceptive agents. Unfortunately, this pregnancy also ended with a second trimester loss.

Discussion

Neuroblastoma, a tumor of the sympathetic nervous system, is the most common malignant tumor in childhood. It comprises 10% of all solid tumors during adolescence and has an annual incidence of 6–8 per million children under 15 yr of age. Surgery, when possible, is the main therapy for these aggressive tumors. However, chemotherapy and radiation therapy have been used to shrink inoperable tumors and, postoperatively, to treat disseminated disease *(1)*. Jacobsen et al. demonstrated that as these tumors are radiosensitive, the response rate is inversely proportional to age *(2)*.

A significant amount of research has been devoted to the studying the effects of radiation exposure on gonadal function. Testes are highly radiosensitive and, therefore, can be irreversibly damaged by small radiation doses *(4)*; Rowley et al. demonstrated that men treated for Hodgkin's disease are azospermic after an average of 233 rads *(5)*. Ovarian sensitivity is related to age; in women 40 yr and older, an average of 600 rads will cause permanent ovarian damage. In younger women, it is estimated that half will have ovarian failure after 1200 rads and 95% will have failure after 2000 rads *(2)*. Wallace et al. followed 19 prepubertal girls who received between 2000 and 3000 rads of whole abdominal radiation for maligancy. Of these women, 18 did not begin spontaneous pubertal development and were noted to have elevated gonadotropin levels *(5)*.

Premature ovarian failure (POF) has traditionally been used to describe a syndrome consisting of amenorrhea, hypergonadotropinism, and hypoestrogenism in young women under the age of 40 yr *(6)*. However, it has been recognized that POF is not simply early menopause. For example, both Rebar et al. and Connolly and Rebar have demonstrated that half of POF patients have hormonal or pathologic evidence of follicular activity *(7,8)*. In a prospective study, Nelson et al. demonstrated ovulation in 20% of patients diagnosed with POF. Clearly, ovarian failure is a misnomer and these patients have some ovarian function; thus, it may be better to designate affected women as having primary hypogonadism or hypergonadotropic hypogonadism. However, because ovarian steroidogenesis is intermittent and unpredictable, ERT should be initiated. As illustrated in this case, ERT can be delayed until the mid-teens when the young woman is emotionally ready for pubertal development. Estrogen should be administered with slowly increasing doses to maximize linear growth and attempt to mimic normal pubertal development. Later, oral contraceptive pills (OCPs) can be administered to provide an adequate estrogen dose; OCPs also provide progestin that protects these women against the development of endometrial cancer.

Several case studies have reported spontaneous pregnancies occurring in patients with POF *(9,10)*. Pregnancies have even occurred in patients without any ovarian follicles noted on biopsy *(8)*. Interestingly and unexplainably, patients, such as this case, have conceived when taking OCPs or other estrogens *(11)*. However, ovulation induction is generally unsuccessful *(2,4,12)*. It appears that perhaps 25% of these women ovulate after the diagnosis of POF is made and 6–8% conceive regardless of the therapy.

In addition to ovarian failure, abdominal radiation therapy has been associated with an increase in perinatal morbidity and spontaneous abortion. Li et al. retrospectively analyzed the pregnancy outcomes of 99 women cured of childhood Wilm's tumors with and without radiotherapy. Those treated with radiation had a fourfold increased risk of low-birth weight infants and a nearly eightfold increased risk of perinatal morbidity in resulting pregnancies *(13)*. In the series by Wallace, no women carried beyond the second trimester *(4)*. Anatomic changes in the uterus and endometrium have been suggested as etiologic. Pridjian et al. published a case report of a patient conceiving 16 yr after treatment with 7000 rad of external beam radiation therapy for clear cell sarcoma *(14)*. This patient required a hysterectomy for placenta percreta diagnosed after a 13-wk spontaneous abortion.

This lends support to the hypothesis that radiation damage affects the uterine micro-structure. MRI has been used to study the immediate and long-term effects of radiation therapy on the uterus *(15)*. Atrophic and fibrotic changes in the myometrium and endometrium can be seen as early as one month after therapy. Radiation exposed premenopausal women had significantly decreased uterine volumes when compared to unexposed controls. Critchley et al. compared the uterine structure of ten women with radiation-induced POF with 22 women with POF unrelated to radiation *(16)*. They treated these women with 28 d of exogenous estrogen therapy and measured uterine length, mean endometrial thickness, and uterine blood flow. All parameters were significantly decreased in the radiation-exposed women. It can be assumed from these studies that radiation therapy can affect pregnancy by disturbing placentation, uterine blood flow, or uterine distensibility.

Interestingly, our patient was also noted to have a uterine septum. This is the first report of a müllerian duct abnormality in a woman with a neuroblastoma as well. Whereas this may be an incidental finding unrelated to her malignancy, Morales et al. previously reported the occurrence of a solitary pelvic kidney and neuroblastoma in a child. In addition, neuroblastoma has been associated with several developmental defects of nonuro-genital origin *(17)*. The incidence of this abnormality is difficult to assess because it may be found in women with normal reproductive outcomes. Tho et al. reported finding a septum in 10% of women with recurrent spontaneous abortion *(18)*. Several authors have demonstrated that, in this set of patients, the surgical removal of the septum significantly decreases pregnancy loss and improves pregnancy outcome *(19–21)*.

As this patient has conceived several times, it is possible that she may conceive again. However, the likelihood of her maintaining a pregnancy is very low. Contraception, therefore, would be recommended. Hormonal contraception, as mentioned earlier, would not be effective for this patient. Recommendations include barrier contraception or an intrauterine device.

REFERENCES

1. Ninane J, Pearson ADJ. Neuroblastoma. In: Pinkerton CR, Plowman PN, eds. Paediatric Oncology. Clinical practice and controversies, 2nd edition. Chapman and Hill Medical, London, UK, 1997, pp. 443–483.
2. Jacobson GM, Sause WI, O'Brien RT. Dose response analysis of neuroblastoma to megavoltage radiation. Am J Clin Oncol 1984;7:693.
3. Lushbaugh CC, Casarett GW. The effects of gonadal irradiation in clinical radiation therapy: a review. Cancer 1976;37:1111–1120.
4. Rowley MJ, Leach DR, Warner GA, Heller CG. Effect of graded doses of ionizing radiation on the human testis. Radiat Res 1972;6:1–6.
5. Wallace WH, Shalet SM, Crowne EC, Morris-Jones PH. Gattameneni HR. Ovarian failure following abdominal irradiation in childhood: natural history and prognosis. Clin Oncol 1989;1:75–79.
6. Morales-Ruehsen M de, Jones GS. Premature ovarian failure. Fertil Steril 1967;18:440.
7. Rebar RW, Erickson GF, Yen SSC. Idiopathic premature ovarian failure: clinical and endocrine characteristics. Fertil Steril 1982;37:35–41.

8. Rebar RW, Connolly HV. Clinical features of young women with hypergonadotropic amenorrhea. Fertil Steril 1990;53:804–810.

9. Kalantaridou SN, Davis SR, Melson LM. Premature ovarian failure. Endocrinol Metab Clin North Am 1998;27(4):989–1006.

10. Rebar RW, Cedars MI. Hypergonadotropic form of amenorrhea in young women. Endocrinol Metab Clin North Am 1992;21(1):173–191.

11. Wright CSW, Jacobs HS. Spontaneous pregnancy in a patient with hypergonadotropic ovarian failure. Br J Obstet Gynaecol 1979;86:389–392.

12. Van Kateren YM, Hoek A, Schoemaker J. Ovulation induction in proemature ovarian failure: a placebo controlled randomized trial combining pituitary suppresion with gonadotropin stimulation. Fertil Steril 1995;64:273–278.

13. Li FP, Gimbrere K, Gelber RD, Sallan SE, Flamant F, Green DM, Heyn RM, Meadows AT. Outcome of pregnancy in survivors of Wilms Tumor. JAMA 1987;257:216–219.

14. Pridjian G, Rich NE, Montag AG. Pregnancy hemoperitoneum and placenta percreta in a patient with previous pelvic irradiation and ovarian failure. Am J Obstet Gynecol 1990;162:1205–1206.

15. Arrivé L, Chang Y, Hricak H, Brescia RJ, Auffermann W, Quivey JM. Radiation-induced uterine changes: MR imaging. Radiology 1989;170:55–58.

16. Critchley HO, Wallace WH, Shalet SM, et al. Abdominal irradiation in childhood; the potential for pregnancy. Br J Obstet Gynaecol 1992;99:392–394.

17. Morales L, Rovira J, Mongard M, Baeta E, Querol FX. Solitary pelvic kidney and neuroblastoma in a child. J Urol 1981;126:249–250.

18. Tho PT, Byrd JR, McDonough PG. Etiologies and subsequent reproductive performance of 100 women with recurrent abortion. Fertil Steril 1979;32:389.

19. Jones HW, Wheeless CR. Salvage of the reproductive potential of women with anomalous development of the Müllerian ducts: 1868:1968:2068. Am J Obstet Gynecol 1969;104:348–364.

20. March CM, Israel R. Hysteroscopic management of recurrent abortion caused y septate uterus. Am J Obstet Gynecol 1987;156:834–842.

21. Goldenberg M, Sivan E, Sharabi Z, Mashiach S, Lipitz S, Seidman DS. Reproductive outcome following hysteroscopic management of intrauterine septum and adhesions. Hum Reprod 1995;10:2663–2665.

CASE #4: HYPOTHALAMIC AMENORRHEA

Case Description

This 28-yr-old Asian-American female presented for the evaluation of secondary amenorrhea at age 24. Menarche began at 13 yr of age and was followed by several years of irregular periods. At age 16, her menses stopped and she remained amenorrheic until her presentation. She denied any significant change in lifestyle or activity. There was no antecedent weight loss or illness. She was not depressed and denied a history of eating disorders or anosmia. Her examination was significant for Tanner stage 4 breast development and Tanner stage 5 axillary and pubic hair development. Her vagina, however, was severely atrophic, suggesting long-term hypoestrogenism. There was no indication of other endocrine disorders.

Serum FSH was <5 mIU/mL, LH was 6 mIU/mL, TSH was 4.1 μU/mL, and prolactin was 18 ng/dL. Because the low gonadotropins suggested a hypothalamic–pituitary abnormality, an MRI was performed to image her sella turcica and this was within normal limits.

Dynamic pituitary testing was performed with 100 μg of GnRH and 25 g of arginine. FSH, LH, prolactin, and growth hormone (GH) responses were within normal limits. Therefore, functional hypothalamic amenorrhea (FHA) was diagnosed. She was placed on a daily dose of 1.25 mg of conjugated equine estrogens (CEE) and a cyclic dose of 10 mg of medroxyprogesterone acetate for days 1–12 of each month. Normal menstrual flow was established with this dose regimen.

The patient remained on estrogen replacement for 6 yr. She returned to the office, with her husband, at age 29 to discuss ovulation induction. After a long discussion, the couple opted for stimulation with intravenous pulsatile GnRH. An intravenous line was placed and attached to a small infusion pump that delivered a dose of 3 mcg of GnRH every 90 min. After 10 d of stimulation, an ultrasound was performed. Several small follicles were noted, but no dominant follicle was seen. Stimulation was continued for an additional 3 wk. Although her endometrial lining thickened (0.9 cm), indicating adequate levels of estrogen, no mature follicles were noted. Therapy was discontinued and menses was induced with progestin therapy. A second course of GnRH infusion was performed. As with the first attempt, growth of multiple follicles was noted without a mature dominant follicle.

Further options for ovulation induction were discussed. These options included continuation of the GnRH pump with adjustment of the amplitude and/or frequency of the pulse, the addition of an opioid inhibitor (i.e., naltrexone) to the pump regimen, and the use of injectable gonadotropins. The couple opted for gonadotropin therapy and began daily injections of 150 mIU of purified urinary gonadotropin. The patient had excellent ovarian stimulation and had three mature follicles on cycle day 12. She was given human chorionic gonadotropin (10,000 IU) to trigger ovulation and instructed to have intercourse the following evening. The couple conceived triplets.

Discussion

This patient had a long-standing history of amenorrhea and a severely atrophic vagina suggesting hypoestrogenism. Because there were no signs of another endocrine disorder, and no history to suggest an anatomic abnormality, the differential diagnosis was primarily limited to disease processes of the hypothalamic–pituitary–gonadal axis. The differential diagnosis included premature ovarian failure (POF), a lesion of the hypothalamic–pituitary region, and hypothalamic chronic anovulation. POF describes a syndrome of hypergonadotropic hypogonadism in women under the age of 40 (1). The diagnosis is easily distinguished from the other causes of estrogen deficiency because FSH is significantly elevated. Treatment for these patients must include hormone replacement therapy (HRT). Although this can be accomplished with "traditional" menopausal replacement regimens, young women will often require higher doses of estrogen to alleviate symptoms such as vaginal dryness. Therefore, replacement with oral contraceptives is often preferred.

Hypogonadotropic hypogonadism is due to abnormalities of the pituitary or hypothalamus. The most common pituitary aberrations are neoplasms and the empty sella syndrome. Prolactin secreting adenomas, the most common pituitary tumor, have been estimated to cause approximately 7.5% of all cases of secondary amenorrhea (2). These tumors arise from clonal expansion of a single lactotrope (3), and the hyperprolactinemia is thought to increase hypothalamic dopamine release through activation of short-loop feedback pathways. Dopamine inhibits GnRH secretion directly through dopamine receptors on the GnRH secreting neuronal cells (4) and indirectly by increasing opioid-dependent inhibition (5). Other pituitary or hypothalamic tumors may result in amenorrhea either by interfering with hormonal feedback mechanisms or by mechanically interfering with the hypothalamus and pituitary.

Hypothalamic amenorrhea is the result of alterations in the hypothalamic secretion of GnRH. GnRH is produced by specialized neuronal cells found in the arcuate nucleus of the hypothalamus. Embryologically, these cells originate from epithelium in the olfactory pit and migrate from the nasal region to the medial basal hypothalamus. GnRH is secreted in a pulsatile fashion, via the tuberoinfundibular tract, into the portal venous system connecting the hypothalamus to the pituitary. Because its half-life is approximately 2 min, and because very little hormone is present in the peripheral circulation, direct measurement is impractical. However, because GnRH stimulates the pulsatile release of FSH and LH, measurements of peripheral LH pulses have provided estimates of GnRH pulse frequency and amplitude. In the follicular phase of the normal menstrual cycle, the frequency is approximately one pulse every 90 min; in the luteal phase, pulse frequency decreases and the amplitude of the pulse increases *(6)*.

Amenorrhea also may result from congenital or destructive lesions of the hypothalamus. Kallmann's syndrome results from the failure of the GnRH neurons to migrate from the olfactory placode to the medial basal hypothalamus. Patients have an eunuchoid habitus, incomplete development of secondary sexual characteristics, and amenorrhea *(7)*. Because of its association with the olfactory placode, these patients frequently present with anosmia. Hand–Schüller–Christian disease, also known as Langerhans' cell histiocytosis, is a rare cause of hypothalamic destruction by eosinophillic granulomas resulting in panhypopituitarism. These patients present with a myriad of symptoms, often including diabetes insipidus, visual disturbances, growth deficiency, obesity, and hypersomnolence. Similarly, injuries to the hypothalamus may present with a number of symptoms depending on the extent of damage and the age of the patient at the time of injury.

Functional hypothalamic amenorrhea (FHA) occurs in women without any apparent organic abnormality of the hypothalamus, pituitary or ovaries. Although studies have shown that GnRH pulsatility is slowed in these women, the etiology of this slowed pulse frequency in unclear *(8)*. Because the disease is associated with stress and exercise, researchers have investigated the role of opioids on hypothalamic–pituitary–ovarian function. During stress, the hypothalamus produces increased quantities of corticotropin releasing hormone (CRH) that stimulates the increased release of β-endorphins from the pituitary. These endogenous opiates may affect menstrual regulation by stimulating the release of prolactin and inhibiting the release of TSH. To investigate the role of this pathway in hypothalamic amenorrhea, several investigators have administered naloxone, an inhibitor of μ and ε opioid receptors, to women with FHA and have demonstrated that naloxone is effective in restoring normal menstrual function in some (but not all) subjects *(9)*. Similarly, dopamine blockade will restore normal LH pulse frequency in some women with FHA *(10)*. These studies strongly support a role of the opioidergic and dopaminergic systems in these patients; however, because all patients do not respond, these studies also suggest that FHA is a heterogeneous process with multiple etiologies. Affected hormones may include gonadotropins, prolactin, and TSH that are subtly decreased and cortisol and growth hormone which are subtly increased *(11)*.

The diagnosis of FHA is a diagnosis of exclusion. Therefore, patients should be evaluated for organic causes of hypothalamic–pituitary dysfunction. The history should inquire about symptoms of endocrine disorders, neurologic changes, antecedent illnesses, changes in weight, changes in activity, and major life events. A careful assessment should be made to evaluate the individual for depression and eating disorders. The physical examination should include a neurologic and fundoscopic assessment and a survey for signs of endocrine diseases.

Imaging and laboratory studies should be used to confirm the suspicion of hypothalamic amenorrhea. An MRI is the preferred method to assess for structural lesions of the hypothalamus and pituitary gland. In addition to its ability to image this area with remarkable detail, an MRI can identify developmental defects of the olfactory placode associated with Kallmann's syndrome. Measurement of FSH, LH, TSH, and prolactin is essential. If hypogonadotropinism is present, dynamic pituitary testing may be helpful.

The treatment of infertility is accomplished with ovulation induction. Possible therapies include the use of pulsatile GnRH and injectable gonadotropin therapy. Pulsatile GnRH is generally thought to be safer because the risk of inducing multiple follicles is much smaller. Several studies, using a wide range of dosing regimens, have evaluated the use of intravenous (iv) and subcutaneous (SC) GnRH therapy to induce ovulation. Subcutaneous administration results in a slow absorption and a slow rise of gonadotropin. An iv administration is more physiologic and is more successful in inducing ovulation when compared to SC administration (~90% vs ~75%). Nonetheless, rates of conception are very similar. Intravenous dosages range from 1 μg to 100 μg. Miller et al. demonstrated that an intravenous pulse of 1 μg corresponds to the lower range of pituitary portal blood concentrations *(12)*. Using this dose, Liu and Yen reported an 82% ovulation rate and 24.4% pregnancy rate per cycle *(13)*. Miller et al. demonstrated that a dose of 75 ng/kg (~3–4 μg) improved the ovulation induction to 95% and found no benefit to higher doses *(14)*. However, higher doses may be necessary when using the SC route. It should be noted that the FDA has only approved pulsatile GnRH therapy for iv administration.

The major complication associated with the use of GnRH therapy is the potential for infection of the indwelling catheter. Hopkins et al., in a prospective study of iv GnRH therapy, found that 11% catheter tips were colonized with bacteria and 2% of women had positive blood cultures. However, with the exception of local inflammation, there were no cases of clinical sepsis *(15)*. Hyperstimulation has never been reported with the use of low-dose GnRH therapy and most pregnancies are singleton.

Patients who conceive with GnRH will need luteal support for their pregnancy until the placenta begins to make adequate levels of hCG. GnRH pulses can be continued during this time period, hCG can be given, or intramuscular progesterone (50 mg/d) can be given. These techniques are identical with regard to their efficacy.

The etiology of the failure of GnRH pump therapy in this patient is unclear. Some follicular development occurred, suggesting that gonadotropins were stimulated. Therefore, changing the pulse frequency to 60 min or increasing the dose to 5 μg may have been effective. This patient has a strong family history of PCOS. It is interesting that, when GnRH pulses were established, she developed polycystic appearing ovaries. Because PCOS has a strong hereditary component, it is conceivable that she has an underlying endocrinopathy similar to PCOS. This may also be further supported by her vigorous response to injectable gonadotropins.

Clomiphene citrate is often ineffective because it acts at the hypothalamus. However, because patients with FHA have low levels of GnRH production (as opposed to no production), clomiphene induction of ovulation may be possible for some affected women. The patient had extremely low levels of gonadotropins; therefore, we would not expect her to respond to clomiphene. Opioid and dopamine antagonists have been utilized to induce ovulation in FHA patients. Although several investigators report success with these drugs in select groups of patients, these results have not been consistent. These agents are not typically used in clinical practice.

REFERENCES

1. Morales-Ruehsen M de, Jones GS. Premature ovarian failure. Fertil Steril 1967;18:440–461.
2. Reindollar RH, Novak M, Tho SPT, McDonough PG. Adult-onset amenorrhea: a study of 262 patients. Am J Obstet Gynecol 1986;155:531–543.
3. Shimon I, Melmed S. Genetic basis of endocrine disease. Pituitary tumor pathogenesis. J Clin Endocrinol Metab 1997;82:1675–1681.
4. Cook CB, Nippoldt, TB, Kletter GB, Kelch RP, Marchall JC. Naloxone increases the frequency of pulsatile lutenizing hormone secretion in women with hyperprolactinemia. J Clin Endocrinol Metab 1991; 73:1099–1105.
5. Quigley ME, Sheehan KL, Casper RF, Yen SSC. Evidence for increased dopaminergic and opioid activity in patients with hypothalamic hypogonadotropic amenorrhea. J Clin Endocrinol Metab 1980; 50:949–954.
6. Filicori M, Santoro N, Merriam GR, Crowley WF. Characterization of the physiological pattern of episodic gonadotropin secretion throughout the human menstrual cycle. JCEM 1986;62:1136–1144.
7. Liu JH. Hyptholamic amenorrhea: clinical perspective, pathophysiology and management. Am J Obstet Gynecol 1990;163:1732–1736.
8. Reame NE, Saunder SE, Case GD, Kelch RP, Marshall JC. Pulsatile gonadotropin secretion in women with hypothalamic amenorrhea: evidence that reduced frequency of gonadotropin-releasing hormone secretion is the mechanism of persistent anovulation. J Clin Endocrinol Metab 1985;61:851–858.
9. Khoury SA, Reame NE, Kelch RP, Marshall JC. Diurnal patterns of pulsatile lutenizing hormone secretion in hypothalamic amenorrhea: reproducibility and responses to opiate blockade and an α_2-adrenergic agonist. J Clin Endocrinol Metab 1987;64:755–762.
10. Quigley ME, Judd SJ, Gilland GB, Yen SSC. Effects of a dopamine antagonist on the release of gonadotropin and prolactin in normal women and women with hyperprolactinemic anovulation. J Clin Endorcrinol Metab 1979;48:718–720.
11. Berga S, Mortola JF, Suh GB, Laughlin G, Pham P, Yen SSC. Neuroendocrine aberrations in women with functional hypothalamic amenorrhea. J Clin Endocrinol Metab 1989;68:301–308.
12. Miller DS, Reid RR, Cetel NS, Rebar RW, Yen SSC. Pulsatile administration of low dose gonadotropin-releasing hormone: ovulation and pregnancy in women with hypothalamic amenorrhea. JAMA 1983; 250:2937–2941.
13. Liu JH, Yen SSC. The use of gonadotropin-releasing hormone for the induction of ovulation. Clinic Obstet Gynecol 1984;27:975–982.
14. Martin K, Santoro, N, Hall, J, Filicori M, Wierman M, Crowley WF. Management of ovulatory disorders with pulsatile gonadotropin releasing hormone. J Clin Endocrinol Metab 1990;71:1081A–1081G.
15. Hopkins CC, Hall JE, Santoro NF, Martin KA, Filicori M, Crowley WF. Closed intravenous administration of gonadotropin-releasing hormone: safety of extended peripheral intravenous catheterization. Obstet Gynecol 1989;74:267–270.

15

Endocrine Problems in Pregnancy

Lisa P. Purdy, MD, CM and Boyd E. Metzger, MD

CONTENTS

CASE #1: A PREGNANT WOMAN WITH ADDISON'S DISEASE AND HYPOTHYROIDISM

Case Description

A 34-yr-old Caucasian female was managed by her primary physician for a history of Addison's disease and hypothyroidism. She was admitted in August with a 4 d history of generalized weakness, postural lightheadedness, and a marked increase in muscle cramping.

She had been diagnosed with Addison's disease at age 17 and subsequently treated with prednisone. She had not been treated with fludrocortisone, but had always craved salt and had numerous admissions for Addisonian crises over the previous several years with no clear precipitants. She described increasing myalgias over a 5-mo period. Four days prior to admission, she presented to her primary physician with increasing fatigue and muscle weakness. As she appeared Cushingoid, her prednisone was decreased from 5 mg tid to 5 mg bid and she was started on fludrocortisone 0.1 mg daily. She experienced increasing muscle weakness and cramping over the subsequent 4 d prior to her admission. She denied abdominal pain, nausea, or diarrhea.

Hypothyroidism had been diagnosed at age 19. She was treated with levothyroxine 0.1 mg daily, but had experienced progressive weight gain, dry skin, brittle nails, hair loss, cold intolerance, and constipation over the previous year. The levothyroxine dose

From: *Contemporary Endocrinology: Challenging Cases in Endocrinology*
Edited by: M. E. Molitch © Humana Press Inc., Totowa, NJ

was increased to 0.125 mg daily 2 mo prior to admission when her thyroid stimulating hormone (TSH) was found to be 9.13 μU/mL. TSH normalized to 0.63 μU/mL, but she experienced little symptomatic improvement.

Her menarche was at age 12 with regular menses, originally. She experienced oligomenorrhea with the onset of her Addison's disease, with only two cycles per year. No investigations were initiated, and no treatment was given. Despite ongoing oligomenorrhea, she became pregnant at age 32, and had a therapeutic abortion because of worsening of her Addison's disease. Her last menstrual period was 2 mo prior to admission, and she denied sexual activity during that interval.

She had a history of hyperlipidemia (cholesterol 294 mg/dL, triglycerides 366 mg/dL, HDL 54 mg/dL, and LDL 167 mg/dL) and was originally treated with simvastatin, but complained of myalgias. Four months prior to admission, she was switched to cholestyramine 4 g bid, taken 1 h after her other medications. The myalgias did not improve with the discontinuation of the simvastatin or with the increase in her levothyroxine and normalization of her TSH.

Her family history was significant for thyroid disease in her sister and paternal grandfather, systemic lupus erythematosus (SLE) in her father, and ischemic heart disease in her father in his 50's.

On examination, her BP was 90/60 mmHg with a 20-mm orthostatic drop, and a supine heart rate of 115 and regular. She was Cushingoid with central obesity, preauricular, supraclavicular, and cervical fat pads, and pigmented striae on her breasts and abdomen. She had diffusely increased skin pigmentation, particularly on the buccal mucosa, areolae, and perineum. There was only minimal sexual hair in her axillae and pubic areas. She had proximal muscle girdle weakness but normal reflexes.

Laboratory values on admission included a sodium of 125 mEq/L, potassium 4.8 mEq/L, chloride 87 mEq/L, and bicarbonate 19 mEq/L, glucose 91 mg/dL, BUN 10 mg/dL, creatinine 0.7 mg/dL, and magnesium 1.1 mEq/L. She was treated with methylprednisolone 40 mg IV + 4 L of 0.9 NaCl and 2 g MgSO4. She was found to be 9 wk pregnant.

After resolution of the crisis, her electrolytes required frequent monitoring during the pregnancy. Her sodium fell as low as 134 mEq/L and potassium rose to 4.4 mEq/L with a bicarbonate of 20 mEq/L. She required steadily increasing doses of fludrocortisone up to 0.6 mg/d, in order to stabilize her electrolytes in the normal range throughout the final half of her pregnancy. Her Cushingoid appearance and proximal muscle girdle weakness resolved, despite requiring hydrocortisone 40 mg daily, which she took in a tid dosing of 20/10/10. She did not exhibit peripheral edema or hypertension throughout her pregnancy. She was given stress doses of hydrocortisone during labor and at delivery, which occurred without complication. Postpartum, her Addison's disease was managed with prednisone 5 mg bid and fludrocortisone 0.1 mg daily, which maintained her potassium levels in the normal range.

She remained euthyroid with a TSH of 0.9 to 1.12 μU/mL on levothyroxine 0.15 mg daily throughout the pregnancy. Her magnesium ranged from 1.3 to 1.5 mEq/L on magnesium oxide 64 mg qid.

A 1 h postbreakfast glucose was noted to be elevated at 181 mg/dL. At 19 wk gestational age, she had a 3-h 100 g glucose tolerance test. Results were: fasting glucose 120 mg/dL, 1-h 297 mg/dL, 2-h 332 mg/dL, and 3-h 320 mg/dL. She was treated with diet and a mixed-split insulin regimen of regular and NPH. By term, she required more than 120 U/d in divided doses. Her glucose levels were well controlled in the 61 to 92 mg/dL range prior to meals. She delivered a boy at 39 wk gestational age, weighing 3410 g. Her post-partum 75-g OGTT revealed a fasting glucose of 67 mg/dL with a 2 h value of 80 mg/dL.

One year subsequent to her pregnancy, she developed premature menopause, which was treated with conjugated estrogen 0.625 mg/mcdroxyprogesterone 5 mg daily. She developed alopecia of her eyebrows, eyelashes, axillary and pubic hair. In addition, she was diagnosed with systemic lupus erythematosus, involving her skin and joints. She experienced a 35-lb. weight loss over 14 mo associated with large volume diarrhea with steatorrhea. Endoscopic biopsy was negative for celiac disease.

Discussion

Multiple changes occur in adrenal steroid metabolism during normal pregnancy. Corticotropin releasing hormone (CRH) levels, primarily of placental origin, increase substantially and modulate both maternal and fetal adrenal axes (1). Unlike the hypothalamic-pituitary-adrenal axis, increasing glucocorticoid levels provide a positive feedback on placental CRH production, which does not exhibit a circadian rhythm (2). A CRH-binding protein is present in maternal plasma and in the amniotic fluid, binding CRH with high affinity and reducing its bioactivity (3). The levels of CRH-binding protein are similar to those found in the nonpregnant woman until the third trimester of pregnancy, when they fall to one-third the previous levels (4). The unbound fraction of CRH stimulates maternal adrenocorticotropic hormone (ACTH) secretion, contributing to the relative hypercortisolism of pregnancy.

ACTH levels increase progressively during the second and third trimesters as a result of both pituitary and placental secretion, and are not suppressed by rising glucocorticoid levels. Despite the increase in placental ACTH, the normal maternal circadian rhythm of ACTH secretion is maintained throughout pregnancy (2).

The fetoplacental unit has a marked capacity for steroidogenesis, which provides the precursors for placental estrogen production, and plays a role in fetal lung maturation and in the onset of labor. At the same time, maternal cortisol levels increase two- to three-fold throughout pregnancy (5,6). The maternal zona fasciculata hypertrophies (7), and maternal cortisol production increases mildly, though still maintaining a diurnal variation. There is an estrogen-stimulated increase in circulating transcortin, resulting in an increase in total cortisol levels and a decreased rate of cortisol clearance (8). Free cortisol levels also increase, in part because of displacement of cortisol from transcortin by progesterone (5).

The renin-angiotensin-aldosterone system demonstrates numerous changes as well. Despite the increase in plasma volume with pregnancy, plasma renin activity increases four-fold and plateaus at 20 wk gestational age (9), in part mediated by the pregnancy rise in PGI2. Angiotensin II levels increase approximately three-fold by term, although there is resistance to its pressor effects (10). Plasma mineralocorticoid levels increase five- to seven-fold during gestation (6,9), although the zona glomerulosa does not enlarge (7). Whereas aldosterone levels increase, its secretion continues to respond normally to physiologic stimuli and varies inversely to changes in volume or dietary salt (11). The increase in aldosterone secretion correlates with the pregnancy increase in GFR and with progesterone (12), which competitively inhibits sodium retention by aldosterone at the distal renal tubules. Progesterone also demonstrates an antikaliuretic effect (11), and there has been a report of amelioration of hypokalemia during pregnancy in a woman with primary aldosteronism *(13)*.

Autoimmune Addison's disease generally causes no problems with fetal development, as the fetoplacental unit largely controls its own steroid milieu. Maternal antiadrenal autoantibodies may cross the placenta, but usually not in sufficient quantities to cause fetal or neonatal adrenal insufficiency *(14)*. Although Osler observed intrauterine growth retardation in offspring of women with Addison's disease *(15)*, this observation has not been supported in most subsequent case series.

Many clinical features of Addison's disease are found in normal pregnancies, including weakness, lightheadedness, syncope, nausea, vomiting, and increased pigmentation. Addisonian hyperpigmentation may be distinguished from chloasma of pregnancy by its presence on the mucous membranes, on extensor surfaces, and over nonexposed areas. The adrenal insufficiency is associated with laboratory findings of hyponatremia, hyperkalemia, hypoglycemia, eosinophilia, and lymphocytosis. Plasma total cortisol levels may fall in the normal "nonpregnant" range as a result of the increase in transcortin concentrations but free cortisol levels are low.

Maternal replacement doses of corticosteroids usually are not different from those required in the nonpregnant state, except during the course of "morning sickness" or during labor and delivery. Mineralocorticoid replacement requirements usually do not change during gestation, though some clinicians have decreased fludrocortisone intake in the third trimester in an attempt to treat Addisonian patients who develop preeclampsia *(16)*. The patient described in this case report was atypical in her requirement for increased fludrocortisone in order to avoid hyponatremia and hyperkalemia during gestation. This was presumed to be a progesterone effect.

The adrenal crisis experienced by the patient when she presented in the first trimester of pregnancy may have several etiologic factors. These include increasing hormonal requirements secondary to her pregnancy, the heat of August, and the potential for decreased absorption of her hormone replacement in the presence of cholestyramine therapy.

This patient had polyglandular autoimmune syndrome, which continued to manifest in the postpartum period. Appropriate therapy is defined by the individual conditions that are present and the awareness of potentially silent disorders, such as pernicious anemia. During gestation, she required a mild increase in her thyroid-hormone replacement, as expected. The gestational diabetes did not appear to be related to the polyglandular syndrome, as her hyperglycemia totally resolved postpartum. Islet cell antibody and glutamic acid decarboxylase (GAD) antibody levels were unmeasureable.

REFERENCES

1. Goland RS, Wardlaw SL, Stark RE, et al. High levels of corticotropin-releasing hormone immunoactivity in maternal and fetal plasma during pregnancy. J Clin Endocrinol Metab 1986;63:1199–1203.
2. Magiakou MA, Mastorakos G, Rabin D, et al. Placental CRH secretion and the maternal hypothalamic-pituitary-adrenal axis in human pregnancy. Clin Endocrinol 1996;44:419–428.
3. Suda T, Iwashita M, Tozawa F, et al. Characterization of corticotropin-releasing hormone binding protein in human plasma by chemical cross-linking and its binding during pregnancy. J Clin Endocrinol Metab 1988;67:1278–1283.
4. Linton EA, Perkins AV, Woods RJ, et al. Corticotropin releasing hormone-binding protein (CRH-BP): plasma levels decrease during the third trimester of normal human pregnancy J Clin Endocrinol Metab 1993;76:260–262.

5. Demey-Ponsart E, Foidart JM, Sulon J, et al. Serum CBG, free and total cortisol and circadian patterns of adrenal function in normal pregnancy. J Steroid Biochem 1982;16:165–169.

6. Dorr HG, Heller A, Versmold HT, et al. Longitudinal study of progestins, mineralocorticoids, and glucocorticoids throughout human pregnancy. J Clin Endocrinol Metab 1989;68:863–868.

7. Whiteley HJ, Stoner HB. The effect of pregnancy on the adrenal cortex. J Endocrinol 1957;14:325.

8. Rosenthal HE, Slaunwhite WR, Sandberg AA. Transcortin, a corticosteroid-binding protein of plasma: Cortisol and progesterone interplay and unbound levels of these steroids in pregnancy. J Clin Endocrinol Metab 1969;29:352–367.

9. Wilson M, Morganti AA, Zervoudakis I, et al. Blood pressure, the renin-aldosterone system and sex steroids throughout normal pregnancy. Am J Med 1980;8:97–104.

10. Gant NF, Daley GL, Chand S, et al. A study of angiotensin II pressor response throughout primigravid pregnancy. J Clin Invest 1973;52:2682–2689.

11. Ehrlich EN, Lindheimer MD. Effect of administered mineralocorticoids or ACTH in pregnant women. Attenuation of kaliuretic influence of mineralocorticoids during pregnancy. J Clin Invest 1972;51:1301–1309.

12. Jones KM, Lloyd-Jones R, Riondel A, et al. Aldosterone secretion and metabolism in normal men and women and in pregnancy. Acta Endocrinol 1959;30:321.

13. Biglieri EG, Slaton Jr, PE. Pregnancy and primary aldosteronism. J Clin Endocrinol Metab 1967;27:1628–1632.

14. Gamlen TR, Aynsley-Green A, Irvine WJ, McCallum CJ. Immunological studies in the neonate of a mother with Addison's disease and diabetes mellitus. Clin Exp Immunol 1977;28:192–195.

15. Osler M. Addison's disease and pregnancy. Acta Endocrinol 1962;41:67.

16. Normington EM, Davies D. Hypertension and oedema complicating pregnancy in Addison's disease. Br Med J 1972;1:148–149.

CASE #2: PREGNANCY IN A PATIENT WITH *MEN-2*

Case Description

A 21-yr-old Caucasian woman with known uterine didelphys (double uterus and cervix) was sent for an obstetrical ultrasound at 22 wk gestational age. During the course of the ultrasound, the pregnancy was noted to be in the left uterine cavity and a left adrenal mass was detected. Fetal growth was measured at the 41st percentile for gestational age.

The patient had a 2 yr history of daily "panic attacks" associated with an abrupt onset of anxiety, palpitations, occasional chest tightness, lightheadedness to the point of pre-syncope, headache, and diaphoresis. These symptoms resolved over the course of several minutes. She described occasional symptoms of mild postural lightheadedness. She had no documentation of hypertension during the course of her pregnancy.

Her family history revealed that her father died during a motor vehicle accident and was discovered on autopsy to have bilateral pheochromocytomas. Family history was also positive for colon carcinoma in her maternal grandmother and lung cancer in her maternal grandfather. Her paternal grandparents had "thyroid problems" of unknown type. Four paternal aunts and her father had SLE. A paternal aunt had diabetes mellitus.

On examination, her vital signs included a supine BP of 100/70 mmHg with a heart rate of 90 and regular, with standing BP of 90/60 mmHg with a heart rate of 118 and regular. There was no evidence of neurofibromatosis or café-au-lait spots. Thyroid examination was normal. She had a II/VI systolic ejection murmur on cardiac auscultation. The rest of her examination was unremarkable except for a gravid uterus of appropriate fundal height. Fetal heart rate was in the 140s.

An MRI revealed a markedly enlarged left adrenal gland containing a large cystic structure, 7 cm in diameter surrounded by a rind of adrenal tissue, with high signal on T2 weighted sequences. She also had right adrenal enlargement of $4.2 \times 4 \times 3.8$ cm with a heterogeneous appearance. There also appeared to be a 1.2×0.6-cm left paraaortic lymph node on T2 weighted imaging. A 24-h urine collection showed that VMA was elevated at 21.4 mg (normal <8), with normetanephrine 4.6 ng (normal <0.89), metanephrines 10.0 ng (normal <0.39), and total metanephrines 14.6 ng (normal <1.2). She was treated with lactated Ringer's for volume replacement and started on phenoxybenzamine therapy, titrating up to 60 mg bid. Her blood pressure ranged from 93/43 to 116/61 with mild postural tachycardia. Eventually she required propranolol 10 mg tid to control tachycardia, and her phenoxybenzamine dose was decreased to 40 mg bid. She remained normotensive with no postural changes. Her symptoms of panic attacks resolved for the first time in 2 yr.

Her 1 h oral glucose challenge at 26 wk gestational age was normal at 102 mg/dL. In view of her family history of pheochromocytoma, she had a screening calcitonin level of 37 pg/mL (normal 0–6.3) and an ionized calcium of 4.9 mg/dL (normal 4.75–5.20). A total calcium was measured at 9.4 mg/dL with an intact PTH of <2.7 pg/mL (normal 0–55).

As she was stable on the phenoxybenzamine and propranolol therapy, definitive therapy for her pheochromocytoma was deferred until after delivery. In view of the uterine didelphys, premature labor was a risk. Therefore, operative delivery of the fetus, a frank breech presentation, was scheduled after confirmation of fetal lung maturity. The patient underwent a low transverse caesarean section at 36 4/7 wk gestational age under an epidural anesthetic. A live female infant weighing 2728 g, Apgars 9 and 9, was delivered from the left uterine horn without fundal pressure and without incident. Maternal blood pressure remained in the 110–128/72–82 mmHg range intraoperatively. Postoperative pain management included the regional anesthetic and PCA pump. Phenoxybenzine and propranol were continued.

Two weeks later, she underwent bilateral adrenalectomy using an anterior subcostal approach. Both adrenals contained encapsulated masses. The left adrenal mass was 10 cm in maximal diameter and had central cystic necrosis. Her right adrenal was 6.5 cm in maximal diameter with a rim of normal adrenal tissue. The retroperitoneal lymph node was not identified. Her blood pressure was well controlled throughout the surgery. She was discharged on hydrocortisone 20 mg qam and 10 mg qpm. At the time, she was normotensive with a BP of 122/58 mmHg (without medication) and a heart rate of 72, and had no further postural complaints. A repeat MRI of the abdomen revealed no evidence of hyperintensity on T2 weighted images 6 mo postoperatively.

Postpartum, her calcitonin level remained elevated at 44 pg/mL (nomal 0–4.6). *RET* protooncogene testing revealed a mutation in exon 11 at codon 634, changing cysteine to arginine. She had a total thyroidectomy, which revealed 2 foci of medullary carcinoma measuring 0.5 and 0.3 cm, with bilateral satellite foci of C-cell hyperplasia. Postoperatively, her calcitonin was unmeasurable.

Discussion

Pheochromocytoma in pregnancy is associated with a dramatic increase in maternal and fetal morbidity and mortality, particularly if the diagnosis is unrecognized prior to delivery. The typical presentation of exacerbation of hypertension is frequently mistaken for pregnancy-induced hypertension or preeclampsia *(1)*. Potential maternal complications include hemorrhage into the neoplasm, hemodynamic collapse, myocardial infarction, cardiac arrhythmias, congestive heart failure, and cerebral hemorrhage. These risks may increase with increasing gestational age as the enlarging uterus and actively moving fetus may compress the neoplasm.

There is minimal placental transfer of catecholamines (2,3), likely resulting from high placental concentrations of catechol-O-methyltransferase and monoamine oxidase (2,4). Adverse fetal effects are a result of catecholamine-induced uteroplacental vasoconstriction and placental insufficiency (5–7), and of maternal hypertension, hypotension, or vascular collapse.

As always, diagnosis of pheochromocytoma requires a high index of suspicion. Preconception screening of families known to have *MEN-2* or familial paraganglioma is optimal. Availability of *RET* protooncogene testing has simplified this process in the former group. In addition, patients with *MEN*-2A are more likely to have paroxysmal hypertension and have higher rates of bilateral neoplasms than those with sporadic pheochromocytoma (8). Genetic testing for families with a paraganglioma history are being developed. Of interest is the inheritance pattern found in such families. Approximately half of the families involved demonstrate paternal transmission of this condition, associated with particular gene mutations (9). Individuals with neurofibromatosis (10), von Hipple-Lindau disease (11), or retinal angiomatosis should also be screened. Pheochromocytoma also should be considered in pregnant women with severe or paroxysmal hypertension, particularly when occurring in the first half of gestation or in association with episodic symptoms of palpitations, anxiety, diaphoresis, or headaches. Orthostatic hypotension is a common finding. Symptoms may present or worsen during pregnancy because of the increased vascularity of the tumor and mechanical factors such as pressure from the expanding uterus or fetal movement (6).

Biochemical diagnosis of pheochromocytoma is unchanged from the nonpregnant state, as catecholamine metabolism is not altered by pregnancy *per se* (12). Urinary catecholamines may be modestly elevated in preeclampsia and other serious pregnancy complications requiring hospitalization, though they remain normal in mild preeclampsia or pregnancy-induced hypertension (13). Catecholamine levels normally rise at the onset of labor until the second day postpartum (14). If possible, methyldopa and labetolol should be discontinued prior to the biochemical investigation, as these agents may interfere with the quantification of the catecholamines and VMA (15). Provocative testing should be avoided because of the increased risk of maternal and fetal mortality. Tumor localization with MRI, with high intensity signals noted on T_2-weighted images, provides the best sensitivity without exposure to ionizing radiation. Metaiodobenzylguanidine (MIBG) scans are contraindicated in pregnancy.

Initial medical management involves α blockade, with phentolamine, phenoxybenzamine, prazosin, or labetolol. Phenoxybenzamine is considered the preferred agent as it provides long-acting, stable, noncompetitive blockade (6). Metyrosine has also been used to reduce catecholamine synthesis in a pregnancy complicated by malignant pheochromocytoma (16). β blockade is reserved for treating maternal tachycardia which persists after full α blockade and volume repletion. Placental transfer of phenoxybenzamine occurs (17), but is generally thought to be safe (18,19). β blockers may be associated with fetal bradycardia and with intrauterine growth retardation, when used early in pregnancy (12,20). These potential fetal risks are small compared to the risk of fetal wastage from unblocked high maternal levels of catecholamines.

The optimal timing of surgical excision of the neoplasm is uncertain, but may depend on the success of the medical management. Hemorrhage into the tumor, pressure from the uterus, motion of the fetus, and labor contractions are all stimuli that may lead to an acute crisis and potential maternal and fetal mortality. In the first half of pregnancy, surgical excision may proceed once adequate α blockade is established, although there is a higher risk of miscarriage with first-trimester surgery. In the early second trimester, abortion is less likely and the size of the uterus will not make excision difficult. If the pheochromocytoma is not recognized until the second half of gestation, increasing uterine size makes surgical exploration difficult. Successful laparoscopic excision of a pheochromocytoma has been described in the second trimester of pregnancy *(21)*. Other options include combined cesarean delivery and tumor resection or delivery followed by tumor resection at a later date. If possible, delivery is delayed until the fetus reaches sufficient maturity to reduce postpartum morbidity, providing successful medical management exists. As this patient was well controlled on her medical therapy, delivery was delayed until fetal lung maturity was confirmed with an amniocentesis.

Although successful vaginal delivery has been reported *(22)*, it is thought to be associated with higher risk of maternal mortality than cesarean section. Labor may result in uncontrolled release of catecholamines secondary to pain and uterine contractions *(23)*. Severe maternal hypertension may lead to placental ischemia and fetal hypoxia. However, intensive pain management with epidural anesthesia and avoidance of mechanical compression, employing techniques of passive descent and instrumental delivery, may make vaginal delivery a possibility for patients that are well controlled with medical therapy. As this patient was nulliparous with a frank breech presentation of the fetus, vaginal delivery was not an option nor was version of the fetus, owing to the risk of potentiating catecholamine release. Premature labor was likely in view of her uterine didelphys. Therefore, a cesarean section was scheduled upon confirmation of fetal lung maturity.

There is no available information regarding the impact of maternal use of phenoxybenzamine on the nursing neonate. In this case, the patient pumped and discarded her breast milk until the excision of her pheochromocytomas, then initiated breastfeeding. Her daughter will be assessed with *RET* protooncogene testing.

Neither clinical nor histologic criteria may distinguish benign from malignant pheochromocytoma. Therefore, lifetime follow-up of all cases is required, particularly during future pregnancies.

Calcitonin levels may be elevated in individuals with pheochromocytoma, and normalize after excision of the neoplasm *(24,25)*. Studies of calcitonin levels in pregnancy provide variable results. Some have found no significant change *(26)*, whereas other investigators report increased concentrations longitudinally through gestation *(27,28)*. The supposition is that the calcitonin may protect the maternal skeleton from excessive resorption *(27)*. In this case, the elevation in calcitonin persisted postpartum and postoperative excision of the pheochromocytoma. This finding and the subsequent positive result of her *RET* protooncogene testing confirmed the diagnosis of *MEN-2*, requiring thyroidectomy for treatment of her medullary carcinoma.

REFERENCES

1. Freier DT, Thompson NW. Pheochromocytoma and pregnancy: the epitome of high risk. Surgery 1993; 114:1148–1152.

2. Saarikoski S. Fate of noradrenaline in the human fetoplacental unit. Acta Physiol Scand 1974;421 (Suppl):1–84.

3. Dahia PLM, Hayashida CY, Strunz C, Abelin N, Toledo SPA. Low cord blood levels of catecholamine from a newborn of a pheochromocytoma patient. Eur J Endocrinol 1994;130:217–219.

4. Barzel US, Barlian Z, Runmery G, et al. Pheochromocytoma and pregnancy. Am J Obstet Gynecol 1964; 89:519–521.

5. Bakri YN, Ingemansson SE, Ali A, Parikh S. Pheochromocytoma and pregnancy: report of three cases. Acta Obstet Gynecol Scand 1992;71:301–304.

6. Harper MA, Murnaghan GA, Kennedy L, Hadden DR, Atkinson AB. Phaeochromocytoma in pregnancy: five cases and a review of the literature. Br J Obstet Gynaecol 1989;96:594–606.

7. Combs CA, Easterling TR, Schmucker BC. Hemodynamic observations during paroxysmal hypertension in a pregnancy with pheochromocytoma. Obstet Gynecol 1989;74:439–442.

8. Falterman CJ, Kreisberg R. Pheochromocytoma: clinical diagnosis and management. South Med J 1982;75:321–328.

9. Baysal BE, Willett-Brozick JE, Lawrence EC, et al. Genetic heterogeneity in hereditary paraganglioma (PGL): SDHD is the primary locus in imprinted PGL pedigrees. Am J Hum Genet 2000;66(Suppl):385f.

10. Kalff V, Shapiro B, Lloyd R, et al. The spectrum of pheochromocytoma in hypertensive patients with neurofibromatosis. Arch Intern Med 1982;142:2092–2098.

11. Kothari A, Bethune M, Manwaring J, Astley N, Wallace E. Massive bilateral phaeochromocytomas in association with von Hippel Lindau syndrome in pregnancy. Aust NZ J Obstet Gynaecol 1999;39:381–384.

12. Freier DT, Eckhauser FE, Harrison TS. Pheochromocytoma. Arch Surg 1980;115:388–391.

13. Pederson EB, Rasmussen AB, Christensen NJ, et al. Plasma noradrenaline and adrenaline in pre-eclampsia, essential hypertension in pregnancy and normotensive pregnant control subjects. Acta Endocrinol (Copenh) 1982;99:594–600.

14. Zuspan FP. Urinary excretion of epinephrine and norepinephrine during pregnancy. J Clin Endocrinol Metab 1970;30:357–360.

15. Sheps SG, Jiang NS, Klee GC. Diagnostic evaluation of pheochromocytoma. Endocrinol Metab Clin North Am 1988;17:397–415.

16. Devoe LD, O'Dell BE, Castillo RA, Hadi HA, Searle N. Metastatic pheochromocytoma in pregnancy and fetal biophysical assessment after maternal administration of alpha-adrenergic, beta-adrenergic, and dopamine antagonists. Obstet Gynecol 1986;68(Suppl 3):15S–18S.

17. Santeiro ML, Stromquist C, Wyble L. Phenoxybenzamine placental transfer during the third trimester. Ann Pharmacother 1996;30:1249–1251.

18. Lyons CW, Colmorgen GHC. Medical management of pheochromocytoma in pregnancy. Obstet Gynecol 1988;72:450–451.

19. Ahlawat SK, Jain S, Kumari S, Varma S, Sharma BK. Pheochromocytoma associated with pregnancy: case report and review of the literature. Obstet Gynecol Surv 1999;54:728–737.

20. Chatterjee TK, Parekh U. Phaeochromocytoma in pregnancy. Aust NZ J Obstet Gynaecol 1985;25:290–291.

21. Finkenstedt G, Gasser RW, Hofle G, et al. Pheochromocytoma and sub-clinical Cushing's syndrome during pregnancy: diagnosis, medical pre-treatment and cure by laparoscopic unilateral adrenalectomy. J Endocrinol Invest 1999;22:551–557.

22. Schenker JG, Granat M. Phaeochromocytoma and pregnancy—An updated appraisal. Aust NZ J Obstet Gynaecol 1982;22:1–10.

23. Schenker JG, Chowers I. Pheochromocytoma and pregnancy: review of 89 cases. Obstet Gynecol Surv 1971;26:739–747.

24. Raue F, Bayer JM, Rahn KH, et al. Hypercalcitoninaemia in patients with pheochromocytoma. Klin Wochenschrift 1978;56:697–701.

25. Heath H, Edis AJ. Pheochromocytoma associated with hypercalcemia and ectopic secretion of calcitonin. Ann Intern Med 1979;91:208–210.

26. Kato T, Seki K, Matsui H, Sekiya S. Monometric calcitonin in pregnant women and in cord blood. Obstet Gynecol 1998;92:241–244.

27. Pitkin RM. Calcium metabolism pregnancy: a review. Am J Obstet Gynecol 1985;151:99.

28. Okah FA, Tsang RC, Sierra R, Brady KK, Specker BL. Bone turnover and mineral metabolism in the last trimester of pregnancy: effect of multiple gestation. Obstet Gynecol 1996;88:168–173.

CASE #3: 31-YR-OLD WOMAN
WITH POORLY CONTROLLED TYPE 1 DIABETES, MULTIPLE
DIABETIC COMPLICATIONS, AND HYPEREMESIS GRAVIDARUM
Case Description

A 31-yr-old nulliparous Caucasian woman with a 17 yr history of type 1 diabetes mellitus presented at 9 6/7 wk gestational age in an unplanned pregnancy. She had never known good diabetic control, was taking Lente insulin 40 U daily in the AM and did not monitor her glucose. Her diabetes was complicated by proliferative retinopathy, requiring photocoagulation 7 and 4 yr previously. She was legally blind in the right eye and had diminished visual acuity in the left eye. She also had bilateral cataracts. She was unaware of any renal complications from her diabetes. She had a 4 yr history of paresthesias and numbness in the lower extremities and had frequent symptoms of lightheadedness with postural changes. For the year prior to her pregnancy, she experienced frequent episodes of nausea and heartburn as well as constipation. She had no recent weight loss, heat intolerance, tremor, palpitations, muscle weakness, or insomnia.

She was admitted to a peripheral hospital for nausea and vomiting and was found to be pregnant. For the next 2 wk, she was treated with fluids and antiemetics, and then was discharged on a 1900 kcal ADA diet and an insulin regimen of 8R/38L before breakfast and 4R before supper. She was seen 2 wk later in the emergency room for nausea and vomiting, was treated with intravenous (iv) fluids, and was referred to maternal fetal medicine at a tertiary care center.

At 15 4/7 weeks gestational age, she weighed 55.7 kg at 162.6 cm. Her recumbent blood pressure was 158/100 with a heart rate of 92. It fell to 126/60 mmHg with a heart rate of 100 upon standing. Her pupils responded sluggishly to light, and funduscopy revealed laser scars bilaterally. She had no thyroid eye findings. Her thyroid was normal to palpation. Her skin was dry. Her patellar and Achilles tendon reflexes were absent, and she demonstrated diminished proprioception, light touch, and pin-prick sensation below the knees. She had a small healing ulcer on the left great toe.

Laboratory values included a hemoglobin A1c of 10.3%, sodium 134 mEq/L, potassium 4.8 mEq/L, chloride 104 mEq/L, bicarbonate 25 mEq/L, BUN 23 mg/dL, creatinine 0.9 mg/dL, total protein 5.6 g/dL, albumin 3.0 g/dL, and hemoglobin 11.1 g/dL. Her creatinine clearance was 52 mL/min with a 24-h urine protein of 2.5 g. Her TSH was 0.12 µU/mL with a free T_4 of 1.56 ng/dL (normal 0.70–1.48).

She experienced recurring episodes of nausea and emesis and was treated with chlorpromazine suppositories and metoclopramide 10 mg 30 min prior to meals. The emesis continued, and she developed a Mallory-Weiss tear with hemoccult positive emesis and a drop in hemoglobin to 8.5 g/dL. After bowel rest and iv fluids, a pureed diet was gradually attempted. She kept the head of her bed elevated, remained upright for 2 h after feeding, and was given a sliding scale of insulin doses, with regular insulin prior to each meal and Lente given at breakfast and dinner. She experienced frequent hypoglycemia with glucose levels varying from 39–380 mg/dL. During a 2 wk admission, she lost 1.6 kg.

Over the next 3 mo, she was readmitted three times for persistent severe nausea and emesis. Despite dietary manipulation, prokinetic, antiemetic, and H_2-blocker therapy, her nutritional intake remained poor. It was estimated that she consumed only 54% of her caloric needs and 76% of her protein requirements. She continued to demonstrate markedly labile glucose levels and experienced two severe hypoglycemic episodes, including one marked by a seizure with decerebrate posturing. She was started on total parenteral nutrition with insulin in the infusate and her blood glucose profile became consistent with glucose levels in the 65 to 100 mg/dL range. Her TSH was now 0.5 μU/mL.

She developed a "pill roll" tremor and Parkinsonian facies, requiring discontinuation of the metoclopramide and phenothiazines. Her renal status deteriorated and her hypertension became more difficult to manage. Her creatinine rose to 2.1 mg/dL with a creatinine clearance of 27 mL/min and 24-h urine protein of 5.1 g. Her serum albumin fell to 1.9 g/dL with a total protein of 4.2 g and she became severely edematous.

She developed preterm labor at 34 2/7 wk gestational age, and delivered a 1780 g male neonate by C-section because of late variable decelerations and fetal acidosis on monitoring. She continued to experience nausea and emesis postpartum, but gradually improved to the point where oral nutrition could be reestablished, and she was discharged 24 d postpartum with a serum creatinine of 1.3 mg/dL, creatinine clearance 45 mL/min, 24-h urine protein 15.7 g, and a serum albumin of 2.9 g/dL.

Discussion

Hyperemesis gravidarum is defined as intractable nausea and vomiting during early gestation, which can result in nutritional deficiencies, ketosis, dehydration, and electrolyte imbalance. It starts at 6–9 wk gestation, and usually resolves by 18–20 wk gestation. It is generally idiopathic, but on occasion may be associated with an underlying pathology. Possibilities of maternal hyperthyroidism and diabetic gastroparesis must be considered in this case.

Graves' disease occurs in 0.1–0.2% of pregnancies *(1)*, and must be considered in this patient with a preexisting autoimmune disease. Autoimmune thyroid disease is approximately twice as likely to occur in individuals with type 1 diabetes mellitus as those without diabetes *(2,3)*. Hyperthyroidism may also complicate the management of diabetes mellitus, contributing to erratic glucose control and increased insulin requirements. Graves' disease must be distinguished from the most common cause of hyperthyroidism found in pregnancy, transient gestational hyperthyroidism of nonautoimmune origin. The latter diagnosis requires no pharmacologic intervention and is secondary to high levels of hCG. It is frequently found in conjunction with hyperemesis gravidarum *(4–6)*. Even in normal pregnancy, hCG may stimulate the thyroid and cause a decline in the TSH level because of the structural homology between the TSH and hCG molecules and their receptors *(7)*. However, hCG molecules are heterogeneous, and modifications of its oligosaccharide side chain alters its TSH-like activity. Deglycosylated and desialylated forms have the greatest thyrotropic effect, and are more often isolated from women with hydatidiform moles and women with hyperemesis gravidarum *(8)*.

Distinguishing between autoimmune thyrotoxicosis and transient hyperthyroidism of hyperemesis gravidarum (THHG) may be difficult, as pregnancy is a hypermetabolic state associated with increased cardiac output, tachycardia, systolic flow murmurs, warm skin, and heat intolerance. Patients with THHG have few manifestations of thyrotoxicosis, have no goiter, and their hyperthyroxinemia is generally transient and resolves by 18 wk gestation without antithyroid drug therapy *(9)*. Both the hyperemesis gravidarum and the suppressed TSH appear to be tied to the elevation in hCG *(6)*. The elevation in hCG contributes to an elevation in estradiol levels that may contribute to the nausea and emesis. Serum TSH levels decline and free T_4 levels rise in response to the thyroid stimulation by hCG *(6,10)*. Total T_4 levels are further elevated by the rise in TBG caused by the hyperestrogenemia of pregnancy. Antithyroid therapy should be considered for women with a prepregnancy history suggestive of hyperthyroidism, overt manifestations of Graves' disease, or with persistent hyperemesis and hyperthyroxinemia past 20 wk gestation.

Diabetic gastroparesis is a likely possibility in this patient with a known history of autonomic neuropathies and her one year history of episodic nausea *(11)*. Diabetic gastroparesis is linked to vagal autonomic neuropathy and is exacerbated by hyperglycemia, which disrupts myoelectric activity *(12,13)*. Severe gastroparesis may result in significant maternal and fetal morbidity. Early satiety, nausea, and postprandial emesis may be exacerbated by the "morning sickness" of early pregnancy, and by the mechanical compression of the stomach by an enlarging uterus in the latter half of pregnancy. Intractable vomiting may result in maternal and fetal malnutrition, hypoalbuminemia, dehydration, and an increased risk of aspiration. The fetal malnutrition may not only result in intrauterine growth retardation and increased neonatal morbidity and mortality, but may have a longer impact on the child including increased risk for cardiovascular disease and type 2 diabetes mellitus *(14,15)*.

Erratic blood sugar control caused by a mismatch of insulin administration with nutrient delivery to the small bowel is a hallmark of diabetic gastroparesis, and may be the only manifestation of this autonomic neuropathy. Most of the diagnostic techniques to confirm gastroparesis can not be used during pregnancy *(13)*. Therapeutic interventions include dietary manipulation, prokinetic agents, and specialized insulin regimens. As lipids and indigestible fibers delay gastric emptying, frequent, small meals which are mechanically soft and low in fat and insoluble fiber are consumed *(16)*. Prokinetic agents such as metoclopramide and antiemetics are classified as Category B, but may be of use in improving gastric emptying. An attempt at euglycemia is not only critical to pregnancy outcome, but may improve gastric motility. Rapidly absorbed insulins, such as Lispro, allow the administration of "meal" boluses after the blood glucose concentration starts to rise, indicating nutrient delivery to the small bowel. Intensive glucose monitoring both pre- and postprandially is required to institute such a regimen. This can be done on a baseline of intermediate or long acting insulins, or in the setting of insulin pump therapy.

In a patient with severe gastroparesis which compromises nutrition over a prolonged period, hyperalimentation becomes essential to provide positive nitrogen balance. Enteral hyperalimentation would be the preferred method, so long as the feeding tube could be placed beyond the gastric outlet and the risk of aspiration were minimized. Total parenteral nutrition is also an option *(17–19)*, although the impact of the amino acid composition and the fat emulsion on fetal brain development and well-being has not been adequately studied in humans. The use of this modality also facilitates a more predictable requirement for insulin, thereby improving glycemic control.

Other autonomic neuropathies may also contribute to significant maternal morbidity in pregnancy. Orthostatic hypotension is an infrequent complication of diabetic pregnancies. Symptoms of severe orthostatic hypotension may be ameliorated by the volume expansion of pregnancy *(20)*, or may worsen with the normal decline in blood pressure accompanying pregnancy. Bladder dysfunction, with urinary retention and overflow incontinence, could increase the risk of urinary tract infections. These should be screened for and treated aggressively. Constipation would be exacerbated by pregnancy, and should be managed with increased water intake and sugar-free bulking agents.

This patient demonstrated no worsening of her retinopathy during the pregnancy. However, a number of studies have demonstrated an association between retinopathy progression during pregnancy and the severity of hyperglycemia at enrollment, as well as the degree of improvement in control achieved in the first half of gestation *(21–23)*. Analysis of the pregnancies that occurred during the DCCT *(24)* demonstrates that pregnancy itself adds independently to the risk of retinopathy progression.

This patient did demonstrate a worsening of her diabetic nephropathy, with worsening proteinuria and hypertension. Numerous studies have shown that women with mild degrees of nephropathy generally go through pregnancy with little permanent effect on renal function despite transient but substantial increases in proteinuria *(25,26)*. However, patients with moderate or severe nephropathy in early pregnancy may demonstrate an accelerated decline in renal function that may continue postpartum *(27,28)*. Pregnancy itself may contribute to this decline, in addition to such factors as hypertension control, urinary tract infections, and inability to use angiotensin converting enzyme inhibitors. The worsening edema which she experienced as a result of her hypoalbuminemia, secondary to poor nutritional intake and increasing proteinuria, may reduce subcutaneous insulin absorption and contribute to poor control *(29)*.

REFERENCES

1. Mestman JH. Hyperthyroidism in pregnancy. Endocrinol Metab Clinics N Am 1998;27:127–149.
2. Goldstein DE, Drash A, Gibbs J, Blizzard RM. Diabetes mellitus: the incidence of circulating antibodies against thyroid, gastric, and adrenal tissue. J Pediatr 1970;77:304–306.
3. Bech K, Hoier-Madsen M, Feldt-Rasmussen U, et al. Thyroid function and autoimmune manifestations in insulin-dependent diabetes mellitus during and after pregnancy. Acta Endocrinologia 1991;124:534–539.
4. Bouillon R, Naesens M, Van Assche FA, et al. Thyroid function in patients with hyperemesis gravidarum. Am J Obstet Gynecol 1982;143:922–926.
5. Chin RK, Lao TT. Thyroxine concentrations and outcome of hyperemetic pregnancies. Br J Obstet Gynaecol 1988;95:507–509.
6. Goodwin TM, Montoro M, Mestman JH, Pekary AE, Hershman JM. The role of chorionic gonadotropin in transient hyperthyroidism of hyperemesis gravidarum. J Clin Endocrinol Metab 1992;75:1333–1339.
7. Yoshimura M, Hershman JM. Thyrotropic action of human chorionic gonadotropin. Thyroid 1995;5:425–434.
8. Tsuruta E, Tada H, Tamaki H, et al. Pathogenic role of asial human chroionic gonadotropin in gestational thyrotoxicosis. J Clin Endocrinol Metab 1995;80:350–355.
9. Goodwin TM, Montoro M, Mestman JH. Transient hyperthyroidism and hyperemesis gravidarum: clinical aspects. Am J Obstet Gynecol 1992;167:648–652.
10. Glinoer D, DeNayer P, Bourdoux P, et al. Regulation of maternal thyroid during pregnancy. J Clin Endocrinol Metab 1990;71:276–287.
11. Merio R, Festa A, Bergmann H, et al. Slow gastric emptying in type I diabetes: relation to autonomic and peripheral neuropathy, blood glucose and glycemic control. Diabetes Care 1997;20:419–423.
12. Barnett JL, Owyang C. Serum glucose concentration as a modulator of interdigestive gastric motility. Gastroenterology 1988;94:739–744.
13. Hornbuckle K, Barnett JL. The diagnosis and work-up of the patient with gastroparesis. J Clin Gastroenterol 2000;30:117–124.
14. Barker DJP, Gluckman PD, Godfrey KM, et al. Fetal nutrition and cardiovascular disease in adult life. Lancet 1993;341:938–941.
15. Barker DJP, Hales CN, Fall CHD, Osmond C, Phipps K, Clarke PMS. Type 2 (non-insulin-dependent) diabetes mellitus, hypertension and hyperlipidaemia (syndrome X): Relation to reduced fetal growth. Diabetologia 1993;36:62–67.
16. Rabine JC, Barnett JL. Management of the patient with gastroparesis. J Clin Gastroenterol 2001;32:11–18.
17. Lavin Jr JP, Gimmon Z, Miodovnik M, von Meyenfeldt M, Fischer JE. Total parenteral nutrition in a pregnant insulin-requiring diabetic. Obstet Gynecol 1982;59:660–664.
18. Zibell FD, Jen KL, Rick J. Use of parenteral nutrition to maintain adequate nutritional status in hyperemesis gravidarum. J Perinatol 1990;10:390–395.

19. Kirby DF, Fiorenza V, Craig RM. Intravenous nutritional support during pregnancy. J Parentr Enteral Nutr 1988;12:72–80.
20. Scott AR, Tattersall RB, McPherson M. Improvement of postural hypotension and severe diabetic autonomic neuropathy during pregnancy. Diabetes Care 1988;11:369–370.
21. Phelps RL, Sakol P, Metzger BE, Jampol LM, Freinkel N. Changes in diabetic retinopathy during pregnancy. Correlations with regulation of hyperglycemia. Arch Ophthalmol 1986;104:1806–1810.
22. Chew EY, Mills JL, Metzger BE, et al. Metabolic control and progression of retinopathy: The Diabetes In Early Pregnancy Study. Diabetes Care 1995;18:631–637.
23. The Kroc Collaborative Study Group: Blood glucose control and the evolution of diabetic retinopathy and albuminuria. N Engl J Med 1984;311:365–372.
24. Diabetes Control and Complications Trial Research Group. Pregnancy increases the risk of complications in the DCCT. Am J Obstet Gynecol 2000.
25. Reece EA, Coustan DR, Hayslett JP, et al. Diabetic nephropathy: pregnancy performance and feto-maternal outcome. Am J Obstet Gynecol 1988;159:56–66.
26. McCance DR, Traub AI, Harley JM, Hadden DR, Kennedy L. Urinary albumin excretion in diabetic pregnancy. Diabetologia 1989;32:236–239.
27. Biesenbach G, Stöger H, Zazgornik J. Influence of pregnancy on progression of diabetic nephropathy and subsequent requirement of renal replacement therapy in female type I diabetic patients with impaired renal function. Nephrol Dial Transplant 1992;7:105–109.
28. Purdy LP, Hantsch CE, Molitch ME, et al. Effect of pregnancy on renal function in patients with moderate-to-severe diabetic renal insufficiency. Diabetes Care 1996;19:1067–1074.
29. Ariza-Andraca CR, Altamirano-Bustamante E, Frati-Munari AC, Altamirano-Bustamante P, Graef-Sanchez A. Delayed insulin absorption due to subcutaneous edema. Arch Investig Med 1991;22:229–233.

CASE 4: 33-YR-OLD PREGNANT WOMAN WITH GRAVES' DISEASE AND AN ENLARGING THYROID NODULE

Case Description

A 33-yr-old Caucasian woman with a strong family history of thyroid disease in her three sisters, paternal aunt, and paternal great aunt was diagnosed with Graves' disease 5 mo after she delivered a macrosomic infant (10 lbs., 10 oz.) at term. She complained of a 1 mo history of heat intolerance, diaphoresis, irritability, tremor, lightheadedness, insomnia, and palpitations. Her thyroid was three times normal size on palpation. TSH was suppressed and her 24-h ^{123}I uptake was elevated at 74% with a normal scan. She was treated with propylthiouracil (PTU). Subsequently, her primary care physician managed her Graves' disease until she presented 3 yr later at 7 wk gestational age. At that time, she was symptomatically euthyroid on PTU 150 mg bid with a TSH of 0.58 µU/mL and total T_3 201 ng/dL (normal nonpregnant values 80–180). Her PTU was decreased to 100 mg bid, and her subsequent laboratory findings included a TSH of 0.43 µU/mL with a T_3 of 268 ng/dL and free T_4 0.8 ng/dL. A 3×2-cm smooth, mobile nodule was found in the thyroid isthmus, with no associated lymphadenopathy. Over the subsequent 2 mo, the nodule grew to 4 cm in size with no obstructive complaints. At 16 wk gestational age, a fine-needle aspiration was performed. The cytology was consistent with papillary carcinoma. A near total thyroidectomy at 20 wk gestational age under a general anesthetic was planned. In view of her Graves' disease, the surgeon desired a 10 d preoperative preparation with iodide therapy.

Discussion

Thyrotoxicosis occurs in approximately 0.2% of pregnancies (1). In general, hyperthyroidism is easier to control during pregnancy, perhaps because of the immunology of pregnancy (1,2), which allows the successful allograft of foreign tissue, namely the fetus.

This decline in immune surveillance includes a decrease in the $CD4^+/CD8^+$ ratio *(3)*, a depression of both humoral and cell-mediated immunity, and a decrease in thyroid antibodies *(4)*. The transplacental passage of soluble factors produced by activated fetal suppressor T cells may also cause a transient decrease in the intensity of Graves' disease during pregnancy. The loss of these fetal suppressor T cells at delivery could result in the clinically recognized postpartum exacerbation of Graves' disease *(5)*.

Untreated hyperthyroidism increases the risk of maternal congestive heart failure, severe preeclampsia, preterm delivery, low birthweight infants, and perinatal mortality *(6,7)*. Maintenance of maternal free-T_4 concentrations in the range of the upper normal limit may be optimal for fetal thyroid function *(8)*. Pregnant women with thyrotoxicosis should be maintained on as low a dose of PTU as possible to avoid fetal hypothyroidism or fetal goiter. Pregnant women tolerate mild degrees of hyperthyroidism without much difficulty.

It is controversial as to whether patients with Graves' disease are more vulnerable to thyroid cancer *(9)*. Occult thyroid cancers appear to occur at the same rate as found in the general population *(10,11)*. The incidence of thyroid cancer in palpable cold nodules approaches 25% in a patient with Graves' disease *(10)*. The thyroid carcinoma may be more aggressive *(11–14)*, suggesting a role for thyroid stimulating immunoglobulin *(15)*.

Except in areas of marginal iodine intake, thyroid nodularity does not increase with parity *(16)*. The effect of pregnancy on the natural history of thyroid carcinoma is controversial *(17)*. Some have found no apparent effect *(18–20)*, whereas others studies suggest there is an increased risk of malignancy in nodules which develop during pregnancy *(21–23)* and that the cancer may be more aggressive *(24)*. The intrinsic TSH-like activity of hCG has been postulated to play a role in the progression of cancers found early in gestation *(24)*. Current recommendations are that patients with nodules less than 2 cm in size could delay the fine-needle aspiration and any needed surgery until postpartum.

Surgery is delayed until after the first trimester, as the spontaneous abortion rate is highest during that time. The risks of thyroid surgery in the second trimester are not well described in the recent literature, though fetal loss may still occur. After 24 wk gestation, surgery may increase the risk of premature labor. Following a near total thyroidectomy, thyroid hormone administration to suppress the TSH substantially below the normal range may increase fetal risk *(21)*. Radioactive iodine is absolutely contraindicated during pregnancy. Induction of hypothyroidism for adjuvant radioiodine therapy or scanning is delayed until the postpartum period, to avoid the fetal risks associated with maternal hypothyroidism. As iodine is concentrated by the breast *(25,26)* and excreted into breast milk, radioactive ^{131}I administration should be delayed if breastfeeding is desired as the radioactive iodine may be detected in the breast milk for several months *(27)*. Furthermore, the ^{131}I dose should not be given for at least 3 mo after breastfeeding is discontinued to avoid an excessive exposure to radiation in the lactating breasts that may potentially increase the risk of breast cancer *(28)*.

There have been numerous reports that describe the safety and efficacy of using propranolol to prepare hyperthyroid patients for thyroid surgery *(29,30)*. Despite this, surgeons believe that iodine administration will reduce the vascularity of the gland, minimizing intraoperative blood loss *(31)*. Studies have not supported the putative benefits of adding iodine to hyperthyroid patients prepared with propranolol *(32)*, or to patients rendered euthyroid with antithyroid drug therapy *(33)*.

Because the surgical benefits of preoperative iodine administration are questionable, what are the potential effects of maternal iodine therapy on the fetus? Iodine deficiency is considered the leading cause of intellectual deficiency in the world *(34)*. The recent NHANES III report indicates that iodine intake has declined 50% in the United States since the NHANES I report was completed *(35)*. As a consequence, the percentage of individuals with iodine deficiency has increased more than four-fold, and now comprises 6.7% of pregnant women and 14.9% of women of child-bearing age *(35)*. In areas with mild to moderate iodine deficiency, maternal supplementation of iodine throughout pregnancy apparently improved the thyroid function of the offspring, with normal thyroid volumes seen in the newborns *(36,37)*. A more recent study with supplementation given at term found higher cord levels of TSH, suggesting an inhibitory effect of iodine supplementation on the fetal thyroid *(38)*. This same picture has been seen in offspring of iodine-deficient mothers who are exposed to iodine-containing disinfectants at delivery *(39,40)*. This fetal thyroid inhibition does not occur when iodine is given to iodine-replete mothers *(41)*. In the past, iodine therapy given to pregnant women with Graves' disease was associated with the development of fetal goiter *(42)*. This complication has not been seen in the offspring of pregnant women with milder forms of Graves' disease who were treated with iodine alone during their pregnancies *(43)*. Although prolonged courses of iodine could potentially cause a fetal goiter, a short 7 d preoperative course, if it is necessary, should not cause problems.

REFERENCES

1. Burrow G. Thyroid function and hyperfunction during gestation. Endocrinol Revs 1993;14:194–202.
2. Mestman JH. Hyperthyroidism in pregnancy. Clin Obstet Gynecol 1997;40:45–64.
3. Stagnaro-Green A, Roman SH, Cobin RH, el-Harazy E, Wallenstein S, Davies TF. A prospective study of lymphocyte-initiated immunosuppression in normal pregnancy: evidence of a T-cell etiology for postpartum thyroid dysfunction. J Clin Endocrinol Metab 1992;74:645–653.
4. Burrow GN. Thyroid diseases. In: Burrow GN, Duffy TP, eds. Medical Complications During Pregnancy, 5th edition. WB Saunders, Philadelphia, PA, 1999, pp. 135–161.
5. Sridama V, Pacini F, Yang SL, Moawad A, Reilly M, DeGroot LJ. Decreased levels of helper T cells: a possible cause of immunodeficiency in pregnancy. N Engl J Med 1982;307:352–356.
6. Millar LK, Wing DA, Leung AS, Koonings PP, Montoro MN, Mestman JH. Low birth weight and preeclampsia in pregnancies complicated by hyperthyroidism. Obstet Gynecol 1994;84:946–949.
7. Davis LE, Lucas MJ, Hankins GD, Roark ML, Cunningham FG. Thyrotoxicosis complicating pregnancy. Am J Obstet Gynecol 1989;160:63–70.
8. Gardner DF, Cruikshank DP, Hays PM, Cooper DS. Pharmacology of propylthiouracil (PTU) in pregnant hyperthyroid women: correlation of maternal PTU concentrations with cord serum thyroid function tests. J Clin Endocrinol Metab 1986;62:217–220.
9. Hales IB, McElduff A, Crummer P, et al. Does Graves' disease or thyrotoxicosis affect the prognosis of thyroid cancer? J Clin Endocrinol Metab 1992;75:886–889.
10. Pacini F, Elisei R, Di Coscio GC, et al. Thyroid carcinoma in thyrotoxic patients treated by surgery. J Endocrinol Invest 1988;11:107–112.
11. Belfiore A, Garofalo MR, Giuffrida D, et al. Increased aggressiveness of thyroid cancer in patients with Graves' disease. J Clin Endocrinol Metab 1990;70:830–835.
12. Behar R, Arganini M, Wu TC, et al. Graves' disease and thyroid cancer. Surgery 1986;100:1121–1127.
13. Pellegriti G, Belfiore A, Giuffrida D, et al. Outcome of differentiated thyroid cancer in Graves' patients. J Clin Endocrinol Metab 1998;83:2805–2809.
14. Ozaki O, Ito K, Kobayashi K, et al. Thyroid carcinoma in Graves' disease. World J Surg 1990;14:437–441.
15. Filetti S, Belfiore A, Amir SM, et al. The role of thyroid-stimulating antibodies of Graves' disease in differentiated thyroid cancer. N Engl J Med 1988;318:753–759.
16. Struve CW, Haupt S, Ohlen S. Influence of frequency of previous pregnancies on the prevalence of thyroid nodules in women without clinical evidence of thyroid disease. Thyroid 1993;3:7–9.

17. McTiernan AM, Weiss NS, Daling JR. Incidence of thyroid cancer in women in relation to reproductive and hormonal factors. Am J Epidemiol 1984;120:423–435.
18. Akslen LA, Nilssen S, Kva'le G. Reproductive factors and risk of thyroid cancer: a prospective study of 63,090 women from Norway. Br J Cancer 1992;65:772–774.
19. Herzon FS, Morris DM, Segal MN, Rauch G, Parnell T. Coexistent thyroid cancer and pregnancy. Arch Otolaryngol Head Neck Surg 1994;120:1191–1193.
20. Mestman JH, Goodwin M, Montoro MM. Thyroid disorders of pregnancy. Endocrinol Metab Clin N Am 1995;24:41–71.
21. Rosen IB, Walfish PG. Pregnancy as a predisposing factor in thyroid neoplasia. Arch Surg 1986;121:1287–1290.
22. Rosen IB, Walfish PG, Nikore V. Pregnancy and surgical thyroid disease. Surgery 1985;98:1135–1140.
23. Hay I. Nodular thyroid disease diagnosed during pregnancy: how and when to treat. Thyroid 1999;9:667–670.
24. Kobayashi K, Tanaka Y, Ishiguro S, Mori T. Rapidly growing thyroid carcinoma during pregnancy. J Surg Oncol 1994;55:61–64.
25. Eskin BA, Parker JA, Bassett JG, George DL. Human breast uptake of radioactive iodine. Obstet Gynecol 1974;44:398–402.
26. Tazebay UH, Wapnir IL, Levy O, et al. The mammary gland iodide transporter is expressed during lactation and in breast cancer. Nat Med 2000;6:871–878.
27. Dydek GJ, Blue PW. Human breast milk excretion of iodine-131 following diagnostic and therapeutic administration to a lactating patient with Graves' disease. J Nucl Med 1988;29:407–410.
28. Doody RE, Becker DV, Brill AB, et al. Cancer mortality following treatment for adult hyperthyroidism. Cooperative Thyrotoxicosis Therapy Follow-up Study Group. JAMA 1998;280:347–355.
29. Toft AD, Irvine WJ, McLeod DAD, Seth J, Cameron EHD, Lidard GP. Propranolol in the treatment of thyrotoxicosis by subtotal thyroidectomy. J Clin Endocrinol Metab 1976;43:1312–1316.
30. Caswell HT, Marks AD, Channick BJ. Propranolol for the preoperative preparation of patients with thyrotoxicosis. Surg Gynecol Obstet 1978;146:908–910.
31. Marigold JH, Morgan AK, Earle DJ, Young AE, Croft DN. Lugol's iodine: its effect on thyroid blood flow in patients with thyrotoxicosis. Br J Surg 1985;72:45–47.
32. Marmon L, Au FC. The preoperative use of iodine solution in thyrotoxic patients prepared with propranolol. Is it necessary? Am Surg 1989;55:629–631.
33. Kaur S, Parr JH, Ramsay ID, Hennebry TM, Jarvis KJ, Lester E. Effect of preoperative iodine in patients with Graves' disease controlled with antithyroid drugs and thyroxine. Ann R Coll Surg Engl 1988;70:123–127.
34. Delange F. Administration of iodized oil during pregnancy: a summary of the published evidence. Bull WHO 1996;74:101–108.
35. Hollowell JG, Staehling NW, Hannon WH, et al. Iodine nutrition in the United States. Trends and public health implications: iodine excretion data from National Health and Nutrition Examination Surveys I and III (1971–1974 and 1988–1994). J Clin Endocrinol Metab 1988;83:3401–3408.
36. Glinoer D, De Nayer P, Delange F, et al. A randomized trial for the treatment of mild iodine deficiency during pregnancy: maternal and neonatal effects. J Clin Endocrinol Metab 1995;80:258–269.
37. Klett M, Ohlig M, Manz F, Troeger J, Heinrich U. Effect of iodine supply on neonatal thyroid volume and TSH. Acta Paediatr Suppl 1999;432:18–20.
38. Nohr SB, Laurberg P. Opposite variations in maternal and neonatal thyroid function induced by iodine supplementation during pregnancy. J Clin Endocrinol Metab 2000;85:623–627.
39. Weber G, Vigone MC, Rapa A, et al. Neonatal transient hypothyroidism: aetiological study. Arch Dis Child Fetal Neonatal Ed 1998;79:F70–F72.
40. Danziger Y, Pertzelan A, Mimouni M. Transient congenital hypothyroidism after topical iodine in pregnancy and lactation. Arch Dis Child 1987;62:295–296.
41. Brown RS, Bloomfield S, Bednarek FJ, Mitchell ML, Braverman LE. Routine skin cleansing with povidone-iodine is not a common cause of transient neonatal hypothyroidism in North America: a prospective controlled study. Thyroid 1997;7:395–400.
42. Senior B, Chernoff HL. Iodide goiter in the newborn. Pediatr 1971;47:510–515.
43. Momotani N, Hisaoka T, Noh J, Ishikawa N, Ito K. Effects of iodine on thyroid status of fetus *versus* mother in treatment of Graves' disease complicated by pregnancy. J Clin Endocrinol Metab 1992;75:738–744.

16 Type 1 Diabetes Mellitus

J. Woody Sistrunk, MD
and Bruce R. Zimmerman, MD*

CONTENTS

CASE #1: CORONARY ARTERY DISEASE

Case Description

A 53-yr-old woman was diagnosed with type 1 diabetes mellitus in 1960 at the age of 15. She initially presented with weight loss, frequent urination, and an increased appetite. She has been treated with insulin since her initial diagnosis, having been started on a multiple daily injection (MDI) program in June 1992. Her diabetes was under good control with her glycosylated hemoglobin ranging from 7.4–8.6% (normal range 4–7%) after the MDI program was instituted.

Complications related to diabetes to date include microalbuminuria and mild peripheral neuropathy. Concomitant medical problems include mitral valve prolapse and fibromyalgia. She was on no other medications besides insulin, particularly no estrogen replacement. She has had intermittent chest pain previously, including a hospital admission in 1992 with dyspnea and a positive electrocardiogram (ECG). Follow-up exercise thallium perfusion study was unremarkable; therefore, symptoms were attributed to an acute panic attack.

In September 1995, her father died. At this time, she began experiencing significant chest discomfort. She was given the diagnosis of pleurisy and coexistent gastroesophageal reflux. She was transiently treated with a nonsteroidal without benefit. The reflux was treated with an H2 blocker and then omeprazole without relief. This discomfort was evaluated with a computed tomography (CT) scan of the chest (routine, without iv contrast) in October 1995, which showed mild emphysematous changes (known smoker) in the upper lungs, as well as coronary artery calcification.

*Deceased.

From: *Contemporary Endocrinology: Challenging Cases in Endocrinology*
Edited by: M. E. Molitch © Humana Press Inc., Totowa, NJ

By December 1995, she was referred to a cardiologist. Her ECG showed normal sinus rhythm, ventricular rate of 78 bpm, and a nonspecific T-wave abnormality. Her chest discomfort basically had three components. First, cold-induced pain that usually lead to upper anterior chest burning. Often, this chest discomfort would lead to belching and vomiting. She had one episode of severe discomfort that was relieved by breathing warm steam. Second, heartburn that was clearly exacerbated when supine, consistent with gastroesophageal reflux. This symptom was relieved by over-the-counter antacids. Third, pleurisy that had improved since September 1995. Despite these findings and symptoms, as well as her risk factors for coronary artery disease, including type 1 diabetes mellitus and previous smoking history [no history of hypertension, hyperlipidemia [LDL-107] or family history of coronary artery disease (CAD)], the cardiologist stated that her pain was atypical and not likely to be cardiac related. At this same time, she underwent pulmonary function testing that yielded a positive methacholine challenge and otherwise was within normal limits. She was subsequently started on an albuterol meter dose inhaler.

On the same day, she saw a gastroenterologist in consultation. She described symptoms of excessive vomiting and the inability to keep food down. She would basically vomit whatever she ate without any retention features. Her symptoms also included nausea, wretching, and heartburn, which was described as substernal radiating to the intrascapular area. Previous upper endoscopy was unremarkable. Ultrasonography of the upper abdomen was unremarkable. The cause of her vomiting was unclear, but she was given another therapeutic trial of omeprazole and the promotility agent, cisapride. The gastroenterologist felt that further studies would be necessary if relief was not achieved on this regimen, considering the possible diagnosis of diabetic gastroparesis.

When she returned in April 1996, she continued to complain of difficulty breathing and wheezing. Her nausea and vomiting had improved on the cisapride and omeprazole. She was referred to an allergist for further evaluation of asthma. The allergist thought her symptoms were consistent with asthma, so inhaled corticosteroids were added in addition to the albuterol inhaler. She also achieved improvement on this regimen.

During follow-up with her endocrinologist in April 1996, she stated that she was having episodes of diffuse upper anterior chest tightness followed by heaviness and neck tightness. She was also bothered by numbness of the upper arms. Her vomiting had improved significantly by this time. These persistent symptoms lead to referral for dobutamine stress echocardiogram. Findings suggested ischemia in a multivessel coronary artery distribution. This was followed with a coronary artery angiogram that showed three vessel disease. She was then referred for a coronary artery bypass graft (CABG).

Following her CABG, her symptoms of nausea/vomiting and asthma essentially abated. She no longer required the use of H2 blockers, proton pump inhibitor, β agonists nor inhaled corticosteroids.

Discussion

This case illustrates the vast and atypical nature of CAD in patients with diabetes. CAD remains the most prevalent cause of morbidity and mortality in women with diabetes. Historically, this has been well documented in women with type 2 diabetes, but it also applies to type 1 diabetes. The clinical symptomatology of women with CAD is inherently different than men. On average, women are approximately 10 yr older at the time of initial presentation (1). In general, a woman's chest pain is more likely to be associated with abdominal pain, dyspnea, nausea, and fatigue. The diagnosis of CAD can also be clouded by concomitant problems such as osteoarthritis and fibromyalgia (as in our case). It has been stated that women with CAD have better-defined risk factors such as diabetes, hypertension, hypercholesterolemia, and a family history of CAD *(1)*. In our case, a confounding factor was our patient's smoking history, her having recently quit.

In a recent prospective study by Galcera-Tomas et al., the prognostic significance of diabetes in relation to gender was assessed. Diabetic women were noted to be usually older and had a more prevalent history of hypertension and congestive heart failure. Also noted was the higher incidence of heart failure and mortality in hospitalized diabetic women with CAD *(2)*.

Atypical presentations of CAD are often associated with/ attributed to diabetes. Because of a high index of suspicion, the clinician is more likely to err on the side of further investigation in these patients with diabetes. In a study regarding diabetes and hospital admissions, diabetes was not associated with a higher rate of acute myocardial infarction (MI), but was associated with a higher hospitalization rate. The study concluded that physicians have a "lower threshold" to admit patients with diabetes for further work-up *(3)*. This "lower threshold," in addition to the atypical presentation of diabetic women, and the increased prevalence of hypertension and congestive heart failure in this population could certainly account for the higher rate of heart failure and mortality in diabetic women during hospitalization, compared to diabetic men *(4)*.

A recent study by Nesto et al. analyzed the incidence of silent MI assessed in 30 patients with diabetes mellitus and peripheral vascular disease by dipyridamole thallium scintigraphy. Eleven patients had a prior clinically silent MI. Seventeen of the 30 patients had reversible thallium defects, compatible with ischemia. Of note, the abnormalities were primarily seen in patients with concomitant hypertension and cigarette smoking *(4)*.

This case also illustrates the importance of choices in assessment of women with CAD. Despite a previously positive ECG, exercise thallium scintigraphy was negative. Thallium scanning in women does pose some testing error, particularly by breast tissue causing anterior perfusion artifacts *(1)*. Recall that our patient had a previously negative exercise thallium study that predated her symptoms. Dobutamine echocardiography, which led to a diagnosis in our patient, is a useful test in women unable to exercise. The chronotropic and inotropic effects lead to increased demand on the myocardium, subsequently yielding visible wall motion abnormalities *(1)*. However, pharmacologic stress (e.g., dobutamine) echocardiography can be limited because of poor acoustic windows. This is especially difficult in women. Stress echocardiography is also highly dependent on the experience of the echocardiographer *(5)*.

The ADA Consensus Statement on Coronary Heart Disease asked the question, "What are the most appropriate tests to detect the presence of coronary heart disease?" The first step in this decision tree should be deciding whether plans are to detect the presence of CAD vs probability of a future event. Historically, patients with diabetes are not able to satisfactorily complete a standard treadmill test; however, this would be a reasonable test, if screening is desired, to begin an exercise program in addition to review of risk factors and a resting ECG. If the patient has "typical or Q-waves on a resting ECG," (or an atypical anginal equivalent, as in our patient) a perfusion study would be the best choice, combining the ability to both assess ventricular function and provide quantitation of perfusion abnormality *(5)*.

Table 1
Indications for Cardiac Testing in Diabetic Patients
Case 1*

Testing for CAD is warranted in patients with the following:

1. Typical or atypical cardiac symptoms.
2. Resting electrocardiograph suggestive of ischemia or infarction.
3. Peripheral or carotid occlusive arterial disease.
4. Sedentary lifestyle, age ≥ 35 yr, and plans to begin a vigorous exercise program.
5. Two or more of the risk factors listed below in addition to diabetes:
    a. total cholesterol ≥ 240 mg/dL, LDL cholesterol > 160 mg/dL, or HDL cholesterol 35 ≤ mg/dL;
    b. blood pressure > 140/90 mmHg;
    c. smoking;
    d. family history of premature CAD;
    e. positive micro/macroalbuminuria test.

*From (5) with permission.

Of late, electron-beam computed tomography (EBCT) is becoming established as a screening tool for CAD. Many studies of EBCT to date have conflicting data regarding predictability of events. Some relationships have been seen between calcification and coronary events, yet significant stenosis can exist despite the absence of calcification (5). Although our patient had coronary artery calcification on a routine chest CT, the clinical suspicion of CAD, considering our patient's symptoms, was low.

Aspirin therapy was instituted after her bypass surgery. At present, the current recommendation of the American Diabetes Association regarding primary prevention with aspirin include patients with a family history of CAD, smokers, hypertension, obesity (BMI > 27.3 females, > 27.8 males), abnormal lipids (total cholesterol > 200 mg/dL, LDL > 100 mg/dL, HDL < 45 mg/dL (men)—< 55 mg/dL women, triglycerides > 200), age > 30 yr. In previous studies, it has been shown that aspirin in doses as low as 75 mg/d are effective in reducing thromboxane synthesis (6). The Early Treatment Diabetic Retinopathy Study (ETDRS) has established that aspirin is even safe in patients with known retinopathy, stating "aspirin neither prevented the development of high-risk proliferative retinopathy nor increased the risk of vitreous hemorrhage…" (7).

In the Bypass Angioplasty Revascularization Investigation (BARI) Study, a comparison was made between the 5 yr clinical outcome between CABG and percutaneous transluminal coronary angioplasty (PTCA). Although the overall 5 yr survival rates were similar, survival in the diabetic subgroup was higher in the CABG group (80.6%) vs the PTCA Group (65.5%) (8).

In a recent case-control study by Kaplan et al., postmenopausal estrogen use and risk of incident MI was studied. Of the 122 patients, 8.5% of case and 13.9% of control subjects were estrogen users. The risk of MI was noted to decrease with the length of time estrogen was used. This study suggested that use of postmenopausal estrogen replacement does not increase the risk of MI in women with diabetes and prolonged use may be of benefit (9).

The American Diabetes Association (ADA) Consensus Development Conference helped define risk factors that warrant further cardiac testing (Table 1) (5).

In summary, this case illustrates many salient facets in prevention, diagnosis, and treatment of CAD in diabetes, especially in women. Careful history taking, risk factor stratification, and modification (including cessation of smoking, treatment of hyperlipidemia,

Table 2
Current ADA Consensus Statement Definitions
for Abnormalities in Testing for Albumin Excretion
Case 3*

Category	24-h collection (mg/24h)	Timed collection (µg/min)	Spot collection (µg/mg creatinine)
Normal	<30	<20	<30
Microalbuminuria	30-300	20-200	30-300
Clinical albuminuria	>300	>200	>300

Because of variability in urinary albumin excretion, two of three specimens collected within a 3- to 6-mo period should be abnormal before considering a patient to have crossed one of these diagnostic thresholds. Exercise within 24 h, infection, fever, congestive heart failure, marked hyperglycemia, and marked hypertension may elevate urinary albumin excretion over baseline values.

*From (14) with permission.

and treatment of hypertension) as well as other modes of primary prevention (estrogen replacement therapy (ERT) and daily aspirin therapy) should be considered in patients with diabetes.

REFERENCES

1. Redberg RF. Coronary artery disease in women: understanding the diagnostic and management pitfalls. Medscape Women's Health 1998;3:1.
2. Galcera-Tomas J, Melgarejo-Moreno A, Garcia-Alberola A, Rodriguez-Garcia P, Lozano-Martinez J, Martinez-Hernandez J, Martinez-Fernandez S. Prognostic significance of diabetes in acute myocardial infarction. Are there differences linked to female gender? Int J Card 1999;69:289–298.
3. Lopez-Jimenez F, Goldman L, Johnson PA, Polanczyk CA, Cook EF, Fleishmann KE, Orav EJ, Lee TH. Effects of diabetes mellitus on the presentation and triage of patients with acute chest pain without known coronary artery disease. Am J Med 1998;105:500–505.
4. Nesto RW, Watson FS, Kowalchuk GJ, Zarich SW, Hill T, Lewis SM, Lane SE. Silent myocardial ischemia and infarction with peripheral vascular disease: Assessment by dipyridamole thallium-201 scintigraphy. Int J Card 1999;69:289–298.
5. American Diabetes Association. Consensus Development Conference on the Diagnosis of Coronary Heart Disease in People with Diabetes: 10–11 Feb. 1998, Miami, FL. Diabetes Care 1998;21:1551–1559.
6. American Diabetes Association Position Statement—Aspirin Therapy in Diabetes. ADA Clinical Practice Recommendations—2000. Diabetes Care 2000;23:S61–S62.
7. Early Treatment Diabetic Retinopathy Study (ETDRS) Investigators. Aspirin effects on mortality and morbidity in patients with diabetes mellitus-ETDRS report 14. JAMA 1992;68:1292–1300.
8. The Bypass Angioplasty Revascularization Investigation (BARI) Investigators. Comparison of coronary bypass surgery with angioplasty in patients with multivessel disease. N Engl J of Med 1996;335:217–225.
9. Kaplan RC, Heckbert SR, Weiss NS, Wahl PW, Smith NL, Newton KM, Psaty BM. Postmenopausal estrogens and risks of myocardial infarction in diabetic women. Diabetes Care 1998;21:1117–1121.

CASE #2: LATENT AUTOIMMUNE DIABETES IN ADULTS

Case Description

This fit, 75-yr-old male flight engineer was initially diagnosed with type 2 diabetes mellitus at the age of 73. At the time of diagnosis in November 1997, he was hospitalized with a deep-seated staphylococcus aureus infection following arthroscopic left rotator cuff repair. He was initially treated with insulin at the time of diagnosis, but later was switched to the combination of metformin and troglitazone by his primary physician. With failure of these agents to provide adequate glycemic control, in June 1999 he was started on insulin. At the time of referral, he was taking NPH, 10 U q AM and 10 U q PM and Rosiglitazone 4 mg daily (added 2 wk prior to presentation and subsequently discontinued).

Concomitant other medical problems included hypertension and hyperlipidemia diagnosed in 1996.

His family history was significant for his mother having type 2 diabetes mellitus, and dying at age 82 of cardiovascular complications. There was no family history of type 1 diabetes mellitus.

Laboratory results referral included a glycosylated hemoglobin of 10.4% (normal range 4.0–7.0 %). Fasting glucose was 79 mg/dL. His creatinine was 1.2 mg/dL. Lipid profile yielded total cholesterol of 243 mg/dL, triglycerides of 116 mg/dL, HDL of 78 mg/dL, and LDL of 142 mg/dL. Spot test for microalbuminuria (ratio of albumin/creatinine) was 72 µg/mg (normal range- <30 µg/mg).

A recent ophthalmology examination showed no evidence of diabetic retinopathy. Subjectively, he noted some changes in sensation in his right hand (known right carpal tunnel syndrome), but otherwise no numbness, tingling, or pain consistent with diabetic neuropathy.

On examination, his blood pressure was 134/70 mmHg, pulse 60. He was a thin, tanned, white male. Other vital signs included: height 175 cm, weight 70.1 kg, and body mass index (BMI) of 22.9 kg/m^2. There was no evidence of acanthosis nigricans. He had Dupuytren's contractures bilaterally. There was no evidence of structural abnormality of the feet. He had normal reflexes bilaterally and normal sense of vibration bilaterally. The remainder of his exam was normal.

Because his presentation was somewhat atypical for type 2 diabetes mellitus, the decision was made to check C-peptide and glutamic acid decarboxylase (GAD) antibodies. His C-peptide was 150 pmol/L (normal range 170–190 pmol/L). GAD65 antibody assay was 237 nmol/L (positive value defined as ≥0.03 nmol/L) (1).

Discussion

Historically GAD antibodies have been associated with the Stiff-man (Moersch–Woltman) Syndrome as well as type 1 diabetes mellitus (1). An early case report involved GAD antibodies in a patient who had the Stiff-man syndrome, epilepsy, and diabetes mellitus (2). The further investigation by Baekkeskov et al. lead to identification of the 65-kd isoform of GAD as an autoantigen in type 1 diabetes in 1990 (3).

Latent autoimmune diabetes in adults (LADA) has been characterized by patients ≥25 yr, "masquerading " as nonobese type 2 diabetes, initial control with diet or oral hypoglycemic agents, and eventual insulin dependency occurring within months to years (4).

In an attempt to characterize LADA, Tuomi et al. studied a population in Finland (5). In this study, the prevalence of GAD antibody was 9.3% in type 2 patients, 3.6% in patients with impaired glucose tolerance, and 4.4% in control subjects. Of the patients with GAD antibody negative, islet cell antibodies were detected in 0.5%. This study defined some clinical features of patients with GAD antibodies. First, these patients had a lower fasting C-peptide concentration and a decreased insulin response to oral glucose. These patients were also noted to have lower systolic and diastolic blood pressures, lower serum triglycerides, and lower waist-to-hip ratios (primarily in men). This study concluded with a formal definition for LADA—"GAD Ab positivity (>5 relative units) in patients older than 35 yr at the onset of type 2 diabetes (5)."

GAD antibodies have been cited as a possible mechanism in the secondary failure of oral sulfonylurea agents. In a recent study from Japan, 11% of patients with secondary failure of diet and/or sulfonylurea agents were found to have anti-GAD. Of great interest in the same study, 23.8% of nonobese, insulin deficient patients were found to have anti-GAD *(6)*. This has also been well described in an Italian cohort of lean, newly diagnosed patients with diabetes *(7)*.

In the United Kingdom Prospective Diabetes Study (UKPDS) 25, islet cell antibodies (ICA) and GAD antibodies decreased with increasing age at diagnosis *(8)*. In addition, patients with GAD antibodies or ICA had a higher HbA_{1c} and a lower BMI than those without antibodies *(8)*.

GAD antibody testing may help in identifying patients at risk for developing type 1 diabetes mellitus in the near future. To date, it remains unclear whether anti-GAD positivity in nondiabetic patients represents slow β-cell destruction or whether it can be attributed to part of the normal aging process *(9)*. Of great interest, a recent report from the Netherlands showed a low prevalence of anti-GAD in 50–80 yr olds with both normal and abnormal glucose tolerance, somewhat refuting concerns regarding decreased positivity in relation to increased age *(10)*.

Hatziagelaki et al. showed that "islet cell antibody status, BMI, and presence of thyroid and adrenal antibodies showed no significant correlation to insulin requirement (<2 yr after diagnosis)." In this same study, GAD 65 antibodies were found to be associated with insulin dependency less than 2 yr after diagnosis *(11)*.

Whittingham et al. studied stored sera of pregnant Finnish women who were eventually diagnosed with diabetes and showed the long latency of seropositivity of GAD antibodies in women before the development of insulin dependent diabetes mellitus. The study also showed the presence of anti-GAD in noninsulin dependent diabetes mellitus, which the authors presumed, represented an NIDDM phase of autoimmune insulitis *(12)*.

The question to whether early diagnosis of type 1 diabetes mellitus makes a long-term difference in the care of these patients is answered by the Diabetes Control and Complications Trial (DCCT). In the DCCT, patients with type 1 diabetes mellitus were studied to evaluated β-cell function with a stimulated C-peptide level following a standard, mixed meal. A portion of the patients showing an elevated C-peptide level were started on intensive insulin therapy. Patients with elevated, stimulated C-peptide level on an intensive insulin program were found to maintain β-cell function as evidenced by yearly C-peptide levels. The intensive therapy helped sustain the endogenous insulin secretion, lowering the risk of hypoglycemia and improving metabolic control. The DCCT also confirmed the importance of intensive therapy in reducing retinopathy progression and preventing microalbuminuria *(13)*.

Another question to address is whether all patients with the propensity to develop type 1 diabetes have GAD antibodies. In a study by Littorin et al. the predictive value of islet cell antibody (ICA) and GAD65 antibody (GADA) was studied in young adults 6 yr following diagnosis of either type 2 or unclassified diabetes mellitus. Of great interest, the sensitivity for eventual insulin treatment was 74% with the presence of ICA or GADA, but with both ICA and GADA the specificity was 100% *(14)*.

This patient presented with atypical features of type 2 diabetes mellitus, particularly his lean body habitus and minimal response to an oral hypoglycemic regimen, prompting GAD antibody testing. This case illustrates the need to carefully classify the type of diabetes, as well as the potential advantages of identifying patients who are antibody positive and really have type 1 diabetes. By early classification, a more effective treatment regimen can be embarked upon and the complications associated with poor glycemic control may be avoided. With early insulin treatment, islet cell functioning may also be preserved to some extent. The residual insulin secretory ability may make glucose fluctuations more stable and insulin management and glycemic control easier.

REFERENCES

1. Walikonis JE, Lennon VA. Radioimmunoassay for glutamic acid decarboxylas (GAD65) autoantibodies as a diagnostic aid for stiff-man syndrome and a correlate of susceptibility to type 1 diabetes mellitus. Mayo Clinic Proc 1998;73:1161–1166.
2. Solimena M, Folli F, Denis-Donini S, Comi GC, Pozza G, De Camilli P, Vicari AM. Autoantibodies to glutamic acid decarboxylase in a patient with stiff-man syndrome, epilepsy, and type 1 diabetes mellitus. N Engl J Med 1998;318:1012–1020.
3. Baekkeskov S, Aanstoot H-J, Christgau S, Reetz A, Solimena M, Cascalho M, et al. Identification of the 64K autoantigen in insulin-dependent diabetes as the GABA-synthesizing enzyme glutamic acid decarboxylase. Nature 1990;347:151–156.
4. Zimmet P, Turner R, McCarty D, Rowley M, Mackay I. Crucial points at diagnosis. Type 2 diabetes or slow type 1 diabetes. Diabetes Care 1999;22:59B–64B.
5. Tuomi T, Carlsson A, Li H, Isomaa B, Miettinen A, Nilsson A, et al. Clinical and genetic characteristics of type 2 diabetes with and without GAD antibodies. Diabetes 1999;48:150–157.
6. Fukui M, Nakano K, Shigeta H, Yoshimori K, Fujii M, Kitagawa Y, et al. Antibodies to glutamic acid decarboxylase in Japanese diabetic patients with secondary failure of oral hypoglycaemic therapy. Diabetic Med 1997;14:148–152.
7. Bruno G, De Salvia A, Arcari R, Borra M, Grosso N, Carta Q, Trovati M, Veglio M, Pagano G. Clinical, immunological, and genetic heterogeneity of diabetes in an Italian population-based cohort of lean newly diagnosed patients aged 30-34 years. Piedmont Study Group for Diabetes Epidemiology. Diabetes Care 1999;22:50–55.
8. Turner R, Sratton I, Orton V, Manley S, Zimmet P, Mackay IR, et al. for UK Prospective Diabetes Study (UKPDS) Group. UKPDS 25: autoantibodies to islet-cell cytoplasm and glutamic acid decarboxylase for prediction of insulin requirement in type 2 diabetes. Lancet 1997;350:1288–1293.
9. Yliharsila H, Tuomilehto J, Mackay IR, Zimmet P, Tuomilehto-Wolf E, Rowley MJ, Nissinen A. GAD Antibodies in elderly men in different categories of glucose tolerance. Diabetes Care 1999;22:996–997.
10. Ruige JB, Batstra MR, Aanstoot HJ, Bouter LM, Bruining GJ, de Neeling JN, Heine RJ. Low prevalence of antibodies to GAD65 in a 50- to 74-year-old general Dutch population. The Hoorn Study. Diabetes Care 1997;20:1108–1110.
11. Hatziagelaki E, Jaeger C, Maeser E, Bretzel RG, Federlin K. GAD 65 antibody but not ICA positivity in adult-onset diabetic patients is associated with early progression to clinical insulin dependency. Acta Diabetologica 1996;33:291–294.
12. Whittingham S, Byron SL, Tuomilehto J, Zimmet PZ, Myers MA, Vidgren G, et al. Autoantibodies associated with presymptomatic insulin-dependent diabetes mellitus in women. Diabetic Med 1997;14:678–685.
13. The Diabetes Control and Complications Trial Research Group. Effect of intensive insulin therapy on residual beta-cell function in patients with type 1 diabetes in the diabetes control and complication trial: a randomized control trial. Ann Intern Med 1998;128:517–523.
14. Littorin B, Sundkvist G, Hagopian W, Landin-Olsson M, Lernmark A, Ostman J, et al. Islet cell and glutamic acid decarboxylase antibodies present at diagnosis of diabetes predict the need for insulin treatment: a cohort study in young adults whose disease was initially labeled as type 2 or unclassifiable diabetes. Diabetes Care 1999;22:409–412.

CASE #3: CHANGING INSULIN REGIMEN

Case Description

This 44-yr-old man was diagnosed with type 1 diabetes mellitus at the age of 27, when he presented with weight loss, frequent urination, and increased appetite. He was started on insulin at the time of diagnosis. There was no family history of diabetes mellitus. His only concomitant medical problem is hyperlipidemia. He has no history of background diabetic retinopathy (yearly ophthalmology visits dating back to 1983) or diabetic nephropathy.

Three years and 11 mo following the diagnosis of type 1 diabetes mellitus, he was enrolled in the Diabetes Control and Complications Trial (DCCT). In the DCCT, he was randomized to the "experimental" arm of the trial that included beginning an intensive insulin regimen of three shots of regular insulin and one shot of ultralente each day. (multiple daily injection [MDI] program). At entry into the DCCT (March 1987), his hemoglobin A_{1c} (HbA$_{1c}$) was 7.8% (normal range 4.0–6.3%). Despite randomization to the intensive insulin regimen, his HbA$_{1c}$ at the time of completion of the trial was 8.3%. The lowest HbA$_{1c}$ achieved during the trial was 7.2%. The patient was quite compliant with the intensive therapy. He experienced hypoglycemia usually two times per week. Despite the study and intervention, his HbA$_{1c}$ did not improve.

In 1994, he was enrolled in the Epidemiology of Diabetes Intervention and Complications (EDIC) Study. At the time of enrollment, he was taking regular insulin 6 U before breakfast, 6 U before lunch, and 17 U before dinner with Ultralente 26 U. His average reflectance meter glucose (RMG) was 137 mg/dL, and his glycosylated hemoglobin prior to enrollment was 10.3% (normal range 4.0–7.0%).

He was begun on lispro insulin in September 1996, soon after its release. His dose was lispro 7 U before breakfast, lispro 7 U before lunch, and lispro 17 U before dinner (with proper supplementation) and ultralente 35 U with the evening meal. After starting lispro, there was some improvement in glycosylated hemoglobin, from 9.9% to 9.3%. With continued modifications to his regimen between December 1996 and September 1999, his glycosylated hemoglobin ranged from 8.8 to 10.3%.

No long-term sequelae of his diabetes have been noted, including no significant background diabetic retinopathy and no microalbuminuria. No significant CAD has been noted, but his risk factors include a 25-pack-yr smoking history and hyperlipidemia.

Despite close follow-up, he continued to have elevated blood sugars, particularly overnight, checking RMG at 3 AM. He had no defined exercise program, but leads an active lifestyle as a farmer. His current laboratory profile includes a fasting glucose of 234 mg/dL and a glycosylated hemoglobin of 10.5%. A lipid profile showed a total cholesterol of 240 mg/dL, an HDL cholesterol of 51 mg/dL, an LDL cholesterol of 148 mg/dL, and triglycerides of 60 mg/dL. His creatinine was 0.9 mg/dL. His examination was essentially normal with no evidence of diabetic neuropathy or diabetic retinopathy. In January 2000, he was started on an insulin infusion pump.

Discussion

This case presents a complicated therapeutic dilemma and illustrates the considerations to be made in modification of the intensive insulin regimen. Despite intensive treatment of this patient, including being one of the original study subjects in the intensive treatment arm of the DCCT, he continued to have elevated HbA$_{1c}$ values. Modifications to his insulin program, including the substitution of lispro insulin for regular insulin, made little impact on the control of his type 1 diabetes mellitus. Even during the DCCT, the endocrinologist following the patient questioned whether the HgbA$_{1c}$ was correct, considering the RMG readings were well documented within a satisfactory range. The decision to switch him to an insulin infusion pump was made with hopes of decreasing glycemic excursions and providing more predictable treatment of postprandial hyperglycemia.

Lispro insulin is a short-acting insulin analog that has the sequence of the β chain inverted at amino acids 28 and 29. In initial studies, lispro proved to have faster action than regular insulin, virtually eliminating the previous waiting period postadministration, prior to eating (1). In an MDI program, when compared to regular insulin, lispro insulin gives a more physiologic profile and tends to lower glycemic excursions (2). Another study by Colombel et al. not only supported the findings of decreased blood glucose fluctuations and reduced hypoglycemia, it also confirmed that patients actually preferred the lispro regimen (3).

Lougheed et al. confirmed the stability of lispro in infusion systems (4). In a 1996 study by Zinman et al. of continuous subcutaneous insulin infusion (CSII), the 1-h postprandial blood glucose was significantly improved on lispro versus regular (5). In 1998, Melki ct al. showed that lispro insulin could be effectively used in CSII and provided better glycemic control than regular insulin without any significant change in the frequency of hypoglycemic episodes. This study also verified that postprandial blood glucose levels were particularly improved on CSII with lispro insulin (6). This is quite applicable to this patient as it was suspected that he was having significant postprandial hyperglycemia as evidenced by a high glycosylated hemoglobin, yet with relatively normal preprandial reflectance meter readings.

As described in the DCCT, both CSII and MDI are effective means of improving glycemic control. In the DCCT, subjects were not randomly assigned to MDI. Patients were first assigned to intensive treatment, and then the treatment team and the patient decided the choice of MDI vs CSII (7). CSII-treated patients maintained a HbA_{1c} of 6.8% while patients with MDI maintained a HbA_{1c} of 7.0%. Complications of hypoglycemia with coma and seizure and diabetic ketoacidosis were reported to be modestly higher with CSII vs MDI (7). CSII therapy requires some specific aspects of care. First and foremost, both the physician and the healthcare team need to have a clear understanding of pump function, appropriate patient selection, and preparedness for specific issues. According to the American Diabetes Association (ADA) Position Statement, "… candidates for CSII must be strongly motivated to improve glucose control and willing to work with their health care provider in assuming substantial responsibility for their day to day care. They must also understand and demonstrate use of the insulin pump, self-monitoring of blood glucose, and use of data so obtained (8)."

Appropriate choice of candidates is essential considering both the costs of a CSII device and the inherent risks and possible morbidity in patients without proper education. Indeed, glycemic control with CSII can be poor or even unpredictable in the unprepared patient, subsequently leading to risks of ketoacidosis and worsening of microvascular disease. The ADA position statement also comments, "Factors to be considered in choosing an insulin pump should include safety features, durability, availability of service by manufacturer, ability of supplier to provide training, ease of use, clinically desirable features, and cosmetic attractiveness to the user (8)."

Other benefits from CSII include findings from a study by Bode et al. which found that severe hypoglycemia could be reduced in patients on CSII. This study basically switched patients from an established MDI program to a CSII program after a minimum of 12-mo time. The incidence of severe hypoglycemia declined from 138 to 22 events per 100 patient yr. $HgbA_{1c}$ remained essentially unchanged between the two modes of therapy, but in patients who entered into the CSII portion of the study with a $HgbA_{1c}$ of ≥8.0%, reductions in $HgbA_{1c}$ were noted (9).

This case essentially parallels the advances that have been made in the past decade in intensive insulin therapy. Despite involvement in the DCCT that confirmed the significance of tighter glycemic control in preventing microvascular complications, the patient had consistently elevated HbA_{1c} values. Even during the study, the patient's primary physician did not believe the lab values. His story exemplifies a complicated problem, i.e., postprandial hyperglycemia seen in the type 1 population. Reasonable modifications were made to his program, including changing the short-acting insulin to lispro with modest benefit. This case confirms the necessity of careful follow-up and decision making with intensive insulin regimens as well as considerations for appropriate use of CSII. With the addition of CSII, his glycemic control has improved significantlpy.

REFERENCES

1. Howey DC, Bowsher RR, Brunelle RL, Woodworth JR. [Lys(B28), Pro(B29)]-Human insulin a rapidly absorbed analogue of human insulin. Diabetes 1994;43:396–402.
2. Jacobs MAJM, Keulen ETP, Kanc K, Casteleijn S, Scheffer P, Deville W, Heine RJ. Metabolic efficacy of preprandial administration of Lys(B28), Pro(B29) human insulin analog in IDDM patients: a comparison with human regular insulin during a three-meal test period. Diabetes Care 1997;20:1279–1286.
3. Colombel A, Murat A, Krempf M, Kuchly-Anton B, Charbonnel B. Improvement of blood glucose control in type 1 diabetic patients treated with lispro and multiple NPH injections. Diabetic Med 1999;16:319–324.
4. Lougheed WD, Zinman B, Strack TR, Janis LJ, Weymouth AB, Bernstein EA, Korbas AM, Frank BH. Stability of insulin lispro in insulin infusion systems. Diabetes Care 1997;20:1061–1065.
5. Zinman B, Tildesley H, Chiasson J, Tsui E, Strack T. Insulin lispro in CSII: results of a double-blind crossover study. Diabetes 1997;46:440–443.
6. Melki V, Renard E, Lassmann-Vague V, Boivin S, Guerci B, Hanaire-Broutin H, et al. Improvement of HbA_{1c} and blood glucose stability in IDDM patients treated with lispro insulin analog in external pumps. Diabetes Care 1998;21:977–982.
7. Diabetes Control and Complications Research Group. Implementation of treatment protocols in the Diabetes Control and Complications Trial. Diabetes Care 1995;18:361–376.
8. American Diabetes Association. Position statement—continuous subcutaneous insulin infusion. (Clinical Practice Recommendations 2000). Diabetes Care 2000;23:S90.
9. Bode B, Steed DR, Davidson PC. Reduction in severe hypoglycemia with long-term continuous subcutaneous insulin infusion in type I diabetes. Diabetes Care 1996; 19:324–327.

CASE #4: PROGRESSIVE DIABETIC NEPHROPATHY

Case Description

This 39-yr-old woman was diagnosed with type 1 diabetes mellitus at the age of 7 yr, during an evaluation for chicken pox. Presenting symptoms included weight loss and frequent urination and was found to be in ketoacidosis. Complications from diabetes at present include neuropathy, nephropathy, and proliferative retinopathy. Her only other medical problem is hypertension.

Her proteinuria was initially diagnosed in 1980 (age 20) on a routine urinalysis when hospitalized for a staphylococcal infection following a spider bite. A 24 urine for protein was 2.16 g. Her serum creatinine and iothlamate clearance were 0.8 mg/dL and 111 mL/min/1.73 m^2, respectively.

During this time, the patient was changed from a one injection daily insulin regimen to a two injection daily lente program. Despite this change, her hyperglycemia persisted, and her physician added regular insulin (LR-0-LR-0 program). In 1983, she was started on an MDI program, leading to improvement in glycemic control with a glycosylated hemoglobin of 8.3%. Monthly blood pressure measurements remained below 140/90 mm Hg.

In October 1981, she first noticed right ankle edema. She was initially treated with hydrochlorothiazide and later was switched to furosemide. Follow-up testing in 1986 showed a creatinine of 1.7 mg/dL, an increase from previous measurements of 1.5 mg/dL (1984) and 1.4 mg/dL (1985). In 1987, enalapril therapy was initiated for persistent proteinuria and mild hypertension. With the combination of furosemide and enalapril, her blood pressure control improved. In 1991, her creatinine remained stable at 1.9 with an iothalamate clearance of 45 mL/min/1.73 m^2.

She returned in the mid-1990s after some time lost to follow-up because she married and moved. She had remained on the combination of enalapril and furosemide. From 1995 to the present, she has remained on these two agents. Over this time period, her mean glycosylated hemoglobin was 8.4%, blood pressure remained within normal range (108/74–126/82 mmHg), and her urinary albumin levels fluctuated from 418 to 1116 mg/24 h. Her level of renal function has remained relatively constant with iothalamate clearances of 47 mL/min/1.73 m^2 in 1997 and 45 mL/min/1.73 m^2 in 1999.

Discussion

This case also parallels the changes in the standards of care in of diabetes. Nephropathy related to diabetes is quite common. According to the United States Renal Data System (USRDS) Report, 40% of end-stage renal disease from 1993–1997 was directly attributed to diabetes [1]. The cost of treatment of diabetic patients with end-stage renal disease was estimated in 1991 to be 2 billion dollars per year [2].

Diabetic Nephropathy can be defined by five distinct stages.

STAGE 1—THE HYPERTROPHY-HYPERFUNCTION STAGE

This stage occurs at the initial onset of type 1 diabetes mellitus. The glomerular filtration rate (GFR) is increased because of hyperfiltration. In addition, overall kidney size is increased and glomerular hypertrophy is demonstrated on renal biopsy. Because of hyperfiltration, microalbuminuria may be present but is reversible with better glucose control [3].

STAGE 2—THE "RENAL-LESION-WITHOUT-CLINICAL-SIGNS STAGE"

As early as 2 yr after onset of disease, mesangial expansion and thickening of glomerular basement membranes are evident on a microscopic level. During this stage, microalbuminuria is only present with poor metabolic control, ketosis and strenuous exercise. Otherwise, urinary albumin excretion is usually normal. With blood glucose levels below 250 mg/dL, the GFR remains elevated, but higher glucose levels are associated with a decline in GFR [4].

STAGE 3—EARLY NEPHROPATHY WITH PERSISTENT MICROALBUMINURIA AND HYPERTENSION

This usually occurs after 10–15 yr of disease. Blood pressure elevation is associated with microalbuminuria and may first be noted in this stage. In the kidney, glomerular histologic changes continue to progress. With years of experience showing that microalbuminuria is a predictor of renal disease progression, intervention is essential at or before this stage [3].

STAGE 4—OVERT NEPHROPATHY

The GFR begins to decrease, typically at a rate of 10 mL/min/yr. On renal biopsy, diabetic nephropathy is classically characterized by nodular glomerulosclerosis, but more commonly the diagnosis is based on clinical findings. Microalbuminuria has progressed to albuminuria by this stage (0.3 g/24 h), and the majority of patients have hypertension. The decline in GFR may be slowed with appropriate antihypertensive therapy and possibly better glucose control (3).

STAGE 5—END STAGE RENAL DISEASE (ESRD)

In diabetic patients, renal replacement therapy with dialysis or renal transplantation is generally recommended once the GFR falls below 15 mL/min. In the past, this typically would occur a mean of 15 yr from the development of proteinuria in patients with type 1 diabetes mellitus (3).

Treatment and prevention of diabetic nephropathy should be a *two-tiered approach* from the initial diagnosis of diabetes. First and foremost, stringent control of blood glucose levels is vital. Second, early identification and treatment of microalbuminuria, along with management of blood pressure, complete this strategy.

The importance of glycemic control was clearly illustrated in the Diabetes Control and Complications Trial (DCCT) (5). In this study, intensive insulin therapy either by multiple daily injections (MDI) or continuous subcutaneous insulin infusion (CSII) was compared with usual insulin therapy. The occurrence of microalbuminuria (defined as ≥40 mg/24 h) decreased by 39%, and albuminuria (urinary albumin excretion ≥300 mg/24 h) decreased by 54% (5). The continuation of the DCCT, the Epidemiology of Diabetes Interventions and Complications (EDIC) study, showed that despite some increases in hemoglobin A_{1C} in the Diabetes Control and Complications Trial study groups, the reduction of risk of nephropathy and retinopathy in patients on intensive insulin treatment persisted (6).

The second essential approach is the addition of an ACE inhibitor. In 1993, the Collaborative Study Group reported a randomized, multicenter, placebo-controlled investigation showing that captopril had "kidney-protecting properties" (7). Although previous small studies showed that ACE inhibitors could decrease the rate of progression from microalbuminuria to clinical albuminuria, this study, performed in type 1 patients with overt nephropathy, showed that captopril was able to delay progression of renal disease as measured by a fall in creatinine clearance. This was one of the first major investigations to clearly show that ACE inhibitors protected against deterioration in renal function above and beyond the antihypertensive effect of this class of drugs (7). In 1994, Hebert et al. reported additional supporting data from the Collaborative Study showing that remission of nephrotic range proteinuria was an attainable goal in the long-term care of type 1 diabetes mellitus (8). In the long-term follow-up of The Collaborative Study involving 409 patients with diabetic nephropathy, 108 patients randomized to captopril therapy and control of blood pressure (mean SBP = 135 ± 6 mmHg, Mean DBP = 78 ± 4 mmHg), eight of these patients had remission of diabetic nephropathy, and to date, six of these patients remain in remission of nephrotic syndrome (9). Data from The Collaborative Study and others have drastically changed the approach and standard of care in the prevention and treatment of diabetic nephropathy.

Further benefits from the use of ACE inhibitors continue to be reported. The HOPE Study (Heart Outcomes Prevention Evaluation) and Micro-HOPE Study demonstrated that with the use of the ACE inhibitor ramipril, not only was nephropathy decreased, but there was also a lower risk of MI, stroke, cardiovascular death, a need for coronary revascularization, and overall mortality *(10)*. Currently, angiotensin subtype 1 receptor antagonists (AT_1RA) remain under investigation, but early studies show that they exert equivalent effects to ACE inhibitors in both reducing blood pressure and proteinuria. Although not considered first-line therapy at present, it has been suggested that AT_1RA could be used in patients intolerant of ACE inhibitors *(11)*. Of interest, the combination of an ACE inhibitor and a nondihydropyridine calcium antagonist has recently been reported to reduce proteinuria greater than either agent alone *(12)*.

The current American Diabetes Association position statement entitled "Standards of Care For Patients With Diabetes Mellitus," includes testing for microalbuminuria in pubertal and postpubertal patients with disease duration of at least 5 yr and in all patients with type 2 diabetes mellitus. In the absence of previously documented microalbuminuria, the current recommendation is yearly testing. The three currently accepted methods for evaluation of microalbuniria include: 1) Spot urine collection, measuring albumin-to-creatinine ratio; 2) 24-h urine collection of albumin and creatinine (allowing the additional measurement of creatinine clearance); and 3) other timed interval collection *(13)*.

In a recent review, Molitch summed up our present knowledge of diabetic nephropathy stating, "The natural history of diabetic nephropathy has been clarified to a great extent over the past 25 years, allowing identification of patients with nephropathy at a point very early in their course, often 15–25 years before they might develop ESRD *(15)*."

This case illustrates the importance of early recognition and aggressive management in preventing progression of diabetic nephropathy. In this case, early recognition of nephropathy, intensive insulin therapy, aggressive control of blood pressure, and the addition of an ACE inhibitor have made a significant impact on slowing the progression of diabetic nephropathy.

REFERENCES

1. United States Renal Data System: USRDS 1999 Annual Data Report. National Institute of Health, National Institutes of Diabetes and Digestive and Kidney Disease. Bethesda, MD. Apr. 1999.
2. Nelson RG, Knowler WC, Pettitt DJ, Bennett PH. Kidney diseases in diabetes. In: Harris MI, ed. Diabetes in America. 2nd ed., NIH Publ No. 95-1468, 1995, pp. 349–400.
3. Mauer M, Mogensen CE, Friedman EA, Diabetic nephropathy. In: Schrier RW, Gottschalk CW, ed. Diseases of the Kidney, 6th ed., vol. III, Little, Brown and Company, 1997, pp. 2019–2062.
4. Vora JP, Chattington PD, Ibrahim H. Clinical manifestations and natural history of diabetic nephropathy. In: Johnson RJ, Feehally J, ed. Comprehensive Clinical Nephrology, Mosby, London, UK, 2000, p. 6.34.3.
5. The Diabetes Control and Complications Trial Research Group. The effect of intensive treatment of diabetes on the development and progression of long-term complications in insulin-dependent diabetes mellitus. N Engl J Med 1993;329:977–986.
6. The Diabetes Control and Complications Trial/ Epidemiology of Diabetes Interventions and Complications Research Group. Retinopathy and nephropathy in patients with type 1 diabetes four years after a trial of intensive therapy. N Engl J Med 2000;342:381–389.
7. Lewis EJ, Hunsicker LG, Bain RP, Rohde RD, for the Collaborative Study Group. The effect of angiotensin-converting-enzyme inhibition on diabetic nephropathy. N Engl J Med 1993;329:1456–1462.
8. Hebert LA, Bain RP, Verme D, Cattran D, Whittier FC, Tolchin N, Rohde RD, Lewis EJ, for the Collaborative Study Group. Remission of nephrotic range proteinuria in type I diabetes. Kidney Int 1994; 46:1688–1693.
9. Wilmer WA, Hebert LA, Lewis EJ, Rohde RD, Whittier F, Cattran D, Levey AS, Lewis JB, Spitalewitz S, Blumenthal S, Bain RP. Remission of nephrotic syndrome in type 1 diabetes: long-term follow-up of patients in the captopril study. Am J Kidney Dis 1999;34:308–314.

10. Heart Outcomes Prevention Evaluation (HOPE) Study Investigators. Effects of ramipril on cardiovascular and microvascular outcomes in people with diabetes mellitus: results of HOPE study and MICRO-HOPE substudy. Lancet 2000;355:253–259.
11. Taal MW, Brenner BM. Renoprotective benefits of RAS inhibition from ACEI to angiotensin II antagonists. Kidney Int 2000;57:1803–1817.
12. Bakris GL, Weir MR, DeQuattro V, McMahon FG. Effects of an ACE inhibitor/calcium antagonist combination on proteinuria in diabetic nephropathy. Kidney Int 1999;54:1283–1289.
13. Amercan Diabetes Association. Position statement—standards of medical care for patients with diabetes mellitus. Diabetes Care 2000;23:S32–S42.
14. American Diabetes Association: Position statement—diabetic nephropathy. Diabetes Care 2000;23:S69–S72.
15. Molitch ME. Management of early diabetic nephropathy. Am J Med 1997;102:392–398.

17

Type 2 Diabetes Mellitus

Neelima V. Chu, MD *and Robert R. Henry,* MD

CONTENTS

CASE #1: 40-YR-OLD OBESE MAN WITH PROGRESSIVE POLYDIPSIA, POLYURIA, WEIGHT LOSS, AND HYPERGLYCEMIA

Case Description

A 40-yr-old African American male presents to the emergency room with a 2 wk history of upper-respiratory infection (URI) symptoms, progressively increasing polydipsia, polyuria, polyphagia, fatigue, nausea, vomiting, blurred vision, and a 10-lb. weight loss. Three weeks prior to admission, his primary care physician started him on a sulfonylurea for elevated blood sugars.

His past medical history is only significant for fungal infection in the groin area for which he is using clotrimazole cream for the last 2 mo. His family history is significant for diabetes mellitus (type 2) and hypertension in both grandparents, parents, and brother. He works as a security guard and has smoked one-half pack cigarettes per day for 10 yr. He is married and has two children. On review of systems, he denies any chest pain or short-ness of breath. He reports a voracious appetite, and has been drinking 10 regular sodas per day because of excessive thirst. In spite of eating and sleeping well, he feels very tired and unable to concentrate at his work.

His physical examination reveals the following: weight 107 kg, height 180 cm, body mass index (BMI) 33 kg/m^2, temp 38.5°C, blood pressure 139/74 mmHg, heart rate 110, respiratory rate 14 breaths/min. Head and neck examination reveals poor dentition with significant periodontal disease. Eye examination shows pupils that are normal and equally reactive. Extraoccular movements are intact and funduscopic exam shows flat discs. The

From: *Contemporary Endocrinology: Challenging Cases in Endocrinology*
Edited by: M. E. Molitch © Humana Press Inc., Totowa, NJ

chest and cardiac examinations are normal. His abdominal exam is remarkable for mild central obesity. The genital examination reveals evidence of tinea in the inguinal folds. The extremities demonstrate normal strength and sensation, with good pedal pulses, warm to touch, scant tinea between the toes and no cutaneous ulcers.

The laboratory examination is notable for a white cell count of 17,000 cells per cubic centimeter with 72% neutrophils, 22% lymphocytes, 3% monocytes, 3% eosinophils, a blood glucose of 580 mg/dL, an anion gap of 28, an aretrial pH of 7.30, serum ketones positive at 1:16 dilution, HbA_{1c} 13.2%, cholesterol 174 mg/dL, triglyceride 400 mg/dL. Antibodies done as an outpatient after discharge when the glucose was stable were positive for GAD and ICA.

Discussion

Diabetic ketoacidosis (DKA) is defined as a metabolic acidosis caused by significant insulin deficiency. The physiologic abnormalities present with DKA include: 1) Chronic hyperglycemia and glucose toxicity (glucose of 300–800 mg/dL); 2) acidosis caused by catabolism of fat and buildup of ketone bodies (pH 6.8–7.3 and HCO3 <15 meq/L); 3) low blood volume secondary to dehydration; and 4) hyperosmolarity is resulting from renal water loss and dehydration from sweating, nausea and vomiting *(1)*.

DKA results from an absolute or relative deficiency of insulin. In patients with type 1 diabetes, there is a total lack of insulin. In patients with type 2 diabetes, there is relative insulin deficiency; circulating insulin is present, but there is an excessive secretion of glucagon, catecholamines, cortisol, and growth hormone (counterregulatory hormones) and insulin secretion cannot increase sufficiently to counter their effects *(2)*. According to the above criteria, this patient appears to be in mild DKA. He has all the key features: glucose of 580 mg/dL, anion gap 28, and pH 7.30. He may be dehydrated as evidenced by the tachycardia but with well maintained blood pressure.

So, does this patient have type 1 or type 2 diabetes? It is possible that this patient may have type 1 diabetes. However, he has several factors in his history and presentation that suggest that he has type 2 diabetes. The patient is 40 yr old. The incidence of type 1 diabetes in this age group is 17.2/100,000 person years vs 155.2/100,000 persons per year for type 2 diabetes *(3)*. He is also obese and has a significant family history of type 2 diabetes *(4)*. The history of a prolonged course of polydipsia and polyuria is more consistent with type 2 diabetes. Patients with type 1 diabetes usually present with a short duration of symptoms before the onset of acidosis.

Individuals with type 2 diabetes can also present with DKA under certain conditions. Those conditions include either poor nutrition that contributes to dehydration, severe physiologic stress [i.e., infection, myocardial infarction (MI)], or chronic poor metabolic control which further contributes to decreased insulin secretion, decreased peripheral glucose uptake and increased hepatic glucose production with greater hyperglycemia *(1)*. The relative lack of insulin and excess of glucagon favors lipolysis with increased circulating free fatty acids, which serves as a substrate for ketone body formation. This hormonal imbalance also converts the liver to a ketogenic organ, using free fatty acids to produce ketone bodies with resulting acidemia *(2)*.

This patient has an elevated white blood cell count with fever and URI symptoms, which all point toward a probable underlying infection that precipitated the metabolic decompensation. He also has many signs and symptoms of poor glycemic control. Polyuria and polydipsia are symptoms of hyperglycemia leading to osmotic diuresis, hypertonicity, and dehydration. Both periodontal and candida skin infections may be signs of poor glycemic control *(5,6)*. Of course, drinking 10 regular sodas a day does not improve and likely worsens the hyperglycemia. Nonspecific symptoms such as lethargy, headaches, myalgia, and weakness are common under these circumstances. The gastrointestinal symptoms of nausea and vomiting maybe related to ketosis and acidosis *(2)*.

Regardless of the cause of the DKA, the cornerstones of therapy are to identify and treat underlying precipitating events, administer fluids and insulin. First priority is fluid replacement. Insulin therapy is only effective if fluid is given rapidly and in the early stages. The total water deficit usually ranges from 50 to 100 mL/kg of body weight. Isotonic saline (0.9%) should be given at the rate of 1.0 L in the first hour, then 1.0 L in 2 h, and then 1.0 L every 4 h until the patient is well hydrated. Once the blood glucose has fallen below 250 mg/dL, iv fluids are changed to 5% dextrose with 0.45% NaCl *(2,7)*. Potassium, phosphate, and bicarbonate replacement may also be necessary for certain patients, depending on the severity of DKA. Aggressive therapy is not usually necessary in type 2 diabetes. Most patients with type 2 diabetes can be treated successfully with frequent (every 3–4 h) injections of regular insulin subcutaneously (5–15 U). Alternatively, an insulin drip can be started at 5 U/h with adjustments based on frequent glucose monitoring. The insulin infusion can be discontinued and intermediate acting NPH can be started when the HCO3 is >15 meq/L and the patient can eat light foods and drink liquids. If a source of infection is found, antibiotic therapy should be initiated early *(1)*.

Why did the patient fail sulfonylurea therapy? Prolonged high levels of glucose have a deleterious effect on β-cell secretory ability *(8)*. Sustained elevation of the plasma glucose also leads to an impairment of insulin action. The phenomenon is referred to as glucose desensitization or toxicity *(9)*. The result is often a temporary and usually reversible inability of the patient to respond to sulfonylurea therapy. Ideally, insulin should be used as initial treatment in newly diagnosed type 2 diabetes mellitus where there is ketosis and acidosis, severe hyperglycemic symptoms or weight loss from prolonged hyperglycemia. Some improvement in insulin secretion and action is likely to occur with normalization of the blood glucose and reversal of glucose toxicity. After a finite period of near normal glycemic control (1–3 wk), the patient's exogenous insulin requirements will probably decrease and reinstitution of therapy with an oral agent may be attempted with a reasonable likelihood of success.

To make the more definitive biochemical diagnosis of type 2 diabetes, measurements of c-peptide and insulin levels may be required. Patients with type 2 diabetes often have normal or elevated c-peptide and insulin levels *(9)*. However, these measurements must be done after the patient recovers from the acute illness, when the blood sugars normalize and the patient is off insulin.

Why does he have positive antibodies to GAD and ICA? Although islet cell antibodies (ICA) and glutamic acid decarboxylase antibodies (GAD) are markers of autoimmune β-cell damage and are present at onset in 70–80% of patients with type 1 diabetes, they can also occur in a subset of adults with type 2 diabetes mellitus *(10)*. A 10-yr followup study by Niskanen et al. *(11)* showed that GAD antibody and ICA positivity at the time of diagnosis was 9.0 and 3.8% in type 2 diabetic patients and 1.6 and 0% in the control population. During the 10-yr follow-up, 2.3% and 7.5% of the diabetic patients developed absolute and relative insulin deficiency, respectively. Of these patients, GAD antibody has a higher sensitivity in predicting the progression to absolute or relative insulin deficiency. Another study *(10)* showed that among young adults with type 2 diabetes, the phenotype of those with ICA or GAD antibodies was similar to that of classic type 1. They also demonstrated that in older adults, the phenotype was closer to that of classic type 2 diabetic patients without antibodies. The presence of antibodies only predicted an increase likelihood of exogenous insulin requirement. Therefore, a positive screening for GAD could be used in patients aged younger than 45 yr at the time of diagnosis to indicate who has an increased risk of requiring insulin therapy. Among GAD antibody positive patients, the presence of ICA increases the likelihood that insulin will be required at an earlier stage.

There are also other features that are common to the GAD antibody positive type 2 patients. They differ with respect to β- cell function, features of the metabolic syndrome, and type 1 susceptibility genes. GAD antibody positive type 2 patients tend to have lower c-peptide concentrations, insulin responses to oral glucose loads, systolic and diastolic blood pressures, triglyceride concentrations, and waist-to-hip ratios, and increased frequencies of HLA-DQB1* 0201/0103 compared to GAD antibody negative patients *(12)*. However, the frequency of genotypes comprising the *0302 allele was significantly lower in GAD antibody type 2 diabetes than in type 1 diabetes.

During the hospitalization, this patient was well controlled on NPH and sliding scale regular insulin. He was instructed on proper diet and given training on home glucose measurements. The fungal infection was treated by topical antifungal cream. The patient switched to diet sodas and began to exercise regularly. When he returned to the clinic 1 mo after discharge, he had lost 5 lb. and was requiring small amounts of subcutaneous insulin. He was then started on Metformin, and the dose gradually titrated upward as insulin was slowly weaned off. He will need to be followed closely to determine if insulin will be required in the future.

REFERENCES

1. Edelman SV, RR Henry. Diagnosis and management of type 2 diabetes. 3rd Edition Professional Communications Inc., Caddo, OK, 1999, pp. 163–172.
2. George K, Alberti MM. Diabetic acidosis, hyperosmolar coma, and lactic acidosis. In: Becker KL, ed. Principals and Practice of Endocrinology and Metabolism, 2nd ed., J.B. Lippincott, Philadelphia, PA, 1995, pp. 1316–1329.
3. Melton LJ, Palumbo PJ, Chu C. Incidence of diabetes mellitus by clinical type. Diabetes Care 1983;6: 75–86.
4. Krolewski AS, Warram JH. Natural history of diabetes. In: Becker KL, ed. Principles of Endocrinology and Metabolism, 2nd ed., J.B. Lippincott, Philadelphia, PA, 1995, pp. 1216–1217.
5. Genco RJ. Current view of risk factors for periodontal disease. J Periodontol 1996;67:1041–1049.
6. Paron NG, Lambert PW. Cutaneous manifestations of diabetes mellitus. Primary Care 2000;27:371–382.
7. Kitabchi A. Consequences of insulin deficiency. In: Korenman SG, ed. Atlas of Clinical Endocrinology, vol. 2. Current Medicine Inc., Philadelphia, PA, 2000, pp. 29–44.
8. Rossetti L, Giaccari A, De Fronzo RA. Glucose toxicity. Diabetes Care 1990;13:610–630.
9. DeFronzo RA, Bonadonna RC, Ferrannini E. Pathogenesis of NIDDM. A balanced overview. Diabetes Care 1992;15:318–368.
10. Turner R, Startton I, Horton V, Manley S, Zimmet P, Mackay IR, Shatton M, Bottazzo GF, Holman R. UKPDS 25: autoantibodies to islet-cell cytoplasm and glutamic acid decarboxylase for prediction of insulin requirement in type 2 diabetes. Lancet 1997;350:1288–1293.
11. Niskanen LK, Tuomi T, Karjalainen J, Groop LC, Uusitupa MIJ. GAD antibodies in NIDDM: ten year follow-up from the diagnosis. Diabetes Care 1995;18:1557–1565.
12. Tuomi T, Carlsson A, Li H, Isomaa B, Miettinen A, Nilsson A, et al. Clinical and genetic characteristics of type 2 diabetes with and without GAD antibodies. Diabetes 1999;48:150–157.

CASE #2: 52-YR-OLD MAN WITH LIPID ABNORMALITIES AND CORONARY ARTERY DISEASE

Case Description

A 52-yr-old Caucasian male with recently diagnosed type 2 diabetes presented to the emergency room with crushing chest pain radiating to the left side. His past medical history is significant for obesity and hypertension for 4 yr. He has been taking glyburide 10 mg BID and fosinopril 20 mg QD for 6 mo.

He has a strong family history of hypercholesterolemia and coronary artery disease. His father had a myocardial infarction (MI) at the age of 50 and his uncle had diabetes and died of an inferior wall MI at the age of 56. His older sister also has hypertension and is taking medications for hypercholesterolemia. The patient has smoked two packs of cigarettes per day for 20 yr. He works as a computer analyst and spends a significant number of hours sitting at his desk. He does not exercise or follow any dietary restrictions. On review of systems, he notes shortness of breath while walking. He denies any previous history of chest pains.

His physical examination reveals the following: weight 121 kg, height 181 cm, BMI 36.9 kg/m^2, blood pressure 149/95 mmHg, heart rate 93, respiratory rate 12. His skin is without any rashes. Funduscopic examination reveals no evidence of retinopathy. He does not have thyromegaly or carotid bruits. Chest and cardiovascular examinations are normal. He has abdominal obesity with a waist circumference of 48 in. Examination of the lower extremities reveals decreased vibratory sensation, 1+ posterior tibial and dorsalis pedis pulses, and no ulcers.

Laboratory examination is notable for a fasting glucose of 190 mg/dL, HbA$_{1c}$ 8.6%, total cholesterol 233 mg/dL, HDL cholesterol 27 mg/dL, LDL cholesterol 150 mg/dL, and triglycerides of 280 mg/dL. TSH, LFT'S, BUN, and creatinine are all within normal limits, but a spot urine for albumin:creatinine ratio is increased at 0.15 g/g (normal range: 0–0.03 g/g). An ECG shows 2 mm ST-T elevations across the anterior leads. A chest X-ray reveals evidence of congestive heart failure with an enlarged heart and interstitial edema.

Discussion

This case illustrates a common cluster of traits in patients with type 2 diabetes mellitus. This patient has multiple risk factors for coronary heart disease. He is a male, hypertensive, diabetic who is older than 50 yr, has abdominal obesity, is a heavy smoker, has high LDL cholesterol and triglyceride levels, has a markedly low HDL cholesterol level, and has a strong family history of premature coronary artery disease (CAD) *(1,2)*. Furthermore, he has microalbuminuria. Proteinuria is an important marker for diabetic nephropathy, but may also be a surrogate marker for advanced atherosclerosis.

Lipid abnormalities that accelerate atherosclerosis and increase the risk of cardiovascular disease are significantly more common in patients with type 2 diabetes than in nondiabetic individuals. In addition, central obesity and the presence of microalbuminuria in association with type 2 diabetes are risk factors for coronary heart disease. This combination of cardiovascular risk factors result in substantially increased cardiac morbidity and mortality in patients with type 2 diabetes. The Framingham Study found that the presence of diabetes doubled the age-adjusted risk for cardiovascular disease in men and tripled the risk in women *(3)*. In addition to increased risk, retrospectively analyzed data on diabetic patients undergoing percutaneous transluminal coronary angioplasty (PTCA) showed frequent evidence of multivessel disease. Furthermore, these diabetic patients had less likelihood of remaining free of infarction or additional revascularization at 5 yr and as a result were more likely to have a worse outcome *(4)*. Diabetic patients also have a higher risk of developing postinfarction angina. A cause of these complications maybe a lack of collateral blood flow *(5)*.

As seen in this case, during an acute MI, patients with diabetes present with pulmonary edema more commonly than do nondiabetic patients, suggesting that in spite of equivalent infarct size and left ventricular ejection fraction, the diabetic ventricle tolerates infarction poorly *(6)*. A number of theories have been postulated for this increased susceptibility and include diabetic cardiomyopathy resulting in diastolic dysfunction, reduced ejection fraction and diminished systolic function, abnormal diastolic function, impaired left ventricular diastolic relaxation, autonomic neuropathy, and decreased insulin sensitivity resulting in a shift from anaerobic metabolism of glucose to fatty acid metabolism with an increase in myocardial oxygen utilization *(6)*.

Although this patient presented with symptoms, another important clinical finding in diabetics is the lack of apparent chest pain, often resulting in silent ischemia *(7)*. Silent ischemia is thought to be caused by an alteration of the afferent and efferent limbs of the autonomic nervous system *(8–10)*. Autonomic dysfunction can promote the development of ischemia and infarction by increasing the resting heart rate and myocardial demand, as well as increasing the vascular tone, causing decreased blood flow.

The general treatment of MI in patients with diabetes is similar to that of nondiabetic patients. However, special considerations have to be taken into account, including the use of thrombolytic therapy, revascularization with bypass surgery or angioplasty, therapeutic management of elevated glucose levels, use of β blockers, ACE inhibitors, and of course, lipid lowering therapy. The International Study of Infarct Survival-II (ISIS-II) trial *(11)* has shown that diabetic patients derive the same benefits from thrombolytic therapy as nondiabetic patients. However, another large study (GUSTO-I) has shown that although they respond similarly with thrombolytic therapy in infarct related arterial patency rates, the mortality is higher among the diabetic patients at 30 d and at 1 yr *(12)*. In the past, the presence of diabetic retinopathy was thought to be an absolute contraindication for thrombolytic therapy owing to the risk of retinal hemorrhage. However, the GUSTO-I trial showed that out of 6011 patients with diabetes only one patient had ocular hemorrhage during thrombolytic therapy *(13)*. Therefore, retinopathy should not be considered a contraindication in the thrombolytic therapy of acute MI in diabetic patients with retinopathy.

The role of coronary artery bypass graft (CABG) in diabetics was investigated in the Bypass Angioplasty Revascularization Investigation (BARI) trial. The results showed that in diabetic patients on insulin or oral anti-diabetic agents, reduction in mortality after an MI was significantly greater with CABG compared to angioplasty *(14)*.

There has always been concern regarding the use of β blockers in diabetic patients because of the possibility of masking the symptoms of hypoglycemia and worsening glucose and lipid levels. However, studies have shown that β blockers after MI lower mortality by reducing the extent of infarction, recurrent ischemia, and sudden death in people with diabetes similarly to those without diabetes, without any increased risk of readmission with diabetic complications *(15)*. Thus, β blockers can and should be used following an acute MI in a diabetic patient. However, caution may be needed in patients with type 1 diabetes who are prone to hypoglycemia.

Recently, the Heart Outcomes Prevention Trials (HOPE) trial has shown that ramipril lowered the incidence of the combined endpoint of any cardiovascular event (cardiovascular death, MI, or stroke) in high-risk patients, including people with diabetes by 25% despite minimal effects on blood pressure *per se* *(16)*. This data suggests that ACE inhibitors have a direct vascular effect in diabetics that is independent of their hypertensive activity.

The role of glycemic control in reducing mortality during the acute MI remains uncertain. However, the diabetes mellitus insulin-glucose infusion in acute MI (DIGAMI) study has shown that the intensive treatment of diabetic patients in the periinfarct period (insulin-glucose infusion for 24 h followed by subcutaneous insulin four times daily for ≥3 mo) had lower mortality at one year and at 3.4 yr *(17)*.

Aside from acute intervention for the MI, this patient also needs long-term management of his dyslipidemia. This patient has the classic diabetic dyslipidemia associated with insulin resistance that includes hypertriglyceridemia, usually owing to elevated triglyceride rich, very low-density lipoprotein (VLDL) particles and a decrease in high-density lipoprotein (HDL) levels *(18)*. Low-density liporpotein (LDL) levels can be low, normal, or elevated in diabetic patients but qualitative changes in LDL with excessive amounts of small, dense low-density lipoprotein and intermediate-density lipoprotein (IDL) particles usually exist. Increased amounts of small dense LDL may increase the risk of atherosclerosis, even if absolute concentrations of LDL cholesterol are not significantly increased *(19,20)*. In addition, the oxidation of lipoproteins, in particular LDL, is enhanced in people with diabetes and oxidized LDL is cytotoxic to the vascular endothelial and smooth muscle cells, probably contributing to atherogenesis *(21)*.

Conventional risk factors, as described above, only partly explain the excess risk of developing atherosclerosis in diabetes mellitus. It has become apparent that type 2 diabetes is commonly associated with many novel cardiovascular risk factors that occur largely as a result of insulin resistance, hyperinsulinemia, and hyperglycemia. Hyperglycemia and advanced glycation endproduct (AGE) formation may also contribute to vascular injury. Both traditional and nontraditional risk factors may play integral roles in activating artery wall endothelial cells, smooth muscle cells, and peripheral/tissue monocytes. These events may, in turn, promote local and systemic inflammation contributing to elevated levels of risk factors including plasminogen activator inhibitor-1 (PAI-1), fibrinogen, and C-reactive protein.

This patient's lipid abnormalities, particularly hypertriglyceridemia, also probably reflect poor glycemic control. Therefore, the first treatment approach to the hyperlipidemia in type 2 diabetes should be to optimize glycemic control with diet, exercise, and pharmacologic therapy as needed. Glycemic control improves diabetic dyslipidemia (especially hypertriglyceridemia), whether it is achieved with sulfonylureas, insulin, acarbose, metformin, or thiazolidinediones *(22)*. As glycemic control improves, lipid levels may also improve particularly when insulin resistance is the underlying metabolic abnormality responsible for the lipid disorder. Aside from the changes in plasma glucose concentrations and body weight, the insulin sensitizing thiazolidinediones and metformin both have effects on diabetic dyslipidemia. The thiazolidinediones have been shown to lower triglycerides levels by up to 15–20% *(23,24)* and increase HDL cholesterol levels by 5–8% *(23)*. Troglitazone use has also been associated with an increase in LDL particle size, which is more buoyant and less prone to oxidative modification *(23,25)*. Some of the thiazolidinediones have also shown to have modest blood pressure lowering effects and can decrease PAI-1 levels *(23,26)*. The lipid modifying effects of metformin have also been well established. Metformin has been shown to reduce the plasma triglyceride levels by 20–25% and PAI-1 levels *(27)*. Reductions in total cholesterol and LDL cholesterol are more modest at 5–10% *(27)*. Plasma HDL is usually unchanged *(27)*.

Along with better glycemic control, initial steps in treatment are nonpharmacologic lifestyle changes. The single most important change this patient should make is the cessation of cigarette smoking *(28)*. He should also be counseled on ways to restrict his caloric intake to attain a more desirable body weight and less abdominal obesity. Limiting calories and saturated fat intake can be highly effective at improving, but not usually normalizing, the dyslipidemia of type 2 diabetes. Increased intake of soluble fiber, particularly from oat and bean products, has been shown to reduce LDL cholesterol levels *(29)*. The fat intake of the diet should be less than 30% of the total calories with less than 7% from saturated fats. The daily dietary cholesterol should be limited to less than 200 mg/d. If triglycerides are higher than 1000 mg/dL, all dietary fats should be drastically reduced to lower circulating chylomicrons (dietary fat particles) *(29)*. Alcohol intake should be limited to not more than two equivalents of an alcohol beverage once or twice a week.

Regular physical exercise should be incorporated into his weekly routine, as it has benefits on glucose levels, insulin sensitivity, dyslipidemia, and weight maintenance *(29)*. The current ADA recommendation includes a plasma cholesterol of <200 mg/dL, triglycerides <200 mg/dL, LDL <100 mg/dL, and HDL >45 mg/dL (55 mg/dL in women) *(30)*.

Often, when the lipid profile does not normalize in response to diet, exercise, and efforts to improve glycemic control, lipid-lowering pharmacologic agents are necessary. The first choice of drugs for LDL cholesterol reduction in diabetic patients are HMG-CoA reductase inhibitors (statins) *(31,32)*. The first choice of drugs for elevated triglyceride levels are fibric acids derivatives. HDL cholesterol is a powerful predictor of coronary heart disease in diabetic patients *(22)*. However, it is difficult to raise HDL cholesterol levels without pharmacologic intervention. Unfortunately, one of the most effective agents for raising the HDL levels, nicotinic acid, is relatively contraindicated in patients with type 2 diabetes because of its adverse effects on glycemic control and insulin resistance. Behavioral interventions (weight loss, smoking cessation, increased physical activity) may increase HDL cholesterol *(30)*. In some cases of combined hyperlipidemia, the first choice of therapy is improved glycemic control in combination with a statin. It should be noted that statins may be moderately effective at reducing triglyceride levels as well as LDL cholesterol. Fenofibrate, a recently approved fibric acid derivative, may have a greater LDL lowering effect than previous agents of this class and may also be useful in diabetic patients with combined hyperlipidemia *(30)*. In some cases, combined lipid therapy may be necessary. Several options are available. A combination of statins with gemfibrozil or fenofibrate can be very effective, but has been associated with increased risk of myositis. The combination of statins with nicotinic acid is also extremely effective in modifying diabetic dyslipidemia but the combination may significantly worsen hyperglycemia. This combination should be used with extreme caution: use low doses of nicotinic acid with frequent monitoring of glucose levels *(30)*.

This patient ruled in for a myocardial infarction and was given thrombolytic therapy. During the hospitalization, he was started on an ACE inhibitor, enteric coated aspirin, simvastatin 10 mg daily and his hyperglycemia was controlled with insulin. The rest of the hospital course was unremarkable and he was discharged home after 5 d of hospitalization. After going home, he started on a diet and a graded exercise program. He was able to lose 30 pounds. With the weight loss, his glycemic control improved significantly. He was also started on metformin with the dose titrated up to 1000 mg BID. He is tolerating the medications well without any notable side effects. Despite joining a smoking cessation class, he has not yet been able to quit smoking.

REFERENCES

1. Wingard DL, Barrett-Connor E, Cirqui MH, Suarez L. Clustering of heart disease risk factors in diabetic compared to nondiabetic adults. Am J Epidemiol 1983;117:19–26.
2. Jarrett RJ, McCartney P, Keen H. The Bedford Study: ten year mortality rates in newly diagnosed diabetics, borderline diabetics and normoglycemic controls and risk indices for coronary heart disease in borderline diabetics. Diabetologia 1982;22:79–84.
3. Kannel W, Mc Gee D. Diabetes and cardiovascular risk factors: The Framingham Study. Circulation 1979;59:8–13.
4. Stein B, Weintraub W, King S. Influence of diabetes mellitus on early and late outcome after percutaneous transluminal coronary angioplasty. Circulation 1995;91:979–989.
5. Abaci A, Oguzhan, A Kahraman, S Eryol NK, Unal S, Arinc H, Ergin A. Effect of diabetes mellitus on formation of collateral vessels. Circulation 1999;99:2239–2242.
6. Nesto RW. Congestive heart failure in diabetes mellitus. In: Rose, BD, ed. Up to date, vol 7. Wellesley, MA, 2000, pp. 1–3.
7. Niakan E, Harati Y, Rolak L, Comstock JP, Rokey R. Silent myocardial infarction and diabetic cardiovascular autonomic neuropathy. Arch Intern Med 1986;146:2229–2230.
8. Watkins PJ, Mackay JD. Cardiac denervation in diabetic neuropathy. Ann Intern Med 1980;92:304–307.
9. Faerman I, Faccio E, Milei J, Nunez R, Jadzinsky M, Fox D. Autonomic neuropathy and painless myocardial ischemia in diabetic patients: histologic evidence of their relationship. Diabetes 1977;26:1147–1158.
10. Lloyd-Mostyn R, Watkins P. Defective innervation of heart in diabetic autonomic neuropathy. BMJ 1975;25:15–17.
11. ISIS-2 Collaborative Group. Randomized trial of intravenous streptokinase, oral aspirin, both, or neither among 17,187 cases of suspected acute myocardial infarction: ISIS-2. Lancet 1988;2:349–360.
12. Woodfield SL, Lundergan CF, Reiner JS, Greenhouse SW, Thompson MA, Rohrbeck SC, Deychak Y, Simoons ML, Califf RM, Topol EJ, Ross AM for the GUSTO-I Angiographic Investigators. Angiographic findings and outcome in diabetic patients treated with thrombolytic therapy for acute myocardial infarction: The GUSTO-I experience. J Am Coll Cardiol 1996;28:1661–1669.
13. Mahaffey KW, Granger CB, Toth CA, White HD, Stebbins AL, Barbash GI, Vahanian A, Topol EJ, Califf RM for the GUSTO-I Investigators. Diabetic retinopathy should not be a contraindication to thrombolytic therapy for acute myocardial infarction: review of ocular hemorrhage incidence and location in the GUSTO-I trial. J Am Coll Cardiol 1997;30:1606–1610.
14. Detre KM, Lombardero MS, Brooks MM, Hardison RM, Holubkov R, Sopko G, Frye RL, Chaitman BR. The effects of previous coronary-artery bypass surgery on the prognosis of patients with diabetes who have acute myocardial infarction. Bypass Angioplasty Revascularization Investigation Investigators. N Engl J Med 2000;342:989–997.
15. Chen J, Marciniak TA, Radford MJ, Wang Y, Krumholz HM. Beta-blocker therapy for secondary prevention of myocardial infarction in elderly diabetic patients. Results from the National Cooperative Cardiovascular Project. J Am Coll Cardiol 1999;34:1388–1394.
16. The Heart Outcomes Prevention Evaluation Study Investigators. Effects of an angiotensin-converting enzyme inhibitor, ramipril, on cardiovascular events in high risk patients. N Engl J Med 2000;342:145–153.
17. Malmberg KA, Efendic S, Ryden LE. Feasibility of insulin-glucose infusion in diabetic patients with acute myocardial infarction: a report from the multicenter trail: DIGAMI. Diabetes Care 1994;17:1007–1014.
18. Edelman SV, RR Henry. Diagnosis and management of type 2 diabetes. 3rd ed. Professional Communications, Inc., Caddo, OK, 1999, pp. 186–196.

19. Barakat HA, Carpenter JW, McLendon VD, Khazanie P, Leggett N, Heath J, Marks R. Influence of obesity, impaired glucose tolerance and NIDDM on LDL structure and composition: possible link between hyperinsulinemia and atherosclerosis. Diabetes 1990;39:1527–1531.

20. Austin MA, Breslow JL, Hennekens CHD, Burming JE, Willett WC, Krauss RM. Low density lipoprotein subclass patterns and risk of myocardial infarction. JAMA 1988;260:1917–1921.

21. Holvoet P, Vanhaecke J, Janssens S, Van de Werf F, Collen D. Oxidized LDL and malondialdehyde-modified LDL in patients with acute coronary syndromes and stable coronary artery disease. Circulation 1998;98:1487–1494.

22. Haffner, SM. Management of dyslipidemia in adults with diabetes. Diabetes Care 1998;21:160–178.

23. Saleh YM, Mudaliar S, Henry RR. Metabolic and vascular effects of the thiazolidinedione, troglitazone. Diabetes Revs 1999;7:55–76.

24. Maggs DG, Buchanan TA, Burant CF, Cline G, Gumbiner B, Hsueh WA, Inzucchi S, Kelley D, Nolan J, Olcfsky G, Polonsky KS, Silver D, Valiquett TR, Shulman GI. Metabolic effects of troglitazone monotherapy in type 2 diabetes mellitus: a randomized, double-blind, placebo-controlled trial. Ann Intern Med 1998;128:176–185.

25. Tack CJ, Smits P, Demacker PNM. Troglitazone decreases the proportion of small dense LDL and increases the resistance of LDL to oxidation in obese subjects. Diabetes Care 1998;21:796–799.

26. Ogihara T, Rakugi H, Ikegami H, Mikami H, Mauo K. Enhancement of insulin sensitivity by troglitazone lowers blood pressure in diabetic hypertensives. Am J Hypertension 1995;8:316–320.

27. Cusi K, DeFronzo R. Metforim: a review of its metabolic effects. Diabetes Revs 1998;6:89–131.

28. American Diabetes Association. ADA: Clinical practice recommendations 2000: smoking and diabetes. Diabetes Care 2000;23:S63–S64.

29. American Diabetes Association. ADA: Clinical practice recommendations 2000: diabetes mellitus and exercise. Diabetes Care 2000;23:S50–S54.

30. American Diabetes Association: Clinical Practice Recommendations 2000: position atatement. Management of dyslipidemia in adults with diabetes. Diabetes Care 2000;23:S57–S60.

31. Scandinavian Simvastatin Survival Study Group. Randomized trial of cholesterol lowering in 4444 patients with coronary heart disease: the Scandinavian Simvastatin Study (4S). Lancet 1994;344:1383–1389.

32. Pyoralla K, Pedersen TR, Kjeksus J, Faergerman O, Olsson AG, Thorgeirsson G. Cholesterol lowering with simvastatin improves prognosis of diabetic patients with coronary heart disease: a subgroup analysis of the Scandinavian Simvastatin Survival Study. Diabetes Care 1997;20:614–620.

CASE #3: ELDERLY WOMAN WITH DIABETIC FOOT ULCER

Case Description

A 78-yr-old woman presents to clinic with a 24-yr history of type 2 diabetes mellitus complicated by retinopathy, early nephropathy, and peripheral neuropathy. She was recently started on insulin after a combination of oral medications became ineffective at controlling her blood sugars. She was never in the habit of checking her feet daily, has never seen a podiatrist, and denies any foot problems. At her quarterly continuing-care visit, she reports that her blood glucose control is erratic.

Her physical examination reveals the following: weight: 77.6 kg, height: 174 cm, BMI: 25.5 kg/m^2, and BP: 110/70 mmHg. Examination of the extremities reveals evidence of poor foot hygiene, thickened nails, diminished pedal pulses, absent ankle reflexes, and hammertoe deformities. A deep ulcer penetrating down to the ligaments and muscle without obvious bone involvement or abscess formation is noted on the sole of the left foot. Sensation by monofilament exam is diminished on the dorsum of both feet and absent on the soles of her feet.

Laboratory studies reveal random plasma glucose of 225 mg/dL, HbA$_{1c}$ of 10%, and a white blood cell (WBC) count of 12,500 cells per cubic centimeter with 72% neutrophils, 22% lymphocytes, 3% monocytes, and 3% eosinophils.

Discussion

This patient has all the identifiable risks for foot ulcers and amputation: she has had diabetes for more than 10 yr, poor glucose control, evidence of retinal and renal complications, pedal pulses that are diminished to palpation, evidence of neuropathy, foot deformity, callous formation, and absence of adequate foot care.

It is absolutely critical that all individuals with diabetes have a thorough foot examination by a trained professional at least once a year to identify those with high-risk foot conditions, because foot ulcers and amputations are a major cause of morbidity, disability, and health care costs [1]. Diabetic foot ulcers are a major cause of hospitalizations. Approximately 20% of all diabetic patients enter the hospital because of foot problems [2]. More than half of all nontraumatic amputations in the United States occur in individuals with diabetes and a majority of them could have been prevented with proper foot care [3].

Diabetic foot ulcers result from a combination of peripheral and autonomic neuropathy and peripheral vascular disease [4]. Foot pressure that is abnormally distributed can predispose a neuropathic patient to pressure ischemia and skin breakdown. This patient has diminished sensation in both feet, which may contribute to why she does not feel the need to check her feet on a daily basis. She assumes that because she does not have any pain, there may not be any problems with her feet. However, it is the lack of pain, position, and vibratory sensations caused by neuropathy that facilitates the development of foot lesions [3]. Autonomic neuropathy causes decreased sweating and dry skin that can result in cracked, thickened skin that is susceptible to infection and ulceration.

A thorough history and physical examination can establish the presence and severity of diabetic neuropathy. The patient should be asked about the type of sensation felt in the legs, location, timing, and factors that relieve symptoms. Similarly, the physical exam should include a quantitative somatosensory threshold test, using both the Semmes-Weinstein 5.07 U monofilament [5] and vibration sensation. One study found that failure to detect pressure from this size of monofilament was the single most practical measurement of risk assessment for foot disease [6]. Vibration sense can be quantitatively estimated by Biothesiometer or a tuning fork. The vibration perception threshold increases with age and is a good predictor of future ulceration [7]. In addition the examination should include questions relating to claudication and assessment of pedal pulses and peripheral vascular disease. The physical examination may reveal several abnormalities such as claw toes, Charcot arthropathy, atrophied muscles, prominent metatarsal heads, and reduced or absent foot pulses.

The key to foot care is prevention [1]. People found to have one or more abnormalities of. protective sensation, foot structure and biomechanics, vascular status, and skin integrity should have their feet examined every time they see a health care professional. However, it is crucial to emphasize that daily inspection of their feet can help detect early skin lesions and prescription of proper footwear can minimize the development of foot problems. Use of mirrors can aid patients to view the soles of feet more easily and accurately. Patients should be taught to cut their toe nails straight across, not trim their calluses, and wash their feet with warm water and mild soap. A moisturizing cream should then be applied. They must avoid wearing constricting shoes [3]. Socks should be cotton, loose fitting, and changed every day. It is absolutely imperative that the patients avoid walking barefoot, using heating pads or hot water bottles, or stepping into hot water (i.e., hot tub) without checking the temperature first. Smoking cessation is mandatory.

Diabetic foot ulcers can be graded according to Wagner grade scheme: grade 0- no ulcer in a high-risk foot; grade 1- superficial ulcer involving the full skin thickness, but not underlying tissues, grade 2- deep ulcer, penetrating down to ligaments and muscle, but without bone involvement; grade 3- deep ulcer with cellulitis or abscess formation, with osteomyelitis; grade 4- localized gangrene; and grade 5- extensive gangrene involving the whole foot *(8)*.

The treatment of ulcers depends on the grade of the lesions. Treatment of grade 1 and 2 ulcers usually does not require hospitalization. However, close monitoring is required. Usually a grade 1 or 2 ulcer requires extensive debridement, good local wound care, and relief of pressure on the ulcer. Antibiotics can be started but local extensive debridement also heals ulcers faster and more completely even without antibiotic therapy *(9)*. The most common infections are aerobic gram positive cocci, gram negative bacilli, and anaerobes *(10)*. Broad spectrum coverage is usually necessary to prevent progression.

Management of grade 3 ulcers requires assessment of the peripheral vascular disease by measurement of the brachial ankle index and a work up to rule out osteomyelitis. Treatment usually involves hospitalization, iv antibiotic therapy, and surgical debridement with culture of the tissue. If the ulcer is not healing well, infected bone may need to be removed surgically *(11)*. Grade 4 and 5 ulcers require urgent hospitalization, and surgical consultation for possible amputation.

There are several new approaches that could possibly improve ulcer healing. An example of such therapies include custom-fit semipermeable polymeric membrane dressings and cultured human dermis applied to the ulcer site *(12,13)*. Topical and systemic hyperbaric oxygen have also been used to promote more rapid ulcer healing. By altering the conditions of hypoxia, hyperbaric oxygen facilitates fibroblast proliferation, angiogenesis, and wound healing *(14)*. Electrical stimulation near the ulcer may also help with wound healing *(15)*. A recent study evaluated the use of granulocyte colony-stimulating factor (G-CSF) vs placebo and found that G-CSF therapy was associated with a higher neutrophil count. These neutrophils produced more superoxide, a factor important for neutrophil bacteriocidal activity. These beneficial effects helped eradicate the pathogens earlier and with more rapid resolution of the ulcers *(16)*.

This patient has a grade 2 ulcer and was seen promptly by a podiatrist and underwent local debridement. She was evaluated radiographically and ruled out for osteomyelitis. She was given broad spectrum oral antibiotics and proper footwear. With regular follow-up, the ulcer healed well. She reported understanding the importance of proper foot care, including skin and nail care, and appropriate footwear. She began to monitor her feet on a daily basis. She also had a vascular surgery consultation for the evaluation of poor pedal pulses and possible need of revascularization surgery.

REFERENCES

1. American Diabetes Association. ADA Clinical Practice Recommendations: preventive foot care in people with diabetes. Diabetes Care 2000;23:S55–S56.
2. Mudaliar SR, Henry RR. Management and Prevention of Diabetic Complications. In: Korenman SG, Khan RC, ed. Atlas of Clinical Endocrinology, vol. 2. Current Medicine Inc., Philadelphia, PA, 1999, pp. 83–94.
3. Edelman SV, Henry RR. Diagnosis and Management of Type 2 Diabetes. Professional Communications, 3rd ed., Caddo, OK, 1999, pp. 214–217.
4. Harkless L, Boulton A. The diabetic foot. In: De Fronzo RA, ed. Current Management of Diabetes Mellitus. Mosby Year Book, Inc., St. Louis, MO, 1998, pp. 195–200.

5. Mayfield JA, Reiber, GE Sanders LJ, Janisse D, Pogasch L. Preventive foot care in people with diabetes. Diabetes Care 1998;21:2161–2177.

6. McNeely MJ, Boyko EJ, Ahroni JH, Stensel VL, Reiber GE, Smith DG, Pecoraro RF. The independent contributors of diabetic neuropathy and vasculopathy in foor ulceration: how great are the risk? Diabetes Care 1995;18:216–219.

7. Young MJ, Breedy JL, Veves A, Boulton AJ. The prediction of diabetic neuropathic foot ulceration using vibration perception thresholds. A prospective study. Diabctes Care 1994;17:557–560.

8. Sammarco GJ, Scioli MW. Examination of the foot and ankle. In: Sammarco GJ, ed. The Foot in Diabetes. Lea and Febiger, Philadelphia, PA, 1991, pp. 29–35.

9. Steed DL, Donohoe D, Webster MW, Lindsley L. Effect of extensive debridement and treatment on the healing of diabetic foot ulcers. J Am Coll Surg 1996;183:61–64.

10. Lipsky BA, Pecoraro RE, Larson SA, Hanley ME, Ahroni JH. Outpatient management of uncomplicated lower extremity infections in diabetic patients. Arch Intern Med 1990;150:790–797.

11. McCulloch DK, Hordon LD. Management of diabetic foot lesions. In: Rose, BD, ed. Uptodate vol. 7. Wellesley, MA, 2000, pp. 2–4.

12. Blackman JD, Senseng D, Quinn L, Mazzone T. Clinical evaluation of a semipermeable polymeric membrane dressing for the treatment of chronic diabetic foot ulcers. Diabetes Care 1994;17:322–325.

13. Gentzkow GD, Iwasaki SD, Hershon KS, Mengel M, Prendergast JJ, Ricotta JJ, Steed DP, Lipkin S. Use of dermagraft, a cultured human dermis, to treat diabetic foot ulcers. Diabetes Care 1996;19:350–354.

14. Roth RN, Weiss LD. Hyperbaric oxygen and wound healing. Clinical Dermatol 1994;12:141–156.

15. Baker LL, Chambers R, DeMuth SK, Villar F. Effects of electrical stimulation on wound healing in patients with diabetes ulcers. Diabetes Care 1997;20:405–412.

16. Gough A, Clapperton M, Rolando N, Foster AV, Philpott-Howard J, Edmonds ME. Randomized placebo-controlled trial of granulocyte colony stimulating factor in diabetic foot infection. Lancet 1997;350:855–859.

CASE #4: 47-YR-OLD MAN WITH DIABETIC NEPHROPATHY

Case Description

A 47-yr-old Hispanic man with type 2 diabetes mellitus diagnosed at the age of 32, presents to clinic for a follow-up visit. He has been treated with glyburide 10 mg bid and metformin 1000 mg bid for the last 5 yr. However, during the last visit, the oral medications were discontinued because of poor glycemic control and he was started on a twice-daily regimen of NPH and regular insulin. Two months ago, his yearly ophthalmologic examination revealed bilateral background diabetic retinopathy. Today he reports that his fasting blood sugars range from 160 mg/dL to 180 mg/dL. He complains of numbness and tingling in both feet, especially at night. He runs 1–2 miles per wk and is following a health food high-protein diet. Recently, he underwent an angiogram for evaluation of chest discomfort he experiences during exercise. He does not smoke and denies any significant family history for diabetes and coronary artery disease. Over the course of the last year, his blood pressure has increased from 110/70 mmHg to 140/85 mmHg.

His physical examination reveals the following: weight 80 kg, height 170 cm, BP 140/90 mmHg, and HR 72/min. Funduscopic exam reveals bilateral microaneurysms. Chest and cardiac examinations are unremarkable. His abdominal exam is benign. The lower extremities show normal pulses, but some mild loss of sensation to 10-gram monofilament and vibration.

Laboratory studies prior to the angiogram reveal a fasting glucose of 170 mg/dL and a HbA_{1c} of 9.0%. A chemistry panel shows sodium of 135 meq/L, potassium 4 meq/L, BUN 12 mg/dL, creatinine 1.5 mg/dL and a spot urine specimen showed microalbumin/creatinine ratio of 0.172 g/g (normal range: 0–0.03 g/g). After the contrast study, his creatinine increased to 1.9 mg/dL.

Discussion

Unfortunately for this patient, he already has microvascular complications of diabetes: retinopathy, neuropathy, and now the start of overt nephropathy. He has certain high-risk factors that need to be addressed. Cross-sectional and longitudinal studies have identified elevated blood pressure, HbA_{1c}, cholesterol, smoking, advancing age, insulin resistance, male sex, and possibly high protein intake contributing to the cause of nephropathy *(1)*.

Diabetes has become the single most common cause of end stage renal disease (ESRD) in the U.S. and Europe *(2)*. The cost of treatment for ESRD in diabetes exceeds $2 billion yearly *(2)*. According to reports from the U.S. Renal Data System, there has been a continual increase in ESRD from type 2 diabetes for many years *(3)*. It is particularly more common among the elderly and in Asians, Native Americans, African Americans, and Hispanics *(2)*.

The three major histologic changes in the glomeruli in diabetic nephropathy are mesangial expansion, glomerular basement membrane thickening, and glomerular sclerosis. Glycosylation of tissue proteins may also contribute to the development of diabetic nephropathy. Excess glucose in chronic hyperglycemia combines with the free amino acids and forms irreversible advanced glycosylation end products (AGEs). The net effect is tissue accumulation of AGEs, which may contribute to renal and microvascular complications *(4)*. Recent studies have shown that through several interventions, the onset and course of diabetic nephropathy can be influenced to a significant degree. But these interventions have the greatest effect if they are started early in the course of the disease.

The earliest sign of nephropathy is the appearance of low but abnormal levels (>30 mg/d or 20 µg/min) of albumin in the urine *(2)*. A high proportion of patients may have microalbuminuria at the time of diagnosis because type 2 diabetes is usually present for many years before the diagnosis is actually made. Without specific interventions, 20–40% of type 2 patients progress to overt nephropathy, but 20 yr after onset of overt nephropathy, only 20% will have progressed to ESRD *(2)*. Screening for microalbuminuria should be performed at the time of diagnosis. It can be in the form of an albumin/creatinine ratio in a random spot collection, a 24-h collection with simultaneous measurement of creatinine clearance, or a timed collection of albumin and creatinine over several hours.

Hyperfiltration occurs early in the course of type 2 diabetes. Up to 45% of patients initially have a glomerular filtration rate (GFR) that is more than two standard deviations above that of age-matched nondiabetic and obese controls *(5)*. A study looking at type 2 diabetic Pima Indians found that the GFR was 14% higher in patients with impaired glucose tolerance, 18% higher in newly diagnosed diabetic patients, was normal in patients with microalbuminuria and 35% lower in those with overt proteinuria *(6)*. Overt nephropathy, or clinical albuminuria is defined as urinary protein excretion >0.5 g/24 h or albumin excretion rates >300 mg/24 h *(7)*.

The Diabetes Control and Complications Trial (DCCT) and The United Kingdom Prospective Diabetes Study (UKPDS) have demonstrated that improved glucose control can significantly reduce the risk of the development of microalbuminuria and overt nephropathy in people with diabetes *(8,9)*. Even decreasing $HgbA_{1c}$ from 9.0% to 8.0% will decrease the risk of microvascular complications by 35% *(9,10)*.

In one out of three patients with type 2 diabetes, hypertension is found at the time of diagnosis *(11)*. The hypertension may be related to underlying nephropathy, dysmetabolic syndrome (coexistence of glucose intolerance, hypertension, dyslipidemia, and obesity), or renal vascular disease *per se*. Lowering blood pressure with the goal of <130/85, by any effective means, will decrease the rate of progression *(2)*. A recent report by the National Kidney Association recommends that the new suggested target for blood pressure is 130/80 in diabetic patients *(12)*. Controlling hypertension through aggressive therapeutic intervention can reduce proteinuria and delay the progression of renal insufficiency. ACE inhibitors are not only effective antihypertensive agents but also delay the progression of diabetic nephropathy to ESRD. ACE inhibitors decrease proteinuria by minimizing efferent glomerular vasocontriction and reducing glomerular filtration *(7)*. In cases where the glomerular filtration rate has already declined, ACE inhibitors also can partially reverse or prevent a further decrease. ACE inhibitors should be considered as first line therapy in all normotensive and hypertensive patients with diabetes who have microalbuminuria or macroalbuminuria *(13)*. Angiotensin receptor blockers (ARB), e.g., losartan, valsartan, irbesartan, candesartan, may also be similarly renoprotective and do not cause cough as can occur with ACE inhibitors *(7)*. Although ARBs have been shown to decrease proteinuria, long-term studies documenting a decrease in the rate of progression of the fall of GFR have not yet been completed.

When blood pressure cannot be adequately controlled with the maximum dose of an ACE inhibitor or ARB, additional antihypertensive medications may be needed, such as calcium channel blockers, low-dose diuretics, β-blockers, α-blockers, and centrally acting agents. Patients with renal insufficiency and hypertension often benefit from a diuretic as part of the antihypertensive regimen, because of related sodium and fluid retention. A loop diuretic is often necessary if the creatinine level exceeds 2 mg/dL *(7)*.

Animal studies have shown that restriction of dietary protein intake also reduces hyperfiltration and intraglomerular pressure and retards the progression of several models of renal disease. At this point, the current adult Recommended Dietary Allowance (RDA) of 0.8 g/kg/d should be instituted with the onset of overt nephropathy and protein should be derived from lean animal and vegetable or plant sources *(14)*. However, once the GFR begins to fall, further restriction of 0.6 g/kg/d may prove to be useful in slowing down the decline of GFR in selected patients.

This patient had a marginal serum creatinine level before the angiogram. An important factor to consider with worsening of kidney disease is the use of metformin, which is excreted solely by the kidneys. In patients with decreased renal function (based on measured creatinine clearance), the plasma and blood half life of metformin is prolonged and the renal clearance is decreased in proportion to the decrease in creatinine clearance. Metformin is contraindicated in patients with renal disease or renal dysfunction, i.e., serum creatinine $\geq$1.5 mg/dL (males) and $\geq$1.4 (in females) or abnormal creatinine clearance (<80 mL/min/1.73 m^2). Lactic acidosis is a serious metabolic complication due to metformin accumulation. Lactic acidosis is characterized by elevated blood levels of lactate (>5 mmol/L), decreased pH, electrolyte imbalance with elevated anion gap, and increased lactate/pyruvate ratio. Because of the risk of lactic acidosis, metformin should be promptly withheld in patients with sepsis, dehydration or hypoxemia. Because impaired hepatic function may significantly limit the ability to clear lactate, metformin should generally be avoided in patients with clinical or laboratory evidence of hepatic disease. Patients should be cautioned about excessive alcohol intake, because alcohol potentiates the effects of metformin on lactate metabolism. Intravascular contrast studies with iodinated material can cause alteration in renal function and has been associated with lactic acidosis in patients receiving metformin. Therefore, metformin should to be withheld prior to an iv contrast procedure and for 48 h afterward with reinstitution only after renal function has been checked and found to be normal *(15)*. In this case, because renal function had deteriorated, the metformin was immediately stopped and the patient gently hydrated. After several weeks, the creatinine returned to 1.6 mg/dL, but metformin was not reinstituted.

The administration of sulfonylureas also requires careful attention to dosing and routes of elimination *(16)*. Glyburide has weak active metabolites that are excreted in the urine. Glipizide and tolbutamide are primarily metabolized by the liver and only inactive metabolites are excreted in the urine. Thus, glipizide and tolbutamide are the sulfonylureas of choice in patients with renal failure. Glyburide can be given at reduced doses if GFR is above 50 mL/min but should be avoided in more severe renal disease *(17)*. Repaglinide and nateglinide could also be considered.

Insulin also requires adjustment in chronic renal failure. No adjustment is required if GFR is above 50 mL/min. The insulin dose should be reduced by about 25% when the GFR is between 10–50 mL/min. The dose may need to be reduced as much as 50% when the GFR is less than 10 mL/min *(17)*.

This patient met with the dietician who was able to design better dietary management. He began therapy with an ACE inhibitor for both hypertension and microalbuminuria. He has been followed carefully with repeat urinary albumin:creatinine ratios being checked every 3–6 mo. In general, one can expect up to 50% reduction in the urinary albumin:creatinine ratio or at least a stabilization of the ratio following institution of an ACE inhibitor *(7)*. If worsening is noted, the patient's compliance should be checked and further measures may be required. Referral to a nephrologist should be made when GFR has fallen to either <70 mL/min, the serum creatinine has increased to >2.0 mg/dL, or when difficulties occur in management of hypertension or hyperkalemia.

REFERENCES

1. Ravid M, Broash D, Ravid-Safran D, Levy Z, Rachmani R. Main risk factors for nephropathy in type 2 diabetes mellitus are plasma cholesterol levels, mean blood pressure, and hyperglycemia. Arch Intern Med 1998;11:998–1004.
2. American Diabetes Association. ADA clinical practice recommendations: diabetic nephropathy. Diabetes Care 2000;23:S69–S72.
3. Ritz E, Orth SR. Primary Care: nephropathy in patients with Type 2 diabetes mellitus. N Engl J Med 1999; 341:1127–1133.
4. Rose BD. Risk factors of diabetic nephropathy. In: Rose BD, ed. Up to date 2000; vol 7. Uptodate, Inc. Wellesley, MA, 2000, pp. 1–11.
5. Nowack R, Raum E, Blum W, Ritz E. Renal hemodynamics in recent onset type II diabetes. Am J Kidney Dis 1992;20:342–347.
6. Nelson RG, Bennett PH, Beck GJ, Tan M, Knowler WC, Mitch WE, et al. Development and progression of renal disease in Pima Indians with noninsulin dependent diabetes mellitus. N Engl J Med 1996;335: 1636–1642.
7. Edelman SV, Henry RR. Diagnosis and Management of Type 2 Diabetes. 3rd ed., Professional Communications, Caddo, OK, 1999, pp. 201–206.
8. The Diabetes Control and Complications Trial research Group. The effect of intensive treatment of diabetes on the development and progression of long-term complications in insulin-dependent diabetes mellitus. N Engl J Med 1993;329:977–986.
9. UK Prospective Diabetes Study (UKPDS) Group. Intensive blood glucose control with sulfonylureas or insulin compared with conventional treatment and risk of complications in patients with type 2 diabetes (UKPDS 33). Lancet 1998;352:837–853.
10. American Diabetes Association. Clinical practice recommendations 2000: Position Statement. Standards of medical care for patients with diabetes mellitus. Diabetes Care 2000;23:32–42.

11. White WB, Prisant LM, Wright JT. Management of patients with hypertension and diabetes mellitus: Advances in the evidence for intensive treatment. Am J Med 2000;108:238–245.

12. Bakris GL, Williams M, Dworkin L, Elliot W, Epstein M, Toto R, Tuttle K, Douglas J, Hsueh W, Sowers J. Preserving renal function in adults with hypertension and diabetes: a consensus approach. Am J Kid Dis 2000;36:646–661.

13. Lewis EJ, Hunsicker LG, Bain RP, Rhode RD. The effect of angiotensin-converting enzyme inhibition on diabetic nephropathy. N Engl J Med 1993;329:1456–1462.

14. Mudaliar SR, Henry RR. Management and Prevention of Diabetic Complications. Atlas of Clinical Endocrinology, Current Medicine, Philadelphia, PA, 2000, pp. 83–94.

15. Physicians Desk Reference. Endocrinology Prescribing Guide, 3rd ed. Medical Econom, Montvale, NJ, 2000, pp. 116–124.

16. Skillman TG, Feldman JM. The pharmacology of sulfonylureas. Am J Med 1981;70:361–372.

17. American College of Physicians. Drug Prescribing in Renal Failure. In: Bennett WM, Arnoff GR, Golper TA, Morrison G, Brata DC, Singer I, eds. Dosing Guidelines for Adults, 3rd ed. American College of Physicians, Philadelphia, PA, 1984, p. 92.

CASE #5: 55-YR-OLD MAN WITH LEG WEAKNESS AND PAIN

Case Description

A 55-yr-old African American male with history of type 2 diabetes mellitus for 6 yr complicated by hypertension and coronary artery disease (CAD) presents to clinic with a 6 mo history of persistent left leg cramping and pain. The pain was initially diagnosed as being possibly secondary to simvastatin but persisted despite discontinuation of this medication. The patient describes the pain as a steady ache and cramping without numbness, starting in the lower back and radiating down the left leg like a "stretched sensation" from the hip to the knee with occasional extension down to the calf. In addition he cannot sleep flat and is only able to sleep in a chair sitting upright. He achieves mild relief from acetaminophen with codeine. He is also taking amitriptyline without any significant benefits. He denies any urinary frequency, urgency, or incontinence of stool or urine. He denies any history of back injury or lifting of heavy objects. He does not smoke or drink alcohol. However, he has lost 35 pounds over the last 6 mo. His other medications include insulin 70/30–35 U before breakfast and dinner, glyburide 10 mg bid, fosinopril 40 mg qd, verapamil 240 mg qd, and rosiglitazone 4 mg bid.

Physical examination reveals the following: weight 137 kg, height 193 cm, BMI 36.8 kg/m^2, BP 161/82 mmHg, pulse 72, and respiratory rate 18. He walks into the exam room with the help of the cane and sits in the chair with great hesitation. On neurologic exam, extraocular movements are normal, as are cranial nerves II through XII. There is marked wasting noted of the left quadriceps with decreased muscle tone. Lower extremity strength is decreased to 2/5 in the left quadriceps. Deep tendon reflexes are 1+ and symmetric in the upper extremities but knee and ankle reflexes are absent bilaterally. Toes are down going bilaterally on Babinski testing. No sensory deficits are noted to light touch or pain. The straight leg raise test is negative and there is no tenderness to palpation on the lumbar spine. His prostate exam is normal. His laboratory tests show average fasting glucose levels of 150 mg/dL and a hemoglobin A_{1c} of 7.8%.

X-ray views of the lumbar spine show mild bilateral hip and sacroiliac osteoarthritis. Anterior posterior and lateral views of the spine are normal. A CT scan of the spine does not show any evidence of masses causing compression. An MRI shows left paracentral L5-S1 disk protrusion but no extruded fragments.

Discussion

Involvement of the peripheral and autonomic nervous system is one of the most common complications of diabetes. Diabetic polyneuropathy is the most common cause of neuropathy in the Western world *(1)*. The prevalence varies with the duration and severity of the hyperglycemia. The Diabetes Control and Complications Trial has shown that strict control of glucose levels decreased the incidence and slowed the progression of the neuropathy *(2)*. Neuropathy, retinopathy, and nephropathy all increase during the first 10–15 yr of diabetes and patients who present with one complication are more likely to have another. The high rate of neuropathy results in increased risk for lower extremity infections, ulcerations, and amputations.

Diabetic neuropathy is characterized into distinct syndromes according to the distribution of the neurologic deficit, each syndrome having a characteristic presentation and course. The most commonly encountered neuropathies include: 1) distal symmetric polyneuropathy; 2) autonomic neuropathy; 3) mononeuropathies (cranial and peripheral); and 4) polyradiculopathies.

Distal symmetric polyneuropathy is the most commonly recognized complication of diabetes *(3)*. Neurologic impairment usually begins in the feet or toes and may progress proximally up the lower and upper extremities. It has the classic "stocking-glove" sensory loss. Histologic and nerve conduction studies show that it is characterized by sensory axon loss and in severe forms by motor weakness and axon loss *(4)*. The complications of this neuropathy are neuropathic foot ulceration, neuroarthropathy (Charcot joint), and diabetic neuropathic cachexia *(1)*.

Autonomic dysfunction is often a diagnosis of exclusion. It is frequently unnoticed by the patient and the physician because of the insidious onset and multiorgan involvement. Clinical characteristics include neuropathic sexual dysfunction, gastroparesis, enteropathy with constipation and/or diarrhea, postural hypotension and exercise intolerance with pulse invariability *(1)*.

Mononeuropathies commonly manifest as cranial nerve palsies, which can be recurrent or bilateral. The cranial nerves most frequently involved are the third, sixth and fourth, respectively and, in most cases, the palsy resolves spontaneously in weeks or months. The most common peripheral mononeuropathies in people with diabetes involve the median nerve at the wrist, radial nerve in the upper arm, ulnar nerve at the elbow, lateral cutaneous nerve at the thigh, and peroneal nerve at the femoral head *(5)*.

Polyradiculopathy presents with dermatomal pain and diminition of cutaneous sensation, followed by hyperesthesias or parathesias. Polyradiculopathy usually involves the lumbar and thoracic areas and is often misdiagnosed as acute intrathoracic or intraabdominal emergencies, such as myocardial infarction, cholecystitis, peptic ulcer, or appendicitis *(1)*. The most common type of polyradiculopathy is frequently called diabetic amyotrophy or diabetic neuropathic cachexia.

This patient had an extensive work-up before a diagnosis was made. First, it was important to rule out any obvious lumbar spine damage or any malignancy causing a spinal cord compression-like syndrome, resulting in weakness and pain. Once the malignancy work-up was negative, the patient had an electromyogram (EMG), which confirmed the diagnosis of diabetic amyotrophy.

Diabetic amyotrophy is an infrequent complication of type 2 diabetes, the prevalence being about 1.1% *(6)*. Burns initially described it in 1890 as "neuritic paralysis in diabetes mellitus". Since then, numerous other names have been given to this primarily motor disturbance in diabetic patients. The primary distinguishing features of diabetic amyotrophy are a subacute or acute development of moderate to marked weakness of the lower extremities, often with wasting of pelvifemoral muscles, accompanied by pain but without sensory impairment *(6)*. There may be an antecedent weight loss of 10–30 pounds *(7)*. The onset is usually in middle age or later.

As with this patient, symptoms usually include difficulty walking, standing, or stair climbing. It may be symmetrical, asymmetrical or unilateral. The progression of weakness may continue for months to more than 1yr especially in more symmetrical variants *(8)*. A severe, diffuse, deep aching or sharp pain in the thigh or the lumbosacral region usually accompanies weakness but occasionally it can be painless *(9)*.

Physical examination reveals muscle involvement in the quadraceps femoris but simultaneous involvement of the gluteal, hamstring, adductor, and iliopsoas muscles often occur *(6)*. Straight leg raising does not aggravate the pain *(10)*. Quadriceps reflexes are usually diminished or absent in proportion to the quadriceps weakness and the ankle reflexes may be normal or diminished. Absence of sensory impairment is characteristic, but some individuals may experience dysesthesias, mild distal impairment of light touch and pin prick sensation in the legs.

Diabetic amyotrophy often occurs in patients with a concomitant, preexisting distal sensorimotor polyneuropathy. It is usually clearly distinguishable from other diabetic neuropathies. The predominantly proximal motor involvement is in clear contrast to the distal, predominantly sensory "stocking" distribution typical of the common diabetic polyneuropathy. The widespread proximal muscle involvement and lack of significant associated sensory loss indicates that diabetic amyotrophy is neither a femoral mononeuropathy nor a lumbosacral monoradiculopathy due to disc herniation.

Nerve conduction studies and needle EMG's are the most useful tests in diabetic amyotrophy to confirm the diagnosis and exclude other possibilities. Nerve conduction studies generally demonstrate evidence of a typical diabetic sensorimotor axonal polyneuropathy *(4)*. EMG reveals abnormalities of ongoing denervation. The fibrillation potentials and positive sharp waves are usually present at the time of medical presentation. The motor units are polyphasic, prolonged and large in amplitude *(6)*. The most commonly affected muscles are the vasti, thigh adductors, and iliopsoas. Lumbar paraspinous muscles are more frequently involved than thoracic paraspinous muscles. Distal leg musculature is less frequently involved. Additional testing, such as MRI or CT, can be done to rule out lumbosacral polyradiculopathy, plexopathy, inflammatory, or neoplastic processes in the subarachnoid space.

Light and electron microscopic examination of the intramuscular nerve filaments in the vastus medialis muscle usually demonstrates axonal degeneration. Motor point biopsies show evidence of denervation and reinnervation of the myoneural junctions, characterized by beaded, thickened terminal axons, spherical axonal swellings, collateral ramification, ultraterminal sprouts, and multiple endplates *(6)*. In a study by Krendel et al. 7 of the 10 patients with either diabetic neuropathy or mononeuritis multiplex had perivascular chronic inflammatory cells and three had arterial occlusion with inflammation *(11)*.

The exact pathogenesis of polyradiculopathy is still unknown. The classic debate of ischemia versus metabolic etiology continues. Metabolic theory causes include hyperglycemia, sorbitol pathway products, deficiency of nerve myoinositol and acceleration of nonenzymatic glycosylation. The theory of ischemia is supported by evidence of endoneural hypoxia *(12)* and lack of improvement in the symptoms with improvement of glycemic control. In addition, pathology findings suggest a possible role for infiltrative T cells in the pathogenesis *(13)*. A recent sural nerve biopsy study in patients with proximal diabetic neuropathy found that all had CD8+ T-cell infiltration of the nerve *(13)*. The pathogenesis of diabetic amyotrophy may involve both ischemia and metabolic components. Those patients with proximal and symmetrical symptoms may be caused by metabolic dysfunction, whereas those neuropathies that are asymmetrical and with rapid onset might be resultant from primary nerve ischemia.

The exact localization of the disease process is still controversial. Originally, it was thought to be because of anterior horn cell involvement. However, clinical involvement of the proximal muscles in the distribution of a particular nerve with relative sparing of distal muscles sharing the same radicular innervation makes it difficult to ascribe the clinical manifestations to anterior horn cell dysfunction with any certainty *(6)*. Some studies, based on clinical analysis and muscle biopsy findings, suggest muscle as the primary site of the lesion. However, the vast majority of muscle, nerve, and motor point biopsy, as well as electromyography studies clearly indicate a neuropathic process and thereby exclude myopathy as the primary pathogenetic locus. The localization within the peripheral nerve is also a subject of debate. Diabetic amyotrophy may result from involvement of multiple sites, such as lumbosacral anterior horn cells, motor roots, plexus, or motor axons to pelvifemoral muscles *(6)*.

The natural course and treatment is variable. There may be gradual and incomplete improvement. Even if strength improves, muscle wasting may persist. As aforementioned, improvement is not related to glycemic control. The severe pain usually abates several months after onset but residual pain may last for years. Analgesics and anti-inflammatory drugs are usually helpful for pain control. Amitriptyline, desipramine, phenytoin, and carbamazapine have been shown to be efficacious for treatment of pain *(6)*. Transcutaneous nerve stimulation has been beneficial in an occasional patient *(14)*. Recent studies have suggested a role of immunomodulating agents *(13)*. Intravenous immunoglobulin (IVIG) at 2 g/kg total body weight over 5 d then monthly for 3 mo *(15)* has been associated with decreased pain and improved strength.

This patient was started on neurontin 300 mg bid. After 1 yr of physical therapy and management in the chronic pain clinic, he is beginning to feel some improvement. He has gained 20 pounds and is able to ambulate with the assistance of the cane. His glycemic control has improved with a HgbA$_{1c}$ of 7.2%. His mood and general feeling of well being has improved tremendously.

REFERENCES

1. Greene DA, Gelber DA, Pfeifer MA, Carroll PB. Diabetic neuropathy. In: Becker, et al., eds. Principles and Practice of Endocrinology and Metabolism, 2nd ed., J.B. Lippincott, Philadelphia, PA, 1995, pp. 1270–1280.
2. The Diabetes Control and Complications Trial Research Group. The effect of intensive treatment of diabetes on the development and progression of long term complications in insulin dependent diabetes mellitus. N Engl J Med 1993;329:977–986.
3. Greene DA, Pfeifer MA. Diabetic Neuropathy. In: Olefsy JM, Sherwin RS, eds. Contemporary Issues in Endocrinology and Metabolism, vol. 1. Diabetes Mellitus, Management and Complications. Churchill Livingston, New York, 1985, p. 233.
4. Feldman EL. Classification of diabetic neuropathy. In: Rose BD, Up to date 2000; vol 7. Wellesley, MA, 2000, pp. 1–6.
5. Vinik A. Diabetic neuropathies. In: Khan RC, Korenman SG, eds. Atlas of Clinical Endocrinology, vol. 2, Current Medicine, Philadelphia, PA, 2000, pp. 163–177.

6. Sander HW, Chokraverty S. Diabetic amyotrophy: current concepts. Sem Neurol 1996;16:173–178.
7. Lev-Ran A, Raskin L. Spontaneous recovery of severe weight loss in diabetic amyotrophy. Diabetes Care 1999;22:1906–1907.
8. Subramony SH, Wilbourn AJ. Diabetic proximal neuropathy. J Neurol Sci 1982;53:293–304.
9. Chokraverty S, Reyes MG, Rubino FA, Tonaki H. The syndrome of diabetic amyotrophy. Ann Neurol 1977;2:181–184.
10. Thomas PK, Brown MJ. Diabetic polyneuropathy. In: Dyck PJ, Thomas PK, Asbury AK, et al., eds. Diabetic Neuropathy. WB Saunders, Philadelphia, PA, 1987, pp. 1219–1250.
11. Krendel DA, Costigan DA. Hopkins LC. Successful treatment of neuropathies in patients with diabetes mellitus. Arch Neurol 1995;52:1053–1061.
12. Dyck PJB, Norell JE, Dyck PJ. Microvasculitis and ischemia in diabetic lumbosacral radiculoplexus neuropathy. Neurology 1999;53:2113–2121.
13. Younger DS, Rosoklija G, Hays AP, et al. Diabetic peripheral neuropathy: a clinicopathologic and immunohistochemical analysis of sural nerve biopsies. Muscle Nerve 1996;19:722–727.
14. Chokraverty S, Sander HW. AAEM case report #13: Diabetic amyotrophy. Muscle Nerve 1996;19:939–945.
15. Krendel DA, Costigan DA, Hopkins, LC. Successful treatment of neuropathies in patients with diabetes mellitus. Arch Neurol 1995;52:1053–1061.

18

Hypoglycemia

Neena Natt, MD and F. John Service, MD, PhD

CONTENTS

CASE #1: NON-HYPOGLYCEMIC SPELLS

Case Description

A 38-yr-old woman was referred to our institution for evaluation of hypoglycemia. Over the past year, she had experienced frequent episodes of hunger, leg tremors, and dizziness occurring up to eight times per day. These symptoms resolved within 15–45 min following the ingestion of food. Symptoms occurred at any time of the day and appeared to be unrelated to food ingestion. Snacks eaten every 2 h did not improve or help prevent symptoms. She had not experienced confusion or loss of consciousness. Self-monitored blood glucose levels up to 15 times per day during symptoms were associated with "low" glucose levels, the lowest value being 52 mg/dL. Her highest blood glucose value was approximately 200 mg/dL, taken shortly after a meal, but she could not recall whether she had symptoms at that time. There was no record of venipuncture plasma glucose values while symptomatic.

Physical examination revealed a lean, somewhat frail-looking woman. Medications included lansoprazole 15 mg daily, atenolol 12.5 mg daily, and alprazolam 6.25 mg. She had a medical history of supraventricular tachycardia, hypertension, Crohn's disease, depression, and anxiety. She had undergone resection of 30 cm of the terminal ileum for localized Crohn's disease 4 yr earlier. There was a strong family history of diabetes (her father and brother were treated with insulin, and her mother and sister were treated with oral agents). Baseline studies, while asymptomatic, revealed a fasting plasma glucose of 75 mg/dL, normal serum cortisol, creatinine, and liver function tests.

From: *Contemporary Endocrinology: Challenging Cases in Endocrinology*
Edited by: M. E. Molitch © Humana Press Inc., Totowa, NJ

Table 1
Case #1: End-of-Fast β-Cell Polypeptide and Insulin Surrogate Levels

Plasma glucose (mg/dL)	Insulin (μU/mL)	C-peptide (pmol/L)	β-Hydroxybutyrate (mmol/L)	*Δ plasma glucose (mg/dL)	Plasma sulfonylurea screen
42	2.1	140	6.9	17	negative

* Following glucagon administration (peak value within 30 min of the injection minus end-of-fast value).

She underwent a 72 h fast according to protocol. Fifty-two hours into the fast she developed mild nausea, fatigue, and leg tremors with concurrent plasma glucose of 57 mg/dL. The fast was continued as the symptoms and signs were considered mild and nonspecific. Seventy hours into the fast she developed diaphoresis, pallor, clammy hands, and leg tremors. Pulse rate was 150 beats per minute. There were no symptoms or signs of neuroglycopenia. Plasma glucose was 42 mg/dL and the fast was terminated. Glucagon 1 mg was administered intravenously. Although, the events were not well documented in the medical record, it appears that her symptoms resolved slowly over the next hour or so despite concomitant blood glucose levels within the normal range. She had a small emesis and managed to eat only a small portion of her meal because of a sensation of bloating and "gagging." Biochemical data obtained at the end-of-fast are shown in Table 1.

Discussion

This case illustrates some of the difficulties that can be encountered during the evaluation of a patient who has symptoms attributed to low glucose levels. The patient had frequent symptoms that appeared to be unrelated to food ingestion. While symptomatic, one of her many reflectance meter glucose values was 52 mg/dL, prompting further evaluation for possible hypoglycemia.

When presented with a patient with symptoms suggestive of a hypoglycemic disorder, it is essential to verify a low plasma glucose level at the time that symptoms occur (either spontaneously or during a supervised 72 h fast) and to demonstrate that symptoms are relieved through correction of the low glucose value (Whipple's triad). Demonstration of Whipple's triad is crucial because symptoms of hypoglycemia are varied and nonspecific. In addition, reflectance meter glucose measurements taken by a patient are likely to be unreliable. Patients are usually not experienced in this technique, the measurements are often obtained under adverse circumstances when the patient is symptomatic, and the method may not provide an accurate measurement of glucose levels in the hypoglycemic range (1).

The 72 h fast is the classic diagnostic test for fasting-state hypoglycemia. The test may be conducted to establish Whipple's triad (as in this patient) or to determine the mechanism of hypoglycemia when Whipple's triad has previously been documented. A fast conducted for the latter purpose may be terminated when plasma glucose is ≤ 55 mg/dL (with or without symptoms) as β-cell polypeptide levels can be expected to be suppressed at and below this plasma glucose level. Diagnostic criteria for hyperinsulinemia at the time of hypoglycemia (plasma glucose ≤ 55 mg/dL), whether induced by the fast or occurring spontaneously, are: plasma insulin level ≥ 6 μU/mL [radioimmunoassay (RIA)]; plasma C-peptide level ≥ 200 pmol/L (ICMA); and plasma proinsulin level ≥ 5 pmol/L (ICMA) *(2)*. An immunochemiluminometric assay for insulin with a sensitivity of less than 1 μU/mL is available at some medical centers. Experience at our institution with this assay suggests that hyperinsulinemia is present at a level of 3 μU/mL or higher.

Markers of insulin action such as plasma β-hydroxybutyrate concentration and plasma glucose response to intravenous glucagon are also measured at the end of the fast (or during a spontaneous hypoglycemic episode). The rationale for measuring these insulin surrogates reflects the antiketogenic and antiglycogenolytic/glycogenic properties of insulin. Thus, normal individuals fasted for 3 d demonstrate elevated plasma ketone levels and depletion of liver glycogen stores (because plasma insulin levels are appropriately suppressed). In contrast, a patient with insulin-mediated hypoglycemia will have suppressed plasma ketone levels and exhibit a generous glucose response to glucagon administration when hypoglycemic. Our experience has been that patients with insulin-mediated hypoglycemia have β-hydroxybutyrate concentrations of less than 2.7 mmol/L, whereas normal individuals or those with noninsulin mediated hypoglycemia have higher levels. Following glucagon administration, patients with insulin-mediated hypoglycemia exhibit a maximal increase in plasma glucose of 25 mg/dL or greater above the terminal glucose in the fast (peak minus end-of-fast value). Both insulin surrogates are applicable when the plasma glucose is 60 mg/dL or lower at the end of the prolonged fast *(3)*.

The purpose of the prolonged fast in this patient was to demonstrate Whipple's triad. She developed her usual symptoms experienced in ordinary life when her plasma glucose level was within the hypoglycemic range. However, recovery from symptoms appeared to be prolonged despite restoration of plasma glucose to the normal range, suggesting that symptoms and low plasma glucose were not causally related. Symptoms can be confidently attributed to hypoglycemia only when Whipple's triad is fulfilled. However, the less than comprehensive documentation in the medical record at a crucial point in the fast (i.e., the patient's response to elevation of plasma glucose into the normal range) hindered our interpretation of the fast. This, and the fact that the patient was symptomatic when plasma glucose was significantly low prompted us to review her case in more detail for other possible explanations.

The exclusion of an insulin-mediated hypoglycemic disorder was straightforward. β-cell polypeptide levels were appropriately suppressed (i.e., below the recommended diagnostic criteria) when plasma glucose was in the hypoglycemic range. End-of-fast plasma β-hydroxybutyrate concentration and maximal plasma glucose response to glucagon administration supported this conclusion. Could this patient have a hypoglycemic disorder not induced by insulin? Probably not, as there was no evidence of an illness or use of medications known to be associated with the risk for low plasma glucose *(4)*.

An unusual feature of this case was the nature of the patient's symptoms. Hypoglycemia-related symptoms have been classified into two major groups: those resulting from autonomic nervous system discharge (e.g., sweating, trembling, and anxiety) and those reflecting neuroglycopenia (e.g., confusion, difficulty speaking, and inability to concentrate) *(5)*. In a retrospective analysis of 60 patients with hypoglycemia caused by insulinomas, 85% had various combinations of diplopia, blurred vision, sweating, palpitations, and weakness; 80% had confusion or abnormal behavior; 53% had amnesia or were in a coma during the episode; and 12% had generalized seizures *(6)*. This patient's symptoms were exclusively in the autonomic subgroup. There is no convincing evidence for the existence of a hypoglycemic disorder characterized solely by autonomic symptoms in our opinion. Although some episodes in persons with true hypoglycemic disorders may be sufficiently mild to generate only autonomic symptoms, eventually episodes of neuro-glycopenia will occur. Another confounding factor in this case was the patient's history of supraventricular tachycardia. It is conceivable that she developed a transient episode of this arrhythmia during the fast with associated autonomic response unrelated to her low plasma glucose value. Thus the attribution of her symptoms to hypoglycemia was not clear-cut.

The decision to end a fast may not be easy and requires considerable judgment on the part of the supervising physician. Plasma glucose values may not be immediately available and the bedside reflectance meter may have to serve as a guide to glucose levels. Some patients may develop symptoms when plasma glucose levels are in or slightly above the hypoglycemic range. In such situations it may be difficult to attribute symptoms to hypoglycemia. Other patients may have plasma glucose values in the hypoglycemic range but remain asymptomatic. A fast terminated solely on the basis of a low plasma glucose value should be interpreted with caution because some young, healthy women undergoing prolonged fasting may achieve plasma glucose levels of 40 mg/dL or less without the accompanying symptoms (7). In addition, there is no diagnostic glucose level for insulinoma clearly distinct from that of healthy persons. Unnecessary prolongation of the fast may also be a problem. Symptoms and signs indicative of neuroglycopenia may be subtle and not readily appreciated by the supervising physician. Careful examination for cognitive function at regular intervals throughout the fast when plasma glucose is near or in the hypoglycemic range is therefore essential.

In conclusion, this patient's symptoms could not be confidently attributed to hypoglycemia for several reasons. Despite the problem with incomplete documentation, it appeared that her symptoms did not resolve in a timely manner with correction of plasma glucose. Thus Whipple's triad was not fulfilled. Also, the exclusively autonomic symptoms experienced in everyday life and during the fast were not suggestive of a true hypoglycemic disorder. We suspect that the patient represents one of the well-recognized persons capable of achieving a low plasma glucose after prolonged fasting, and that her autonomic-type symptoms were unrelated. Although the diagnosis or exclusion of a hypoglycemic disorder tends to be relatively straightforward, difficult cases such as this are encountered from time to time. In such situations, there is no substitute for punctilious assessment and documentation of the timing and nature of symptoms and signs that develop during the 72 h fast in relation to plasma glucose values.

REFERENCES

1. American Diabetes Association. Consensus statement on self-monitoring of blood glucose. Diabetes Care 1987;10:95–99.
2. Service FJ. Hypoglycemic disorders. N Engl J Med 1995;32:1144–1152.
3. O'Brien T, O'Brien PC, Service FJ. Insulin surrogates in insulinoma. J Clin Endocrinol Metab 1993; 77:449–451.
4. Service FJ. Diagnostic approach to adults with hypoglycemic disorders. In: Endocrinology and Metabolism Clinics of North America 1999;28(3):519–532.
5. Towler DA, Havlin CE, Craft S, et al. Mechanism of awareness of hypoglycemia. Diabetes 1993;42:1791–1798.
6. Service FJ, Dale AJD, Elveback LR, et al. Insulinoma: clinical and diagnostic features of 60 consecutive cases. Mayo Clinic Proc 1976;51:417–429.
7. Merimee TJ, Fineberg S. Homeostasis during fasting. Hormone substrate differences between men and women. J Clin Endocrinol Metab 1973;37:698–702.

CASE #2: NONINSULINOMA
PANCREATOGENOUS HYPOGLYCEMIA SYNDROME

Case Description

A 72-yr-old man experienced intermittent episodes of lightheadedness, diplopia, diaphoresis, perioral paraesthesiae, and tremor. These symptoms occurred 1–2 h after eating, often up to three times per day. He had had similar symptoms for many years previously but to a much milder degree and less frequently (once monthly). Over the past 2 mo, his symptoms increased in severity and frequency to such a degree that he ate frequently and carried food in his car. His symptoms resolved within 15 min of carbohydrate ingestion. Medications included ranitidine 150 mg twice daily and primidone 125 mg daily. Past medical history included prostate carcinoma and laryngeal carcinoma. Physical examination was normal.

During a spontaneous episode 2 h following a light lunch, plasma glucose was 40 mg/dL and plasma insulin was 21 µU/mL. He was given intravenous (iv) dextrose and promptly recovered. During a subsequent episode 4 h after breakfast, plasma glucose was 36 mg/dL, plasma was insulin 960 µU/mL, C-peptide was 5600 pmol/L, proinsulin was 190 pmol/L and plasma sulfonylurea screen was negative for first- and second-generation agents. He recovered after the administration of oral carbohydrate.

He underwent a 72 h fast by protocol throughout which he remained asymptomatic with no signs of neuroglycopenia (end-of-fast plasma glucose value was 82 mg/dL). Ninety minutes into a mixed meal test, plasma glucose was 49 mg/dL with concurrent plasma insulin and plasma C-peptide levels of 9 µU/mL and 390 pmol/mL, respectively. Spiral computed tomography (CT) scan and transabdominal ultrasound of the pancreas were negative. A selective arterial calcium stimulation test showed a more than twofold increase in hepatic vein insulin values following calcium injection into the splenic artery and to a lesser extent the gastroduodenal artery.

The patient underwent pancreatic exploration. Intraoperative ultrasound and careful palpation of the pancreas failed to localize a tumor. Gradient guided subtotal distal pancreatectomy was performed. Pathology of the resected pancreas showed histological features consistent with nesidioblastosis (islet cell enlargement and β cells budding off ducts). No insulinoma was identified. To date, he has remained symptom-free, 3 yr following surgery.

Discussion

This case illustrates a new clinical entity termed noninsulinoma pancreatogenous hypoglycemia syndrome (NIPHS). Several aspects of the case serve to differentiate it from insulinoma. The patient experienced symptoms only in the postprandial state. Although fasting hypoglycemia is the rule in insulinoma, some insulinoma patients may have a combination of fasting and postprandial symptoms. Postprandial symptoms alone, however, are extremely rare *(1)*. The patient's history therefore might have led to a diagnosis of "reactive" hypoglycemia and recommendation for diet therapy by some. Confirmation of a history of postprandial hypoglycemia may be obtained during a mixed meal test. Although this test is considered positive if the plasma glucose falls to 50 mg/dL or lower, it is important to recognize that standards have not been generated for the interpretation of the mixed meal test. The 5-h glucose tolerance test should not be used as a diagnostic test for hypoglycemia because a substantial percentage of healthy persons may have a plasma glucose nadir of 50 mg/dL or lower *(2)*.

A negative 72 h fast in a patient with an insulinoma is an extraordinarily rare occurrence. Over the past 25 yr, insulinomas have been removed from 205 patients at the Mayo Clinic. Among these, 171 underwent the 72 h fast. All except two patients had a positive fast. In one patient, the fast remained negative when fasting was extended to 96 h. In most situations, a negative fast would halt further evaluation of hypoglycemia. The presence of neuroglycopenic symptoms and prior demonstration of autonomous β-cell function during hypoglycemia in this patient, however, prompted further evaluation despite the negative 72 h fast. The criteria of endogenous hyperinsulinemia during hypoglycemia apply whether the hypoglycemia is induced by fasting or occurs spontaneously, even in the postprandial state.

The rationale for the selective intraarterial calcium stimulation test is based on the observation that insulinomas respond to calcium injection by releasing insulin, whereas normal β cells do not. The test may be used to localize insulinomas before surgery when more conventional methods have been unsuccessful. With the intraarterial injection of calcium, a step-up of insulin in the venous effluent regionalizes the hyperinsulinemia primarily to the head of the pancreas for the gastroduodenal artery, the uncinate primarily for the superior mesenteric artery, and the body or the tail for the splenic artery. A greater than twofold increase in insulin values from baseline in the right hepatic vein is considered a positive response and indicative of insulinoma in the vascular artery of the territory studied *(3)*. This patient had an increase in insulin following injection into the splenic artery and to a lesser extent the gastroduodenal artery, indicating a nonfocal process.

Over the past 5 yr, NIPHS has been recognized in 10 patients at our institution (age range: 16–78 yr; 7 males, 3 females) *(4,5)*. The disorder is characterized by the following clinical features: neuroglycopenic symptoms primarily in the postprandial state; endogenous hyperinsulinemic hypoglycemia; normal 72 h fast; negative sulfonylurea screen; negative radiologic localizing studies of the pancreas (spiral CT, transabdominal ultrasound, celiac angiography and intraoperative ultrasound); and positive response to the selective arterial calcium stimulation test. In all patients careful mobilization and palpation of the pancreas at surgical exploration failed to detect an insulinoma. Histologic examination of resected pancreatic tissue showed evidence of nesidioblastosis (islet cell enlargement and β cells budding off ducts).

Nesidioblastosis has been observed in rare cases of adults with hyperinsulinemic hypoglycemia and has also been reported in pancreatic tissue resected from hypoglycemic patients who had concurrent insulinoma, and in other clinical syndromes such as Zollinger-Ellison syndrome. The attribution of nesidioblastosis to the syndrome of hyperinsulinemic hypoglycemia in adults without insulinoma is therefore controversial. The finding of subtle histologic changes characteristic of nesidioblastosis in one third of autopsy cases in one series *(6)* has led some authors to conclude that the histologic features of nesidioblastosis may represent a normal variant. Although this may be the case, the positive responses to the selective arterial calcium stimulation test in NIPHS is indicative of some form of diffuse islet cell dysfunction. Abnormalities in *kir6.2* and *SUR1* genes, which encode the subunits of the pancreatic adenosine triphosphate (ATP)-sensitive potassium channel responsible for glucose induced insulin secretion, have been observed in some cases of familial persistent hyperinsulinemic hypoglycemia of infancy *(7)*. No disease-causing mutation of these genes was detected in the patients with NIPHS.

In summary, this patient was diagnosed with the newly recognized clinical disorder of NIPHS. This diagnosis should be considered in those patients with a history of post-prandial neuroglycopenia (confirmed either during a spontaneous episode or during a mixed meal test) and a negative 72 h fast. These patients should undergo the calcium stimulation test. In a patient with a negative response to this procedure, other mechanisms to explain the postprandial hypoglycemia should be explored. Nuclear gastric emptying studies to detect accelerated transit as a cause of postprandial hypoglycemia should be considered.

REFERENCES

1. Connor H, Scarpello JHB. An insulinoma with reactive hypoglycaemia. Postgrad Med J 1979;55:735–738.
2. Lev-Ran A, Andresen RW. The diagnosis of postprandial hypoglycemia. Diabetes 1981;30:996–999.
3. Doppman JL, Miller DL, Chang R, et al. Insulinoma localization with selective intraarterial injection of calcium. Radiology 1991;178:327–241. (Erratum, Radiology 1993;187:880).
4. Service FJ, Natt N, Thompson GB, et al. Noninsulinoma pancreatogenous hypoglycemia. A novel syndrome of hyperinsulinemic hypoglycemia in adults independent of mutations in kir6.2 and SUR1 genes. J Clin Endocrinol Metab 1999;84:1582–1589.
5. Thompson GB, Service FJ, Natt N, et al. Noninsulinoma pancreatogenous hypoglycemia syndrome: an update in 10 surgically treated patients. Surgery 2000;128:937–944.
6. Karnauchow PN. Nesidioblastosis in adults without insular hyperfunction. Am J Clin Path 1981;78:511–513.
7. Dunne MJ, Kane C, Shepherd RM, et al. Familial persistent hyperinsulinemic hypoglycemia of infancy and mutations in the sulfonylurea receptor. N Engl J Med 1997;336:703–706.

CASE #3: FACTITIOUS HYPOGLYCEMIA

Case Description

A 37-yr-old woman was evaluated at an outside institution with a 1 yr history of episodic blurred vision, tremor, fatigue, diaphoresis, and perioral paresthesiae. On two occasions she lost consciousness and drove her car off the road. Repeated emergency room visits documented plasma glucose levels ranging between 15 and 20 mg/dL. She reported that symptoms occurred at any time during the day with no apparent relationship to the ingestion of food. Symptoms occurred almost daily and were relieved within 15 min of ingestion of orange juice.

Physical examination was normal. Past medical history included depression. There was no family history of diabetes. Medications included amitriptyline 75 mg at night. Prior to referral to our institution, she presented to an emergency room in an obtunded state. At that time, plasma glucose was 42 mg/dL, insulin 16 µU/mL, and C-peptide 600 pmol/L. A diagnosis of hypoglycemia secondary to an insulinoma was made. Preoperative abdominal CT and ultrasound of the abdomen were negative. Exploratory laparotomy was performed. Although palpation suggested slight thickness of the pancreatic head, intraoperative ultrasonography was negative. No further surgical intervention was made. She was diagnosed with an occult insulinoma and referred to our institution for further evaluation.

She underwent a 72 h fast by protocol. Twenty-one hours into the fast she developed blurred vision, diaphoresis, and dull mentation. Laboratory data at the time of these symptoms are shown in Table 2.

Table 2
Case #3: End-of-Fast β-Cell Polypeptide and Insulin Surrogate Levels

Glucose (mg/dL)	Insulin (μU/mL)	C-peptide (pmol/L)	β-Hydroxybutyrate (mmol/L)	Δ plasma glucose (mg/dL)
33	40	1600	0.2	50

She was on medical assistance and extremely concerned, as she was unable to pay for her medical bed or hospital evaluation. She also could not afford to pay for a hotel should she have to undergo outpatient evaluation. Social services were contacted to help deal with this issue. In view of the patient's financial concerns and the fact that outside pre-operative localization studies were negative, a selective arterial calcium stimulation test was performed to expedite the evaluation. While waiting for the results of this test, the plasma sulfonylurea screen was reported positive for glipizide. Subsequently, results of the calcium stimulation test were available and showed a flat insulin response.

The patient was told that glipizide had been detected in her blood. She could offer no explanation for this and steadfastly denied taking the medication. She had not brought her medications with her. She declined psychiatric evaluation and was dismissed with a diagnosis of factitious hypoglycemia secondary to sulfonylurea use.

Discussion

This case of factitious hypoglycemia illustrates several potential pitfalls in the evaluation of a patient with hypoglycemia. Sulfonylurea agents produce hypoglycemia by liberating preformed insulin from beta cells by a direct action. Thus in the presence of sulfonylurea-induced hypoglycemia, insulin and C-peptide levels are inappropriately elevated (as demonstrated in this patient). Because the pattern of beta cell polypeptides and insulin surrogate parameters obtained when a patient is hypoglycemic from use of sulfonylureas is identical to that observed in insulinoma, differentiation of sulfonylurea-induced hypoglycemia from insulinoma is impossible without analysis for sulfonylureas in the same blood sample drawn for the other measurements.

The evaluation of insulinoma traditionally involves a two-step approach that requires biochemical confirmation of the presence of endogenous hyperinsulinemia in a sulfonyl-urea-negative patient, followed by an attempt to localize the tumor preoperatively. Indeed the major purpose of conducting the 72 h fast in this patient was to determine the mechanism of hypoglycemia, as Whipple's triad had been demonstrated previously. We were influenced by the financial concerns voiced by this patient and hence did not strictly follow the recommended approach for the evaluation of the patient with hyperinsulinemic hypoglycemia. Measurement of plasma sulfonylurea is an essential component of the 72 h fast and the results should be available before pursuing localization procedures. At our institution liquid chromatography tandem mass spectrometry can detect both first- and second-generation agents and repaglinide at low concentration.

It is important to recognize that misuse of sulfonylureas may be deliberate or unintended e.g. a dispensing error. In addition, accidents may occur if the patient or an elderly partner becomes confused as to the medication to be taken. Because of the potential for drug errors, the physician or pharmacist should identify all medications taken by the patient.

Occasionally it is necessary to perform a little "detective work" to determine the types of medications kept in the patient's house.

The true incidence of factitious hypoglycemia is unknown and likely to be under-reported. The clinical history may be indistinguishable from that obtained in a case of insulinoma and may extend over a period of many years sometimes with a long remission. The use of sulfonylurea agents must therefore be considered in the differential diagnosis of all patients who present with a hypoglycemic disorder. It is not unusual for patients with factitious hypoglycemia to have undergone one or more pancreatic explorations in search for an occult insulinoma (1). Management of the patient with factitious hypoglycemia is difficult. Patients often deny surreptitious sulfonylurea use even in the face of overwhelming evidence and are unwilling to undergo psychiatric treatment. Little information is available on the long-term treatment and outcome of patients with factitious hypoglycemia. A small number of follow up studies indicate a poor long-term prognosis (2).

REFERENCES

1. Klonoff DC, Barrett MJ, Nolte MS, et al. Hypoglycemia following inadvertent and factitious sulphonylurea overdosages. Diabetes Care 1995;18:563–567.
2. Roy M, Roy A. Factitious hypoglycemia: an 11-year follow-up. Psychosomatics 1995;36:64–65.

CASE #4: REOPERATIVE INSULINOMA

Case Description

A 38-yr-old woman had episodes of confusion over a 3 yr period. The first episode occurred in the late morning while at home recovering from influenza. Her husband telephoned her from work and was concerned to find her incoherent. Their 5-yr-old son came on the phone and told his father that mother was yelling at him and behaving abnormally. On arrival at home he found his wife confused, sitting in a chair with a strange look on her face. While waiting for the paramedics to arrive, he gave her some juice and her condition improved. In the emergency room her blood glucose was 36 mg/dL. She fully recovered following intravenous (iv) dextrose administration. She was dismissed with no follow-up evaluation. Her symptoms were attributed to influenza. Following this episode she noticed that she was slow to wake up in the morning and found it difficult to focus. She felt better after eating breakfast. Her husband described that she was often incoherent and confused in the morning. On routine testing a fasting plasma glucose level was 32 mg/dL. She was referred to an endocrinologist for further evaluation.

The following biochemical results were obtained during a spontaneous episode of confusion: plasma glucose 40 mg/dL, insulin 10 µU/mL, C-peptide 888 pmol/L, and negative sulfonylurea screen. The patient was diagnosed with an insulinoma and underwent preoperative portal venous sampling. This revealed a step-up in insulin levels in the region of the head of the pancreas. On the basis of this result, she underwent exploratory laparotomy. At surgery, palpation of the pancreas and intraoperative ultrasound failed to reveal a tumor. A Whipple's procedure was performed. Pathological examination was negative for insulinoma. Postoperatively, she continued to have low plasma glucose values and 3 mo later symptoms recurred. Once again she found it difficult to wake up fully in the morning and was unable to process information. Her husband stated that she would look drunk and wander aimlessly around the house. Drinking orange juice or eating chocolate relieved these symptoms within 15 min of ingestion. On occasion she would resist food

Table 3
Case #4: End-of-Fast β-Cell Polypeptide and Insulin Surrogate Levels

Plasma glucose (mg/dL)	Insulin (µU/mL)	C-peptide (pmol/L)	Proinsulin (pmol/L)	β-Hydroxybutyrate (mmol/L)	Δ plasma glucose (mg/dL)
48	9	400	17	0.5	50

presented to her. Further localization studies for insulinoma were performed. No tumor was seen on angiography and repeat portal venous sampling was nondiagnostic. CT scan of the abdomen was negative. She was treated with diazoxide 100 mg twice daily, which successfully prevented symptoms of hypoglycemia.

Six mo later, the patient was evaluated at our institution having been instructed to discontinue her diazoxide 5 d prior to her appointment. She developed neuroglycopenic symptoms 5 h into a fast conducted in our outpatient endocrine testing center. Concurrent biochemical data was as follows in Table 3.

The sulfonylurea screen was negative for first- and second-generation agents. Review of the outside CT scan of the abdomen suggested a 3-cm lesion in the left lobe of the liver. A selective arterial calcium stimulation test was performed primarily to determine whether the hepatic lesion was secreting insulin, i.e., was a metastatic lesion. This test showed a flat insulin response following injection into all relevant arteries. Transabdominal ultrasound revealed a 0.5-cm lesion in the body of the pancreas. Spiral CT scan of the abdomen demonstrated a small hepatic cyst and a very subtle 0.5-cm enhancing area in the anterior portion of the body of the pancreas corresponding to the abnormality seen on ultrasound. The patient underwent exploratory laparotomy. Intraoperative ultrasound confirmed the presence of a 0.7-cm lesion in the anterior portion of the body of the pancreas. Palpation of this area revealed a thin small nodule that was difficult to differentiate from scar tissue. The area was enucleated. No hepatic tumor was identified. Pathology of the resected pancreatic tissue confirmed a 0.7-cm islet cell adenoma consistent with insulinoma. To date, the patient has remained symptom-free.

Discussion

This case of reoperative insulinoma illustrates several important points in the preoperative localization and surgical management of a patient with insulinoma. Before proceeding to further evaluation, the diagnosis of insulinoma should be reconfirmed in all cases of hypoglycemia persisting after surgical exploration

Surgical failures occur primarily as a result of surgical inexperience, multicentric disease, malignant tumors or improper diagnosis, such as factitious disorders (1). On rare occasions, an occult solitary adenoma is missed by even the most experienced surgeon supported by intraoperative ultrasound. Despite the use of CT, ultrasound and magnetic resonance imaging (MRI), the localization of insulinomas smaller than 2 cm remains a problem. Even in the best of hands, transabdominal ultrasound and spiral CT may detect only about 60% of insulinomas (2). Accurate preoperative localization of insulinoma is desirable because in the hands of some surgeons as many as 10% of insulinomas remain occult to palpation at the time of surgery (3). Experts differ in their preferred approaches to radiologic localization, most likely because of differences in their expertise. Our preferred approach is to obtain transabdominal ultrasound then spiral CT of the pancreas. The selective calcium stimulation test is reserved for some patients with negative imaging studies, and other complex cases. Intraoperative ultrasound (IOUS) is utilized at the time of surgical exploration to confirm the location of the tumor and aid in its excision.

This patient underwent portal vein sampling as her initial localization study for insulinoma. This method can regionalize a tumor to the head-uncinate or body-tail regions. We do not use portal venous sampling because it is highly invasive and rarely offers useful information over that obtained with more conventional preoperative localization methods and IOUS. The calcium stimulation test was performed in this patient primarily to elucidate the nature of the hepatic lesion seen on an outside CT scan. The insulin response to calcium stimulation of the pancreas likely showed a flat response due to the altered vasculature caused by the initial surgery.

It is generally accepted that IOUS provides the highest success rate in the localization of insulinomas. The technique can occasionally localize insulinomas that remain undetected by surgical exploration *(4)* and appears to be particularly valuable for the detection of deep-seated tumors within the pancreas (particularly those located in the head which are usually more difficult to palpate). IOUS can not only reveal the location of an insulinoma but also provides useful information about the precise relationship of the tumor to surrounding vital structures especially the pancreatic duct. This information can help the surgeon choose appropriate surgical procedures such as enucleation or pancreatic resection. Although complete mobilization and palpation of the pancreas by an experienced surgeon in combination with IOUS performed by a skilled radiologist is successful in localizing almost all insulinomas, information gained from preoperative radiologic studies remains desirable as it allows the surgeon to plan the surgical approach ahead of time and facilitates explanation to the patient regarding the anticipated extent of surgery.

Blind distal resection of the pancreas at the time of initial exploration in the hope of excising an occult tumor is not recommended for several reasons. Insulinoma is distributed evenly throughout the pancreas: thus the failure rate for successful resection of these tumors is unacceptably high. Surgery results in scarred tissue planes and a pancreas that is firmer than usual, making it difficult for the surgeon to palpate a small tumor at reoperation. In addition, completion pancreatectomy with its attendant serious consequences may be the only therapeutic option at the time of reoperation.

In summary, this patient presented with an occult insulinoma. We recommend preoperative localization studies in both initial explorations for insulinoma and reoperative cases. In skilled hands, IOUS is the most sensitive method for detecting an insulinoma and may aid the surgeon in resection of the tumor. The patient in whom an insulinoma is not located at first operation should be referred to a center with considerable experience in the management of these fascinating tumors.

REFERENCES

1. Thompson GB, Service FJ, van Heerden JA, et al. Reoperative insulinomas, 1927 to 1992: an institutional experience. Surgery 1993;114:1196–206.
2. Stark DD, Moss AA, Goldberg HI, et al. Computed tomography and nuclear magnetic resonance imaging of pancreatic islet cell tumors. Surgery 1993;94:1024–1027.
3. Fedorak IJ, Ko TC, Gordon D. Localization of islet cell tumors of the pancreas: a review of current techniques. Surgery 1993;113:242–249.
4. Jian-Cun Huai, Zhengzhou Henan, Wel Zhang, et al. Localization and surgical treatment of pancreatic insulinomas guided by intraoperative ultrasound. Am J Surgery 1997;175:18–21.

19

Disorders of Lipoprotein Metabolism

Ira J. Goldberg, MD and Phillip Bukberg, MD

CONTENTS

CASE #1: DIABETES WITH FAMILIAL COMBINED HYPERLIPIDEMIA

Case Description

A 59-yr-old man presented with the diagnosis of type 2 diabetes. He was in good health until 5 yr ago when he presented to the emergency room (ER) with an episode of chest pain and numbness in his jaw that occurred as he was walking up stairs. He was admitted to the hospital, and although an acute myocardial infarction (MI) was ruled out, an exercise stress test was positive. Coronary angiography revealed triple-vessel disease, and a coronary bypass operation was performed. Risk factors for coronary disease included the following: family history—his father died of an MI at age 52, mild hypertension −145/88, cigarette smoking—1 pack per day × 20 yr. He works as a bus driver and is 5 ft 9 in and 180 lbs. A lipid profile taken 2 mo postoperatively was as follows: cholesterol 250 mg/dL, triglyceride 180 mg/dL, HDL 30 mg/dL, and LDL 184 mg/dL. Liver, renal, and thyroid functions were normal.

The patient was begun on a β-blocker, aspirin, and 20 mg/d of simvastatin. A subsequent evaluation one month later included cholesterol 210 mg/dL, triglyceride 240 mg/dL, HDL 28 mg/dL, LDL 144 mg/dL.

His primary care physician followed the patient for the next 3 yr with no change in his medications and no new symptoms. Two weeks prior to his visit, he was seen for a routine evaluation. He now weighs 210 lbs. His cholesterol was 240 mg/dL, triglycerides 600 mg/dL, HDL 25 mg/dL, and LDL was not estimated. You order several additional tests including Lp(a), small dense LDL measurement, glucose and HA_{1c}. Lp(a) was less than 30, LDL was pattern B (more small dense LDL), fasting glucose was 160, and HbA_{1c} was 8.0%.

From: *Contemporary Endocrinology: Challenging Cases in Endocrinology*
Edited by: M. E. Molitch © Humana Press Inc., Totowa, NJ

Discussion

As is not uncommon, patients with prediabetes often present first with clinical evidence of coronary artery disease. These patients often have a constellation of risk factors that include low HDL, small dense LDL, hypertension, and insulin resistance *(1)*. Although this latter finding was not assessed in this patient, insulin levels are often elevated in this situation.

In the course of treatment for his anginal syndrome, this man was appropriately given β-blockers and a cholesterol-lowering medication, simvastatin. Although β-blockers have been reported in one study to be associated with increased development of diabetes *(2)*, their positive effects to reduce cardiac death make their usage in this situation appropriate. It should also be noted that, as in this patient, β-blockers can increase triglyceride and reduce HDL levels *(3)*.

Another issue is the measurement of cardiac risk factors other than a lipid profile. A number of other blood tests have been associated with increased risk in several studies. These include homocysteine, Lp(a) in Caucasians, but not blacks, and measurements of inflammation such as C-reactive protein, tumor necrosis factor, and Interleukin-6 (IL-6). A number of investigations have suggested that LDL particle size is associated with greater cardiovascular risk; however, this effect seemed to be limited to subjects who also had increased apoB levels—owing to either increased LDL or hypertriglyceridemia—or reduced HDL *(4,5)*. In other studies this measurement did not seem to add additional information *(6)*. In addition to hypertriglyceridemia, other predictors of small dense LDL include abdominal obesity and, presumably, insulin resistance *(7)*. Therefore, clinical assessment might be as informative as direct measurement of this LDL subfraction in this patient.

The current problem is hypertriglyceridemia. Although the β-blocker may have contributed to this, the likelihood is that the diabetes is the primary reason for the triglyceride elevation. Occasional patients with mild hypertriglyceridemia will become severely hypertriglyceridemic with the onset of diabetes mellitus; some of these patients have a heterozygous defect in lipoprotein lipase, the rate-limiting enzyme for triglyceride removal *(8)*. This may be the case in this patient. Although that enzyme can be measured in the blood after a heparin injection and the patient's gene can be sequenced, neither evaluation will alter the clinical approach to the disorder.

The role of hypertriglyceridemia as a risk factor for cardiovascular disease has been debated for several decades *(9)*. Except for hypertriglyceridemia associated with estrogens or alcohol, these patients invariably have reduced HDL owing to transfer of VLDL triglyceride for HDL cholesterol, a reaction mediated by the cholesteryl ester transfer protein *(10)*. Although a primary prevention trial of triglyceride-lowering agents has not been done, a recent study in VA patients with established cardiovascular disease and low HDL demonstrated that gemfibrozil reduces the incidence of recurrent events in a lower HDL population *(11)*. Gemfibrozil reduced triglycerides 25% and increased HDL 7%— the lipid change responsible for the beneficial effect of the drug cannot be ascertained because both changes occurred. Although the subjects in this VA study were not as hypertriglyceridemic as our patient, it is likely that triglyceride reduction would be of benefit. Moreover, because triglyceride levels over 500 mg/dL are at a level associated with saturation of lipoprotein lipase, there is concern that dietary indiscretion or worsening diabetes might lead to an acute, rapid increase in triglyceride leading to pancreatitis.

The primary approach to this patient is life-style modification and diabetes management. Without control of his diabetes, the hypertriglyceridemia is unlikely to resolve.

Weight reduction and exercise can sometimes lead to dramatic reductions in triglyceride; this alone may well correct the problem. Diets should avoid alcohol completely, free sugars and simple carbohydrates should be reduced, and fats that will exacerbate postprandial lipemia should be limited. After introduction of diabetes therapy, triglyceride-lowering medications should be considered. In this situation, fibric acids—gemfibrozil and fenofibrate—are probably the first line therapy. Occasionally, the improved glycemic control will fully correct the triglycerides; sometimes the LDL will increase and the patients may then benefit most by a statin. Alternatively, combination therapy may be needed, however, with the patient's statin therapy there is an increased the risk of development of myositis. The patient needs to be warned to stop his medications and inform his physician if he develops myalgias. Niacin in low dose may be effective, but it may exacerbate glucose intolerance. High-dose statins and fish oil also may be useful.

REFERENCES

1. Haffner SM, Stern MP, Hazuda HP, Mitchell BD, Patterson JK. Cardiovascular risk factors in confirmed prediabetic individuals. Does the clock for coronary heart disease start ticking before the onset of clinical diabetes? JAMA 1990;263:2893–2898.
2. Gress TW, Nieto FJ, Shahar E, Wofford MR, Brancati FL. Hypertension and antihypertensive therapy as risk factors for type 2 diabetes mellitus. Atherosclerosis Risk in Communities Study. N Engl J Med 2000;342:905–912.
3. Kasiske BL, Ma JZ, Kalil RS, Louis TA. Effects of antihypertensive therapy on serum lipids. Ann Intern Med 1995;122:133–141.
4. Lamarche B, Tchernof A, Mauriege P, Cantin B, Dangenais GR, Lupien PJ, Despres JP. Fasting insulin and apolipoprotein B levels and low-density lipoprotein particle size as risk factors for ischemic heart disease. JAMA 1998;279:1955–1961.
5. Grundy S. Small LDL, atherogenic dyslipidemia, and the metabolic syndrome. Diabetologia 1997;40:512–520.
6. Stampfer MJ, Krauss RM, Ma J, Blanche PJ, Holl LG, Sacks FM, Hennekens CH. A prospective study of triglyceride level, low-density lipoprotein particle diameter, and risk of myocardial infarction. JAMA 1996;276:882–888.
7. Lemieux I, Pascot A, Couillard C, Lamarche B, Tchernof A, Almeras N, Bergeron J, Gaudet D, Tremblay G, Prud'homme D, Nadeau A, Despres J-P. Hypertriglyceriemic Waist: A Marker of the Atherogenic Metabolic Triad (Hyperinsulinemia; Hyperapolipoprotein B; Small, Dense LDL) in Men? Circulation 2000;102:179–184.
8. Wilson DE, Hata A, Kwong LK, Lingam A, Shuhua J, Ridinger DN, Yeager C, Kaltenborn KC, Iverius PH, Lalouel JM. Mutations in exon 3 of th elipoprotein lipase gene segregating in a family with hypertriglyceridemia, pancreatitis, and non-insulin-dependent diabetes. J Clin Invest 1993;92:203–211.
9. Miller M. Current perspectives on the management of hypertriglyceridemia. Am Heart J 2000;140:232–240.
10. Tall AR, Jiang X, Luo Y, Silver D. 1999 George Lyman Duff memorial lecture: lipid transfer proteins, HDL Metabolism, and atherogenesis. Arterioscler Thromb Vasc Biol 2000;20:1185–1188.
11. Rubins HB, Robins SJ, Collins D, Fye CL, Anderson JW, Elam MB, Faas FH, Linares E, Schaefer EJ, Schectman G, Wilt TJ, Wittes J. Gemfibrozil for the secondary prevention of coronary heart disease in men with low levels of high-density lipoprotein cholesterol. Veterans Affairs High-Density Lipoprotein Cholesterol Intervention Trial Study Group. N Engl J Med 1999;341:410–418.

CASE #2: LOW CHOLESTEROL SYNDROME

Case Description

A 72-yr-old man presented with a complaint of increased fatigue developing over several months, and low blood cholesterol levels. He had a history of cigarette smoking, two packs per day for 40 yr, until age 60 when he was hospitalized for a nontransmural

MI. At that time he was 5 ft 9 in and weighed 210 lbs. His lipids prior to this event were cholesterol 175 mg/dL, triglycerides 300 mg/dL, HDL 25 mg/dL, and LDL 90 mg/dL. Family history was significant for a mother with type II diabetes and death in her 50s from pneumonia and a father who died of a stroke at age 72. He was not hypertensive and did not have diabetes at this time.

Subsequent to this episode, the patient was primarily followed by his cardiologist and was treated with aspirin and β-blockers. He took sublingual nitroglycerin approximately 4–6 times per week for typical exercise-related angina that occurred with rapid walking, ascending stairs, and in cold weather. Both his cardiogram and chest X-ray indicated cardiomegaly, but the patient refused additional work-up stating that his symptoms were not severe enough for him to agree to either surgical intervention or angioplasty. Lipid profiles taken over this period of time showed a total cholesterol of 150–170 mg/dL, triglyceride of 200–350 mg/dL and HDL from 23–30 mg/dL.

At the current visit, the patient notes that walking even a block was associated with marked fatigue. Although he had had mild pedal edema in the past, this had not changed. In addition, he noted no dyspnea. Surprisingly, no angina had occurred for the past 3 mo. His physical exam was unchanged and showed obesity, cardiomegaly, and clear lungs.

His Hct was 27% with normal indices. His chemistry profile and iron indices were normal. His total cholesterol was 80 mg/dL, triglycerides 150 mg/dL, HDL 20 mg/dL, and calculated LDL 30 mg/dL.

Discussion

Low levels of plasma cholesterol and LDL occur as a primary genetic disorder or, as in this case, as an acquired problem. Low levels of apoB, the major protein in LDL and VLDL, leads to hypobetalipoproteinemia. This occurs with genetic abnormalities in this protein including truncations, deletions, and base substitutions. Homozygous or compound heterozygous patients with complete absence of apoB have not been described. Homozygous knockout of apoB in mice is an embryonic lethal; this suggests that apoB has an important, but unclear, role in development. Humans with hypobetalipoproteinemia have no obvious medical problems and they have a very low risk of cardiovascular disease. This genetic experiment suggests that such low levels of LDL are safe. These LDL levels are lower than those achieved with any lipid-lowering medication.

The second genetic cause of very low LDL is a defect in microsomal triglyceride transfer protein (MTP). This protein is required to add lipid to apoB within cells and is the protein that is defective in abetalipoproteinemia *(1)*. These patients are unable to assemble apoB-containing lipoproteins (chylomicrons, VLDL, and LDL) in either the gut or liver. This leads to defective absorption of fat-soluble vitamins and the clinical presentation of these children is as vitamin deficiency syndromes *(2)*.

Secondary causes of very low cholesterol occur in several settings. Malnutrition and chronic disease lead to low cholesterol; this does not appear to be the problem in this patient. Acute inflammatory conditions such as MI and pneumonia also reduce plasma cholesterol levels.

In a more chronic situation such as this case, there are several disorders that can reduce LDL to these levels. Such dramatic LDL decreases are found in myeloproliferative disorders including polycythema vera and myelofibrosis. This man was found to have chronic myelomonocytic leukemia; his white blood count (WBC) was 28,000 and his bone marrow biopsy done as part of his anemia work-up was diagnostic. The etiology of the cholesterol reduction appears to be increased uptake of lipoproteins in the organs of the reticuloendo-thelial system such as bone marrow and spleen *(3)*. In some chronic leukemias, the activ-ity of the disease can be correlated with cholesterol, presumably more neoplastic disease is associated with increased uptake of circulating lipoproteins by the neoplastic cells *(4)*.

The physicians attending this man assumed that his decrease in angina symptoms were because of fatigue and reduced exercise, especially because anemia would have been expected to lead to more angina. An alternative explanation for the decrease in angina is that the reduction in LDL cholesterol led to an improvement in either endothelial function or his atherosclerotic plaque burden. In support of this, is the recent observation that over 40% of patients with mild angina had a symptomatic improvement when LDL was reduced to, on average, 77 mg/dL *(5)*.

REFERENCES

1. Wetterau JR, Aggerbeck LP, Bouma ME, Eisenberg C, Munck A, Hermier M, Schmitz J, Gay G, Rader DJ, Gregg RE. Absence of microsomal triglyceride transfer protein in individuals with abetalipo-protein-emia. Science 1992;258:999–1001.
2. Rader DJ, Brewer HB Jr. Abetalipoproteinemia. New insights into lipoprotein assembly and vitamin E metabolism for a rare genetic disease [clinical conference]. JAMA 1993;270:865–869.
3. Ginsberg H, Goldberg IJ, Wang-Iverson P, Gitler E, Le NA, Gilbert HS, Brown WV. Increased catabo-lism of native and cyclohexanedione-modified low density lipoprotein in subjects with myeloprolifera-tive diseases. Arteriosclerosis 1983;3:223–241.
4. Gilbert HS, Ginsberg H. Hypocholesterolemia as a manifestation of disease activity in chronic myelo-cytic leukemia. Cancer 1983;51:1428–1433.
5. Pitt B, Waters D, Brown WV, van Boven AJ, Schwartz L, Title LM, Eisenberg D, Shurzinske L, McCormick LS. Aggressive lipid-lowering therapy compared with angioplasty in stable coronary artery disease. Atorvastatin versus Revascularization Treatment Investigators. N Engl J Med 1999;341:70–76.

CASE #3: FAMILIAL HYPERCHOLESTEROLEMIA

Case Description

A 50-yr-old woman with a history of coronary artery disease (CAD) and familial hypercholesterolemia presents with a recent exacerbation of her lipid disorder. At age 35, this woman was admitted to the hospital with an episode of substernal chest pain asso-ciated with ST depression in the lateral precordial leads. At that time, she gave a family history of cardiac disease; her mother died at age 42 after several years of chest pain on exertion and an older sister had a sudden death at age 37. She was rapidly evaluated during this first hospitalization and underwent bypass surgery for LAD and right coro-nary lesions of >70%. Postoperatively, she had a total cholesterol of 350 mg/dL, HDL 32 mg/dL, triglyceride 140 mg/dL, and LDL 290 mg/dL. She related that her cholesterol had been as high as 450 mg/dL in the past. Her examination was significant for large xanthomas on both Achilles tendons.

The patient had three children, ages 5, 9, and 11. None of her children had increased cholesterol. She had never taken hormonal contraceptives. She was begun on lovastatin that was gradually increased and then switched to 80 mg/d of simvastatin. This reduced her cholesterol to 220 mg/dL and her LDL to 160 mg/dL. Cholestyramine, 4 scoops per day, was then added and led to a further reduction in LDL to 130 mg/dL and total choles-terol to 190 mg/dL. Regular niacin 1 g three times a day was eventually included and LDL decreased to 105 and HDL increased to 38 mg/dL. Over the past 15 yr, her total cholesterol has remained between 170 and 220, depending on her compliance. One year prior to this visit she was seen by her cardiologist and complained at that time of fatigue and non-exercise related substernal aching. An exercise tolerance test was normal and a cardiac catheterization done because of her high-risk status showed full patency of her grafts and no critical lesions. The chest syndrome subsequently has subsided, but did not entirely leave. It is an aching in the substernal region that is not related to either food or exercise.

At this visit she is perimenopausal and having periods once every 3 mo. Her cholesterol has risen to 250 mg/dL despite continued compliance with her medications. Her weight has increased 10 lbs over the year despite her adherence to a low fat/low cholesterol diet.

Discussion

Although the principal cause of death in women, as in men, is atherosclerotic cardio-vascular disease, this usually occurs at a later age. In premenopausal women, the development of CAD is distinctly unusual but is found in association with collagen-vascular disease, diabetes, and, as in this case, familial hypercholesterolemia.

This patient gives a classic presentation of familial hypercholesterolemia. This disorder is due to defective LDL receptors, leading to a reduction in hepatic removal of LDL cholesterol from the bloodstream. Both her mother and sister are likely to have also had this disorder. It is an autosomal dominant disease and heterozygous carriers have markedly elevated cholesterol levels and premature coronary artery disease that begins in early adulthood. The rare homozygous carriers have LDL levels that are twice as high as was found in this patient and often develop vascular disease in childhood *(1)*. Each of this patient's children has a 50% chance of inheriting this defective gene; therefore, screening is required to identify carriers so they can received cholesterol-lowering treatment prior to adulthood. Fortunately, none of the three children of this patient was affected. Although neither genetic screening nor assessment of LDL receptors was performed in this patient, the presence of Achilles xanthomas is virtually diagnostic for this disease. A second molecular defect that can cause hypercholesteralemia is an abnormality of apoB, the major protein of LDL, that leads to a defect in the LDL receptor-binding region of this protein; the ligand rather than the receptor is defective. This defect termed "familial defective apoB" leads to the same lipoprotein abnormality. Although techniques are available to define both of these defects on a molecular level, such information does not alter the treatment of these patients and is therefore not usually obtained.

This woman's very premature heart disease is because of her elevated LDL and the low HDL level that she also inherited. The initial cholesterol of 350 mg/dL was obtained post-operatively and was lower than that obtained previously. Postoperative stress and inflammatory conditions such as MI, stroke, and infectious disease will reduce cholesterol. Patients with familial hypercholesterolemia usually require multiple lipid-lowering medications. This patient was originally started on lovastatin on a "compassionate use" protocol prior to introduction of statin drugs to the market. She obtained the expected effect of those medications leading to a greater than 45% decrease in LDL. It should be noted that all statin medications tend to have their greatest effect using the starting dosage. Thereafter, doubling the dose leads to an additional 7% reduction in LDL. Addition of resin, cholestyramine or colestipol, can reduce LDL 20% more. This woman was instructed to eat a high roughage diet including bran cereal each morning to prevent constipation from the resin. Some patients find it most convenient to only take the resin with their largest meal, usually dinner. The ingestion of two scoops of resin in juice or water has the added benefit of appetite suppression for many people.

Niacin leads to a similar LDL reduction as resin and it has the most beneficial effect on HDL; an increase of 25% is not unusual. Lp(a) is also reduced 35% by niacin (2). Lesser increases in HDL are found with fibric acid drugs. These drugs do increase the chances of myositis and because this patient does not have concomitant hypertriglyceridemia fibric acids are not appropriate in this situation.

This patient took regular over-the-counter niacin, 1 g with each meal. Niacin is associated with a number of side effects most prominent of which is hepatitis, dyspepsia, exacerbation of peptic ulcer disease, and worsening glucose tolerance in diabetes-prone patients. Most dramatic is the cutaneous vasodilatation leading to flushing, a sunburn-like reddening of the skin. This is transient, and is reduced by aspirin. Flushing occurs more if the niacin is taken on an empty stomach, with hot beverages, or with alcohol. A number of slow release forms of niacin are also available and a once-a-day form, Niaspan, that is only taken at night.

Once a patient is on a stable dose of medication plasma lipoprotein profiles usually do not change dramatically. The increase in this patient, therefore, requires some investigation. One possibility is a change in diet. The weight gain suggests that this could have occurred, however, a review of the patient's 7 d food record did not suggest a major deviation from a diet low in saturated fat and cholesterol. A second possibility is reduced compliance with medications. Except for history and pharmaceutical records this is often hard to determine. Niacin therapy tends to raise plasma levels of uric acid and this measurement is sometimes an indication of niacin use, or in this case nonuse. A third possibility is menopause. Although LDL cholesterol levels generally rise after menopause, those changes are usually less than 10% (3). Finally, a new disorder that could lead to increased LDL may have developed. In this case, the patient was found to have an elevated TSH of 15 µU/mL, and LDL decreased to previous levels after initiation of thyroid replacement therapy. Even mild hypothyroidism is associated with increased LDL cholesterol (4).

A final issue, as this woman approaches menopause, is the decision to use hormone replacement therapy (HRT). Although epidemiologic and experimental data had suggested that estrogen replacement was beneficial for heart disease protection, randomized clinical trial data have not supported this (5). For this reason, the primary rationale for choosing HRT is relief of intolerable menopausal symptoms. This can be done with either oral or transdermal estrogen with progesterone.

REFERENCES

1. Goldstein JL, Brown MS. The LDL receptor defect in familial hypercholesterolemia. Implications for pathogenesis and therapy. Med Clin N Amer 1982;66:335–362.
2. Illingworth DR, Stein EA, Mitchel YB, Dujovne CA, Frost PH, Knopp RH, Tun P, Zupkis RV, Greguski RA. Comparative effects of lovastatin and niacin in primary hypercholesterolemia. A prospective trial. Arch Intern Med 1994;154:1586–1595.
3. Matthews KA, Meilahn E, Kuller LH, Kelsey SF, Caggiula AW, Wing RR. Menopause and risk factors for coronary heart disease. N Engl J Med 1989;321:641–646.
4. Danese MD, Ladenson PW, Meinert CL, Powe NR. Clinical review 115: effect of thyroxine therapy on serum lipoproteins in patients with mild thyroid failure: a quantitative review of the literature. J Clin Endocrinol Metab 2000;85:2993–3001.

5. Hulley S, Grady D, Bush T, Furberg C, Herrington D, Riggs B, Vittinghoff E. Randomized trial of estrogen plus progestin for secondary prevention of coronary heart disease in postmenopausal women. Heart and estrogen/progestin replacement study (HERS) research group. JAMA 1998;280:605–613.

CASES #4 AND #5: UNUSUAL LEVELS OF HDL CHOLESTEROL

Case Descriptions

CASE #4: LOW HDL

A 29-yr-old man is referred to your office for evaluation of cardiac risk and low HDL. He works for a publishing company and, although he avoids high fat/ high cholesterol foods, he does not exercise regularly. In high school, he was a runner on the track team; at college he played intramural sports. He weighed 150 pounds when he graduated from college.

His family history, and the reason for this consultation, is remarkable for the sudden death of his father at age 34 on a tennis court. Although he was a child at the time of his father's death, he recalls that his father was overweight and a cigarette smoker.

The patient has a regular girlfriend, is contemplating marriage in the near future, and would like any information that about potential genetic problems that may have caused his father's death.

His physical examination is unremarkable. He is 5'10" and weighs 170 pounds. His pulse was 54 and regular and his blood pressure was 115/68 mmHg. He has no tendon or palmer xanthomas, no xanthalasmas, and normal fundi. He is bradycardic, but has no murmurs or gallops. Liver and spleen are not palpable and his neurological exam is normal.

Laboratory examination shows a normal chemistry profile. The total cholesterol is 200 mg/dL, HDL 27 mg/dL, triglyceride 90 mg/dL, and calculated LDL 165 mg/dL. Lp(a) is 45 and homocysteine is not elevated. Because of his family history, he is evaluated by a cardiologist who performs an exercise tolerance test and an echocardiogram. The stress test is negative, and the echocardiogram shows a normal sized heart and no valvular pathology.

Exercise programs are discussed and he agrees to begin a three-time per week program of cardiovascular fitness (treadmill) at a gym that he attends with his girlfriend. He is seen by a nutritionist and loses 3 lbs over the next 6 wk. A repeat lipid profile shows a 10 mg/dL decrease in his total cholesterol and no change in his HDL. At this point you begin statin therapy. 2 mo later on 20 mg/d of simvastatin, his LDL is reduced to 95 mg/dL, HDL is 32 mg/dL, and triglycerides are 80 mg/dL.

Two weeks later the patient calls to inform you that he has investigated low HDL syndromes on the Internet. The use of niacin had been mentioned and he is now prepared to try this. You have him purchase niacin from the local health store and begin with 250 mg with each meal. Although he develops flushing during the first week, thereafter he has flushing only for the 2 d when the dose is increased and when he drinks alcohol. For this reason, he agrees to stop drinking his usual nightly glass of wine until the niacin therapy is adjusted. Increasing 250 mg each week, he is able to reach a dose of 1 g per meal. The patient returns in 2 mo complaining of fatigue. His cholesterol is now 120, HDL 32, triglyceride 50, and LDL 78. ALT, AST, and bilirubin are elevated. The niacin is stopped and his liver functions and lipid profile return to pretreatment levels.

CASE #5: ELEVATED HDL AND LDL

A 32-yr-old woman is referred for a "second opinion" regarding the need for lipid-lowering medication. A recent lipid profile showed a total cholesterol level of 278 mg/dL, triglycerides 55 mg/dL, HDL 72 mg/dL, and LDL 195 mg/dL. Her past medical history is negative for serious illness. She exercises 4–5 d/wk at a local health club, workouts consisting of a combination of treadmill, cross-country skiing machine, and/or "stepper" apparatus for a total of 45–60 min. A review of her diet indicates that it is well within "prudent" guidelines.

Her family history is significant for her father having died of an acute MI at age 59, after having had stable angina for a number of years. Her mother is alive and well at age 65. Both of her grandmothers lived into their late 80s.

Her physical examination is unremarkable. Her weight is 116 lb (height 64"). No tendon xanthomas are noted.

The patient's primary care physician had suggested to her that she start on statin therapy to lower her LDL-cholesterol. The patient is extremely reluctant to take medication, and feels that her excellent level of HDL-cholesterol is sufficiently protective against ischemic heart disease in the future.

Discussion

These two cases of unusual levels of HDL present two similar types of management issues. Although the relationship between HDL and cardiovascular risk is well established within the population, extremes in HDL may not represent the same pathophysiological risk as found within the normal distribution.

Several diseases are associated with very low levels of HDL, lower than that found in Case 4. These include LCAT (lecithin acyl transferase) deficiency, genetic mutations in apoAI, including apoAI Milano, and Tangier Disease. Although apoAI deficiency is often associated with premature heart disease, apoAI Milano is not *(1)*. The risks of heart disease with the other defects are variable. Similarly, although elevated HDL is usually associated with less cardiovascular risk, increased HDL owing to a mutation of CETP (cholesteryl ester transfer protein) or hepatic lipase is not associated with protection from CAD *(2)*. CETP is responsible for the transfer of cholesterol from HDL into triglyceride-rich lipoproteins and the very large HDL produced with CETP deficiency may be defective in returning cholesterol to the liver. CETP deficiency is primarily found in the Japanese population. Hepatic lipase deficiency is associated with increased concentrations of circulating remnant lipoproteins; presumably this is the reason for the increased CAD risk despite the elevated HDL.

The reasons for the low HDL in Case 4 are not clear. The level of HDL in most people correlates with the rate of removal of apoAI, the major HDL protein, from the bloodstream. Thus, HDL production is not usually impaired. HDL is formed as a nascent particle that is relatively depleted in lipids. It then acquires lipid from peripheral tissues and the cholesterol is converted to a hydrophobic form, cholesteryl ester, via the actions of LCAT. HDL also acquires lipids from the surface of triglyceride-rich lipoproteins (VLDL and chylomicrons) during their intravascular lipolysis. HDL metabolism involves removal of the entire lipoprotein from the bloodstream or selective removal of only lipid in the liver followed by renal degradation of the small lipid depleted particles. Liver (and adrenal gland) HDL lipid uptake is mediated by the scavenger receptor B-I (SRB-I).

Case 4 might have a heterozygous genetic deficiency of some of the enzymes responsible for HDL production. Heterozygous mutation in lipoprotein lipase may, especially in younger people, present as a low HDL syndrome *(3)*. This is because of reduced transfer of lipid to the HDL and also loss of HDL lipid due to the CETP reaction. Less commonly, mutations in HDL proteins are found. Very low levels of HDL, below 15 mg/dL, are associated with lipid deposits in the tonsils and spleen, a condition known as Tangier Disease. This disease is due to a defect in an ATP binding cassette (ABC) transporter that is required for cholesterol efflux from cells *(4)*. These patients are unable to effect the process of reverse cholesterol transport. A number of mutations of this transporter have been found. Studies have also demonstrated that heterozygous defects in ABC1 are associated with low cholesterol syndromes *(5)*. A recent study of low HDL syndromes found that increased hepatic lipase was often found in patients with HDL in this range *(6)*. Hepatic lipase is involved in the pathway of lipid uptake into the liver; higher levels of hepatic lipase reduce HDL levels by increasing its catabolic rate.

Although in the future, it is likely that the genetic tools to diagnose the etiology of this man's HDL defect will be available, such analyses are currently limited to the research setting. Although his father had several additional risk factors (obesity and cigarette smoking), prudent management assumes that this patient has a high likelihood of having increased risk because of his low HDL syndrome. Although, not always necessary in an active young man, because of the bradycardia and the lack of recent exercise, the cardiac evaluation was performed. In the future, asymptomatic coronary atherosclerosis might instead be evaluated using noninvasive imaging *(7)*.

This man's lifestyle is not uncommon. He is well educated, aware of premature CAD in his family, and attempts to eat a prudent diet. Like many busy people, exercise and weight maintenance are more difficult. A good approach is to resume previous exercise patterns, i.e., having runners run and swimmers swim. Another option is to perform exercise with a buddy or spouse. A third option, especially in patients who have very limited time to exercise, is to do home exercise such as running or bicycling when watching the evening news.

One sure method to reduce this man's cardiac risk is to lower his LDL. This approach was beneficial in a group of middle-aged subjects with HDL below 50 mg/dL and LDL of approximately 150 mg/dL *(8)*. It is, therefore, likely that a similar approach would be useful in this man. It should be noted, however, that because there are no randomized clinical trials with patients whose HDL levels are at the extremes of these two cases; this is not evidence-based medicine.

Because of the widespread information about cardiac risk factors, patients often obtain information from multiple sources; a request to try additional methods of HDL elevation is common. Over-the-counter niacin preparations are a reasonable approach. Nicotinamide is a vitamin preparation that is ineffective as a lipid-altering medication. The flushing that occurs is more akin to a sunburn than to a menopausal hot flash; the skin vasodilates, but core body temperature does not increase and there is no sweating. Flushing is reduced by taking the niacin with meals (this also reduces the gastrointestinal (GI) upset) and may be decreased even further by aspirin. Patients who are averse to taking "medication" are often attracted to niacin, and this is useful for the clinician trying to convince a patient to accept pharmacologic therapy, the clinician needs to emphasize to the patient that doses of niacin that are used for lipid-lowering are well beyond the "vitamin" range. Niacin therapy has been somewhat simplified by use of the newer timed-release preparations (i.e., Niaspan), and this might be an attractive option for this patient.

Although this man took his niacin appropriately, he returned with fatigue and a marked reduction in cholesterol because of hepatitis. He recovered after stopping the niacin. This side effect is dose related, but because the benefit of therapy in this situation is unclear, the niacin was not restarted.

Case 5 is the mirror image of the first, a patient with a family history of longevity, relatively elevated LDL, but high HDL. This patient presents a somewhat unusual, but not rare, management problem. The question as to whether a markedly elevated HDL-cholesterol exerts "blanket" protection against cardiovascular disease, regardless of the LDL-cholesterol level, has long been debated. The answer is that the elevated LDL does carry independent risk, and the authors have seen a number of patients with distinctly elevated LDL-cholesterols who have developed CAD despite very high levels of HDL. Some of these patients have had HDL >100 mg/dL; the LDL was also elevated.

This patient's lipid abnormalities are almost certainly genetic, because her LDL-cholesterol remained elevated despite an excellent diet, optimal body weight, and regular exercise. Conversely, her HDL-cholesterol is almost certainly too high to be attributed simply to her exercise program. In terms of her family history, one would be tempted to assume that she has independently inherited her hyperalphalipoproteinemia from her mother and the hypercholesterolemia from her father. The elevation of her LDL is not in the range typical for heterozygous familial hypercholesterolemia, but is most likely of the "polygenic" variety.

The patient is clearly quite health-conscious, and not atypical for this type of individual, is reluctant to embark on "artificial" (i.e. pharmacologic) methods of cholesterol lowering. Because the need for medication will almost certainly be life-long, one can understand her potential doubts about the long-term safety of statin therapy, even though such drugs have now been in use for nearly 20 yr without any evidence for "silent" deleterious effects. It might, therefore, be counterproductive to "push" her too hard to accept such therapy especially at this age when the risk of disease is relatively low. Rather, this case may be a situation where the use of the "prestatin" therapies (i.e., resins or niacin) might be considered. Both of these agents are distinctly less potent than statins, but the degree of cholesterol lowering required in this patient is easily achievable with either of these agents. Given her single cardiac risk factor of a positive family history for CAD, her target LDL-cholesterol would be 160 mg/dL.

In patients who are concerned about potential toxicity (short-term or long-term) from statin therapy, resins have the attraction of their long-term safety record, as well as their lack of systemic toxicity; it can be pointed out to patients that resins are inherently safe because they are not absorbed from the intestinal tract. Resins are, of course, associated with GI side effects, but this may not be a problem at the modest doses that would likely be sufficient in this patient (10–15 g of colestid or 8–12 g of cholestyramine per day). The other options for this patient are niacin and statins *(9)*.

REFERENCES

1. Franceschini G, Sirtori CR, Capurso AD, Weisgraber KH, Mahley RW. A-IMilano apoprotein. Decreased high density lipoprotein cholesterol levels with significant lipoprotein modifications and without clinical atherosclerosis in an Italian family. J Clin Invest 1980;66:892–900.

2. Zhong S, Sharp DS, Grove JS, Bruce C, Yano K, Curb JD, Tall AR. Increased coronary heart disease in Japanese-American men with mutation in the cholesteryl ester transfer protein gene despite increased HDL levels. J Clin Invest 1996;97:2917–2923.

3. Nordestgaard BG, Abildgaard S, Wittrup HH, Steffensen R, Jensen G, Tybjaerg-Hansen A. Heterozygous lipoprotein lipase deficiency: frequency in the general population, effect on plasma lipid levels, and risk of ischemic heart disease. Circulation 1997;96:1737–1744.

4. Hobbs HH, Rader DJ. ABC1: connecting yellow tonsils, neuropathy, and very low HDL. J Clin Invest 1999;104:1015–1017.

5. Brooks-Wilson A, Marcil M, Clee SM, et al. Mutations in ABC1 in Tangier disease and familial high-density lipoprotein deficiency [see comments]. Nat Genet 1999;22:336–345.

6. Cohen JC, Wang Z, Grundy SM, Stoesz MR, Guerra R. Variation at the hepatic lipase and apolipoprotein AI/CIII/AIV loci is a major cause of genetically determined variation in plasma HDL cholesterol levels. J Clin Invest 1994;94:2377–2384.

7. O'Rourke RA, Brundage BH, Froelicher VF, Greenland P, Grundy SM, Hachamovitch R, Pohost GM, Shaw LJ, Weintraub WS, Winters WL Jr, Forrester JS, Douglas PS, Faxon DP, Fisher JD, Gregoratos G, Hochman JS, Hutter AM Jr, Kaul S, Wolk MJ. American College of Cardiology/American Heart Association Expert Consensus document on electron-beam computed tomography for the diagnosis and prognosis of coronary artery disease. Circulation 2000;102:126–140.

8. Downs JR, Clearfield M, Weis S, Whitney E, Shapiro DR, Beere PA, Langendorfer A, Stein EA, Kruyer W, Gotto AM Jr. Primary prevention of acute coronary events with lovastatin in men and women with average cholesterol levels: results of AFCAPS/TexCAPS. Air Force/Texas Coronary Atherosclerosis Prevention Study. JAMA 1998;279:1615–1622.

9. Stone NJ. Lipid management: current diet and drug treatment options. Am J Med 1996;101:40S–48S.

20

Disorders of Puberty

Dennis M. Styne, MD

CONTENTS

INTRODUCTION

A knowledge of the normal range of pubertal development and the normal physical changes of puberty is a prerequisite for the evaluation of disorders of puberty. Indeed, many children are inappropriately referred for evaluation of abnormal puberty when they are still within the normal range of pubertal development. On the other hand, among the patients detailed in this chapter is one boy in which evaluation was delayed far beyond the normal upper limit of the onset of puberty.

The very question of which age represents precocious puberty remains controversial and practice patterns have recently changed. Data on the normal variation in pubertal development in the United States were sparse and did not span the possible range of ages of normal pubertal development *(1–3)*. Thus, previous ranges of normal pubertal development were partially derived from the United States data and partially extrapolated from data from other countries, predominantly from the studies of Tanner et al. in Britain *(4,5)*. A recent longitudinal study of Caucasian boys and girls was meticulously carried out, but started at 9.5 yr of age *(6)*. While it aids the determination of the mean age of attainment of stages of puberty and the upper limits of pubertal development, it starts too late to determine the lower normal limit of pubertal development *(6)*. A large cross-sectional study of 17,070 girls visiting the office of 225 specially trained pediatricians across the United States started at 3 yr of age of the girls, but ended at 12 yr of age and so excludes a proportion of normal children who enter puberty at a later age *(7)*. The mean age of breast development of Caucasian girls in this later study was 9.96 yr with +/– 2.5 SD limited by 6.3 to 13.5 yr whereas the mean age for African-American girls was 8.9 yr with −2.5 SD at 5 yr and +2.5 SD at 12.7 yr. Remarkably, 3.0% of apparently normal

From: *Contemporary Endocrinology: Challenging Cases in Endocrinology*
Edited by: M. E. Molitch © Humana Press Inc., Totowa, NJ

Caucasian girls had stage 2 breast development by 6 yr and 5.0% by 7 yr whereas 6.4% of African-Americans had stage 2 breast development by 6 yr and 15.4% by 7 yr. It is clear that guidelines previously published of the normal age of puberty of 8–13 yr in North American girls must be modified or too many girls will undergo evaluation for normal variation and too many parents will be unnecessarily worried.

A practical compromise reached by combining the various sources of information from United States children in recent years is generally (but not universally) accepted. Thus, the range of ages of normal onset of puberty in Caucasian girls is 7–13 yr and for African-American girls is 6–13 yr. While African-American girls have an earlier onset of pubertal development of about 1 yr, their average age of menarche in the cross-sectional study was only 0.7 mo different (12.2 yr for African Americans and 12.9 yr for Caucasians). It is notable that the average age of menarche for the United States has not changed in the last 30 yr in spite of media references to the contrary (12.8 yr in 1970s vs the newer ages of 12.2–12.9 yr noted above) *(1–8)*. Thus, there are no data to prove that these earlier guidelines for pubertal development in United States girls are due to a change in the biology of puberty; the revisions of the limits of normal puberty are necessary because we have not previously had data spanning this range of ages. Further, the height of children in the United States at any given age has not changed in the last 30 yr, reflected in the virtual identity of children's heights at various ages on the United States growth charts released in 2000 (found at http://www.cdc.gov/growthcharts/) compared to charts that were presented in the 1970s.

New data for puberty in boys do not extend to such early ages as those for girls, but recent studies *(6)* agree with the ages described in the 1970s *(2)*. Thus, the mean age of onset of puberty in boys is 11 yr with the limits of 2.5 SD at 9 to 13.5 yr of age (14 yr is usually invoked as the upper limit to simplify communication). These figures are similar to those recommended over the last decades.

Care is necessary in choosing candidates for expensive diagnostic tests and long-term therapy, as many of the children that appeared to have mild sexual precocity in the past, may represent normal variation. It is generally inappropriate to extensively study apparently normal girls who enter puberty at ages above these lower limits. Of course, the pubertal ages found in family histories, the rapidity of development, and the presence or absence of symptoms of CNS or other disease must enter into the decision of whether to evaluate children due to fear of significant disease or to simply watch them over time.

Objective description of the stages of puberty improve clinical care and communication with consultants and colleagues. The stages popularized by Tanner are used internationally and are variously called Tanner Stages or Sexual Maturity Ratings (Tables 1 and 2) *(4,5)*.

REFERENCES

1. MacMahon B. Age at menarche. National Health Survey. DHEW Publication No. (HRA) 74-1615, Series 11, No. 133. Washington, DC, 1973.
2. Harlan WR, Harlan EA, Grillo GP. Secondary sex characteristics of girls 12 to 17 years of age: the U.S. Health Examination Survey. J Pediatr 1980;96:1074–1078.
3. Harlan WR, Grillo GP, Cornoni-Huntley J, Leaverton PE. Secondary sex characteristics of boys 12 to 17 years of age: the U.S. Health Examination Survey. J Pediatr 1979;95:293–297.
4. Marshall WA, Tanner JM. Variations in pattern of pubertal changes in girls. Arch Dis Child 1969;44:291–303.
5. Marshall WA, Tanner JM. Variations in the pattern of pubertal changes in boys. Arch Dis Child 1970;45:13–23.

Table 1
Normal Stages of Pubertal Development in Girls

Breast Development

B1   Prepubertal: elevation of the papilla only.
B2   Breast buds are noted or palpable with enlargement of the areola. (This stage is quite subtle and often missed on casual examination.)
B3   Further enlargement of the breast and areola with no separation of their contours.
B4   Projection of areola and papilla to form a secondary mound over the rest of the breast.
B5   Mature breast with projection of papilla only.

Female Pubic Hair Development

PH1   Prepubertal: no pubic hair.
PH2   Sparse growth of long, straight, or slightly curly minimally pigmented hair, mainly on the labia. (This stage is very subtle.)
PH3   Considerably darker and coarser hair spreading over the mons pubis.
PH4   Thick adult-type hair that does not yet spread to the medial surface of the thighs.
PH5   Hair is adult in type and is distributed in the classic inverse triangle.

Table 2
Normal Stages of Pubertal Development in Boys

Male Genital Development

G1   Preadolescent.
G2   The testes are more than 2.5 cm in the longest diameter, and the scrotum is thinning and reddening.
G3   Growth of the penis occurs in width and length and further growth of the testes is noted.
G4   Penis is further enlarged and testes are larger with a darker scrotal skin color.
G5   Genitalia are adult in size and shape.

Male Pubic Hair Development

P1   Preadolescent: no pubic hair.
P2   Sparse growth of slightly pigmented, slightly curved pubic hair mainly at the base of the penis. This stage is very subtle.
P3   Thicker, curlier hair spread laterally.
P4   Adult-type hair that does not yet spread to the medial thighs.
P5   Adult-type hair spread to the medial thighs.

6. Roche AF, Wallens R, Attia KM, Siervogel RM. The timing of sexual maturation in a group of US white youths. J Pediatr Endocrinol Metab 1995;8:11–18.
7. Herman-Giddens ME, Slora EJ, Wasserman RC, Bourdony CJ, Bhapkar MV, Koch GG, et al. Secondary sexual characteristics and menses in young girls seen in office practice: a study from the Pediatric Research in Office Settings network. Pediatrics 1997;99:505–512.
8. Zacharias L, Rand M, Wurtman R. A prospective study of sexual development in American girls: the statistics of menarche. Obstet Gynecol Surv 1976;31:325–337.

CASE #1: PREMATURE SEXUAL DEVELOPMENT IN A BOY

Case Description

A 2.1-yr-old male was brought in by his mother because of a 6 mo history of coarse pubic hair growth. There has also been scrotal thinning and enlargement and growth of

Table 3
Laboratory Test Results for Case 1

	Patient values	Normal range
Androstenedione	84 ng/dL	(5–40)
Testosterone	443 ng/dL	(2–25)
17-Hydroxyprogesterone	50 ng/dL	(20–80)
DHEA-S	9 ng/dL	(1-40)
LH	<0.1 mIU/mL	(<0.3)
FSH	<0.1 mIU/mL	(<0.3)
Cortisol	9 µg/dL at 10 am	(8–24)
Beta HCG	<2.0 IU/mL	(0–5)
CEA	<0.5	(0–2.5)
Phosphorus	5.8 mg/dL	(3.6–6.8)
Calcium	10.6 mg/dL	(8.8–10.6)

the penis. His stature increased from the 50th to 85th percentile with a corresponding increase in weight. He has not demonstrated aggressive or other abnormal behavior. Prenatal history was normal, and the child was delivered at term with a birth weight of 7 lbs 4 oz. Past medical history was normal. Development was normal, as all milestones were reached at a normal age.

His father had a history of premature pubertal development and early cessation of growth. The father was 5'5" in height. The mother was 5'2" height and had normal onset of puberty and menarche. There were no other children in this family. There were no other related medical problems in the family and no history of infertility in close relatives.

On physical examination, he was a 2.1-yr-old male who was playful, alert, and bright. He was muscular appearing, but his voice was of normal pitch. His vital signs were normal with a height of 37 in (94 cm) (85th%) and a weight of 32 lbs (14.6 kg) (85th%). Head, eyes, ears, nose, and throat examinations were normal, except for mild acne and comedones on his face. There was no moustache, but the facial velus hair appeared increased. The thyroid was not enlarged. Axillae demonstrated no glandular development or hair. His abdomen was soft without masses. He had no café-au-lait spots on his skin. His penis measured 2 × 8 cm. The right testis was 1.5 × 2.5 cm (4 mL), and the left was 1.75 × 3 cm (6 mL), so he was in stage III of genital development. He also had a tuft of coarse pubic hair which extended below the base of the penis and laterally and described the beginning of stage III of pubic hair development by its distribution. The scrotum was thin and tended to be a reddish color. The neurological examination was normal, including optic discs. An ultrasound showed both testes to be homogeneous with the right bigger than the left, but no evidence of tumor. A magnetic resonance imaging (MRI) of the testes demonstrated the same. X-rays of the hand and wrist showed a bone age of 4.6 yr, which was >7 standard deviations above normal. A routine chemistry panel, including liver function tests and a sedimentation rate were normal. Endocrine laboratory test results are shown in Table 3.

Discussion

This boy has the very early appearance of pubic hair, penile enlargement, and other virilizing features. There is small, but definite testicular enlargement, although less than expected, compared to the testosterone level. Furthermore, the testes are not as large as expected for the amount of virilization noted. The fact that the testes are enlarging makes it likely that the testes are the source of the testosterone rather than other sites, such as the adrenal glands. There is no irregularity of the testes suggesting an adenoma or carcinoma as the etiology; this also limits the likelihood of hyperplastic adrenal rests resulting from the increased adrenocorticotropic hormone (ACTH) secretion of congenital adrenal hyperplasia.

The scrum testosterone level is quite high, with no notable elevation of testosterone precursors (androstenedione is only slightly elevated), indicating that direct secretion of testosterone, rather than conversion from a circulating precursor, is the cause of the virilization. The gonadotropins are suppressed, eliminating true central precocious puberty or any central nervous system (CNS) process as the etiology of the testosterone secretion. Serum βhCG is not detectable, eliminating a human chorionic gonadotropin (hCG) producing tumor of the liver, CNS or other area as the source of testicular stimulation. The rather low serum concentrations of adrenal androgens limit the possibilities of congenital adrenal hyperplasia (CAH) or adrenal adenoma as the etiology of the androgens. An ACTH stimulation test was performed; the rise in serum 17-OH Progesterone and DHEA were normal, eliminating the possibility of CAH.

There appears to be a family history of male ancestors manifesting the same condition, indicating an X-linked or sex-limited dominant trait. This boy has *familial male-limited gonadotropin-independent sexual precocity with premature leydig cell and germ cell maturation* (often called *testotoxicosis*), which is a gonadotropin releasing hormone (GnRH) independent form of male isosexual precocity *(1–7)*. Affected boys have secondary sexual development with penile enlargement, which may be present at birth *(3)*, and bilateral enlargement of testes to the early or midpubertal range, but they remain smaller than expected in relation to penile growth. The testes show premature Leydig and Sertoli cell maturation and spermatogenesis and possibly Leydig cell hyperplasia *(2,3,5)*. The normal pubertal enlargement of the testes is mostly caused by seminiferous tubular maturation rather than the enlargement of Leydig cell mass. Thus, in this syndrome, mainly due to luteinizing hormone (LH) receptor effcct, the seminiferous tubules are less affected than the Leydig cells and the testes remain rather small.

Growth rate is rapid and skeletal maturation is advanced, as in all forms of precocious puberty. The level of serum dchydroepiandrosterone-sulfate (DHEA-S), correlates with his chronologic age and adrenarche appears to be years away.

The disorder is because of heterozygous activating mutations of the heterotrimeric Gs protein-coupled LH/CG receptor which transduces the LH/CG signal to the main effector, adenyl cyclase *(8,9)*. The LH receptor in the human is being encoded by a gene localized to chromosome *2p21* (the same as the follicle-stimulating hormone [FSH] receptor) *(10–14)*. More than 11 constitutively activating heterozygous missense mutations, all residing within exon 11, have been reported, mostly between amino acid residues 542 and 581 *(8,9,15–21)*.

In patients with this disorder, there are prepubertal or suppressed basal and GnRH-stimulated gonadotropin concentrations *(3)* whereas plasma testosterone values are in the normal pubertal or adult range *(3)*. Boys with GnRH-independent, pituitary gonadotropin-independent maturation of the testes do not respond to chronic administration of a GnRH agonist with suppression of testosterone secretion because the condition is not gonadotropin dependent *(3,7),* in contrast to the characteristic response in patients with true precocious puberty *(3)*. However, in late childhood or early adolescence, a pattern of pubertal LH secretion in the basal state and in response to GnRH is demonstrable due to the development of secondary GnRH-dependent true precocious puberty *(4)* and the condition then becomes controllable with a GnRH agonist. Fertility may ultimately be achieved, accounting for the multigenerational presentations; this disorder is inherited as a sex-limited autosomal dominant trait *(3–7)*. A kindred with nine generations of affected males has been reported *(4)*; obligatory female carriers of the trait are unaffected *(4,22)*.

Previously, testosterone secretion, height velocity and rate of bone maturation, and aggressive and hyperactive behavior were decreased by treatment with oral or intramuscular medroxyprogesterone acetate *(3,23)*. Newer therapies have come to the fore. Ketoconazole suppresses gonadal and adrenal biosynthesis at several steps *(24)*. In the dosage used in testotoxicosis (200 mg every 8–12 h orally) *(6,25)* ketoconazole mainly inhibits the enzyme cytochrome P-450c17, which regulates both 17-hydroxylation and the scission (17,20 lyase) of 17α-hydroxypregnenolone to dehydroepiandrosterone.

Ketoconazole causes a mild transient decrease in cortisol secretion and interferes with binding of testosterone to TeBG. Ketoconazole can cause hepatic injury, which is usually mild and reversible, but hepatotoxicity may rarely be severe *(24)*. Further, reversible renal injury, rash, and interstitial pneumonia have been reported in a patient who tolerated lower doses, suggesting a dose response effect *(26)*.

A more recent therapeutic approach is use of the antiandrogen (and antimineralocorticoid) spironolactone combined with testolactone, an inhibitor of cytochrome P-450 aromatase (CYP19), the key enzyme in the conversion of androgens to estrogens *(27)*. Thus, the androgen effects are blocked and the bone maturing effects of estrogen are reduced or eliminated. The addition of a GnRH agonist after the development of secondary central precocious puberty is a useful step to suppress pituitary gonadotropin secretion *(19)* later in the course of the condition.

REFERENCES

1. Faggiano M, Criscuolo T, Perrone L, Quarto C, Sinisi AA. Sexual precocity in a boy due to hypersecretion of LH and prolactin by a pituitary adenoma. Acta Endocrinol (Copenhagen) 1983;102:167–172.
2. Schedewie HK, Reiter EO, Beitins IZ. Testicular Leydig cell hyperplasia as a cause of familial sexual precocity. J Clin Endocrinol Metab 1981;52:271–278.
3. Rosenthal SM, Grumbach MM, Kaplan SL. Gonadotropin-independent familial sexual precocity with premature Leydig and germinal cell maturation (familial testotoxicosis): effects of a potent luteinizing hormone-releasing factor agonist and medroxyprogesterone acetate therapy in four cases. J Clin Endocrinol Metab 1983;57:571–579.
4. Egli CA, Rosenthal SM, Grumbach MM, Montalvo JM, Gondos B. Pituitary gonadotropin-independent male-limited autosomal dominant sexual precocity in nine generations: familial testotoxicosis. J Pediatr 1985;106:33–40.
5. Gondos B, Egli CA, Rosenthal SM, Grumbach MM. Testicular changes in gonadotropin-independent familial male sexual precocity. Familial testotoxicosis. Arch Pathol Lab Med 1985;109:990–995.
6. Holland FJ. Gonadotropin-independent precocious puberty. Endocrinol Metab Clin North Am 1991;20: 191–210.
7. Wierman ME, Beardsworth DE, Mansfield MJ, et al. Puberty without gonadotropins. A unique mechanism of sexual development. N Engl J Med 1985;312:65–72.
8. Shenker A, Laue L, Kosugi S, Merendino JJJ, Minegishi T, Cutler GBJ. A constitutively activating mutation of the luteinizing hormone receptor in familial male precocious puberty. Nature 1993;365:652–654.
9. Kremer H, Mariman E, Otten BJ, et al. Cosegregation of missense mutations of the luteinizing hormone receptor gene with familial male-limited precocious puberty. Hum Mol Genet 1993;2:1779–1783.

10. Minegishi T, Nakamura K, Takakura Y, et al. Cloning and sequencing of porcine LH-hCG receptor cDNA. Biochem Biophys Res Comm 1990;172:1049–1054.

11. Dufau ML. The leutinizing hormone receptor. The Leydig Cell. In: Payne AH, Hardy MP, Russell LD, eds. Cache River Press, Vienna, IL, 1994, pp. 334–350.

12. Baldwin JM. Stucture and function of receptors coupled to G protein. Curr Opinion Cell Biol 1994;6: 180–190.

13. Dufau ML. The luteinizing hormone receptor. Curr Op Endo Diabetes 1995;2:365–374.

14. Segaloff DL, Ascoli M. The lutotropin/choriogonadotropin (LH/CG) receptor—4 years later. Endocr Rev 1997;14:324–347.

15. Kawate N, Kletter GB, Wilson BE, Netzloff ML, Menon KM. Identification of constitutively activating mutation of the luteinising hormone receptor in a family with male limited gonadotrophin independent precocious puberty (testotoxicosis). J Med Genet 1995;32:553–554.

16. Kraaij R, Post M, Kremer H, Milgrom E, Epping W, Brunner HG, et al. A missense mutation in the second transmembrane segment of the luteinizing hormone receptor causes familial male-limited precocious puberty. J Clin Endocrinol Metab 1995;80:3168–3172.

17. Latronico AC, Anasti J, Arnhold IJ, et al. A novel mutation of the luteinizing hormone receptor gene causing male gonadotropin-independent precocious puberty. J Clin Endocrinol Metab 1995;80:2490–2494.

18. Yano K, Saji M, Hidaka A, et al. A new constitutively activating point mutation in the luteinizing hormone/choriogonadotropin receptor gene in cases of male-limited precocious puberty. J Clin Endocrinol Metab 1995;80:1162–1168.

19. Laue L, Chan WY, Hsueh AJ, et al. Genetic heterogeneity of constitutively activating mutations of the human luteinizing hormone receptor in familial male-limited precocious puberty. Proc Natl Acad Sci USA 1995;92:1906–1910.

20. Evans BA, Bowen DJ, Smith PJ, Clayton PE, Gregory JW. A new point mutation in the luteinising hormone receptor gene in familial and sporadic male limited precocious puberty: genotype does not always correlate with phenotype. J Med Genet 1996;33:143–147.

21. Yano K, Kohn LD, Saji M, et al. A case of male-limited precocious puberty caused by a point mutation in the second transmembrane domain of the luteinizing hormone choriogonadotropin receptor gene. Biochem Biophys Res Commun 1996;220:1036–1042.

22. Rosenthal IM, Refetoff S, Rich B, et al. Response to challenge with gonadotropin-releasing hormone agonist in a mother and her two sons with a constitutively activating mutation of the luteinizing hormone receptor—a clinical research center study. J Clin Endocrinol Metab 1996;81:3802–3806.

23. Grumbach MM, Kaplan SL. Recent advances in the diagnosis and management of sexual precocity. Acta Paediatr Jpn (Overseas Ed) 1988;30:155–175.

24. Feldman D. Ketoconazole and other imidazole derivatives as inhibitors of steroidogenesis. Endocr Rev 1986;7:409–420.

25. Holland FJ, Fishman L, Bailey JD, et al. Ketoconazole in the management of precocious puberty not responsive to LHRH-analogue therapy. N Engl J Med 1985;312:1023–1028.

26. Babovic-Vuksanovic D, Donaldson MD, Gibson NA, Wallace AM. Hazards of ketoconazole therapy in testotoxicosis. Acta Paediatr 1994;83:994–997.

27. Laue L, Kenigsberg D, Pescovitz OH, et al. The treatment of familial male precocious puberty with spironolactone and testolactone. N Engl J Med 1989;320:496–502.

CASE #2: SMALL TESTES
AND GYNECOMASTIA IN AN ADOLESCENT

Case Description

A 17-yr-old boy presented because of concern about bilateral gynecomastia and small testes, the latter noted on routine physical examination by his local physician. He first noticed pubertal development at about 12 yr of age. He had no complaints about the development or size of his penis or pubic hair.

Past history revealed that his birth weight was 3 kg after a normal pregnancy and delivery. His development was normal, as he started to walk and talk at an average age. His school performance has been problematic, as he was in his sophomore year of high school with average to poor grades. He stated that he reads well and has no speech impediments. He has had no serious accidents or CNS injuries. Surgical history included an orchiopexy for an undescended testis at 2 yr of age. Family history showed his mother to be 167 cm in height and his father to be 180 cm. The mother had her first menstrual period at 14 yr of age. There was no available pubertal history for the father. The patient has a 14-yr-old brother who is healthy and had reportedly normal pubertal development.

Upon physical examination, the patient was generally cooperative. His pulse was 66, blood pressure was 118/60 mmHg, and respiratory rate was 18. His height was 71 in, (180 cm—75th percentile), and his weight was 150 lbs (68.2 kg—50th percentile).

His upper to lower segment ratio was 0.87 (below the mean for a Caucasian male). His arm span was 180 cm (acceptable value for height). HEENT revealed some comedones and some acne. He also had some facial hair. The thyroid gland was not enlarged. His abdomen was soft without masses and his extremities were normal. He had gynecomastia with 4 cm of palpable tissue on the left and 3 cm on the right. He had moderate axillary hair and a history of axillary odor. His phallus measured 2 × 10 cm. His testes measured 1.5 × 2.5 cm (4–6 mL) bilaterally. He had pubic hair stage 4. His neurological exam was normal. Laboratory testing showed elevated levels of LH and FSH at 25 mIU/mL (normal 1.3–13) and 60 mIU/mL (normal 0.9–15 mIU/mL), respectively, a very low testosterone of 10.6 ng/dL (300–1000) and a normal prolactin of 8 ng/mL (2–25).

Discussion

This boy has a history of normal onset of pubertal development, but small testes in midpuberty associated with gynecomastia. This suggests Klinefelter syndrome by physical examination, which is supported by the elevated levels of serum LH and FSH. Serum testosterone is in an acceptable pubertal range, which is found in Klinefelter syndrome, but values may not rise by the end of puberty. Usually, there is a low upper to lower segment ratio, but only a modest or no increase in arm span compared to height, and he fits these characteristics as well. The appropriate next step is a karyotype determination, with the expectation of a 47 XXY or a variant in Klinefelter syndrome. However, the karyotype in this patient returned as 46 XX. This suggests an XX male is the diagnosis. An *Sry* probe revealed the *Sry* gene to be located on the X chromosome indicating that he is an XX male. This manifests in a similar manner to Klinefelter syndrome.

Klinefelter syndrome, or seminiferous tubular dysgenesis, and its variants occur in approximately 1 in 1000 males and are the most common forms of male hypogonadism (1,2). The testes are small and firm (less than 3.5 cm in length), spermatogenesis is impaired, and a male phenotype, usually with gynecomastia and eunuchoid proportions of the legs is characteristic (1). After the onset of puberty, patients have a decreased upper/lower body ratio without an increase in arm span (3). The onset of puberty usually is not delayed, but slow progression or arrest of pubertal changes is due to impaired Leydig cell reserve and low testosterone levels are characteristic. Tall stature for family size is common in this disorder due to the disproportionate growth of the legs.

Prepubertal testes show only subtle histological changes, although the testes are small and the germ cell content is reduced. Hyalinization and fibrosis of the seminiferous tubules and pseudoadenomatous changes of the Leydig cells develop after puberty.

Before the age of 12, gonadotropin concentrations are in the prepubertal range, whereas the characteristic elevated gonadotropin levels are found after the onset of puberty. The plasma concentration of testosterone tends to be in the normal range until about age 14, after which it may fail to rise to normal adult levels because of decreased Leydig cell function *(4,5)*.

Testosterone replacement should be considered when the LH level rises above the normal range of values. New studies have been designed to determine whether there is benefit to early onset of testosterone administration on behavior or mood, but no conclusions are available. Serum estradiol/testosterone ratios and TeBG levels are higher than those in normal males, which indicates an increased estrogen effect and decreased testosterone effect. These factors probably account, at least in part, for the gynecomastia characteristic of Klinefelter syndrome during adolescence *(5–7)*. Testosterone administration does not appear to reduce the gynecomastia, but dihydrotestosterone *(8)* may be effective. If the gynecomastia does not regress, a reduction mammoplasty may be required. Aromatase inhibitors to reduce estrogen production and thus gynecomastia may be useful, but the results of ongoing clinical trials of this approach are not yet available.

Severe mental retardation is uncommon in Klinefelter syndrome, although there is an increased prevalence of speech and learning disorders and adjustment problems in adolescence. Psychopathology is rare in most studies, and a 20 yr follow-up of 47 XXY individuals shows little or no variation from nonaffected controls in employment, social status, mental or physical health, or criminality *(9–11)*.

Klinefelter syndrome is associated with aortic valvular disease and ruptured berry aneurysms (six times the normal rate) *(12)*; breast carcinoma (20 times the rate in normal men and one fifth that of women) *(13)*; other malignancies such as acute leukemia, lymphoma, and germ cell tumors at any midline site *(9)*; systemic lupus erythematosus *(14, 15)*; and osteoporosis (25% are affected) *(16,17)*. There is an increased risk of diabetes mellitus and thyroid disease.

About 20% of mediastinal germ cell tumors are associated with Klinefelter syndrome. These germ cell tumors secrete hCG and can induce sexual precocity. Klinefelter syndrome needs to be considered in boys with hCG-secreting germ cell tumors with or without GnRH-independent sexual precocity, especially if the tumor is located in the mediastinum *(18–20)*. There are also increased incidences of fatigue, varicose veins, and essential tremor.

Most patients have a 47 XXY chromosomal karyotype. The rare 46 XX male has some features of Klinefelter syndrome *(1)*. The *SRY* gene, located at the pseudoautosomal boundary of the Y chromosome, is the testes determining gene in human beings. The bipotential gonad will differentiate into an ovary in most 46 XX individuals without the *SRY* while 46 XY individuals with the *SRY* will develop a testis. If the *SRY* is found on an X chromosome a 46 XX male can result. The prevalence of 46 XX males is 1 in 20,000 phenotypic males. The physical findings are similar to those of Klinefelter syndrome except for a lesser degree of skeletal proportion abnormalities. The etiology of 46 XX males is a balanced translocation of the pseudoautosomal regions of the *p* segments of the X and Y chromosomes that include *SRY*. About 20% of XX males lack the *SRY* gene; these situa-tions presumably arise from mutations of downstream autosomal or X linked genes involved in testes determination.

REFERENCES

1. Grumbach MM, Conte FA. Disorders of sex differentiation. In: Wilson JD, Foster DW, eds. Williams Textbook of Endocrinology. WB Saunders, Philadelphia, PA, 1998, pp. 1303–1425.

2. Klinefelter HF Jr, Reifenstein EC Jr, Albright F. Syndrome characterized by gynecomastia, aspermato-genesis without A-leydigism, and increased excretion of follicle-stimulating hormone. J Clin Endocrinol 1942;2:615–627.

3. Caldwell PD, Smith DW. The XXY (Klinefelter's) syndrome in childhood: detection and treatment. J Pediatr 1972;80:250–258.

4. Sagawa I, Kazama T, Terada T, et al. Hormonal profiles in Klinefelter's syndrome with and without testicular epidermoid cyst. Arch Androl 1988;21:205–209.

5. Salbenblatt JA, Bender BG, Puck MH, et al. Pituitary-gonadal function in Klinefelter syndrome before and during puberty. Pediatr Res 1985;19:82–86.

6. Plymate SR, Leonard JM, Paulsen CA. Sex hormone-binding globulin changes with androgen replace-ment. J Clin Endocrinol Metab 1983;57:645–648.

7. Wieland RG, Zorn EM, Johnson MW. Elevated testosterone-binding globulin in Klinefelter's syn-drome. J Clin Endocrinol Metab 1980;51:1199–1200.

8. Eberle AJ, Sparrow JT, Keenan BS. Treatment of persistent pubertal gynecomastia with dihydrotestos-terone heptanoate. J Pediatr 1986;109:144–149.

9. Kleczkowska A, Fryns JP, Van den Berghe H. X-chromosome polysomy in the male: the Leuven expe-rience 1966-1987. Hum Genet 1988;80:16–22.

10. Nielsen J, Pelsen B. Follow-up 20 years later of 34 Klinefelter males with karyotype 47,XXY and 16 hypogonadal males with karyotype 46,XY. Hum Genet 1987;77:188–192.

11. Sorenson K, Porter ME, Gardner HA, DeFeudis P. Verbal deficits in Klinefelter (XXY) adults living in the community. Clin Genet 1988;33:246–253.

12. Price WH, Clayton JF, Wilson J. Causes of death in X chromatin positive males (Klinefelter's syn-drome). J Epidemiol Community Health 1985;39:330–336.

13. Scheike O, Visfeldt J, Peterson B. Male breast cancer: III Breast carcinoma in association with the Klinefelter sydrome. Acta Pathol Microbiol Scand Suppl 1973;81:352–358.

14. Bizzarro A, Valentini G, DiMartino G. Influence of testosterone therapy on clinical and immunological features of autoimmune diseases associated with Klinefelter's syndrome. J Clin Endocrinol Metab 1987; 64:32–36.

15. Fialkow PJ. Genetic aspects of autoimmunity. Prog Med Genet 1969;6:117–167.

16. Foresta C, Busnardo B, Zanatta G. Lower calcitonin levels in young hypogonadic men with osteoporo-sis. Horm Metab Res 1983;15:206,207.

17. Foresta C, Zanatta GP, Busnardo B. Testosterone and calcitonin plasma levels in hypogonadal osteo-porotic young men. J Endocrinol Invest 1985;8:377–379.

18. Derenoncourt AN, Castro-Magana M, Jones KL. Mediastinal teratoma and precocious puberty in a boy with mosaic Klinefelter syndrome. Am J Med Genet 1995;55:38–42.

19. Von Muhlendahl KE, Heinrich U. Sexual precocity in Klinefelter syndrome: report on two new cases with idiopathic central precocious puberty. Eur J Pediatr 1994;153:322–324.

20. Hasle H, Jacobsen BB, Asschenfeldt P, Andersen K. Mediastinal germ cell tumour associated with Klinefelter syndrome. A report of case and review of the literature. Eur J Pediatr 1992;151:735–739.

CASE #3: PREMATURE APPEARANCE OF PUBIC HAIR IN A GIRL

Case Description

A 16-mo-old girl presented with an enlarged clitoris. Her parents thought she was born with a large clitoris, but this was not reflected in physician records. Birth history revealed a normal vaginal delivery induced at 38 wk. Birth weight was 8 lbs and 14.5 oz. Apgar scores were 10/10 at 1 and 5 min. She had a five- and a-half-year-old brother who was healthy, but slightly short for his age. No medications or substances were used during pregnancy and there were no toxic exposures or other illnesses noted. The mother had no evidence of a virilizing tumor. The girl's development had been normal, sitting up at 5 mo, walking at 13 mo, and speaking 3–4 words at present. She was breast-fed until 14 mo, and at the time, was eating table food bought at an ordinary food store. The family did not engage in food faddism. She took no medications, had no surgery, and had no serious ill-nesses. There were no androgens in the house that the child might have accessed. Family

Table 4
Laboratory Testing in Case 3

	Patient values	Normal range
Sodium	135 mEq/L	(136–145)
Potassium	4.7 mEq/L	(3.3–5.0)
Chloride	104 mEq/L	(95–110)
Bicarbonate	19 mEq/L	(22–32)
BUN	6 mg/dL	(3–7)
Creatinine	0.3 mg/dL	(0.1–0.5)
Glucose	80 mg/dL	(60–105)
LH	<0.02 IU/mL	0.02–1.77
FSH	2.2 mIU/mL	0.68–6.7
DHEA-S	3 ng/dL	(3–24)
17OH-Progesterone	3839ng/dL	(4–115)
Androstenedione	<0.1ng/dL	(5–40)
Cortisol (am)	15 µg/dL	(6–25)
11 Deoxycortisol	159 ng/dL	7–210
Testosterone	12 ng/dL	<12
Free Testosterone	1.3 pg/mL	<0.6

history revealed the mother to be 5 ft 3 in in height. She was of mixed Northern European ancestry. Her menarche occurred at 12.5 yr. The father's height was 6 ft 2 in. He was of Ashkenazi Jewish background. There was no family history of infertility, hirsutism, acne, or other related conditions. There was no history of infertility in the family.

Physical examination revealed this 1 yr 4 mo old to be quite active. Her length measured 74.9 cm (10th percentile), and her weight was recorded at 9.59 kg (25th percentile). Her weight for height ratio was at the mean. She had no increase in muscularity. Her head circumference was 46.5 cm. HEENT examination revealed no comedones, acne, or facial hair. Her voice was of normal pitch. The thyroid was not enlarged. Her abdomen was soft without masses. There was no pubic hair, axillary hair, or axillary odor. Her clitoris was 1.5 cm in length and 0.5 cm in width. There was no labial fusion. Her labia were normal and without rugation or pigmentation. There was no estrogen effect on the vaginal mucosa. Her neurological exam was normal. Her skin was normal. X-rays of her hand and wrist showed a bone age of 2 yr. Laboratory testing is shown in Table 4.

Discussion

This young girl has a large clitoris, but no sign of prenatal virilization, as the vaginal opening was quite normal without posterior fusion. There was no classic ambiguity of the genitalia at birth, although the clitoral size was increased at presentation. She was not growing rapidly by history nor was she tall for the family, so the virilization must have been a new feature. Surprisingly, there were no other signs of virilization, such as pubic or axillary hair, acne, comedones, muscular development, or lowering of the voice, although other changes might follow in the untreated state. The elevated serum 17OH-progesterone suggests the 21 hydroxylase deficient form of congenital adrenal hyperplasia (CAH-p450$_{c21}$) and the age of appearance suggests nonclassical or late onset CAH. Because the basal values already point to this diagnosis, an ACTH stimulation test may

Table 5
ACTH Stimulation Test in Case 3

	Case 3 basal	Normal basal	Case 3 ACTH stimulated	Normal ACTH stimulated
17OHP	3839 ng/dL	4–115	30388	50–350
Androstenedione	65 ng/dL	5–51		
DHEA	30 ng/dL	9–42	65	21–98
Compound S	159 ng/dL	7–210	291	98–360
Cortisol	9 µg/dL	6–25	15	22–40
Testosterone	12 ng/dL	<12		

not be necessary, but is usually performed, and was in this case (Table 5). With hydrocortisone administration, androgen secretion decreased and there were no further signs of virilization.

Classic CAH presents in the newborn period with ambiguous genetalia in girls but no change in appearance in boys *(1)*. In the presence of the *SRY*, a bipotential gonad turns into a testes, which in turn, produces testosterone to bring about virilization of the primitive genital anlage *(2)*. This girl would not have SRY and should have a normal ovary and normal Mullerian derivatives (uterus and vagina). Androgens exert effects of fetal sexual development between 9–13 wk of gestation to determine whether a clitoris versus a penis forms or whether a scrotum versus the labia majora forms. If androgens arise after the 13th wk or in the postnatal period, there is no posterior vaginal fusion of the labia majora or the development of a penile urethra, and this patient did not have such fusion. This patient has only clitoromegaly rather than ambiguous genitalia and so cannot have congenital virilizing adrenal hyperplasia of the classic type. Late onset or nonclassical CAH may present at any time after birth and does not include vaginal fusion or the development of a penile urethra as features *(3,4)*.

The most common type of CAH is 21-hydroxylase deficiency, leading to elevation of 17OH-progesterone as the precursor compound to the 21 hydroxylase enzyme. In late onset cases, the basal value may be high enough to make the diagnosis, as here, but more commonly, an ACTH stimulation test must be invoked to make a firm diagnosis *(5,6)*.

Mutations of the CPY21 gene for 21 hydroxylase are transmitted in an autosomal recessive manner *(7)*. The enzyme is a member of the P450 superfamily of monooxygenases bound to the endoplasmic reticulum. The gene is located on the short arm of chromosome 6 *(6p21.3)* within the human lymphocyte antigen (HLA) locus region. HLA-DR1, B14 occurs more frequently in the nonclassical form. There are two *CPY21* genes, a functional CPY21B gene and a pseudogene CPY21A. The genotype does not always determine the severety of the phenotype *(8)*. Nonclassic CAH results from allelic variations in the same gene causing classic CAH. Nonclassic CAH is found more frequently in the Ashkenazi Jewish population, Hispanics and Yugoslavian individuals *(9–11)*. The disease is the most common disorder in human beings with an overall frequency of 0.01.

Nonclassical CAH presents in girls who had normal female phenotypes at birth. They may develop signs of elevated androgen secretion that present similar to premature adrenarche at first *(2,12–14)* More significant androgen effects include advancement of the bone age with rapid early growth leading to early fusion of the epiphyses of the bones and cessation of growth resulting in short stature if the clinical appearance is well before epiphyseal fusion. In addition, cystic acne and, later in life, male pattern baldness and menstrual irregularity may ultimately occur. Those females with late pubertal or early adulthood onset of symptoms may manifest facial hair, severe acne, amenorrhea, and other findings similar to those found in ovarian hyperandrogenism (polycystic ovarian disease) *(15–17)*.

Remarkably, within the same family manifesting classic 21 OH deficiency are some members with serum androgen and precursor values similar to those of nonclassical CAH patients, but who demonstrate no signs of virilization *(18,19)*. This is cryptic CAH, which may later manifest virilizing symptoms that wax and wane over years.

Treatment of nonclassical CAH presents problems. Patients may have adequate cortisol secretion for daily life and may even mount normal stress responses of cortisol (this patient did not mount an adequate response to ACTH stimulation). The administration of glucocorticoid will suppress the androgen secretion to halt the progression of virilization but will suppress ACTH and cortisol secretion. The patient may be rendered glucocorticoid deficient if glucocorticoid therapy is interrupted or if stress is encountered and the patient does not take a double or triple dose of glucocorticoids at that time. Thus, patients and families must be carefully educated about glucocorticoid management in times of stress. Patients should wear an alert bracelet, or other warning, to inform others about glucocorticoid deficiency in emergencies. In mild cases where one dose per day of glucocorticoids may suppress manifestations, iatrogenic adrenal gland suppression may be avoided *(20)*.

REFERENCES

1. New MI. Diagnosis and management of congenital adrenal hyperplasia. Annu Rev Med 1998;49:311–328.
2. Grumbach MM, Conte FA. Disorders of sexual differentiation. In: Wilson JD, Foster DW, Kroneberg HM, Larsen PR, eds. Willliams Textbook of Endocrinology. WB Saunders, Philadelphia, PA, 1999, pp. 1509–1626.
3. Kohn B, Levine LS, Pollack MS, et al. Late-onset steroid 21-hydroxylase deficiency: a variant of classical congenital adrenal hyperplasia. J Clin Endocrinol Metab 1982;55:817–827.
4. Drucker S, New MI. Nonclassic adrenal hyperplasia due to 21-hydroxylase deficiency. Pediatric Clin N Am 1987;34:1067–1081.
5. New MI, Lorenzen F, Lerner AJ, et al. Genotyping steroid 21-hydroxylase deficiency: hormonal reference data. J Clin Endocrinol Metab 1983;57:320–326.
6. Ibaaanez L, Bonnin MR, Zampolli M, et al. Usefulness of an ACTH test in the diagnosis of nonclassical 21-hydroxylase deficiency among children presenting with premature pubarche. Hormone Res 1995;44: 51–56.
7. New MI, Speiser PW. Genetics of adrenal steroid 21-hydroxylase deficiency. Endocr Rev 1986;7:331–349.
8. Wilson R, Mercado A, Cheng K, et al. Steroid 21-hydroxylase deficiency: genotype may not predict phenotype. J Clin Endocrinol Metab 1995;80:2322–2329.
9. Speiser PW, Dupont B, Rubenstein P, et al. High frequency of nonclassical steroid 21-hydroxylase deficiency. Am J Hum Genet 1985;35:650–667.
10. Temeck JW, Pang S, Nelson C, et al. Genetic defects of steroidogenesis in premature pubarche. J Clin Endocrinol Metab 1987;64:609–617.
11. Balducci R, Boscherini B, Mangiantini A, Morellini M, Toscano V. Isolated precocious pubarche: an approach. J Clin Endocrinol Metab 1994;79:582–589.
12. Silverman SH, Migeon CJ, Rosenberg E, et al. Precocious growth of sexual hair without other secondary sexual development; "premature pubarche," a constitutional variation of adolescence. Pediatrics 1952; 10:426–31.

13. Thamdrup E. Premature pubarche, a hypothalamic disorder? Acta Endocrinol 1955;18:564–567.

14. Grumbach MM, Styne DM. Puberty, Ontogeny, Neuroendocrinology, Physiology, and Disorders. In: Wilson JD, Foster DW, Kronenberg MD, Larsen PR, eds. Williams Textbook of Endocrinology. WB Saunders Company, Philadelphia, PA, 1998, pp. 1509–1625.

15. Miller WL, Auchus RJ, Geller DH. The regulation of 17,20 lyase activity. Steroids 1997;62:133–142.

16. Apter D, Bhtzow T, Laughlin GA, Yen SSC. Metabolic features of polycystic ovary syndrome are found in adolescent girls with hyperandrogenism. J Clin Endocrinol Metab 1995;80:2966–2973.

17. New MI. Nonclassical congenital adrenal hyperplasia and the polycystic ovarian syndrome. Ann NY Acad Sci 1993;687:193–205.

18. Levine LS, Dupont B, Lorenzen F, et al. Cryptic 21-hydroxylase deficiency in families of patients with classical congenital adrenal hyperplasia. J Clin Endocrinol Metab 1980;51:1316–1324.

19. Carrera P, Bordone L, Azzani T, et al. Point mutations in Italian patients with classic, non-classic, and cryptic forms of steroid 21-hydroxylase deficiency. Hum Gen 1996;98:662–665.

20. Rosenfield RL, Ghai K, Ehrmann DA, Barnes RB. Diagnosis of the polycystic ovary syndrome in adolescence: comparison of adolescent and adult hyperandrogenism. J Pediatr Endocrinol Metab 2000; 13(Suppl 5):1285–1289.

CASE #4: DELAYED PUBERTY IN AN 18-YR-OLD BOY

Case Description

An 18-yr-old boy presented because of lack of pubertal development. His mother noted that for much of the last 10 yr, he looked many years younger than his chronological age. He had no pubic hair development, growth of genitalia, or other findings of maturity, according to mother. In addition, he had been moody and had labile emotions. He was doing very well in school, but he had only a few friends. He had no plans for college, in spite of his good grades. He was teased quite a bit because of his youthful appearance. His appetite was good, and he was sleeping about 10 h/d. He had a very poor sense of smell. He was born with undescended testes, which were treated by orchiopexy at 1 yr of age. The mother denied any prenatal substance abuse. There were no prenatal complications. Birth weight was 6 lbs 10 oz.

Family History revealed that his mother's menarche occurred at 14 yr of age. Her height was 5 ft 4 in. His father had puberty at about 13 yr of age. His height was 5 ft 5 in. The rest of the family was of variable height. He had a 12-yr-old brother and a 10-yr-old brother who were apparently doing well. Neither were said to have entered puberty as yet.

On physical examination, this young Caucasian man appeared many years younger than his stated age; he could have easily been considered to be a 12-yr-old. His vital signs were normal. His height was 62 inches (158 cm) (<5th percentile), and weight was 100 lbs (45 kg) (<5th percentile). He was thin and his skin revealed minimal acne and comedones on the face. The thyroid was not enlarged. His abdomen was soft and without masses. He had scoliosis of 5–10°. His penis was 1.5×5.5 cm in length; volume of each testes was 3 mL at most. He had pubic hair present, but it barely qualified as stage II. He had no axillary hair. His neurological exam was normal, with the sole exception that he could not recognize common smells offered to him. Laboratory test results are listed in Table 6. GnRH stimulation produced no significant changes in LH or Testosterone levels. X-rays of the hand and wrist showed a bone age of 15 yr. An MRI of the brain revealed no abnormalities and there were normal olfactory sulci and olfactory bulbs.

Discussion

This boy has characteristics of both constitutional delay in puberty and of hypogonadotropic hypogonadism with hyposmia, which makes Kallmann's syndrome likely. The

Table 6
Laboratory Testing in Case 4

	Patient values	Normal values
Free T4	0.9 ng/mL	0.9–2
TSH	1.77 mIU/L	0.5–5
LH	<0.03 mIU/mL	1.3–13 mIU/mL
FSH	0.5mIU/mL	0.9–15
Testosterone	20 ng/dL	300–1000 ng/dL
DHEAS	120 ng/dL	100–555
IGF 1	450 ng/mL	202–957
IGFBP 3	3.5 mg/L	2.2–4.2

normal CNS MRI directs the diagnosis away from Kallmann's syndrome, but the MRI of the CNS is not always abnormal in Kallmann's syndrome. The short stature could be familial or could be because of constitutional delay in puberty. Thus, both diagnoses should be considered.

Healthy individuals with no complicating conditions who spontaneously enter puberty after the age of 13 for girls and 13.5–14 yr for boys have constitutional delay in growth and adolescence (1,2). They usually are short compared to peers throughout their childhood, although growth velocity and height are usually appropriate for bone age. There is often a family history of the same, with mothers recalling delayed menarche and fathers and siblings noting that they did not enter puberty until 14–18 yr of age. They have a delay in the activation of the GnRH pulse generator and have a functional deficiency of GnRH secretion for chronological age, but since their whole body is physiologically immature, secretion of GnRH is appropriate for the stage of physiological development. Adrenarche and gonadarche occur later in subjects with constitutional (idiopathic) delay in growth and adolescence, whereas adrenarche usually occurs at a normal age in patients with isolated gonadotropin deficiency (3,4).

Patients with constitutional delay in growth and puberty have a retarded bone age at presentation but, on achieving a bone age of approximately 12–14 yr for boys and 11–13 yr for girls, can be expected to show the earliest stages of sexual maturation. In contrast to isolated gonadotropin deficiency, there is no impairment of olfaction and undescended testes are uncommon in constitutionally delayed patients. Plasma gonadal steroid levels may be low at the time of presentation (adrenarche as well as gonadarche is usually delayed). However, as bone age advances, gonadotropin concentrations and pulsatile LH secretion increase (initially at night), and the LH response to GnRH reflects maturation of the hypo-thalamic–pituitary system. Patients with constitutional delay in growth and adolescence will attain full sexual maturity, but the process takes longer than usual. Their final height is in the normal range, but may be lower than expected from family heights.

Uncomplicated hypogonadotropic hypogonadism is often difficult to differentiate from constitutional delay in puberty, as both manifest prepubertal or decreased serum gonadotropins and a prepubertal appearance. If a brain tumor or midline defect is the etiology of hypogonadotropic hypogonadism, other symptoms may be found. However, when there is no associated condition, the diagnosis may rest upon watchful waiting until serum gonadotropins and sex steroids start to rise and secondary sexual development is noted.

The most common genetic cause of hypogonadotropic hypogonadism, Kallmann's syndrome, combines sexual infantilism with hyposmia. Kallmann's syndrome is a genetically heterogeneous disorder in which anosmia or hyposmia resulting from agenesis or hypoplasia of the olfactory lobes and/or sulci is associated with GnRH deficiency (5). Although the extent of the defect in olfaction usually seems to correlate with the degree of GnRH deficiency, even in patients with complete anosmia the GnRH deficiency may be partial (the fertile eunuch syndrome) (6). The magnitude of the GnRH deficiency correlates with the size of the testes (7). Undescended testes and gynecomastia are common in this and all types of hypogonadotropic hypogonadism in boys (7). About one-half of males with Kallmann's syndrome have a micropenis (8). Associated defects include cleft lip, cleft palate, imperfect facial fusion, seizure disorders, short metacarpals, pes cavus, neurosensory hearing loss, cerebellar ataxia, ocular motor abnormalities (9), and unilateral, or rarely bilateral, renal aplasia, or dysplasia that is limited to the X linked form (10). There may be mirror movements of the upper extremities (5,11).

Coronal and axial cranial MRI scans of the olfactory bulbs and sulci may aid diagnosis (12,13). In a review of MRI findings in 64 individuals with Kallmann's syndrome, 56% had bilateral agenesis of the olfactory bulbs (in 2% the agenesis was unilateral); 56% had absent or abnormal olfactory sulci bilaterally (in 17% the abnormality was unilateral) (14). Hence, in Kallmann's syndrome less than 10% of individuals have a normal cranial MRI. Serum LH and FSH may be indistinguishable from prepubertal children except for the lack of or diminished nocturnal pulses of gonadotropin in Kallmann's patients (15).

Kallmann's syndrome may be transmitted as an X-linked, autosomal dominant, or autosomal recessive trait (5). The molecular genetics of only the X-linked form are well established. The KAL-1 gene encodes a 680-amino-acid glycoprotein with characteristics of an extracellular neural adhesion molecule that putatively could function as a pathfinder in the guidance of GnRH neurons to the medial basal hypothalamus. The locus of the KAL-1 gene is Xp22.3, an X-linked gene which escapes X-inactivation and maps 1.5 megabases proximal to the steroid sulfatase gene at the same locus. A variety of deletions and mutations of the KAL gene have been described including large and small (exon) deletions (16–18), point mutations, and a variety of nonsense mutations leading to frameshift and premature stop codons (14,19,20). A small proportion of familial cases in which X-linked inheritance is well documented apparently do not have a mutation in the coding region of the KAL gene; the defect in some of these patients may be located in the promoter region of the KAL gene (21). Contiguous gene deletions in this region of the X chromosome can lead to an association of Kallmann's syndrome with X-linked ichthyosis caused by steroid sulfatase deficiency, mental retardation, and chondroplasia punctata (16,17).

Autosomal dominant inheritance of the phenotype is suggested by some studies (8,22), and this pattern of inheritance is supported by a report of an affected male who fathered an affected son after treatment with hCG (23). Apparent autosomal recessive inheritance characterizes other kindreds (24). Thus, the various forms of Kallmann's syndrome are because of heterogeneous mutations (8,22,24) in which the phenotype can vary.

Hypogonadotropic hypogonadism may be transmitted by autosomal recessive inheritance with none of the other features of Kallmann's syndrome. Males with cerebellar ataxia and deficient gonadotropin production have been reported in kindreds with X-linked inheritance (possibly a variant form of Kallmann's syndrome) and hypogonadotropic hypogonadism may be associated with the multiple lentigenes and basal cell nevus syndromes.

Kallmann's syndrome may be found in the same kindred as constitutional delay in puberty. This suggests that one cause of apparent constitutional delay in puberty is a form fruste of Kallmann's syndrome.

REFERENCES

1. Wilkins L. The diagnosis and treatment of endocrine disorders in childhood and adolescence, 3rd edition. Charles C. Thomas, Springfield, IL, 1965.
2. Prader A. Delayed adolescence. Clin Endocrinol Metab 1975;4:143–155.
3. Sklar CA, Kaplan SL, Grumbach MM. Evidence for dissociation between adrenarche and gonadarche: studies in patients with idiopathic precocious puberty, gonadal dysgenesis, isolated gonadotropin deficiency, and constitutionally delayed growth and adolescence. J Clin Endocrinol Metab 1980;51:548–556.
4. Counts DR, Pescovitz OH, Barnes KM, et al. Dissociation of adrenarche and gonadarche in precocious puberty and in isolated hypogonadotropic hypogonadism. J Clin Endocrinol Metab 1987;64:1174–1178.
5. Kallmann F, Schonfeld WA, Barrera SW. Genetic aspects of primary eunuchoidism. Am J Ment Defic 1944;48:203–236.
6. Wortsman J, Hughes LF. Case report: olfactory function in a fertile eunuch with Kallmann syndrome. Am J Med Sci 1996;311:135–138.
7. Van Dop C, Burstein S, Conte FA, et al. Isolated gonadotropin deficiency in boys: clinical characteristics and growth. J Pediatr 1987;111:684–692.
8. Santen RJ, Paulsen CA. Hypogonadotropic eunuchoidism. I. Clinical study of the mode of inheritance. J Clin Endocrinol Metab 1973;36:47–54.
9. Prager D, Braunstein GD. Editorial: X-chromosome-linked Kallmann's syndrome: pathology at the molecular level. J Clin Endocrinol Metab 1993;76:824–826.
10. Kirk JMW, Grant DB, Besser GM, et al. Unilateral renal aplasia in X-linked Kallmann's syndrome. Clin Genet 1994;46:260–262.
11. Dunek A, Heye B, Schroedter R. Cortically evoked motor responses in patients with Xp22.3-linked Kallmann's syndrome and in female gene carriers. Am J Neuroradiol 1992;31:299–304.
12. Klingmhller D, Dewes W, Krahe T, et al. Magnetic resonance imaging of the brain in patients with anosmia and hypothalamic hypogonadism (Kallmann's syndrome). J Clin Endocrinol Metab 1987;65:581–584.
13. Truwit CL, Barkovich AJ, Grumbach MM, et al. Magnetic resonance imaging of Kallmann syndrome, a genetic disorder of neuronal migration affecting the ofactory and genital systems. Am J Neuroradiol 1993;14:827–838.
14. Quinton R, Duke VM, de Zoysa PA, et al. The neuroradiology of Kallmann's syndrome: a genotypic and phenotypic analysis. J Clin Endocrinol Metab 1996;81:3010–3017.
15. Wu FC, Butler GE, Kelnar CJ, Stirling HF, Huhtaniemi I. Patterns of pulsatile luteinizing hormone and follicle-stimulating hormone secretion in prepubertal (midchildhood) boys and girls and patients with idiopathic hypogonadotropic hypogonadism (Kallmann's syndrome): a study using an ultrasensitive time-resolved immunofluorometric assay. J Clin Endocrinol Metab 1991;72:1229–1237.
16. Ballabio A, Bardoni B, Carrozzo R, et al. Contiguous gene syndromes due to deletions in the distal short arm of the human X chromosome. Proc Natl Acad Sci USA 1989;86:10,001–10,005.
17. Hardelin JP, Levilliers J, Young J, et al. Xp22.3 deletions in isolated familial Kallmann's syndrome. J Clin Endocrinol Metab 1993;76:827–831.
18. Legouis R, Hardelin J-P, Levilliers J, et al. The candidate gene for the X-linked Kallmann syndrome encodes a protein related to adhesion molecules. Cell 1991;67:423–435.
19. Hardelin J-P, Levilliers J, Blanchard S, et al. Heterogeneity in the mutations responsible for X chromosome-linked Kallmann syndrome. Hum Mol Genet 1993;2:373–377.
20. Oliveira LM, Seminara SB, Beranova M, et al. The importance of autosomal genes in Kallmann syndrome: genotype-phenotype correlations and neuroendocrine characteristics. J Clin Endocrinol Metab 2001;86:1532–1538.
21. Cohen-Salmon M, Tronche F, del Castillo, et al. Characterization of the promotor of the human KAL gene responsible for the X-chromosome-linked Kallmann syndrome. Gene 1995;164:235–242.
22. Santen RJ, Paulsen CA. Hypogonadotropic eunuchoidism. II. Gonadal responsiveness to exogenous gonadotropins. J Clin Endocrinol Metab 1973;36:55–63.
23. Merriam GR, Beitins IZ, Bode HH. Father to son transmission of hypogonadism with anosmia. Am J Dis Child 1977;131:1216–1219.
24. White BJ, Rogol AD, Brown KS, et al. The syndrome of anosmia with hypogonadotropic hypogonadism: a genetic study of 18 new families and a review. Am J Med Genet 1983;15:417–435.

CASE #5: DELAYED PUBERTY IN A GIRL
Case Description

A 16-yr-old girl presented with primary amenorrhea. Birth history revealed a full-term labor with a birth weight of 5 lbs. Early childhood was complicated by three ear infections leading to the placement of PE tubes. Otherwise, her health had been good. Her school experience was generally going well, but she was having trouble understanding problems in geometry regarding spatial orientation.

Family history revealed the mother's height to be 5 ft 4 in and her menarche was at 12.5 yr of age. Her father's height was 5 ft 8 in. He could not recall his age of puberty, but it was felt to be average. There was no contributory other family history.

On physical examination the patient was a normal appearing girl who looked younger than her stated age. Vital signs, including blood pressure, were within normal limits. Her height was 5 feet (153 cm—5th percentile), and her weight was 100 lbs (45 kg—25th percentile). HEENT examination showed no acne or comedones. Her mouth appeared normal. Her neck was normal without goiter. Her hair line, wrists, and abdomen were normal. Her lungs and heart were normal. There was no breast tissue noted and the areolae were normal. Pubic hair was at stage 2 and the genitalia were normal in appearance. A neurological examination was within normal limits. Laboratory testing (Table 7) was remarkable for elevated gonadotropins with a low estradiol. A routine chemistry panel and complete blood count (CBC) were normal.

Discussion

The elevated serum concentrations of LH and FSH indicate primary gonadal failure and, without another explanation, Turner's syndrome must be suspected. Her height was in the normal range but even without short stature or other physical features of Turner syndrome, a karyotype is indicated in girls with gonadal failure. Her karyotype was 45 X0/46 XX, indicating mosaic Turner's syndrome.

The most common form of hypergonadotropic hypogonadism in the female is the syndrome of gonadal dysgenesis or Turner's syndrome and its variants *(1,2)*. This group of sporadic disorders has an overall incidence of 1 per 2500 to 10,000 liveborn girls *(2–6)* and is characterized by absence of all or part of the second sex chromosome. The 45 X karyotype is associated with female phenotype, short stature, sexual infantilism, various somatic abnormalities, and frequent fetal demise. Sex chromosome mosaicism or structural abnormalities of an X or Y chromosome may modify the features of this syndrome, although about 40% of the individuals with the five features noted above have mosaicism or structural abnormalities of the X chromosome *(1)*.

Short stature and sexual infantilism are invariable features of 45 X gonadal dysgenesis, or classic Turner's syndrome. This karyotype is found in approximately 60% of cases of Turner's syndrome *(3,7)*. The short stature is owing to loss of a homeobox-containing gene located on the pseudoautosomal region (*PAR 1*) of the short arms of the X (*Xp22*) and *Yp11.3* chro-mosomes *(8,9)* that encodes anosteogenic factor *(9)*. The gene is called *SHOX* (short stature homeobox-containing gene) *(8)* or PHOG (pseudoautosomal homeobox osteogenic gene) *(9)*.

Affected newborn infants may have loose skin folds of the neck that scar down to a webbed neck or manifest lymphedema of the extremities (the Bonneville–Ullrich syn-

Table 7
Laboratory Testing in Case 5

	Patient values	Normal values
LH	45 mIU/mL	0.6–15
FSH	80 mIU/mL	1–9.2
Estradiol	10 pg/mL	20–60
DHEAS	150 ng/mL	100–555

drome). It is important to determine whether coarctation of the aorta and/or a bicuspid aortic valve is present because of the risk of hypertension and aortic rupture or a tendency to valvular infection.

Features noted during childhood are found in various locations in the body. The classic features of Turner's syndrome were not found in this patient, indicating the remarkably variable nature of this condition. Frequent features are distinct facies with micrognathia causing a "fishmouth" appearance, high-arched palate with dental abnormalities, epicanthal folds, ptosis, low-set or deformed ears, short neck with low hairline, and webbing (pterygium colli), and recurrent otitis media, often leading to impaired hearing (7,10). A broad shield-like chest leads to the appearance of wide-spaced nipples; the areolae are often hypoplastic. Skeletal defects include short fourth metacarpals and cubitus valgus (that may develop after birth), Madelung deformity of the wrist, genu valgum, and scoliosis (2,7). The skin demonstrates extensive pigmented nevi, a tendency to keloid formation, and hypoplastic nails (1,7). Lymphatic obstruction leads not only to the infantile puffiness of extremities and pterygium colli, but to a distinctive shape of the ears. Cardiovascular anomalies include coarctation of the aorta (40% also usually have webbing of the neck), aortic stenosis, and bicuspid aortic valves; the latter individuals are at risk for a dissecting aortic aneurysm (11). An echocardiogram of the cardiovascular system must be performed. Abnormal pelvocaliceal collecting systems, abnormal position or alignment of the kidneys, and abnormal vascular supply to the kidney may be encountered and recurrent urinary tract infections are not uncommon (12). Defects of the gastrointestinal system include intestinal telangiectasias and hemangiomatoses that can rarely lead to massive gastrointestinal bleeding. Furthermore, the prevalence of inflammatory bowel disease is increased (13–15). The uterus and fallopian tubes are infantile. Pelvic ultrasonography or MRI usually permits the detection of even a small uterus in these patients and, commonly, streak gonads.

Autoimmune diseases, such as Hashimoto's thyroiditis and Graves' disease, are common. Glucose intolerance resulting from increased insulin resistance is also common after the age of puberty, although in some this may be owing to associated obesity (16,17). Turner's syndrome patients commonly have have elevated serum cholesterol concentrations (18).

IQ is normal when verbal ability including comprehension and vocabulary are considered. However, spatiotemporal processing, visuomotor coordination (19,20), and mathematical ability (particularly in geometry) may be impaired in patients with Turner's syndrome, leading to a decrease in the overall IQ performance (21,22). Difficulties associated with social adjustment and cognition are common (23). 45 X individuals in whom the X is of paternal origin (Xp) show better adjustment and "social cognition" as a group than Xm individuals (24,25). This difference has been attributed to the imprinting of a gene that escapes X-inactivation inherited from the mother located on *Xm*, but that is not imprinted on *Xp* *(24)*. The first example of an imprinted gene on the X chromosome, this locus resides in the pericentric region of the short arm or on the long arm of the X chromosome. Skuse et al. *(24)* postulate that this imprinted gene may play a role in male–female differences in social behavior and developmental disorders. It is useful to monitor the patient's progress in high school mathematics so that assistance may be offered. Gender identity and sexual orientation are female *(21)*.

Patients are usually small at birth because of intrauterine growth retardation, exhibit a relatively normal growth rate until a bone age of about 3 yr, and then a decrease in growth with a profound reduction in growth rate at the time of expected puberty with failure to have a pubertal growth spurt *(26–28)*. Individuals with Turner's syndrome have a mean final height of approximately 142–143 cm *(27)*; but the adult stature of these patients correlates with midparental height so that subjects with tall parents will tend to be taller *(6)*. Their pattern of growth does not suggest that these individuals are GH deficient *(28)*. However, growth hormone in pharmacologic doses is now approved for use in this disorder and increases the mean final height, although to a variable extent. Specific growth curves are available for plotting the growth of affected children *(27,28)*. In a group of girls with Turner's syndrome and spontaneous puberty, height velocity was transiently higher during puberty than in girls with amenorrhea, but final adult heights were not different *(1)*.

Baseline gonadotropin concentrations and peak LH and FSH values after GnRH administration are above normal between birth and 4 yr of age and again after age 10. Baseline values of FSH are 3–10 times higher than LH values. However, between ages 4 and 10, mean gonadotropin concentrations in this syndrome are similar to the mean values in normal girls and are lower than those before age 4 and after age 10 *(29,30)*.

The appearance of pubic hair is often delayed in the syndrome of gonadal dysgenesis, even though adrenarche, as assessed by an increase in concentration of plasma DHEAS, occurs at the normal age *(31)*. The pubic hair of affected individuals is sparse, but estrogen therapy increases the growth of pubic hair despite a lack of increase in adrenal androgen secretion *(32)*. The streak gonads usually result in sexual infantilism, but in about 10% of cases, puberty, menarche, and, even more rarely, pregnancy may occur because the ovaries are not completely affected *(1)*.

The bone density is decreased, at least in part, because of hypogonadism at puberty, and this becomes more severe with age in patients who discontinue or do not receive estrogen replacement therapy (ERT).

REFERENCES

1. Grumbach MM, Conte FA. Disorders of sex differentiation. In: Wilson JD, Foster DW, eds. Williams' Textbook of Endocrinology, 1998, pp. 1303–1425.
2. Turner Syndrome. In: Rosenfeld R, Grumbach, MM, eds. Marcel Decker, New York, 1990.
3. Hook EB, Warburton D. The distribution of chromosomal genotypes associated with Turner's syndrome: livebirth prevalence rates and evidence for diminished fetal mortality and severity in genotypes associated with structural X abnormalities or mosaicism. Hum Genet 1983;64:24–27.
4. Hook EB, Hamerton JL. The frequency of chromosome abnormalitites detected in consecutive newborn studies.Results by sex and severity of phenotypic involvement. In: Hook EB, Porter IH, eds. Population cytogenetics. Academic, New York, 1977, pp. 63–79.
5. Turner HH. A syndrome of infantilism, congenital webbed neck and cubitus valgus. Endocrinology 1938;23:566–574.

6. Massa G, Vanderschueren-Lodeweyckx M, Malvaux P. Linear growth in patients with Turner syndrome: influence of spontaneous puberty and parental height. Eur J Pediatr 1990;149:246–250.

7. Palmer CG, Reichman A. Chromosomal and clinical findings in 110 females with Turner syndrome. Hum Gen 1976;35:35–49.

8. Roa E, Weiss B, Fukami M, et al. Pseudoautosomal deletions encompassing a novel homeobox gene cause growth failure in idiopathic short stature and Turner syndrome. Nature Genet 1997;16:54–62.

9. Ellison JW, Wardak Z, Young M, et al. PHOG, a candidate gene for involvement in the short stature of Turner syndrome. Hum Mol Genet 1997;6:1341–1347.

10. Szpunar J. Middle ear disease in Turner's syndrome. Arch Otolaryngol Head Neck Surg 1968;87:34–40.

11. Lin AE, Lippe BM, Geffner ME, et al. Aortic dilation, dissection, and rupture in patients with Turner syndrome. J Pediatr 1986;109:820–826.

12. Lippe BM, Geffner ME, Dietrich RB, et al. Renal malformations in patients with Turner syndrome: imaging in 141 patients. Pediatrics 1988;82:852–856.

13. Arulanantham K, Kramer MS, Gryboski JD. The association of inflammatory bowel disease and X-chromosomal abnormality. Pediatrics 1980;66:63–67.

14. Knudtzon J, Svane S, Price WH. Turner's syndrome associated with chronic inflammatory bowel disease: a case report and review of the literature A high incidence of chronic inflammatory bowel disease in patients with Turner's syndrome. Acta Med Scand 1979;16:263–266.

15. Price WH. A high incidence of chronic inflammatory bowel disease in patients with Turner's syndrome. J Med Genet 1979;16:263–266.

16. Nielsen J, Johansen K, Yde H. The frequency of diabetes mellitus in patients with Turner's syndrome and pure gonadal dysgenesis. Acta Endocrinol 1969;62:251–269.

17. Forbes AP, Engel E. A high incidence of diabetes mellitus in 41 patients with gonadal dysgenesis, and their close relatives. Metabolism 1997;16:263–266.

18. Ross JL, Feuillan P, Long LM, et al. Lipid abnormalities in Turner syndrome. J Pediatr 1995;126:242–245.

19. Silbert A, Wolffe PH, Lilienthal J. Spatial and temporal processing in patients with Turner's syndrome. Behav Genet 1977;7:11–21.

20. Swillen A, Fryns JP, Kleczkowska A, et al. Intelligence, behaviour and psychosocial development in Turner syndrome. A cross-sectional study of 50 pre-adolescent and adolescent girls (4-20 yr). Genet Couns 1993;4:7–18.

21. Nielsen J. Mental aspects of Turner syndrome and the importance of information and Turner contact groups. In: Rosenfeld RG, Grumbach MM, eds. Turner Syndrome. Marcel Dekker, New York, 1946, p. 451.

22. Garron DC. Intelligence among persons with Turner's syndrome. Behav Genet 1977;7:105–127.

23. Albertsson-Wiklund K, Ranke MB. Turner syndrome in a life span perspective: research and clinical aspects. Elsevier Science BV, Amsterdam, The Netherlands, 1995.

24. Skuse DH, James RS, Bishop DVM, et al. Evidence from Turner's syndrome of an imprinted X-linked locus affecting cognitive function. Nature 1997;387:705–708.

25. McGuffin P, Scourfield J. A father's imprint on his daughter's thinking. Nature 1997;387:652–653.

26. Brook CGD, Murset G, Zachmann M, et al. Growth in children with 45,XO Turner's syndrome. Arch Dis Child 1974;73:789–795.

27. Lyon AJ, Preece MA, Grant DB. Growth curve for girls with Turner syndrome. Arch Dis Child 1985; 60:932–935.

28. Ranke MB, Stubbe P, Majewski F, et al. Spontaneous growth in Turner's syndrome. Acta Paediatr Scand Suppl 1988;343:22–30.

29. Conte FA, Grumbach MM, Kaplan SL, Reiter EO. Correlation of luteinizing hormone-releasing factor-induced luteinizing hormone and follicle-stimulating hormone release from infancy to 19 yr with the changing pattern of gonadotropin secretion in agonadal patients: relation to the restraint of puberty. J Clin Endocrinol Metab 1980;50:163–168.

30. Conte FA, Grumbach MM, Kaplan SL. A diphasic pattern of gonadotropin secretion in patients with the syndrome of gonadal dysgenesis. J Clin Endocrinol Metab 1975;40:670–674.

31. Sklar CA, Kaplan SL, Grumbach MM. Evidence for dissociation between adrenarche and gonadarche: studies in patients with idiopathic precocious puberty, gonadal dysgenesis, isolated gonadotropin deficiency, and constitutionally delayed growth and adolescence. J Clin Endocrinol Metab 1980;51:548–556.

32. Sklar CA, Kaplan SL, Grumbach MM. Lack of effect of oestrogens on adrenal androgen secretion in children and adolescents with a comment on oestrogens and pubic hair growth. Clin Endocrinol 1981;14: 311–320.

CASE #6: GNRH-INDEPENDENT PRECOCIOUS PUBERTY

Case Description

A 3-yr-10-mo-old girl presented with breast development and skin lesions, as well as other endocrine abnormalities. She was born after a 38-wk gestation by normal spontaneous vaginal delivery. Birth weight was 7 lbs 11 oz. There were no complications of pregnancy. Her mother used no substances nor had any illnesses during pregnancy. Abnormal skin pigmentation was noted at birth, and a dermatologist performed a biopsy at 4 mo of age. No diagnosis was established. At 2 yr of age, the mother noted a lump on the child's jaw. A head CT and MRI were performed and, after a biopsy of the lesion, the diagnosis of fibrous dysplasia was made. The additional finding of *café-au-lait* spots led to the diagnosis of McCune–Albright syndrome. Ophthalmologic evaluation revealed no compromise of the optic nerve.

On physical examination, this 3.8-yr-old was quite pleasant, cooperative, and of normal intelligence. Her pulse was 93, blood pressure was 119/71 mmHg, and respiratory rate was 20. Her height was 113.1 cm (>95th percentile), and weight was 19 kg (>95th percentile). HEENT examination revealed normal eyes, pupils equal and reactive to light, and a normal pharynx. A palpable mass, about 2 cm in irregular diameter, was noted on the right jaw. The thyroid gland was enlarged, with a 1.5-cm nodule on the left lobe. The rest of the thyroid was palpable and the isthmus was thickened as well. There were no bruits in the thyroid gland. The areolae were about 2 cm in diameter. The breast buds appeared to be about the same size as the areolae, although the right side was greater than left. Breast development was stage 2. Her abdomen was soft without masses or organomegaly. Her extremities revealed no asymmetry and appeared normal. There was a slight scoliosis (20° to the left) and a small degree of lordosis of the lower back. There was no pubic hair (stage 1). There was clear estrogen affect in the vaginal mucosa based upon the thickness and the pinkish color of the mucosa. There was no axillary hair and no axillary odor. Her left forearm revealed a *café-au-lait* spot of 11 × 6 cm. She had another very large *café-au-lait* spot over the front of her trunk, which crossed the midline, covering 20% of the thorax and some of the neck, as it involved both the right and left sides of the neck. It extended down the left arm as well. She had two *café-au-lait* spots on the back of her leg, lower spine, and shoulder. The neurological exam revealed no deficits of the cranial nerves, and she had normal DTRs and normal mentation.

Laboratory test results are shown in Table 8. A GnRH test showed a suppressed LH (peak of <0.1 mIU/mL) and FSH (peak of <0.1 mIU/mL), but serum estradiol was 50 pg/mL. Because of the increased serum T3 levels, she was begun on propylthiouracil 25 mg tid.

Discussion

This girl has GnRH-independent precocious puberty reflected in the low LH and FSH levels in the face of elevated serum estrogen levels. The skin lesions and skeletal abnormalities in association with precocious puberty, thyroid hyperactivity, and suggestion of autonomous GH secretion noted by the consistently measurable and indeed elevated growth hormone concentrations all point to the McCune–Albright syndrome *(1,2)*.

McCune–Albright syndrome occurs sporadically and for years the cause was unknown. Recent studies demonstrate that it is owing to somatic activating mutations in the gene (*GNAS 1*) encoding the α-subunit of the trimeric guanosine triphosphate (GTP-binding protein (Gαs) that stimulates adenyl cyclase. It is characterized by the triad of

Table 8
Laboratory Results for Case 6

	Patient values	Normal values
Serum T-3	320 ng/dL	105–269
Serum total T4	10.5 µg/dL	7.2–15.7
GH	6–8 ng/mL several occasions	<1.0
TSH	<0.05 mU/L	0.7–6.4
IGF-1	350 ng/mL	17–248
Bone age	5 yr 9 mo	2 SD above the mean

1. irregularly edged hyperpigmented macules (café-au-lait spots);
2. a slowly progressive bone disorder, polyostotic fibrous dysplasia, that can involve any bone and is frequently associated with facial asymmetry and hyperostosis of the base of the skull and is about twice as often in girls than boys;
3. GnRH-independent sexual precocity, which is also more common in girls (3,4).

Autonomous hyperfunction most commonly involves the ovary, but other endocrine involvement includes thyroid (nodular hyperplasia with thyrotoxicosis or, remarkably, with euthyroid status), adrenal (multiple hyperplastic nodules with Cushing syndrome) (5), pituitary (adenoma or mammosomatotrope hyperplasia with gigantism and acromegaly and hyperprolactinemia) (6), and parathyroids (adenoma or hyperplasia with hyperparathyroidism) (3). In addition, hypophosphatemic vitamin D-resistant rickets or osteomalacia can occur in this syndrome, either because of a putative phosphaturic factor, phosphatonin (7), secreted by the bone lesions or an intrinsic renal abnormality leading to the excess generation of nephrogenous cyclic adenosine 5'-monophosphate (AMP) in the proximal tubule with decreased reabsorption of phosphate (8). At least two of the features must be present to consider the diagnosis.

The skin manifestations may not be noted in infancy although they were noted in this case. The café-au-lait macules usually do not cross the midline and often are located on the same side as the main bone lesions and have a segmented distribution (1). In this case, the lesions do cross the midline.

The skeletal lesions in the cortex are dysplastic and are filled with spindle cells with poorly organized collagen support; they take the form of scattered cystic areas of rarefaction on radiography and often result in pathological fractures and progressive deformities (9). Technetium bone scintigraphy has been the most sensitive approach to the detection of bone lesions before they are visible radiographically. If the skull is involved, there may be entrapment and compression of optic or auditory nerve foramina, which can lead to blindness, deafness, facial asymmetry, and ptosis. This patient is being frequently evaluated for these features.

The heterotrimeric guanine nucleotide binding proteins (G proteins) are a subfamily within the large superfamily of GTP-binding proteins and serve to transduce signals from a large number of cell surface receptors with a common structural motif of seven membrane-spanning domains to their intracellular effect; in essence, they couple serpentine cell surface receptors to effectors. For Gs, the stimulatory G-proteins, the effector is adenylyl cyclase that is controlled by Gs and inhibitory (Gi) G-proteins [reviewed in (10–12)].

The heterotrimer is composed of an α-subunit (39–45 kDa) that binds GTP and has intrinsic GTPase activity that converts GTP to GDP, a β-subunit (35–36 kDa), and a smaller (γ sub-unit (7–8 kDa) that are tightly associated with each other. Each of the subunits is encoded by a distinct gene. The G proteins function as "conformational switches." The GDP-liganded α-subunit is bound to the β subunits and is in an inactivated state. When the cell surface receptor is activated by its ligand or agonists, the GDP is catalytically released from the α-subunit and enables GTP to bind. This leads to dissociation of the GTP activated α-subunit, its dissociation from the bound β subunit and the effector adenylyl cyclase is activated. When GTP is hydrolyzed by the intrinsic GTPase activity of the G-α, it and G-β reassociate and the α-subunit is in the off or inactive conformation. The three- dimensional structure of the heterotrimeric G proteins has been determined (13–17).

Recently a mutation in the gene encoding the "α-subunit of the stimulatory G protein of the adenylyl cyclase was identified in tissue of children with the McCune–Albright syndrome (18). This was a single base substitution of arginine with histidine at position 201 of the Gs protein. These activating mutations, which lead to constitutive excess cAMP production and, in some tissues cAMP-induced hyperplasia (16), have a mosaic pattern of hyperactivity and the proportion of mutant to normal cells varies, contributing, at least in part, to varied clinical findings, severity, its sporadic nature, and the discordant occurrence in monozygotic twins. A germ-line mutation that would affect all cells is presumed to be lethal to the embryo. Two gain of function missense mutations have been described in this order, both of which involve the arginine 201 residue of the α-subunit (10), the site of covalent modification by cholera toxin: Arg 201 with either a Cys or His substitution (4,19–21). The arginine 201 residue is critical for α-subunit GTPase activity, and each of the two mutations decreases GTPase activity and causes constitutive activation. These activating mutations have been found in cell tissues affected in the syndrome (22,23), including bone lesions. The involvement of the adrenal cortex can lead to macronodular adrenal hyperplasia and Cushing's syndrome. Thyroid adenomas causing hyperthyroidism along with hepatic involvement associated with hepatobiliary disease and jaundice and pancreatitis can be early manifestations of the McCune–Albright syndrome in infancy (24). Another nonendocrine manifestation is cardiac disease that carries the risk of cardiac arrhythmia and sudden death.

The sexual precocity may begin in the first 2 yr of life and is frequently heralded by menstrual bleeding. It is initially GnRH independent and the ovaries contain multiple follicular cysts, but not corpora lutea and commonly exhibit asymmetrical enlargement as a result of a large solitary cyst that characteristically enlarges and spontaneously regresses only to recur later (3,5,25–27,34). Serum estradiol is elevated (at times to extraordinarily high levels), but initially the LH response to GnRH is prepubertal, and the pubertal pattern of nighttime LH pulses is absent (25,28,29). Later, when the bone age approaches 12 yr, the GnRH pulse generator becomes operative and ovulatory cycles ensue. Thus, an affected girl may progress from GnRH-independent precocious puberty to GnRH-dependent precocious puberty (25,28,30). GnRH agonists are not effective for treatment in the early stages, but are effective when the condition becomes GnRH dependent. Testolactone (40 mg/kg/d orally) (31), a relatively weak aromatase inhibitor, has been of equivocal usefulness (32) and some patients become resistant to the drug (33). Tamoxifen is under clinical study to determine if its antiestrogen effects can help control the advancement of bone age (35).

REFERENCES

1. McCune DJ, Bruch H. Osteodystrophia fibrosa: report of a case in which the condition was combined with true precocious puberty, pathologic pigmentation of the skin and hyperthyroidism, with a review of the literature. Am J Dis Child 1937;54:806–848.

2. Albright F, Butler AM, Hampton AO, et al. Syndrome characterized by osteitis fibrosa disseminata, areas of pigmentation and endocrine dysfunction, with precocious puberty in females. N Engl J Med 1937;216: 727–746.

3. Danon M, Crawford JD. The McCune-Albright syndrome. Ergeb Inn Med Kinderheilkd 1987;55:81–115.

4. Ringel MD, Schwindinger WF, Levine MA. Clinical implications of genetic defects in G proteins. Medicine 1996;75:171–184.

5. Danon MS, Robboy SH, Kin S, et al. Cushing syndrome, sexual precocity and polyostotic fibrous dysplasia. J Pediatr 1975;87:917–921.

6. Feuillan PP, Jones J, Ross JL. Growth hormone hypersecretion in a girl with McCune-Albright syndrome: comparison with controls and response to a dose of long-acting somatostatin analog. J Clin Endocrinol Metab 1995;80:1357–1360.

7. Eons MJ, Drezner MK. Tumor-induced osteomalacia—unveiling a new hormone. N Engl J Med 1994; 330:1679–1681.

8. Zung A, Chalew SA, Schwindinger WF, et al. Urinary cyclic adenosine 3',5'-monophosphate response in McCune-Albright syndrome: clinical evidence for altered renal adenylate cyclase activity. J Clin Endocrinol Metab 1995;80:3576–3581.

9. Keijser LC, Van Tienen TG, Schreuder HW, et al. Fibrous dysplasia of bone: management and outcome of 20 cases. J Surg Oncol. 2001;76:157–166.

10. Spiegel AM, Shenker A, Weinstein LS. Receptor-effector coupling by G proteins: implications for normal and abnormal signal transduction. Endocr Rev 1992;13:536–565.

11. Neer EJ. Heterotrimeric G proteins: organizers of transmembrane signals. Cell 1995;80:249–257.

12. Spiegel AM. The molecular basis of disorders caused by defects in G proteins. Horm Res 1997;47: 89–96.

13. Bourne HR. Trimeric G proteins: surprise witness tells a tale. Science 1995;270:933–934.

14. Clapham DE. The G-protein nanomachine. Nature 1996;379:297–299.

15. Neer EJ, Smith TF. G protein heterodimers: new structures propel new questions. Cell 1996;84:175–178.

16. Coleman DE, Sprang SR. How G proteins work: a continuing story. TIBS 1996;21:41–44.

17. Dhanasekaran N, Heasley LE, Johnson GL. G protein-coupled receptor systems involved in cell growth and oncogenesis. Endocr Rev 1995;16:259–270.

18. Schwindinger WF, Francomano CA, Levine MA. Identification of a mutation in the gene encoding the alpha subunit of the stimulatory G protein of adenylyl cyclase in McCune-Albright syndrome. Proc Natl Acad Sci USA 1992;89:5152–5156.

19. Weinstein LS, Shenker A, Gejman PV, et al. Activating mutations of the stimulatory G protein in the McCune-Albright syndrome. N Engl J Med 1991;325:1688–1695.

20. DeLuch J, Riess W Hanze J, et al. Gs alpha mutation at codon 201 in pituitary adenoma causing gigantism in a 6-year-old boy with McCune-Albright syndrome. J Clin Endocrinol Metab 1996;81:3839–3842.

21. Spiegel AM. Mutations in G proteins and G protein-coupled receptors in endocrine disease. J Clin Endocrinol Metab 1996;81:2434–2442.

22. Shenker A, Weinstein LS, Sweet DE SA. An activating Gs" mutation is present in fibrous dysplasia of bone in the McCune-Albright syndrome. J Clin Endocrinol Metab 1994;79:750–755.

23. Candeliere GA, Gloueux FH, Prud' homme J, et al. Increased expression of the C-fos proto-oncogene in bone from patients with fibrous dysplasia. N Engl J Med 1995;332:1546–1551.

24. Shenker A, Weinstein LS, Moran A, et al. Severe endocrine and nonendocrine manifestations of the McCune-Albright syndrome associated with activating mutations of stimulatory G protein Gs. J Pediatr 1993;123:509–518.

25. Kaplan SL, Grumbach MM. Pathogenesis of sexual precocity. In: Grumbach MM, Sizonenko PC, Aubert ML, eds. Control of the Onset of Puberty. Williams & Wilkins, Baltimore, MD, 1990, pp. 620–660.

26. Carani C, Pacchioni C, Baldini A, Zini D. Effects of cyproterone acetate, LHRH agonist and ovarian surgery in McCune-Albright syndrome with precocious puberty and galactorrhea. J Endocrinol Invest 1988;11:419–423.

27. Reith KG, Comite F, Shawker T, et al. Pituitary and ovarian abnormalities demonstrated by CT and ultrasound in children with features of the McCune-Albright syndrome. Radiology 1984;153:389–393.

28. Foster CM, Comite F, Pescovitz OH, et al. Variable response to a long-acting agonist of luteinizing hormone-releasing hormone in girls with McCune-Albright syndrome. J Clin Endocrinol Metab 1984;59: 801–805.

29. Foster CM, Ross JL, Shawker T, et al. Absence of pubertal gonadotropin secretion in girls with McCune-Albright syndrome. J Clin Endocrinol Metab 1984;58:1161–1165.

30. Pasquino AM, Tebaldi L, Cives C, et al. Precocious puberty in the McCune-Albright syndrome. Progression from gonadotrophin-independent to gonadotrophin-dependent puberty in a girl. Acta Paediatr Scand 1987;76:841–843.

31. Feullian PP, Foster CM, Pescovitz O, et al. Treatment of precocious puberty in the McCune-Albright syndrome with the aromatase inhibitor testolactone. N Engl J Med 1986;315:1115–1119.

32. Hauffa BP, Havers W, Stolecke H. Short term effects of testolactone compared to other treatment modalities on longitudinal growth and ovarian activity in a girl with McCune-Albright syndrome. Helv Paediatr Acta 1987;42:471–480.

33. Feuillan PP, Jones J, Cutler GBJ. Long-term testolactone therapy for precocious puberty in girls with the McCune-Albright syndrome. J Clin Endocrinol Metab 1993;77:647–651.

34. Wierman ME, Beardsworth DE, Mansfield MJ, et al. Puberty without gonadotropins. A unique mechanism of sexual development. N Engl J Med 1985;312:65–72.

35. Eugster EA, Shankar R, Feezle LK, Pescovitz OH. Tamoxifen treatment of progressive precocious puberty in a patient with McCune-Albright syndrome. J Pediatr Endocrinol Metab 1999;12:681–686.

21

Disorders of Growth and Development

Erick J. Richmond, MD
and Alan D. Rogol, MD, PhD

CONTENTS

CASE #1: ACCELERATED GROWTH DUE TO CONGENITAL ADRENAL HYPERPLASIA

Case Description

This 4-yr-4-mo-old boy presented to the local pediatric endocrinologist for evaluation of accelerated growth velocity and development of pubic hair over the past year.

The family history was negative. Parents were healthy and both had normal puberty. Mother's height: 5 ft 6 in, father's height: 5 ft 10 in. He did not have brothers or sisters at that time and there was no history of endocrine disorders. Birth history was unremarkable with an uncomplicated full-term pregnancy, normal vaginal delivery, and birth weight of 3.5 kg. No neonatal problems. His past medical history was remarkable for mild language delay and frequent ear infections.

He was described as a very tall white male who appeared older than his chronological age. His initial physical exam at age 4 yr 4 mo showed: a height of 116.8 cm (well above the 95th percentile), height age 6 yr 3 mo, weight 21.3 kg (50th percentile for weight/height), B/P 80/50 mmHg, pubic hair Tanner III, penile length, 7.5 cm and testicles 1.8 cm (approximately 1 mL), with slightly increased consistency.

The initial laboratory exams showed the following: Na 141 mEq/L, K 4.2 mEq/L, T4 8.3 mcg/dL thyroid-stimulating hormone (TSH) 1.2 µIU/mL, luteinizing hormone (LH) 0.03 IU/L, follicle-stimulating hormone (FSH) 0.38 IU/L, testosterone 83 ng/dL (normal <10 ng/dL), dehydroepi-androsterone sulfate (DHEAS) 281 mcg/dL (normal 5–57 mcg/dL), plasma renin activity 610 ng/dL/h (normal 100–650 ng/dL/h). Bone age 11 yr.

From: *Contemporary Endocrinology: Challenging Cases in Endocrinology*
Edited by: M. E. Molitch © Humana Press Inc., Totowa, NJ

Table 1
Adrenal Steroid Hormone Response to ACTH Stimulation

	Case 0'- Baseline-	Normal baseline range	Case 60'-Stimulated	Normal stimulated range
ACTH	59 pg/mL			
Cortisol	8.1 mcg/dL	3–21 mcg/dL	9.8 mcg/dL	12–36 mcg/dL
17-OH progesterone	3183 ng/dL	3–90 ng/dL	23900 ng/dL	<700 ng/dL
17-OH pregnenolone	525 ng/dL	15–221 ng/dL	2799 ng/dL	45–600 ng/dL
11-deoxycortisol	28 ng/dL	20–155 ng/dL	48 ng/dL	40–300 ng/dL

An adenocorticotropic hormone (ACTH) stimulation test (250 mcg) was performed as shown in Table 1. Based on his tall stature, small testicles, early pubic hair, advanced bone age, and ACTH stimulation test results, he was diagnosed with "late onset" adrenal hyperplasia, 21-hydroxylase deficiency, and started on prednisone 7.5 mg bid for 3 wk and then switched to hydrocortisone 10 mg tid. The initial pediatric endocrinologist referred the patient to our clinic 2 mo after the diagnosis was made because the patient moved to another state. At that time, his only complaint was weight gain (2.7 kg in 2 mo). The physical exam was remarkable for tall stature, pubic hair Tanner III, and small testicles (1–2 mL). Because the laboratory exam showed a 17-OH progesterone level of 122 ng/dL, it was decided to decrease his hydrocortisone dose to 10, 7.5, 10 mg and to change the diagnosis to congenital adrenal hyperplasia due to 21-hydroxlase deficiency, "simple virilizing form" (late diagnosis).

The patient has been followed in our clinic since May 1992. It has been necessary to modify the hydrocortisone dose several times to keep the 17-OH progesterone at an acceptable level, but also to permit normal linear growth. The latest visit was at age 12 yr: height146.3 cm (25–50th percentile); weight 59 kg (>95th percentile weight/height); blood pressure 96/68 mmHg, pubic hair Tanner II, testicles 3 mL. He was receiving hydrocortisone 10, 7.5, 10 mg and the 17-OH progesterone level was 321 ng/dL (see Fig. 1). His bone age was 13 yr.

Discussion

The evaluation of virilization in childhood is always a challenge. In this particular case, we are dealing with a very tall 4-yr-4-mo-old boy with significant pubic hair, an enlarged phallus, and small testicles. First, we need to decide whether it is a variation of a normal or an abnormal condition.

Premature adrenarche is considered a variation of normal. It is the early development of sexual hair, secondary to an increase in adrenal androgenic steroids (1,2). It usually presents after age 6 yr and levels of DHEAS are typically elevated. In contrast with our patient's findings, the growth velocity and bone age are normal or only slightly accelerated and no other secondary sex characteristics are present. Consequently, the likelihood of premature adrenarche in our patient is minimal, and the alternative is that he has an abnormal condition, called sexual precocity.

Sexual precocity can be central [gonadotropic releasing hormone (GnRH)-dependent] or peripheral (GnRH-independent) (3). Central precocious puberty is either idiopathic or secondary to a hypothalamic disease. On the other hand, causes of peripheral precocious

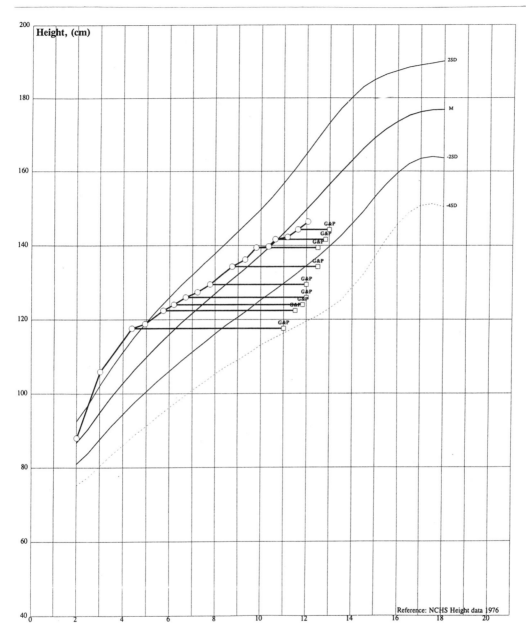

Fig. 1. Growth chart for height for a boy with simple virilizing congenital adrenal hyperplasia. Note the accelerated growth velocity between age 2 and 4 yr before diagnosis. The growth velocity returned to normal after starting hydrocortisone treatment at age 4 yr. The rate of biological (bone age) maturation slowed after initiating treatment. G&P: Greulich and Pyle atlas, a standard bone age method for children and adolescents.

puberty in boys include: congenital adrenal hyperplasia (CAH), adrenal tumors, McCune–Albright Syndrome, testicular tumors, testotoxicosis, and GnRH secreting tumors *(4)*. With the exception of the rare GnRH secreting tumors, all causes of peripheral precocious puberty are associated with small testicles (<2.5 cm) or at least with a testicular size that is inconsistent with the degree of virilization; in contrast, central precocious puberty is associated with pubertal or adult size testicles. Based on the striking virilization in our patient and small testicles, it was thought that peripheral precocious puberty was the most likely cause. Because CAH is by far the most common cause of peripheral precocious puberty, an ACTH stimulation test was performed, the basal and post-ACTH 17-hydroxy-progesterone (17-OHP) levels were consistent with this diagnosis.

CAH is an inherited inability to synthesize cortisol and may be caused by defective transport of cholesterol into mitochondria (5,6) or, more commonly, by mutations in steroidogenic enzymes. More than 90% are caused by a deficiency of the 21-hydroxylase activity required to convert 17-hydroxyprogesterone to 11-deoxycortisol (7,8). CAH, due to 21-hydroxylase deficiency, occurs in a wide spectrum of clinical variants: a severely affected type with a concurrent defect in aldosterone, called "salt wasting form," a type with apparently normal aldosterone biosynthesis: "simple virilizing form," and a mild "nonclassic form" that may be asymptomatic or may be associated with mild signs of androgen excess developing during childhood or at puberty, ["late onset"] (9).

Our patient was diagnosed initially with "late onset" CAH, but we decided to change it to "simple virilizing form" of CAH. Why? Because there is no evidence or history of a salt wasting crisis, it is clear that he does not have the "salt wasting form." He presented with significant virilization early in life, which is a characteristic of the "simple virilizing form," but not of the "late onset form"; moreover, the robust increase in 17 OHP levels after ACTH stimulation is more consistent with the "simple virilizing form" than with the "late onset form" (10,11).

Recently, there has been a tendency to consider CAH owing to 21-hydroxylase deficiency as a continuum of disorders, rather than a disorder with discrete subtypes (12). Several large studies have shown good phenotype-genotype correlations (13,14). Specific mutations in the CYP21 gene (gene that encodes for 21-hydroxylase) have been associated with different phenotypes and enzyme activity. Mutations such as deletions or nonsense mutations that ablate enzyme activity are most often associated with salt-wasting disease. Ile172Asn, a missense mutation (15), yields an enzyme with 1–2% normal activity and is carried predominantly by patients with simple virilizing disease. Mutations such as Val281Leu and Pro30Leu (16,17) produce enzymes with 20–60% of normal activity and are most often associated with the nonclassical disorders.

What would have been the role of neonatal screening in our patient? The diagnosis of 21-OH deficiency can be made in some states in the United States by microfilter paper radioimmunoassay for 17-OH progesterone, similar to the existing screening programs for phenylketonuria and hypothyroidism (12). There are several obvious advantages of neonatal screening for CAH, such as earlier diagnosis, avoidance of salt crisis, and an early correct gender assignment (18). Because our patient is a nonsalt losing male, the only potential benefit of screening would have been the possibility of early diagnosis, although it would have been very difficult to differentiate the salt-wasting form from other forms without other diagnostic complement any tests such as genotyping (19,20). An early diagnosis in our patient would had guaranteed more careful surveillance, and very likely the disadvantages of severe virilization would have been minimized.

The problems associated with the treatment that our patient has had, including weight gain and high glucocorticoid dose illustrate some of the difficulties that most patients with CAH face. Adequate glucocorticoid therapy is needed to prevent signs and symptoms of androgen excess, but also to allow normal growth and pubertal maturation and fertility. In practice, the balance between overtreatment and undertreatment is quite complex. The suggested hydrocortisone dose range has been decreased in recent years to approximately 12–15 mg/m²/d as pediatric endocrinologists have become aware that higher glucocorticoid doses figured prominently in impaired linear growth *(21,22)*.

He has been receiving higher than average glucocorticoid doses for years, mainly because controlling the progression of his bone age and virilization has been a priority. Based on the physical findings and bone age at his last visit, we expect him to progress normally into puberty and to reach a normal adult height, although it is very unlikely that he will reach his mid-parental height (genetic potential). As stated by Blizzard *(23)*, there have been several reports showing that the adult height of patients with salt-wasting CAH and simple virilizing CAH, who are diagnosed early and treated properly are less than ideal or expected. There is some hope that in the near future the treatment for CAH patients will be improved. Several examples of this effort toward a better treatment are the NIH experimental multidrug regimen consisting of low-dose glucocorticoid, mineralocorticoid, androgen blocker (flutamide) and aromatase inhibitor (testolactone) *(24)*, and a recent study using carbenoxolone, an inhibitor of 11 β-hydroxysteroid dehydrogenase [an enzyme important for inactivating cortisol] *(25)*.

REFERENCES

1. Sklar CA, Kaplan SL, Grumbach MM. Evidence for dissociation between adrenarche and gonadarche: studies in patients with idiopathic precocious puberty, gonadal dysgenesis, isolated gonadotropin deficiency, and constitutional delayed growth and adolescence. J Clin Endocrinol Metab 1980;51:548–556.
2. Gell JS, Atkins B, Margraf L. Adrenarche is associated with decreased 3-beta-hydroxysteroid dehydrogenase expression in the adrenal reticularis. Endocr Res 1996;22:723–728.
3. Klein KO. Editorial: precocious puberty: who has it? Who should be treated? J Clin Endocrinol Metab 1999;84:412–414.
4. Kaplan SL, Grumbach MM. Pathogenesis of sexual precocity. In: Grumbach MM, Sizonenko PC, Aubert ML, eds. Control of the Onset of Puberty. Williams & Wilkins, Baltimore, MD, 1990, pp. 620–660.
5. Lin D, Sugawara T, Strauss JF III, Clark BJ, Stocco DM, Saenger P, Rogol A, Miller WL. Role of steroidogenic acute regulatory protein in adrenal and gonadal steroidogenesis. Science 1995;267:1828–1831.
6. Bose HS, Sugawara T, Strauss JF III, Miller WL. The pathophysiology and genetics of congenital lipod adrenal hyperplasia. N Engl J Med 1996;335:1870–1878.
7. White PC, Speiser PW. Congenital adrenal hyperplasia due to 21-hydroxylase deficiency. Endocr Rev 2000;21:245–291.
8. New MI. Diagnosis and management of congenital adrenal hyperplasia. Annu Rev Med 1998;49:311–328.
9. Speiser PW, White PC. Congenital adrenal hyperplasia due to steroid 21-hydroxylase deficiency. Clin Endocrinol 1998;49:411–417
10. Pang S. Congenital adrenal hyperplasia. Endocrinol Metab Clin N Am 1997;26:853–890.
11. New MI, Lorenzen F, Lerner A, et al. Genotyping steroid 21-hydroxylase deficiency: hormonal reference data. J Clin Endocrinol Metab 1983;57:320–325.
12. Therrell B, Berenbaum S, Manter-Kapanke V, et al. Result of screening 1.9 million Texas newborns for 21-hydroxylase deficient congenital adrenal hyperplasia. Pediatrics 1998;101:583–590.
13. Wedell A, Thilen A, Ritzen E, et al. Mutational spectrum of the steroid 21-hydroxylase gene in Sweden: implications for genetic diagnosis and association with disease manifestations. J Clin Endocrinol Metab 1994;78:1145–1152.
14. Krone N, Braun A, Roscher AA, et al. Predicting phenotype in steroid 21-hydroxylase deficiency? Comprehensive genotyping in 155 unrelated, well defined patients from southern Germany. J Clin Endocrinol Metab 2000;85:1059–1065.

15. Amor M, Parker KL, Globerman H, New MI, White PC. Mutation in the CYP21B gene (Ile-172—Asn) causes steroid 21-hydroxylase deficiency. Proc Natl Acad Sci USA 1998;85:1600–1604.

16. Speiser P, New M, White P. Molecular genetic analysis of nonclassic steroid 21-hydroxylase deficiency associated with HLA-B14, DR1. N Engl J Med 1988;90:584–595.

17. Tusie-Luna M, Speiser P, Dumic M, et al. A mutation (Pro-30 to Leu) in CYP21 represents a potential nonclassic steroid 21-hydroxylase deficiency allele. Mol Endocrinol 1991;5:685–692.

18. Thilen A, Nordenstrom A, Hagenfeldt L, et al. Benefits of neonatal screening for congenital adrenal hyperplasia (21-hydroxylase deficiency) in Sweden. Pediatrics 1988;81:866–874.

19. Nordenstrom A, Thilen A, Hagenfeldt L, et al. Genotyping is a valuable diagnostic complement to neonatal screening for congenital adrenal hyperplasia due to steroid 21-hydroxylase deficiency. J Clin Endocrinol Metab 1999;84:1505–1509.

20. Root AW. Editorial: neonatal screening for 21-hydroxylase deficient congenital adrenal hyperplasia-the role of CYP21 analysis. J Clin Endocrinol Metab 1999;84:1503–1504.

21. Girgis R, Winter J. The effect of glucocorticoid replacement therapy on growth, bone mineral density, and bone turnover markers in children with congenital adrenal hyperplasia. J Clin Endocrinol Metab 1997;82:3926–3929.

22. Silva I, Kater C, Cunha C, et al. Randomised controlled trial of growth effect of hydrocortisone in congenital adrenal hyperplasia. Arch Dis Child 1997;77:214–218.

23. Blizzard, R. Adult consequences of pediatric endocrine disease, I: congenital adrenal hyperplasia. Growth Gen Hormones 1999;15:33–41.

24. Merke DP, Keil MF, Jones JV, et al. Flutamide, testolactone and reduced hydrocortisone dose maintain normal growth velocity and bone maturation despite elevated androgen levels in children with congenital adrenal hyperplasia. J Clin Endocrinol Metab 2000;85:1114–1120.

25. Irony I, Cutler G. Effect of carbenoxolone on the plasma renin activity and hypothalamic-pituitary-adrenal axis in congenital adrenal hyperplasia due to 21-hydroxylase deficiency. Clin Endocrinol 1999; 51:285–291.

CASE #2: GROWTH HORMONE DEFICIENCY

Case Description

A 17-yr-old male initially presented to our pediatric endocrinology clinic at age 3.5 yr for the evaluation of short stature. The family history was positive for delayed puberty in both parents: mother's menarche was at age 15 yr and his father described himself as a "late bloomer"; he stopped growing at 21 yr. Father's height: 175 cm, mother's height: 163 cm. His 6-yr-old sister was of average height (50th percentile). There was no family history of endocrine disorders.

The birth history was normal: 40 wk pregnancy, uncomplicated vaginal delivery, APGAR 9-9, birth weight 3.8 kg, length: 50 cm. No neonatal problems; specifically, no history of hypoglycemia. His past medical history was relevant only for mild chronic constipation.

Physical examination at age 3.5 yr showed: height 85 cm (<5th percentile), height age 21 mo, weight 13.5 kg (50th percentile for weight/height), blood pressure 91/62 mmHg. He was described as a short, thin male with an immature face and frontal bossing, normal male genitalia, Tanner stage I, both testes descended.

The initial laboratory tests included: normal biochemistry screen, T4 11.6 mcg/dL, TSH 3.0 μU/mL, exercise growth hormone stimulation test peak = 3.6 ng/mL, insulin-induced hypoglycemia stimulation test peak = 9.8 ng/mL, arginine stimulation GH test peak = 16 ng/mL, bone age 2 yr. These were considered consistent with growth hormone sufficiency and the patient was considered to have constitutional delay of growth; careful follow-up evaluation by his pediatrician was recommended.

The patient was followed by his personal pediatrician, who saw him only occasionally, when he was sick. The growth pattern was not reassessed until age 10 yr, when it was considered abnormal. He was evaluated again for short stature in the pediatric endocrine clinic of the University of Virginia at age 10.6 yr. His mother stated that his growth rate was very slow; she was concerned about psychosocial problems at school because of his short stature (the smallest in class). At that time, his height was 121.0 cm (approximately −3 SD), height age 8 yr, bone age 7.6 yr, IGF1 61 ng/mL, T4 7.1 mcg/dL, TSH 1.96 µU/ mL, clonidine growth stimulation test peak = 11.7 ng/mL. Although he did not fail the growth hormone stimulation test, based on his significant short stature, physical appearance, and body fat distribution consistent with growth hormone deficiency, severely delayed bone age and low insulin-like growth factor 1 (IGF-1) level, it was decided to perform a 6-mo clinical trial with human recombinant growth hormone therapy.

During the 6-mo trial, the patient grew at an accelerated rate of 15.2 cm/yr. Although he did not have significant side effects from the treatment, his mother was concerned with the struggle associated with the daily injections. He started puberty at age 13 yr and his pubertal development has progressed normally. When he was 14 yr there was a 4-mo period of time when his growth velocity decreased significantly, very likely because of noncompliance with the medication.

Growth hormone (GH) therapy was continued for a total of 6 yr when chronological age was 16.9, height was 170.8 cm (virtually his height predicted from the midparental target height), genitalia and pubic hair was Tanner stage V and bone age was 16.9 yr (*see* Fig. 2). We explained to the patient and his parents the importance of being retested for GH deficiency in the near future to decide about the issue of adult GH deficiency. Although he did not seem to be very interested with the possibility of restarting daily injections, his parents did show interest in the metabolic benefits in case of GH deficiency as an adult.

Discussion

The parents of this patient presented with the very common concern of short stature. Interestingly, both parents had significant delayed puberty, which immediately seemed consistent with constitutional delay of growth. Because the patient had some clinical findings consistent with GH deficiency *(1–3)*, namely, frontal bossing, immature face, characteristic fat distribution, delayed bone age, significant short stature, and growth failure, it was decided to perform a GH stimulation test. Discouragingly, the GH stimulation test, as often happens, was not conclusive. Most pediatric endocrinologists use a cutoff level of 10 ng/mL to define a "normal response;" our patient's response was 9.8 ng/mL to insulin and 16 ng/mL to arginine. These were considered "normal," but careful follow-up by his pediatrician was recommended. Unfortunately, he was not formally reevaluated for growth failure until age 10.5 yr when he returned to our clinic.

There are at least two lessons from this patient's presentation. First, the single most important clinical manifestation of GH deficiency of all causes is growth failure. Second, GH testing is not infallible *(4,5)*. Careful documentation of the growth rate is critical to confirming the correct diagnosis. Very likely, with a more careful follow-up, he would have been referred sooner and treatment might have diminished the psychosocial problems of his perception of being extremely small.

The key difficulty of this case was making the diagnosis of GH deficiency. This difficulty results mainly from the lack of appropriate tools to reliably make (or exclude)

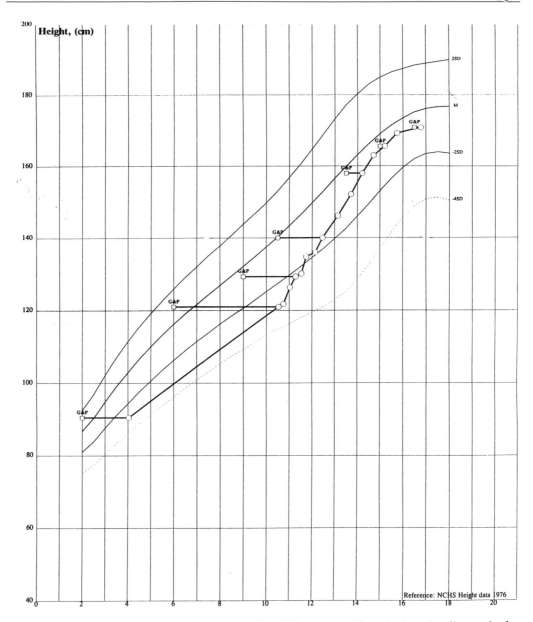

Fig. 2. Height growth chart of a boy "responsive" to GH treatment. Note the "catch up" growth after GH was started at age 10 and 9/12 yr. The growth rate was normal during puberty and the patient attained an adult height (170.8 cm) appropiate for his genetic potential (175 cm). G&P: Greulich and Pyle atlas, a standard bone age method for children and adolescents.

this diagnosis. A consensus view concluded that clinical assessment of the growth-retarded child is the single most useful parameter in diagnosing growth disorders and challenged the status of GH measurements as the diagnostic "gold standard" (6). In general, the diagnosis of impaired GH secretion can be confirmed only if subnormal GH secretion is observed during two tests. Insulin and arginine are the two most widely employed for this purpose *(7)*, exactly the two that we used in our patient. In essence, the issue is not biochemical growth hormone deficiency, but *responsiveness* to GH therapy.

The limitations of provocative GH testing include:

1. they are nonphysiological;
2. the cutoff level of "normal" is arbitrary;
3. they are age dependent, and the role of sex steroid administration has not been adequately defined, although it is known that priming prepubertal and peripubertal subjects with estrogen increases the likelihood that a normal child will have a normal response to a variety of stimuli;
4. they rely on GH assays of variably accuracy;
5. they are expensive, uncomfortable and carry some risks (mainly insulin-induced hypoglycemia);
6. their reproducibility has not been adequately documented *(6)*.

The second time we evaluated the patient, the most striking element was the growth chart; clearly, he was failing to grow. In addition, the bone age was severely delayed and the IGF-1 level was low. Nevertheless, the GH stimulation test was "normal," inconsistent with the clinical picture. Because the medical insurance company considered GH deficiency a biochemical diagnosis, GH therapy was initially denied. The first 6 mo of therapy ("proof of principle" and supported by one of the pharmaceutical manufacturers) convinced the insurance company that the patient was indeed GH responsive.

It is important to note that the psychological difficulties related to being very short, played a relevant role in our patient. Although GH deficiency in children has been associated with difficulties in psychosocial adjustment, including immaturity and difficulty in socializing, and with higher rates of academic underachievement; no specific psychiatric symptoms have been linked to this disorder *(8)*.

Finally, there is the issue of retesting for GH deficiency in the transition from adolescence to adulthood *(9)*. It is understandable that our patient did not like the idea of restarting daily injections, but the potential benefits are significant *(10,11)*. Patients with GH deficiency and congenital hypothalamic–pituitary abnormalities probably do not need to retested, because the condition is generally permanent *(12)*. On the other hand, patients without pathologic (organic) disease should have a stimulation test because a significant percentage will no longer be GH deficient *(13)*. The metabolic effects of GH replacement therapy in adults with GH deficiency include: increase in lean body or fat-free mass, decrease in fat mass, increase in bone mineral density, decrease in total cholesterol, increase in HDL cholesterol, decrease in LDL cholesterol and decrease in triglycerides *(14,15)*; i.e., a more favorable cardiovascular lipid profile.

REFERENCES

1. Wit JM, Van Unen H. Growth of infants with neonatal growth hormone deficiency. Arch Dis Child 1992;67:920–924.
2. Gluckman PD, Gunn AJ, Wray A, et al. Congenital idiopathic growth hormone deficiency associated with prenatal and early postnatal growth failure. J Pediatr 1992;121:920–923.
3. DeLuca F, Bernasconi S, Blandino A, et al. Auxological, clinical and neuroradiological findings in infants with early onset growth hormone deficiency. Acta Paediatr Scand 1995;84:561–565.
4. Reiter E, Martha P. Pharmacological testing of growth hormone secretion. Horm Res 1990;33:121–127.
5. Price DA. GH testing in KIGS: the clinical reality. In: Ranke MB, Wilton P, eds. Growth Hormone Therapy in KIGS-10 Years' Experience. Huthig GmbH, Heidelberg-Leipzig, Germany, 1999, pp. 73–80.

6. Rosenfeld RG, Albertsson-Wikland K, Cassorla F, et al. Diagnostic controversy: the diagnosis of child-hood growth hormone deficiency revisited. J Clin Endocrinol Metab 1995;80:1232–1540.

7. Raiti S, Davis WT, Blizzard RM. A comparison of the effects of insulin hypoglycemia and arginine infusion on release of human growth hormone. Lancet 1967;2:1182–1183.

8. Allen D. Childhood growth hormone (GH) deficiency: statural and psychological effects of long-term GH replacement. The Endocrinologist 1998;8:3S–7S.

9. Van den Broeck J, Hering P, Van de Lely A, et al. Interpretative difficulties with growth hormone provocative retesting in childhood-onset growth hormone deficiency. Horm Res 1999;51:1–9.

10. Kleinberg D, Melmed S. The adult growth hormone deficiency syndrome: signs, symptoms and diag-nosis. The Endocrinologist 1998;8:8S–14S.

11. Ter Maaten J, de Boer H, Kamp O, et al. Long-term effect of growth hormone (GH) replacement in men with childhood-onset GH deficiency. J Clin Endocrinol Metab 1999;84:2373–2380.

12. Maghnie M, Strigazzi C, Tinelli C, et al. Growth hormone (GH) deficiency (GHD) of childhood onset: reassessment of GH status and evaluation of the predictive criteria for permanent GHD in young adults. J Clin Endocrinol Metab 1999;84:1324–1328.

13. Vance M, Mauras N. Growth hormone therapy in adults and children. N Engl J Med 1999;341: 1206–1216.

14. Beshyah S, Henderson A, Niththyananthan R, et al. The effects of short and long-term growth hormone replacement therapy in hypopituitary adults on lipid metabolism and carbohydrate tolerance. J Clin Endocrinol Metab 1995;80:356–363.

15. Baum H, Biller B, Finkelstein J, et al. Effects of physiologic growth hormone therapy on bone density and body composition in patients with adult-onset growth hormone deficiency: a randomized, placebo-controlled trial. Ann Intern Med 1996;125:883–890.

CASE #3: HYPOPITUITARISM FROM SUPRASELLAR MASS

Case Description

This 12-yr-old female presented in December 1998 at age 11 yr to her personal oph-thalmologist with decreased visual acuity of 6 wk duration. She was diagnosed with myopia at age 8 yr when corrective lenses were prescribed for the first time. The myopia had been stable and her glasses were changed only once since the initial prescription. However, her father recently noticed that she was sitting closer to the computer screen, television set, or to a book that she was reading. She had only occasional mild headaches, which resolved after eating. There was no history of vomiting, polyuria, polydipsia, weight gain or loss, behavioral problems, or changes in school performance. The growth rate was considered to be normal.

Family history was unremarkable. Mother's height was 167 cm and she was healthy. Father's height was 183 cm and also was healthy. One brother, 4 yr old, was of average height (50th percentile). There was no family history of endocrine disorders. The birth history was normal: gestational age 40 wk; birth weight 3.4 kg; length 50 cm; no neonatal problems. She was not receiving any medication.

The ophthalmologist found no change in the refractive error, but noticed temporal visual field defects bilaterally, decreased central acuity and optic atrophy. A magnetic resonance imaging (MRI) study of the brain showed an 18 × 19 mm lobular suprasellar mass, with homogeneous contrast enhancement and extension along the anterior and pos-terior segments of the optic nerves. The appearance of the mass was considered consis-tent with a glioma arising in the optic chiasm or hypothalamus. The patient was referred to our pediatric endocrine clinic as part of the preoperative evaluation.

The first visit in our clinic was 1 wk after the ophthalmologist had evaluated her. Physi-cal examination showed: Height 134.6 cm (5th–10th percentile), height age 9.6 yr, weight

30.3 kg (50th percentile for weight/height), and blood pressure 95/57 mmHg. She was very cooperative and interactive. The skin was normal to inspection and without nodules. Lymph nodes in neck, axilla, and groin were not enlarged. Her neck was symmetric and her thyroid was not enlarged. Oropharynx, mouth, nose, and throat were normal. Lungs were clear to auscultation. Her heart had a normal rate and rhythm and no murmurs. Her abdomen was soft, nontender, and without masses. Her extremities were symmetric with normal motion. The neurologic evaluation was normal except for diminished eyesight bilaterally and abnormal confrontational examination consistent with the previous ophthalmologic findings. Breast and pubic hair were Tanner stage I.

The initial laboratory tests included: TSH 7.75 µU/mL, T4 4.6 mcg/dL, T3 uptake 35%, prolactin 28.8 ng/mL, LH <0.5 IU/L, FSH <0.5 IU/L, cortisol <1 mcg/dL, IGF-1 40 ng/mL, α-subunit 0.2 ng/mL. The bone age was 8.10 yr.

Based on the imminent stress associated with surgery and nondetectable levels of cortisol, hydrocortisone acetate (5 mg tid) was started. In January 1999, she underwent surgery (open biopsy) without complications for which she received stress doses of glucocorticoids. During the first week postsurgery, the patient developed diabetes insipidus and hypothyroidism; consequently oral DDAVP (0.1 mg/d) and thyroxine (75 mcg/d) were started.

Histologic exam of the removed tumor tissue was consistent with a hypothalamic germinoma; the patient received both radiation therapy (3600 cGy to the suprasellar region, the "involved field" over 1 mo in 20 fractions) and chemotherapy consisting of vincristine, cisplatin, etoposide, and cyclophosphamide. Six months after surgery, her growth rate was 1.2 cm/yr, IGF-1: 44 ng/mL, and IGFBP3: 1.4 ng/mL. A GH stimulation test (arginine and L-dopa) showed a GH peak of 0.4 mg/mL. The patient was considered growth hormone deficient (now panhypopituitarism) and GH therapy was started.

The most recent visit was at age 12.1 yr; she was free of symptoms and compliant with her medications including: GH (0.3 mg/kg/wk), oral DDAVP (0.05 mg/d), hydrocortisone acetate 5 mg bid, and thyroxine (75 mcg/d). Her general appearance was very good and she was full of energy. Her height was 138 cm (5th–10th percentile), height age 10.5 yr, growth rate 12 cm/yr (based on the last 3 mo), weight 31.2 kg (25th–50th percentile for weight/height), and bone age 10.6 yr. Her physical exam was unremarkable with normal vision and neurological examination. Breast and pubic hair were Tanner stage I. A head MRI was within normal limits.

Discussion

This patient illustrates the differential diagnosis of brain tumors in children and the endocrinological consequences of them. Our patient presented with a frequent manifestation of brain tumors, visual disturbance (1). The differential diagnosis of decreased visual acuity in children is not large and should always include the possibility of brain tumors. Midline supratentorial tumors are more likely to produce vision abnormalities than tumors in other sites (2). Our patient was fortunate that a proper evaluation by her personal physician led to a rapid diagnosis of the suprasellar mass with involvement of the optic nerves and optic chiasm as the cause of her visual complaints. Although the prognosis for pediatric brain tumors, in general, is much better than for adults, the earliest possible diagnosis can be critical to achieving the best outcome (3).

What was the differential diagnosis of this tumor? Midline supratentorial tumors represent approximately 15% of all pediatric brain tumors; among them, the three most common are craniopharyngioma (5%), low-grade glioma (5%) and germ cell tumors (2%) *(4)*. Most children with craniopharyngiomas present with symptoms owing to increased intracranial pressure, including headaches, vomiting and oculomotor abnormalities, as well as growth failure. Usually, the MRI shows cystic and solid components of the tumor *(5)*. Because neither the clinical presentation, nor the radiologic findings were consistent with a craniopharyngioma, it was not considered likely as the initial diagnosis. In this particular patient, the absence of clinically evident diabetes insipidus (the most common presenting abnormality in suprasellar germinomas), statistics and the MRI description favored the possibility of glioma rather than germinoma. However, our current understanding of CNS germinomas may be limited because most of the information is based on historical data that included patients without a histologically confirmed diagnosis. In the past, many institutions utilized a trial of radiation therapy as a means of "radiodiagnosis and treatment," and no tissue for histologic diagnosis was obtained *(6)*.

This patient is a good example that obtaining pathologic confirmation is imperative in the management of pediatric patients with brain tumors. Although some experts consider that most patients with optic chiasmal gliomas present clinical and radiological features sufficiently characteristic to obviate the need of biopsy *(7)*, it would have been a major mistake not to perform a biopsy in our patient. Although the histopathology of a pediatric brain tumor sometimes can be predicted from its appearance and location on diagnostic imaging, at present, the consensus is that tissue diagnosis is required to establish a correct diagnosis and to offer the best treatment possible *(2,4)*.

There are special considerations in a growing child with a suprasellar germinoma. Although germinomas are highly radio-sensitive tumors *(8,9)* and the results with craniospinal irradiation are excellent, with a 10 yr relapse-free survival rates of approximately 90% *(10,11)*; significant concerns regarding late effects of this specific radiation have decreased its utility only to special cases *(12)*. Delayed skeletal growth, impaired neurocognitive skills and hormonal deficiencies can occur as a result of craniospinal irradiation *(13–15)*. Our patient received neoadjuvant chemotherapy followed by "involved field" radiotherapy with the purpose of minimizing the radiation dose and volume. Matsutani et al. *(16)* treated seven patients with intracranial germ cell tumors with three courses of chemotherapy followed by involved-field radiation; all had a complete response following chemotherapy alone. At a median follow-up of 4.3 yr, all patients are alive without recurrence. Other investigators have shown similar outcomes using involved-field radiotherapy combined with chemotherapy *(17–19)*. This protocol is now the first line treatment for intracranial germinomas in most cases.

Although some damage to the hypothalamic–pituitary unit of our patient was likely to be caused by the combination of the biopsy procedure, chemotherapy, and radiation therapy, we have to assume that there was tumor infiltration and damage to this area prior to surgery, since cortisol insufficiency was documented in the preoperative evaluation. Progression of the neuroendocrine dysfunction was expected and careful follow-up permitted replacement of all the pituitary hormones, including GH, soon after surgery. It has been shown that multiple factors contribute to poor growth after treatment of childhood brain tumors, including radiation to the hypothalamic–pituitary axis, spinal irradiation and chemotherapy *(20,21)*. These facts enhance the importance of frequent and accurate measurement of the growth velocity to facilitate early initiation of growth hormone therapy and optimization of adult height in this specific population *(22)*.

Because the patient was 12 yr old at the most recent visit, it would be important to evaluate her hypothalamic–pituitary–ovarian axis soon. If gonadotropins are absent, she will require estrogen therapy to induce feminization. Considering that her bone age is almost the same as her height age, we expect her to reach an adult height close to the 50th percentile. The time at which estrogen is started should be decided after informed discussion with the patient and her parents; however, a reasonable age to start estrogen would be at age 13 yr when her bone age will be close to 11 1/2 yr. Ross et al. *(23)* reported a beneficial psychological role for estrogen replacement therapy initiated at a relatively physiological age (12–14 yr) in patients with Turner syndrome. Conjugated estrogens, if needed, will be started in a low dose (0.15–0.3 mg/d) and increased gradually to a maintenance dose of 0.625 mg/d. Progestin therapy will be added, either when the first breakthrough bleeding occurs or in the second or third year of therapy.

REFERENCES

1. Pollack IF. Brain tumors in children. N Engl J Med 1994;331:1501–1507.
2. Robertson PL. Pediatric brain tumors. Endocrinol Metab Clin N Am 1999;28:323–339.
3. Albright AL. Pediatric brain tumors. Cancer J Clin 1993;43:272–288.
4. Pollack IF. Pediatric brain tumors. Semin Surg Oncol 1999;16:73–90.
5. Freda PU, Post KD. Differential diagnosis of sellar masses. Endocrinol Metab Clin N Am 1999;28:81–117.
6. Kuttesch JF. The Paulino/Wen/Mohideen article reviewed. Oncology 1999;13:529–530.
7. Jacobson DM. Gliomas of the anterior visual pathways. Neurosurg Clin N Am 1999;10:683–698.
8. Paulino AC, Wen BC, Mohideen MN. Controversies in the management of intracranial germinomas. Oncology 1999;3:513–521.
9. Huh SJ, Shin KH, Kim IH, et al. Radiotherapy of intracranial germinomas. Radiother Oncol 1996;38: 19–23.
10. Aoyama H, Shirato H, Kakuto Y, et al. Pathologically-proven intracranial germinoma treated with radiation therapy. Radiother Oncol 1998;47:201–205.
11. Dearnaley DP, A'Hern RP, Whittaker S, et al. Pineal and CNS germ cell tumors: Royal Marsden Hospital experience 1962–1987. Int J Radiat Oncol Biol Phys 1990;18:773–781.
12. Duffner PK, Horowitz ME, Krischer JP, et al. Postoperative chemotherapy and delayed radiation in children less than 3 yr of age with malignant brain tumors. N Engl J Med 1993;328:1725–1731.
13. Ellenberg L, McComb JG, Siegel, SE, et al. Factors affecting intellectual outcome in pediatric brain tumor patients. Neurosurg 1987;21:638–644.
14. Radcliffe J, Packer RJ, Atkins TE, et al. Three-and four-year cognitive outcome in children with non-cortical brain tumors treated with whole-brain radiotherapy. Ann Neurol 1992;32:551–554.
15. Duffner PK, Cohen ME, Voorhess ML, et al. Long-term effects of cranial irradiation on endocrine function in children with brain tumors. A prospective study. Cancer 1985;56:2189–2193.
16. Matsutani M, Sano K, Takakura K, et al. Combined treatment with chemotherapy and radiation therapy for intracranial germ cell tumors. Child's Nerv Syst 1998;14:59–62.
17. Sawamura Y, Shirato H, Ikeda J, et al. Induction chemotherapy followed by reduced-volume radiation therapy for newly diagnosed CNS germinoma. J Neurosurg 1998;66–72.
18. Baranzelli MC, Patte C, Bouffet E, et al. Nonmetastatic intracranial germinoma: the experience of the French Society of Pediatric Oncology. Cancer 1997;80: 1792–1797.
19. Calaminus G, Bamberg M, Baranzelli MC, et al. Intracranial germ cell tumors: a comprehensive update of the european data. Neuropediatrics 1994;25:26–32.
20. Livesey EA, Hindmarsh PC, Brook CG, et al. Endocrine disorders following treatment of childhood brain tumors. Br J Cancer 1990;61:622–625.
21. Donahue B. Short- and long-term complications of radiation therapy pediatric brain tumors. Pediatr Neurosurg 1992;18:207–217.
22. Clarson CL, Del Maestro RF. Growth failure after treatment of pediatric brain tumors. Pediatrics 1999; 103(3):E37.
23. Ross JL, McCauley E, Roeltgen D, et al. Self-concept and behavior in adolescent girls with Turner syndrome: potential estrogen effects. J Clin Endocrinol Metab 1996;81:926–931.

CASE #4: SHORT STATURE OWING TO SARCOIDOSIS

Case Description

A 12 and 5/12-yr-old female with sarcoidosis presented for evaluation of short stature. A definitive diagnosis of sarcoidosis was made at 11 yr of age by histologic examination of a skin biopsy. Between the ages of 3 and 11 yr, she received daily systemic glucocorticoids (prednisone, 10–25 mg/d) to control skin and pulmonary manifestations of this retrospectively diagnosed condition.

At age 6 yr, she developed blurred vision and photophobia, was diagnosed with anterior uveitis and treated with topical corticosteroids. At age 11 yr, she underwent emergency corneal transplant surgery secondary to corneal ulcers. During this admission (corneal transplant), a skin biopsy showed noncaseating granulomas consistent with sarcoidosis; at that time it was also necessary to start antidepressive medication (fluoxetine hydrochloride, Prozac). After age 11 yr she has been receiving inhaled and topical (ocular) glucocorticoids and very occasional short cycles of systemic glucocorticoids for pulmonary exacerbations.

At age 12 yr, she had two tonic-clonic seizures; the evaluation was negative, including a cranial MRI with emphasis on the hypothalamic–pituitary unit. Carbamazepine therapy was started. During this admission, bilateral posterior subcapsular cataracts were documented, likely due to previous steroid use. At age 12 and 5/12 yr, she was referred for evaluation of short stature because her growth rate was only 1.6 cm/yr (over the last 2.5 yr) and she was the shortest adolescent in her class at school.

Her maternal grandmother raised her. Mother's height was 173 cm and she was healthy. No information is available on her father. She does not have brothers or sisters and there is no family history of endocrine disorders. Pregnancy and delivery were reported to be normal.

Physical exam at chronological age of 12 and 5/12 yr showed: height 126.2 cm (<-4 SDS), height age 8 yr, weight 25.7 kg (50th–75th percentiles for weight/height), and blood pressure 92/58 mmHg. She did not have Cushingoid features. Her skin was dry with multiple reddish, flaky macules on her back, chest, and extremities. Bilateral cataracts did not permit a proper funduscopic examination. The heart rhythm was normal and no murmurs were noted but there were mild crackles in both lung bases. Her abdomen was soft and nontender. Breast and pubic hair were Tanner stage I.

Initial laboratory evaluation included: T4 11.0 mcg/dL, TSH 1.6 µU/mL, IGF-1 40 ng/mL, IGFBP-3 1.4 mg/L, LH <0.5 IU/L, FSH 2.3 IU/L, prolactin 12.6 ng/mL, cortisol 9.5 mcg/dL, Na 143 mEq/L, K 4.6 mEq/L. After 7 h of water deprivation, serum osmolality was 285 mOsmol/kg and urine osmolality was 576 mOsmol/kg. The bone age was 6 and 3/12 yr.

A clonidine stimulation test showed a GH peak of 1.7 ng/mL, consistent with GH deficiency. Six months after GH replacement was started, the growth rate was 14 cm/yr, a remarkable "catch up" growth. The TSH was 3.58 µU/mL, and T4 was 4.9 mcg/dL; it was decided to start thyroxine replacement.

She started puberty at age 16 yr, and had menarche at age 18. At that time height was 157.6 cm (10th–25th percentile), and weight was 75.2 kg, and she decided to discontinue GH therapy. Her main concern was excessive weight gain; consequently caloric intake restriction and regular exercise were recommended.

The most recent visit was at age 20 yr; she was free of symptoms and compliant with her medications, including thyroxine (75 mcg/d), carbamazepine (600 mg/d) and Prozac (20 mg/d). Her height was 160.4 cm and her weight was 76.7 kg.

Discussion

This patient illustrates the difficulties in the evaluation of growth in children with chronic diseases receiving glucocorticoids. In general, children with chronic disease have a tendency to be short and to have delayed puberty. On the other hand, any child, including chronically ill patients, with an abnormally slow growth velocity, should be evaluated carefully, and the possibility of GH deficiency must be addressed.

Sarcoidosis is a systemic disorder of unknown etiology. Although our patient had clinical manifestations of sarcoidosis in multiple organs since age 3 yr, the diagnosis was not certain until a skin biopsy was performed. The current recommendation is to confirm by biopsy all suspected cases to exclude infectious or malignant conditions *(1)*. After approximately 8 yr of supraphysiologic glucocorticoid therapy, the patient was referred for evaluation of short stature. The key elements to consider were the effects of a systemic chronic disease and glucocorticoid therapy on growth, but also the possibility of hypo-thalamic–pituitary invasion.

The effects of glucocorticoid therapy on linear growth are well known *(2,3)*, but the pathogenesis of growth suppression is complex and multifactorial. Glucocorticoids inhibit bone formation directly through the inhibition of osteoblast function *(4)* and indirectly by decreasing sex steroid secretion, attenuate GH secretion *(5)*, and inhibit IGF-1 activity *(6)*. In our patient, the glucocorticoids might have contributed to stunted growth. However, between 10 yr and 12 and 1/2 yr her annual growth rate was only 1.6 cm/yr despite not receiving any steroids.

Neurosarcoidosis has been reported to affect between 5–10% of all patients with sarcoidosis *(7,8)*. Hyperprolactinemia and diabetes insipidus are relatively common findings of adults with hypothalamic sarcoidosis, but hypothalamic involvement is uncommon in children *(9)*. However, considering that at age 12 and 5/12 yr the height was <-4 SDS, bone age was 6 and 3/12 yr, the growth velocity was subnormal (1.6 cm/yr) and there was a history of seizures, evaluation of the hypothalamic–pituitary unit was mandatory. The GH stimulation test was consistent with the clinical diagnosis of GH deficiency. Moreover, the robust "catch up" growth after GH therapy was started was proof of GH deficiency. Interestingly, despite indirect evidence of CNS involvement (seizures and growth hormone deficiency), a cranial MRI was reported normal. MRI scanning is highly sensitive, with CNS abnormalities detected in 31 of 34 patients with neurosarcoidosis when two large series are combined *(10,11)*.

Six months after GH therapy, TSH levels increased from 1.6 μU/mL to 3.58 μU/mL, and T4 levels decreased from 11.0 mcg/dL to 4.9 mcg/dL. The discussion at that time was whether to start thyroxine therapy or not. Because our patient had proven neurosarcoidosis and there have been reports of hypothalamic hypothyroidism in patients with neurosarcoidosis *(12)*, the risk-benefit ratio was considered to be in favor of starting treatment. The patient appears to have had a beneficial effect of 75 mcg/d of levothyroxine.

The clinical manifestations of sarcoidosis were more significant between 3–11 yr of age in our patient. It is not known why some patients recover spontaneously, whereas others worsen or relapse even after apparent recovery *(13,14)*. The presence of sarcoidosis in young children as well as seizures are associated with poorer prognosis *(15,16)*; thus, careful long-term follow-up is warranted in our patient.

Although multiple factors influence eating and satiety *(17)*, the excessive weight in our patient may be related with hypothalamic dysfunction, but there is no evidence to support this association. Unfortunately, despite good control of her depression and recommendations to eat healthier and exercise regularly, she continues gaining weight even knowing that her linear growth is virtually finished.

REFERENCES

1. Newman LS, Rose CS, Maier LA. Medical progress: sarcoidosis. N Engl J Med 1997;336:1224–1234.
2. Allen DB. Growth suppression by glucocorticoid therapy. Endocrinol Metab Clin N Am 1996;25:699–717.
3. Hanania NA, Chapman KR, Kesten S. Adverse effects of inhaled corticosteroids. Am J Med 1995;98:196–208.
4. Locascio V, Bonucci E, Imbimbo B. Bone loss in response to long-term glucocorticoid therapy. Bone Miner 1990;8:39–51.
5. Guistina A, Wehrenberg WB. The role of glucocorticoids in the regulation of growth hormone secretion-mechanisms and clinical significance. Trends Endocrinol Metab 1992;3:306–311.
6. Unterman T, Phillips LS. Glucocorticoid effects on somatomedins and somatomedin inhibitors. J Clin Endocrinol Metab 1985;61:618–626.
7. Scott TF. Neurosarcoidosis: progress and clinical aspects. Neurol 1993;43:8–12.
8. Sharma OP, Sharma AM. Sarcoidosis of the nervous system. A clinical approach. Arch Int Med 1991;151:1317–1321.
9. Milman N, Hoffman AL, Big K-E. Sarcoidosis in children. Epidemiology in Danes, clinical features, diagnosis, treatment and prognosis. Acta Pediatr 1998;87:871–878.
10. Sherman JL, Stern BJ, Sarcoidosis of the CNS: comparison of unenhanced and enhanced MR images. AJR 1990;155:1293–1301.
11. Miller DH, Kendall BE, Barter S, et al. Magnetic resonance imaging in central nervous system sarcoidosis. Neurology 1988;38:378–383.
12. Campbell IW, Short AI, Douglas AC. Hypothalamic manifestations of sarcoidosis with particular reference to hypothalamic hypothyroidism. In: Jones Williams W, Davies BH, eds. Sarcoidosis. Alpha & Omega, Cardiff, Wales, 1980, p. 579.
13. Marcille R, McCarthy M, Barton JW, et al. Long-term outcome of pediatric sarcoidosis with emphasis on pulmonary status. Chest 1992;102:1444–1449.
14. DeRemee RA. Sarcoidosis. Mayo Clin Proc 1995;70:177–181.
15. Hafner R, Vogel P. Sarcoidosis of early onset. A challenge for the pediatric rheumatologist. Clin Exp Rheumatol 1993;11:685–691.
16. Chadelat KC, Baculard MD, Grimfeld A, et al. Pulmonary sarcoidosis in children: serial evaluation of bronchoalveolar lavage cells during corticosteroid treatment. Pediatr Pulmonol 1993;16:41–47.
17. Leibowitz SF. Neurochemical-neuroendocrine systems in the brain controlling macronutrient intake and metabolism. Trend Neurosci 1992;15:491–497.

ACKNOWLEDGMENTS

The authors would like to thank Pharmacia & Upjohn for the use of the KIGS program to plot the growth charts.

22 Multiple Endocrine Neoplasia Syndromes

Kelly L. Wirfel, MD, Douglas B. Evans, MD, Jeffery E. Lee, MD, Helmuth Goepfert, MD, and Robert F. Gagel, MD

CONTENTS

CASE #1: WHAT IS THE APPROPRIATE MANAGEMENT OF AN OLDER PATIENT FOUND TO BE AT RISK FOR MEDULLARY THYROID CARCINOMA?

Case Description

An 80-yr-old white man who had been treated for primary hypothyroidism presented for evaluation of possible medullary thyroid carcinoma (MTC). His sister, diagnosed with thyroid cancer in the 1970s, had undergone thyroidectomy for MTC. When the MTC recurred in 1998, she was found to have a germline *RET* protooncogene mutation involving codon 618 (cys→phe, TGC→TTC). Her son and our patient were subsequently found to have the same mutation. Further family history included that of a maternal aunt who died of an unknown thyroid carcinoma.

An ultrasonogram showed a 1.2-cm thyroid nodule without evidence of lymphadenopathy, and fine needle aspiration of the nodule confirmed medullary thyroid carcinoma. Calcium, intact parathyroid hormone (PTH), and 24-h urine analysis for catecholamines and metanephrines were normal, thereby excluding hyperparathyroidism and pheochromocytoma. Carcinoembryonic antigen (CEA) was 5.6 ng/mL (normal range, 0–3 ng/mL). Otherwise healthy for his age, our patient suffered only from mild depression related to

From: *Contemporary Endocrinology: Challenging Cases in Endocrinology*
Edited by: M. E. Molitch © Humana Press Inc., Totowa, NJ

the recent death of his spouse from pancreatic cancer, and symptoms of benign prostatic hypertrophy. His concern about malignancy prompted an initial decision to undergo thyroidectomy, but he later reversed this decision. Subsequently, his daughter had surgery for MTC, and she has tried to persuade him to do the same, as she experienced great relief of anxiety after the tumor was removed.

Discussion

This older patient poses several unique questions. Given his advanced age, what should the treatment recommendations be and what is his risk of dying from MTC? Does this particular mutation hold a higher or lower risk of tumor progression and death than other mutations? What is the optimal evaluation and follow-up in this unusual case?

Addressing these questions may begin with the first point, that an age of 80 yr is no longer unusual. In 1980, the average age of death of white males was 70.9 yr *(1)* and by 1998 it had increased to 74.5 yr *(2)*. The changes in longevity have affected management of a wide spectrum of diseases. One example is the experience with primary hyperparathyroidism. Previously, many older patients were merely observed in the belief that the risk of surgery was higher than the perceived benefits. Given a rising life expectancy, and evidence that surgical treatment increases bone mass and may alleviate other subtle symptoms, recommendations for surgery have changed. Currently, many elderly patients over age 70 yr are treated surgically for hyperparathyroidism with low risk, minimal mortality, high cure rates, and short hospital stays *(3)*. Older patients suffer from more advanced disease, are at higher risk of hypercalcemic crisis, and are affected more commonly than younger patients by mental impairment related to hyperparathyroidism. Therefore, surgical cure may offer them relief of these symptoms.

The opposing viewpoint is that MTC in this patient appears to be a relatively benign process, unlikely to cause death or significant morbidity at his age. Two lines of evidence support the latter viewpoint. The first and most compelling is that germline mutations occur in 6–8% of cases of apparently sporadic MTC, and evaluation of these families has shown numerous examples of individuals with germline mutations who died from other causes *(4)*. A second piece of evidence that argues for limited progression of MTC concerns survival statistics of patients with Multiple Endocrine Neoplasia type 2A (MEN 2A). A number of studies have shown that no more than 20% of patients with MEN 2A actually die from metastatic MTC *(5,6)* (see Figs. 1 and 2). When these observations are combined, an argument can be made that our patient's risk of death from MTC is small.

Our patient is 80-yr-old and in excellent health. Both of his parents died in their nineties, which makes it reasonable to believe that our patient could remain healthy for another 10–15 yr. The major question then becomes; what is the probability that the 1.2-cm focus of MTC in his thyroid will metastasize or cause local-regional symptoms before he dies a natural death?

An important factor in the decision regarding thyroidectomy is the aggressiveness of MTC caused by a codon 618 mutation of the *RET* protooncogene. The discovery of the *RET* protooncogene mutation in 1993 and subsequent analysis of the clinical behavior of specific mutations provides another method for assessing the potential for tumor progression in this patient. For example, there is convincing evidence that a codon 918 mutation, be it germline or acquired through somatic mutation, is associated with the most aggressive MTC *(7)*. Mutations in codons 618, 634, 611, 620, and 891 are considered high risk because metastases have been found in some children with these mutations.

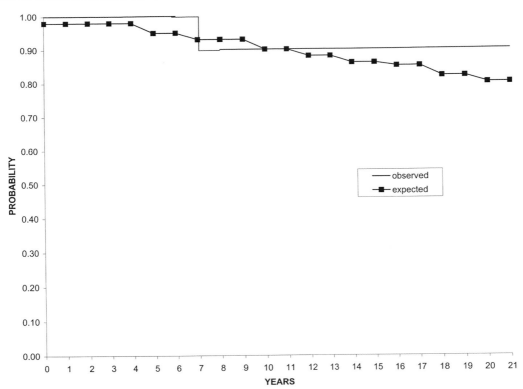

Fig. 1. Survival to last follow-up (death) of 18 patients with multiple endocrine neoplasia type 2A. Statistical analysis according to Kaplan-Meier method. (Adapted from ref. *(6)* with permission from Cancer.)

Intermediate risk has been ascribed to patients with mutations of codons 609, 768, 790, 791, and 804; these tumors have variable biologic behavior but are considered to be the least aggressive mutations (Discussions at the Seventh International Workshop on Multiple Endocrine Neoplasia). Further experience will be necessary to show definitive effects on survival. Our patient's codon 618 mutation appears to have an atypical biologic behavior resulting from his early stage of disease and his advanced age.

A final factor in the decision-making process is the estimated life expectancy of this patient. A life insurance analysis of survival in a normal 80-yr-old man predicts an average survival of 10 yr, a reasonable estimate in this healthy man (see Fig. 3). Given that death related to intrathyroidal MTC in MEN 2A in two large series *(5,6)* rarely exceeded 20% over a 25–30-yr period, one could infer that the risk of death from MTC in this patient before he dies of natural causes is less than 10%. In contrast, as shown in Fig. 2, an individual who is 50 yr old is likely to have a much greater probability of death from a tumor of the same size, simply because of longer life expectancy.

Another consideration is the risk of death or morbidity related to surgery. The risks of anesthesia and surgical mortality of thyroidectomy in elderly patients are difficult to document definitively, but they appear to be low and based on underlying co-morbidities, extent of surgery, and expertise of the surgeon *(8)*. For total thyroidectomy, the risk of recurrent laryngeal nerve injury and/or hypoparathyroidism ranges from 1–14%, but in

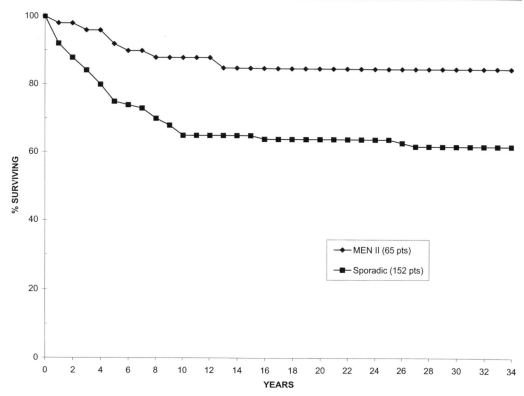

Fig. 2. Survival rate of patients with MTC associated with multiple endocrine neoplasia, type 2 and those with sporadic MTC ($p < 0.005$). (Adapted from ref. 5 with permission from The Endocrine Society.)

major medical centers it is routinely less than 1% *(8–11)*. The incidence of permanent recurrent laryngeal nerve palsy, defined as persistence of paralysis for greater than 6 mo, ranges from 0.5%–4.8% *(10–12)* calculated for nerves at risk but again in major medical centers is less than 0.5% *(8)*.

A reasonable approach, given the low probability that he will die or incur major morbidity from MTC combined with his current reluctance to undergo surgery, is to perform periodic (6–12-mo) ultrasound examinations of the thyroid gland and serial calcitonin and CEA measurements. Because this patient's major concern is local tumor progression, his decision to forego surgery could be reversed if there were evidence of significant growth.

In summary, this case highlights some of the issues involved in the decision to perform surgery for indolent MTC in an older patient. The major determinants include: mutation-specific biologic behavior of the tumor, and the life expectancy of this patient. This is a healthy elderly patient with familial MTC whose particular mutation is in a more aggressive category. However, the overall survival rate of patients with MTC is approximately 90% at 10–20 yr. The risks of surgery in this elderly patient could result in significant morbidity, and, once all factors are considered, the decision depends on the patient's comfort level with observing a cancer. If observation is preferred, reasonable follow-up can be arranged to monitor the tumor's stability and detect changes that may sway the decision toward surgery.

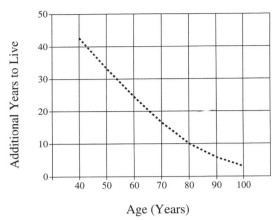

Age (Years)

Fig. 3. Life insurance analysis of estimated survival based on Annuity 2000 Mortality table, National Association of Insurance Commissioners, and created by the Society of Actuaries: http://data.insure. com/life/chances.cfm

REFERENCES

1. Statistical Yearbook. 43rd Issue. United Nations, New York 1999, 79–86.
2. Murphy SL. Deaths: final data for 1998. National Vital Statistics Report 2000;48:1–105.
3. Chen H, Parkerson S, Udelsman R. Parathyroidectomy in the elderly: do the benefits outweigh the risks? World J Surg 1998;22:531–536.
4. Wohllk N, Cote GJ, Bugalho MMJ, et al. Relevance of RET proto-oncogene mutations in sporadic medullary thyroid carcinoma. J Clin Endocrinol Metab 1996;81:3740–3745.
5. Samaan NA, Schultz PN, Hickey RC. Medullary thyroid carcinoma: prognosis of familial versus sporadic disease and the role of radiotherapy. J Clin Endocrinol Metab 1988;67:801–805.
6. Kakudo K, Carney JA, Sizemore GW. Medullary carcinoma of thyroid: biologic behavior of the sporadic and familial neoplasm. Cancer 1985; 55:2818–2821.
7. Zedenius J, Larsson C, Bergholm U, et al. Mutations of codon 918 in the RET proto-oncogene correlate to poor prognosis in sporadic medullary thyroid carcinomas. J Clin Endocrinol Metab 1995;80:3088–3090.
8. Sosa JA, Bowman HM, Tielsch JM, et al. The importance of surgeon experience for clinical and economic outcomes from thyroidectomy. Ann Surg 1998;228:320–330.
9. de Roy van Zuidewijn DB, Songun I, Kievit J, van de Velde CJ. Complications of thyroid surgery. Ann Surg Oncol 1995;2:56–60.
10. Bergamaschi R, Becouarn G, Ronceray J, Arnaud JP. Morbidity of thyroid surgery. Am J Surg 1998;176:71–75.
11. Moulton-Barrett R, Crumley R, Jalilie S, et al. Complications of thyroid surgery. Int Surg 1997;82:63–66.
12. Friedrich T, Steinert M, Kietel R, et al. Incidence of damage to the recurrent laryngeal nerve in surgical therapy of various thyroid gland disease: a retrospective study. Zentralbl Chir 1990;123:25–29.

CASE #2: SPORADIC VS HEREDITARY MEDULLARY THYROID CARCINOMA: IS FAMILY HISTORY A RELIABLE INDICATOR FOR EXCLUDING HEREDITARY DISEASE?

Case Description

A 42-yr-old man presented to his primary physician in 1989 with a mass in the right lobe of the thyroid gland. He subsequently underwent a partial thyroidectomy for a 3-cm medullary thyroid carcinoma. Residual tumor was left adherent to the right trachea, larynx, and

Table 1
Pentagastrin Stimulation Test Case 2

Time (min)	Calcitonin (pg/mL)
Baseline	36
2	313
5	458
10	320

Normal calcitonin increment after 0.5
µg/kg pentagastrin bolus is <106 pg/mL.

strap muscles. During initial evaluation at the M. D. Anderson Cancer Center several months later, he was noted to have focal areas of thallium uptake in the left submandibular and right supraclavicular regions, and in the thyroid bed. Screening at that time and before surgery revealed a normal serum calcium level and a negative 24-h urine for catecholamines and metanephrines. CEA was 6.4 ng/mL (normal range, 0–3 ng/mL). The patient had no knowledge of any family history of thyroid cancer.

He subsequently underwent completion thyroidectomy and right modified radical neck dissection. Pathologic evaluation of the resected specimen demonstrated metastatic disease in 9 of 41 lymph nodes, and residual adherent tumor causing his physicians to recommend external-beam radiotherapy to the neck and upper mediastinum. Following completion of surgery and radiotherapy, the patient's CEA was <1.5 ng/mL. Posttreatment measurements of CEA were normal; basal calcitonin level was 33 pg/mL (normal range, 0–40 pg/mL). A computed tomography (CT) scan of the neck performed 1 yr after reoperative surgery revealed no evidence of recurrence but a pentagastrin stimulation test in late 1992 revealed an abnormal result (see Table 1).

Ultrasonography of the neck at that time showed no evidence of recurrent disease, or lymphadenopathy, and chest roentgenogram was normal. Although additional neck exploration was discussed, the patient hesitated to proceed with repeat explorative surgery, and he has been monitored by periodic screening with basal calcitonin and CEA measurements that have remained normal. Ultrasound and computed tomographic scans of the neck, chest roentgenograms, and physical examinations have also been normal.

During a routine study to detect the frequency of *RET* protooncogene mutations in apparently sporadic MTC, this patient was found to have a codon 609 (cys→tyr, TGC→TAC) mutation *(1)*. Repeat questioning at this time revealed a poorly documented history of an uncle who died of papillary thyroid carcinoma. There was no family history of sudden death nor evidence to suggest a pheochromocytoma. A family member had nephrolithiasis, but no hyperparathyroidism was documented. To exclude germline transmission of the codon 609 mutation, this patient's parents, siblings, and children were tested. Surprisingly many family members were found to be affected. Some members had MTC whereas others had C-cell hyperplasia (see Fig. 4).

Subsequently, a sibling (see patient II-3, Fig. 4) with an elevated serum calcium, and recurrent nephrolithiasis was found to have a 1-cm right thyroid nodule (see laboratory evaluation, Table 2). Total thyroidectomy and cervical neck dissection showed a 2-cm right-lobe MTC, and a 1.5-mm left-lobe MTC with adjacent C-cell hyperplasia, but without metastases to the lymph nodes. A 2-cm left inferior parathyroid adenoma and a small

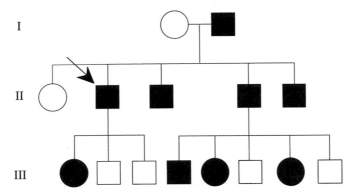

Fig. 4. Case 2 family tree. Arrow indicates the propositus, and darkened figures indicate family members with either MTC or *RET* protooncogene mutations.

Table 2
Laboratory Evaluation for Patient II-3 (Fig. 4), Case 2

Pentagastrin stimulation test		Laboratory results
Time (min)	Calcitonin (pg/mL)	Calcium 10.6 mg/dL (8.9–10.5) 0
0	15	Phosphate 2.4 mg/dL (2.5–4.5)
2	235	Ionized calcium 6.1 mg/dL (4.7–5.2)
5	71	Intact PTH 83 pg/mL (10–65)
10	43	Roche CEA 2.3 (<2.5)
		Urinary calcium 465 mg/24 h
		Normal 24-h urine for
		metanephrines/catecholamines

Normal calcitonin increment after 0.5 μg/Kg pentagastrin bolus is <106 pg/mL.

hyperplastic parathyroid gland were also resected. He has done well and remains free of disease.

Discussion

The finding of hyperparathyroidism in patient II-3 and nephrolithiasis in other family members led to the conclusion that this mutation causes MEN 2A rather than familial MTC (defined as MTC only), a distinction that is important to ensure periodic screening for pheochromocytoma. Further discussion with this family revealed the history of another sibling, also a gene carrier, who was treated for Hirschsprung disease as a child. Hirschsprung disease was first identified in some families with MEN 2A *(2,3)* and subsequent investigations showed that *RET* codon 609, 618, and 620 mutations may be associated with Hirschsprung disease.

This family illustrates several points. The first is the difficulty of differentiating between sporadic and hereditary MTC. Until the mutation was identified, our patient was considered to have sporadic MTC. As events unfolded, it became clear that several important clues, including a death from thyroid carcinoma and a family history of nephrolithiasis, had been underappreciated. A second point is the difficulty of differentiating between familial MTC and MEN 2A. In this family, hyperparathyroidism was proved in only one family member and then only after a *RET* protooncogene mutation was identified. Additionally, there was no evidence of pheochromocytoma, a point supported by earlier data showing the infrequency of pheochromocytoma with a codon 609 mutation *(4)*.

Family history of pheochromocytoma is often lacking or inadequately investigated. Although sudden death caused by cardiac arrest or stroke was common in families with MEN 2A before this syndrome was elucidated in 1961, pheochromocytomas were only rarely identified *(5)*. In family history that focuses on cardiovascular events, the true incidence of pheochromocytoma will be systematically underestimated. The fact that adrenomedullary disease is found in only 12–42% of affected MEN 2A patients *(6)* further reduces the reliability of family history.

Over the years, several studies have documented the difficulty of identifying pheochromocytomas *(7–9)*. Many cases are discovered at autopsy, after patients have died from complications related to the pheochromocytoma. Death during surgery for conditions other than pheochromocytoma carries a significant risk for a patient with undiagnosed pheochromocytoma. A large family in the Netherlands, eventually found to have MEN 2A, lost five young women to hypertensive crises during childbirth before the diagnosis of MEN 2A was established *(7)*. The events in this Dutch family highlight the variability of pheochromocytoma symptoms and signs that may include shaking, anxiety attacks, headache, palpitations, sweating, and hypertension. The absence of symptoms in patients with pheochromocytoma in this family highlights the need for persistent screening. In a series of 100 MEN 2A patients, sudden death occurred in 8.9%, but symptoms suggestive of pheochromocytoma were seen in only 40% of these sudden-death cases. Pheochromocytoma was diagnosed following systematic investigations in 43% after MTC or parathyroid disease was identified *(9)*.

Symptoms consistent with pheochromocytomas are often not given credence. A postmortem study of patients who died of pheochromocytoma, showed that typical symptoms were present for more than 3 mo in 61% of patients before they died, and less than 3 months in 29% of patients *(8)*. The most common symptoms were palpitations, episodic sweating, dyspnea, and headaches. Seventy-three percent of the patients were hypertensive, whereas 10% were hypotensive. Four of 62 patients had some family history of MEN 2 or neurofibromatosis. In 50% of patients who died of pheochromocytomas, the disease was clinically unsuspected, and in 23% of those who died it was suspected but not confirmed. Other series show similar findings *(10,11)*. Given the absence of symptoms and signs in many cases, it is imperative that screening for pheochromocytomas be performed annually on family members with positive results of *RET* protooncogene analysis.

A frequently asked question is whether it is necessary to screen relatives of a patient with MTC and negative *RET* protooncogene results (exons 10,11,13,14,15, and 16) by calcium or pentagastrin stimulation. Use of Bayes' theorem makes it possible to assign a relative probability. A first-degree relative of an affected individual would have a 0.5 (probability of inheriting an autosomal dominant genetic mutation) × 0.07 (the probability of the patient's apparently sporadic MTC having a germline *RET* mutation) × 0.02 (the percentage of families with proven hereditary MTC who do not have a germline *RET* protooncogene mutation) = 0.07% *(12)*. Most family members, when informed of a risk of <0.1%, choose to forego pentagastrin or calcium testing for MTC. For the occasional patient not reassured by this low probability, continued annual pentagastrin testing until age 35 yr could be performed. Therefore, we recommend that all patients with MTC have a germline analysis of the *RET* protooncogene *(1,12)*.

In summary, differentiating between sporadic and hereditary MTC is facilitated by the use of *RET* protooncogene analysis. Before genetic mutational analysis was performed for this family, the absence of an adequately detailed family history essentially excluded the concern about hereditary disease. This family also illustrates that entities such as Hirschsprung disease or symptoms suggestive of pheochromocytoma should lead to further investigation. We suggest that further screening for MEN 2A or familial MTC is not warranted in family members who do not have *RET* protooncogene mutational abnormalities because their risk of developing disease is extremely low.

REFERENCES

1. Wohllk N, Cote GJ, Evans DB, et al. Application of genetic screening information to the management of medullary thyroid carcinoma and multiple endocrine neoplasia type 2. Endocrinol Metab Clin North Am 1996;25:1–25.
2. Verdy M, Weber A, Roy C, et al. Hirschsprung's disease in a family with multiple endocrine neoplasia. J Pediatr Gastroenterol Nutr 1982;1:603–607.
3. Decker RA, Peacock ML. Occurrence of MEN 2A in familial Hirschsprung's disease: A new indication for genetic testing of the *RET* proto-oncogene. J Pediatr Surg 1998;33:207–214.
4. Eng C, Clayton D, Schuffenecker I, et al. The relationship between specific RET protooncogene mutations and disease phenotype in multiple endocrine neoplasia type 2. International RET mutation consortium analysis. JAMA 1996;276:1575–1579.
5. Sipple JH. The association of pheochromocytoma with carcinoma of the thyroid gland. Am J Med 1961; 31:163–166.
6. Howe JR, Norton JA, Wells SA. Prevalence of pheochromocytoma and hyperparathyroidism in multiple endocrine neoplasia type 2A: results of long-term follow-up. Surgery 1993;114:1070–1077.
7. Lips CJM, Landsvater RM, Höppener JWM, et al. From medical history and biochemical tests to presymptomatic treatment in a large MEN 2A family. J Intern Med 1995;238:347–356.
8. Platts JK, Drew PJT, Harvery JN. Death from phaeochromocytomas: lessons from a post-mortem survey. J Royal Coll Phys London 1995;29:299–306.
9. Casanova S, Rosenberg-Bourgin M, Farkas D, et al. Phaeochromocytoma in multiple endocrine neoplasia type 2A: survey of 100 cases. Clin Endocrinol 1993;38:531–537.
10. St John Sutton MG, Sheps SG, Lie JT. Prevalence of clinically unsuspected pheochromocytomas. Review of a 50-year autopsy series. Mayo Clin Proc 1981;56:354–360.
11. Stenstrom G, Svardsudd K. Pheochromocytoma in Sweden 1958-81. Acta Med Scand 1986;220:225–232.
12. Wohllk N, Cote GJ, Bugalho MMJ, et al. Relevance of RET proto-oncogene mutations in sporadic medullary thyroid carcinoma. J Clin Endocrinol Metab 1996;81:3740–3745.

CASE #3: DIFFERENTIAL DIAGNOSES OF COMBINED ISLET CELL TUMOR AND PHEOCHROMOCYTOMA

Case Description

A 29-yr-old man presented to M. D. Anderson Cancer Center with nonspecific gastrointestinal symptoms. An abdominal computed tomogram (CT) showed an 8 × 6-cm nodular right adrenal mass, a vascular pancreatic mass, and renal calculi (see Fig. 5). He had no history of headaches or palpitations. He had a history of hyperparathyroidism, with resection of a 1-g parathyroid adenoma. Biopsy results of two other glands were reported as normal. Additionally, he had type I diabetes mellitus. His father had had a nonsecretory islet cell carcinoma and rectal leiomyomas, but there was no other family history of endocrine tumors, Zollinger-Ellison syndrome, hypoglycemia, kidney stones, pituitary, or other brain tumors. Physical examination showed him to have normal blood pressure and multiple skin lesions over his face and back (see Fig. 6). Table 3 shows the results of his laboratory evaluation. Based on these test results, several preoperative

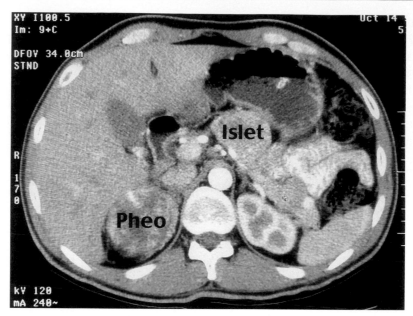

Fig. 5. Computed tomography of abdomen in Case 3 showing large right pheochromocytoma (Pheo) and large islet cell tumor of the head of the pancreas (Islet).

diagnoses were considered, including hyperparathyroidism, pheochromocytoma, and Zollinger-Ellison syndrome.

Before surgery for the adrenal and pancreatic masses, he received α-methyl tyrosine and alpha-blockade. Four variably sized pancreatic tumors were identified and removed (see Figs. 7 and 8). When the right adrenal gland was excised, it showed a pheochromocytoma and several cortical adenomas; the left adrenal was normal.

Biopsy of one facial skin lesion showed an angiofibroma. An ophthalmologic exam was negative for retinal hemangiomas often found in von Hippel-Lindau syndrome (VHL). The patient subsequently underwent two more parathyroid explorations for recurrent hyperparathyroidism.

Discussion

What is this patient's multiple endocrine neoplasia syndrome? The presence of primary hyperparathyroidism, angiofibromas, islet cell tumors, pheochromocytomas, adrenal cortical adenomas, and type I diabetes mellitus does not easily meet Occam's razor for a single diagnosis. Both MEN 1 and VHL are considerations, but neither provides a perfect fit (see Table 4).

The MEN 1 syndrome includes hyperparathyroidism, pancreatic tumors most commonly gastrinomas, and pituitary tumors *(1)*. Additionally, angiofibromas, collagenomas *(2)*, and lipomas are often found, as are thyroid goiters and well-differentiated thyroid carcinomas. Adrenal cortical abnormalities are seen in 36–41% of MEN 1 patients including adrenal adenomas, hyperplasia, nodular hyperplasia, and rarely carcinomas *(3–6)*. Carcinomas have developed in patients with adrenal cortical hyperplasia after many years of stable sized glands *(7)*. Adrenal abnormalities are found only in patients with pancreatic tumors, and the affected adrenal glands do not show the loss of heterozygosity seen in

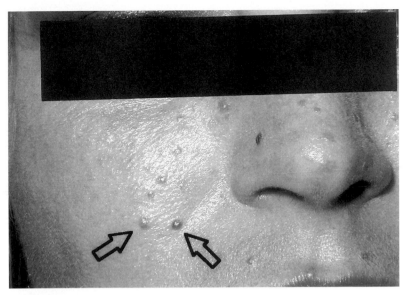

Fig. 6. Representative photograph of angiofibromas shown by arrows.

Table 3
Laboratory Evaluation for Case 3

Gastrin 845 pg/mL (10–100)	Prolactin 12 ng/mL (2–16)
Calcium 11.6 mg/dL (8.9–10.5)	FSH 4 IU/mL (2–9)
Phosphate 2.8 mg/dL (2.5–4.5)	LH 19 IU/mL (1.5–9)
Intact PTH 82 pg/mL (10–65)	Testosterone 1096 ng/mL (350–1030)
Calcitonin 15 pg/mL (<26)	11 am cortisol 13 µg/dL (5–25)
Albumin 4.1 mg/dL (3.5–4.5)	ACTH 37 ng/L (7–51)
DHEAS 119 µg/dL (100–450)	

24-H Urine Results

VMA 10.5 mg/d (0.7–6.8)	Metanephrines 5.0 mg/d (0.3–0.9)
Norepinephrine 133 µg/d (16–125)	Epinephrine 15 µg/d (3–38)
Urinary free cortisol 42 µg/d (11–84)	

VMA-vanillylmandelic acid.

the pancreatic and parathyroid gland tumors, which suggests a mode of proliferation different from that due to mutation of the MEN 1 tumor suppressor gene. Other investigations have excluded the pituitary and the hypothalamic-pituitary-adrenal axis as the etiology of adrenal adenomas in these cases *(7)*.

Pheochromocytomas are not commonly found in MEN 1. However, three recent articles analyzing the incidence of pheochromocytoma and islet cell tumors in MEN 1 found up to 3% of patients presenting with both islet cell tumors and pheochromocytoma *(8)*. Several other case reports have identified pheochromocytomas in MEN 1 patients *(8)*.

VHL syndrome is an autosomal-dominant inherited neoplastic disorder more commonly associated with pheochromocytomas than MEN 1. Twenty-five to thirty-five percent of VHL patients have pheochromocytomas, and 15–20% have pancreatic islet cell

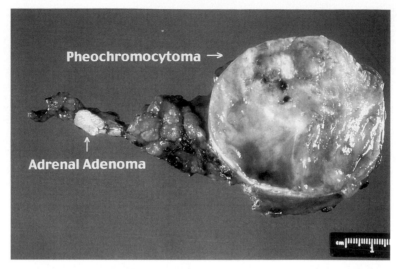

Fig. 7. Adrenal gland from Case 3 showing pheochromocytoma and adrenal cortical adenomas.

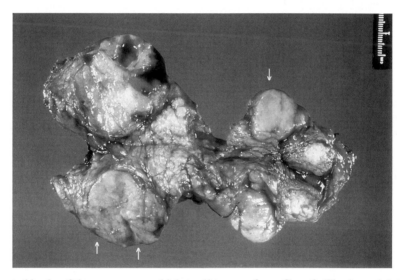

Fig. 8. Bisected body of the pancreas and islet cell tumors from Case 3. The large islet cell tumor (double arrows) and the smaller tumor (single arrow) are visualized in Fig. 5.

tumors *(9,10)*. Renal cell carcinoma affects approximately 70% of patients by the age 60 yr *(11)*. Retinal and cerebellar hemangiomas and testicular tumors are also common findings. The absence or presence of pheochromocytoma permits further categorization of VHL into type 1 (65–75% of total) and type 2 (25–35% of total) respectively. VHL type 2A includes pheochromocytoma without renal cell carcinoma, and type 2B includes both tumors. Islet cell tumors are found predominantly in the type 2 variant. Carney et al. *(12)* described three patients with pancreatic islet cell tumors and pheochromocytoma and suggested the existence of a separate syndrome. However, closer evaluation of these families identified typical features of VHL in other family members.

Table 4
Differential Diagnosis Considerations in Case 3

MEN 1	von Hippel-Lindau	Neurofibromatosis 1
Hyperparathyroidism	Renal cell carcinoma	Neurofibromas
Islet cell tumors	Retinal hemangioma	Café au lait spots
Pituitary adenomas	Cerebellar hemangioma	Hyperparathyroidism
Angiofibromas, lipomas, collagenomas	Islet cell tumors	Somatastatin-producing Carcinoid tumors
Adrenal cortical adenomas	Pheochromocytoma	Pheochromocytoma
Pheochromocytoma	Testicular tumors	Medullary thyroid carcinoma
Carcinoid		
Thyroid nodules/carcinoma		

The *VHL* gene is a tumor suppressor gene that is inactivated by production of a truncated or nonfunctional protein in approximately 70% of cases. The molecular defect in the remaining patients is a missense mutation associated with a higher incidence of pheochromocytoma (VHL type 2) *(13)*.

A less likely diagnosis to consider in this case is neurofibromatosis 1 (NF 1). Approximately 1% of patients with NF 1 develop pheochromocytoma *(14)*. Neurofibromatosis 1 is a multiple endocrine neoplasia syndrome in which rare patients will develop a syndrome characterized by hyperparathyroidism and somatostatin-producing carcinoid tumors. Islet cell tumors are seldom seen in this variant. The absence of neurofibromas and *café au lait* spots and the presence of angiofibromas excludes NF 1. MEN 2 is associated with pheochromocytoma, but there have been no reports of islet cell tumor, which effectively excludes this disorder. Tuberous sclerosis, Sturge-Weber syndrome and other paraganglioma syndromes almost never have the clinical features seen in this patient.

The diagnosis of MEN 1 was proved definitively in this patient by the finding of an inactivating mutation at exon 9 of the *MEN 1* gene *(8)*. His father and an unaffected cousin were also found to carry the same mutation.

In summary, the key points in this patient's differential diagnosis were the presence of multiglandular hyperparathyroidism and cutaneous angiofibromata. Both of these entities are common in MEN 1, but are not seen in VHL or the other less likely possibilities. This case also illustrates the importance of including both pheochromocytoma and cortical adenomas in the differential diagnosis of an adrenal abnormality in MEN 1.

REFERENCES

1. Wermer P. Genetic aspects of adenomatosis of endocrine glands. Am J Med 1954;16:363–371.
2. Marx S, Spiegel AM, Skarulis MC, et al. Multiple endocrine neoplasia type 1: clinical and genetic topics. Ann Intern Med 1998;129:484–494.
3. Ballard HS, Frame B, Hartsock RJ. Familial multiple endocrine adenoma-peptic ulcer complex. Medicine 1964;43:481–516.
4. Crosier JC, Aserad E, Lubetzki J. L'Adénomatose polyendocrinienne. A propos d'une observation personell et revenue de la literature. Semin Hop Paris 1971;47:494–525.
5. Shigematsu S, Shimoyama N, Sato Y, et al. A case of multiple endocrine neoplasia, type 1, with parathyroid adenoma, multinodular adrenal cortical hyperplasia, islet cell tumor and hyperplasia of thyroid with concomitant hypersecretion of gastrin and total glucagons-like immunoreactivity. Nippon Naika Gakki Sasshi 1989;78:357–362.

6. Houdelett P, Chagnon A, Dumotier J, Marthan E. Corticosurrénalome malin dans le cadre d'un syndrome de Wermer. J Chir 1989;126:385–387.

7. Skogseid B, Rastad J, Öberg, K. Multiple endocrine neoplasia type 1 clinical features and screening. Endocrinol Metab Clin North Am 1994;23:1–18.

8. Dackiw APB, Cote GJ, Fleming JB, et al. Screening for MEN1 mutations in patients with atypical endocrine neoplasia. Surgery 1999;126:1097–1104.

9. Neumann HP, Berger DP, Sigmund G, et al. Pheochromocytomas, multiple endocrine neoplasia type 2, and von Hippel-Lindau disease. N Engl J Med 1993; 329: 1531-1538. Erratum, N Engl J Med 1994; 331:1535.

10. Hoff AO, Cote GJ, Gagel RF. Multiple endocrine neoplasias. Annu Rev Physiol 2000;62:377–411.

11. Maher ER, Kaelin WG Jr. Von Hippel-Lindau disease. Medicine 1997;76:381–391.

12. Carney JA, Go VL, Gordon H, et al. Familial pheochromocytoma and islet cell tumor of the pancreas. Am J Med 1980;68:515–521.

13. Chen F, Kishida T, Yao M, et al. Germline mutations in the von Hippel-Lindau disease tumor suppressor gene: Correlations with phenotype. Hum Mutat 1995;5:66–75.

14. Norton JA. Neuroendocrine tumors of the pancreas and duodenum. Curr Probl Surg 1994;31:77–156.

INDEX